Litt's DRUG ERUPTION & REACTION MANUAL

23rd EDITION

Jerome Z. Litt, MD
Case Western Reserve University School of Medicine
Cleveland, Ohio, USA

Neil H. Shear, MD, FRCPC, FACP
Professor of Dermatology and Clinical Pharmacology and Toxicology, University of Toronto
Toronto, Ontario, Canada

CRC Press
Taylor & Francis Group
Boca Raton London New York

CRC Press is an imprint of the
Taylor & Francis Group, an informa business

CRC Press
Taylor & Francis Group
6000 Broken Sound Parkway NW, Suite 300
Boca Raton, FL 33487-2742

Printed at CPI on sustainably sourced paper
Version Date: 20161017

International Standard Book Number-13: 978-1-138-19799-2 (Paperback) 978-1-138-63311-7 (Hardback)

Visit the Taylor & Francis Web site at
http://www.taylorandfrancis.com

and the CRC Press Web site at
http://www.crcpress.com

Printed at CPI on sustainably sourced paper

CONTENTS

To Vel – my Muse

JZL

Editors' introductory notes

Any drug has the potential to cause an adverse reaction. An adverse drug reaction (ADR) is an unwanted, unpleasant, noxious, or harmful consequence associated with the use of a medication that has been administered in a standard dose by the proper route, for the purpose of prophylaxis, diagnosis, or treatment. Death is the ultimate adverse drug event.

ADRs are a major problem in drug therapy. They are the most common of all iatrogenic illnesses that complicate up to 15% of therapeutic drug courses, and are a leading cause of morbidity and mortality in healthcare. ADRs should therefore be considered in the differential diagnosis of a wide variety of medical disorders. Many more people – particularly the elderly – are taking more and more prescription and over-the-counter medications. In addition, new drugs are appearing in the medical marketplace on an almost daily basis. It is unsurprising, then, that more and more drug reactions and cutaneous eruptions are emerging.

Prevention, diagnosis and treatment of adverse drug events are becoming increasingly complex, and it is to be expected that physicians in all specialties are often perplexed by the nature of ADRs. To this end, I now offer a new and improved edition that has evolved from the treasured Drug Eruption Reference Manual of previous editions. I hope that you will find this new edition informative and valuable.

Enjoy!

Jerome Z. Litt, M.D.

"Is it safe?"

In my first chance to acknowledge participation in Litt's outstanding text, I need to address that big question from a patient: "Is it safe?" This text is meant to help all prescribers, dispensers and patients understand what the risk of harm might be; whether it is from a drug reaction or interaction, Litt's is the go-to information source. How does this information help answer the unanswerable? Simply put, safety is a process, not a question. With the right information at hand a safety environment can thrive; the most relevant concerns help peel away background noise from a seemingly infinite number of sources. This new edition adds additional support to a risk managed environment, and we will continue to provide the most up-to-date and relevant information. I look forward to feedback and suggestions. And I thank Jerry Litt for this great opportunity and his trust that we can make his book an on-going success.

Neil H. Shear, M.D., F.R.C.P.C., F.A.C.P.

Litt's Drug Eruption & Reaction Manual – at a glance

This 23rd edition has been revised and updated throughout to present a quick clinical reference guide to adverse drug reactions (ADRs), side effects, drug interactions and other safety information for prescription and over-the-counter medications. There is also material on reactions caused by classes of drugs, enabling you to see at a glance whether a reaction is common to all the drugs in that particular class, or to a majority of them, or only to a significant few.

The aims of this edition remain:

1. To help medical practitioners make informed and safe decisions when diagnosing and prescribing, and also when generally seeking information.
2. To help healthcare professionals remain pharmacovigilant.
3. To provide all physicians, lecturers, educators and pharmacists with an easy-to-use and reliable quick reference tool.

Space in the manual is, unfortunately, constrained, so various generic drugs have been eliminated from this print manual because either they have been withdrawn from the marketplace or they are rarely, if ever, prescribed today. In their place we have included many important new drugs, noted with an asterisk. The full and comprehensive picture – from which our information derives – can be found at our website database (www.drugeruptiondata.com), which is updated continually. All drug profiles (together with all the other information in this book) are available to subscribers on our website.

A note on ADRs

The incidence and severity of ADRs are influenced by a number of factors:

1. Patient-related factors:

- Age – geriatric, pediatric, adolescent . . . older patients are taking more medications—hence more of a possibility of developing reactions; pediatric patients have more delicate skins; hormonal changes occur in adolescents . . . All these factors play roles in the development of possible adverse reactions.
- Gender – male or female – and if the latter, then pregnant/breast-feeding/menopausal . . .
- Disease – not only the disease being treated, but also other pre-existing health conditions and comorbid diseases. For example, atopic patients are at increased risk for serious allergic reactions. Also, there would be an increased risk for hypersensitivity drug reactions if the patient has asthma or lupus erythematosus.
- Genetics – a patient could have abnormal drug metabolism by cytochrome P450 due to inheriting abnormal alleles.
- Geography – patients living in sunny climes could develop photoxicities from photosensitizing drugs more readily than those who inhabit cooler, less sunny climates.

2. Drug-related factors:

- Type/class of drug – for example, there is a heightened risk of hypersensitivity with the use of beta-blockers (see further the tables on class reactions).
- Duration of therapy – the longer a patient maintains the therapy, the greater the possibility that he/she could develop a reaction.
- Dosage – the greater the dosage, the more likely an adverse side effect.
- Bioavailability – the extent to and rate at which the drug enters systemic circulation, thereby accessing the site of action.
- Interactions with other drugs – for example, synergistic QT prolongation can occur when two QT prolonging agents, such as erythromycin + ritonavir, are used together.
- Route of administration – intramuscular, intravenous, subcutaneous, and topical administrations are more likely to cause hypersensitivity reactions; oral medications are less likely to result in drug hypersensitivity.

The terms "drug allergy," "drug hypersensitivity," and "drug reaction" are often used interchangeably. Drug allergy specifically refers to a reaction mediated by IgE; drug hypersensitivity is an immune-mediated response to a drug agent in a sensitized patient; and drug reactions comprise all adverse events related to drug administration, regardless of etiology.

Vigilance at point of care:

While the possibilities for adverse drug reactions seem endless, we must be on the lookout for any new medication(s) the patient might be taking. A thorough, detailed history of all medications must be made in order to elicit any remote possibility that the drug in question might be the culprit for the side effect. People do not often realize that the common over-the-counter analgesics – aspirin, Tylenol, Advil, Motrin, Naprosyn, and others – are actually medications. Herbals and supplements such as St. John's wort, ginkgo biloba, and echinacea can be responsible for various hypersensitivity reactions. For example, St. John's wort, in particular, interacts adversely with SSRIs and tricyclic antidepressants.

Contents of the book, and how to use them

1. **The A–Z**

   The major portion of the manual lists in alphabetical order the 850+ generic drugs, biologics, and supplements, and the adverse reactions that can arise from their use. An asterisk against the entry title indicates this drug is new to this edition. If you do not find a drug in the main A–Z listing under the name you know it by, you can turn to the concordance of synonyms and trade names to find the generic name it will be listed under.

   Trade (Brand) name(s) are then listed alphabetically. When there are many trade names, the ten (or so) most commonly recognized ones are listed.

Following the trade names is – in parentheses – the latest name of the pharmaceutical company that markets the drug. Many of the names of the companies have changed from earlier editions of this manual because of acquisitions, mergers, and other factors in the pharmaceutical industry.

Next appear the Indication(s), the Class in which the drug belongs, and the Half-life of each drug, where known.

Drug interactions: many severe, hazardous drug–drug interactions are recorded. Only clinically significant drug interactions that have been reported to trigger potential harm and that could be life threatening have been included here in the profile. These interactions are predictable and well documented in controlled studies; they should be avoided.

Pregnancy category: for new drugs approved on or after 30 June, 2015 this field gives (where available) a brief summary of the full statement reflecting the risk for pregnant women as given in the prescribing guidelines; health care providers are advised to check the individual label where necessary.

An explanation of the categories for older drugs (A, B, C, D and X) can be found on our website www.drugeruptiondata.com.

Adverse Drug Reactions: under each drug profile is a list of related ADRs. These adverse events have been classified under the following categories: **Skin**, **Hair**, **Nails**, **Mucosal**, **Cardiovascular**, **Central Nervous System**, **Neuromuscular/Skeletal**, **Gastrointestinal/Hepatic**, **Respiratory**, **Endocrine/Metabolic**, **Genitourinary**, **Renal**, **Hematologic**, **Otic**, **Ocular**, **Local**, **Other**.

Within each category, the reactions are listed alphabetically. Thus, the order of listing does not reflect severity or frequency in any way.

The terminology used to list reaction patterns has been simplified as far as possible by eliminating, for the most part, tags such as "like" (as in "-Psoriasis-like"), "-reactivation," "-syndrome," "-dissemination," "-iform," etc.

The number of reports is given for each reaction in square brackets. The incidence of the most important reactions is given in parentheses where indicated (usually from the full prescribing information for the relevant drug). For example, the profile for Amoxicillin begins:

Skin

AGEP [26]
Anaphylactoid reactions/Anaphylaxis [15]
Angioedema (<10%) [5]

This means that we have 26 journal articles referring to occurrence of AGEP (acute generalized exanthematous pustulosis); 15 articles mentioning the occurrence of anaphylaxis; and 5 articles discussing angioedema, as reactions to Amoxicillin within the Skin category. All these articles appear on the website www.drugeruptiondata.com together with links to the article abstracts on PubMed®. Additionally, the incidence of angioedema as a reaction has been reported as up to 10%.

On some occasions, there are very few adverse reactions to a specific drug. These drugs are still included in the manual as there is a positive significance in negative findings.

2. **Important eruptions / reactions**

i) This section of the manual includes a listing of descriptions of important eruption and reaction patterns. Over 40 eruptions/reactions are described here in alphabetical order, from Acanthosis nigricans to Xerostomia.

ii) Following this section are lists of all drugs that have been found to cause these important eruptions/reactions. This section is a quick look-up tool for drugs that cause important reaction patterns.
(Descriptions of several other reactions, and lists of drugs associated with these reactions, can be found on our website – www.drugeruptiondata.com.)

iii) We then have a list of the main classes of drugs, from 5-HT1 agonists to Xanthine alkaloids, as a quick reference guide.

iv) There follow lists of the classes of drugs most likely to cause important interactions with other drugs, with the drugs in those classes.

v) We then have an enlarged section of tables of class reactions, enabling you to see at a glance whether a reaction is common to all the drugs in that particular class, or to a majority of them, or only to a significant few.

3. **The Concordance**

The final part of the manual is a concordance to match synonyms (noted in italic) and trade names with the generic drug name. If you know only the synonym or trade name, you can use this list to find the corresponding generic name to look up in the main A–Z listing section of the book.

Acknowledgements

The editors would like to thank Dr. Mohannad Abu Hilal for his commitment and skill in reviewing the literature and correcting errors that had crept into the final proofs. If there are other errors we missed, please let us know. We want to keep the quality of the Litt's Manual high!

JZL / NS
November 2016

ABACAVIR

Trade names: Epzicom (ViiV), Triumeq (ViiV), Trizivir (ViiV), Ziagen (ViiV)
Indications: HIV infections in combination with other antiretrovirals
Class: Nucleoside analog reverse transcriptase inhibitor
Half-life: 1.5 hours
Clinically important, potentially hazardous interactions with: alcohol, arbutamine, argatroban, arsenic, darunavir, ganciclovir, lopinavir, methadone, phenobarbital, phenytoin, protease inhibitors, ribavirin, rifampin, tipranavir, valganciclovir
Pregnancy category: C
Important contra-indications noted in the prescribing guidelines for: nursing mothers
Note: Epzicom is abacavir and lamivudine; Triumeq is abacavir, dolutegravir and lamivudine; Trizivir is abacavir, lamivudine and zidovudine.
Black Box Warning: HYPERSENSITIVITY REACTIONS, LACTIC ACIDOSIS and SEVERE HEPATOMEGALY, and EXACERBATIONS OF HEPATITIS B

Skin
Anaphylactoid reactions/Anaphylaxis (3%) [3]
Exanthems [2]
Hypersensitivity (8–9%) [69]
Lipoatrophy [2]
Rash (5–7%) [17]
Stevens–Johnson syndrome [2]
Toxic epidermal necrolysis [2]

Cardiovascular
Myocardial infarction [9]

Central Nervous System
Abnormal dreams (10%) [2]
Anxiety (5%)
Chills (6%)
Depression (6%)
Fever (6%) [2]
Headache (7–13%) [3]
Insomnia [2]
Migraine (7%)
Neuropsychiatric disturbances [3]
Sleep related disorder (10%)
Vertigo (dizziness) (6%) [3]

Neuromuscular/Skeletal
Asthenia (fatigue) (7–12%) [2]
Bone or joint pain (5–6%)
Myalgia/Myopathy (5–6%) [2]

Gastrointestinal/Hepatic
Abdominal pain (6%)
Diarrhea (7%) [2]
Gastritis (6%)
Hepatotoxicity [3]
Nausea (7–19%) [4]
Vomiting (2–10%)

Respiratory
Bronchitis (4%)
Cough [2]
Pneumonia (4%)

Endocrine/Metabolic
ALT increased (6%)
AST increased (6%)
Hyperamylasemia (2–4%)
Hypertriglyceridemia (2–6%)

Renal
Fanconi syndrome [2]

Hematologic
Agranulocytosis [3]
Neutropenia (2–5%)

Other
Adverse effects [4]
Infection (5%)

ABATACEPT

Trade name: Orencia (Bristol-Myers Squibb)
Indications: Rheumatoid arthritis, juvenile idiopathic arthritis in pediatric patients 6 years of age and older
Class: Disease-modifying antirheumatic drug (DMARD), T-cell co-stimulation modulator
Half-life: 12–23 days
Clinically important, potentially hazardous interactions with: adalimumab, anakinra, certolizumab, denosumab, echinacea, etanercept, golimumab, infliximab, lenalidomide, live vaccines, natalizumab, pimecrolimus, sipuleucel-T, tacrolimus, TNF antagonists, trastuzumab
Pregnancy category: C
Important contra-indications noted in the prescribing guidelines for: nursing mothers; pediatric patients

---

Skin
Basal cell carcinoma [3]
Eczema [2]
Herpes simplex (<5%) [3]
Herpes zoster [3]
Hypersensitivity [2]
Malignancies [10]
Psoriasis [12]
Rash (4%) [6]
Sjögren's syndrome [4]
Squamous cell carcinoma [5]
Vasculitis [2]

Mucosal
Stomatitis [3]

Cardiovascular
Hypertension (7%) [4]
Hypotension [2]

Central Nervous System
Fever (5%) [2]
Headache (5–18%) [5]
Vertigo (dizziness) (9%) [3]

Neuromuscular/Skeletal
Asthenia (fatigue) [2]
Back pain (7%) [2]
Pain in extremities (3%)

Gastrointestinal/Hepatic
Abdominal pain (5%)
Diarrhea (5%) [3]
Dyspepsia (6%)
Gastroenteritis [5]
Nausea (5%)
Vomiting [2]

Respiratory
Bronchitis (<13%) [4]
Cough (5–8%)
Influenza (5–13%) [2]
Nasopharyngitis (12%) [5]
Pharyngitis [3]
Pneumonia (<5%) [7]
Pulmonary toxicity [2]
Rhinitis (<5%) [2]
Sinusitis (5–13%) [3]
Tuberculosis [2]
Upper respiratory tract infection (>10%) [7]

Genitourinary
Urinary tract infection (5–13%) [10]

Local
Infusion-related reactions [4]
Infusion-site reactions (9%) [5]
Injection-site erythema [3]
Injection-site hematoma [2]
Injection-site pain [3]
Injection-site pruritus [2]
Injection-site reactions (3%) [8]

Other
Adverse effects [24]
Death [2]
Infection (36–54%) [24]

ABIRATERONE

Trade name: Zytiga (Janssen Biotech)
Indications: Metastatic castration-resistant prostate cancer (in combination with prednisone)
Class: CYP17 inhibitor, Enzyme inhibitor
Half-life: 12 hours
Clinically important, potentially hazardous interactions with: atazanavir, carbamazepine, clarithromycin, CYP3A4 inhibitors or inducers, indinavir, itraconazole, ketoconazole, nefazodone, nelfinavir, phenobarbital, phenytoin, rifabutin, rifampin, rifapentine, ritonavir, saquinavir, telithromycin, thioridazine, voriconazole
Pregnancy category: X
Important contra-indications noted in the prescribing guidelines for: nursing mothers; pediatric patients
Note: Contraindicated in women who are or may become pregnant.

Skin
Edema (27%) [18]
Hot flashes (19%) [2]

Cardiovascular
Arrhythmias (7%)
Atrial fibrillation [3]
Cardiac failure (2%)
Cardiotoxicity [4]
Chest pain (4%)
Hypertension (9%) [22]
Tachycardia [3]

Central Nervous System
Headache [2]

Neuromuscular/Skeletal
Arthralgia [5]
Asthenia (fatigue) [10]
Back pain [4]
Bone or joint pain (30%) [7]
Myalgia/Myopathy (26%)
Pain in extremities [2]

Gastrointestinal/Hepatic
Constipation [7]

Diarrhea (18%) [5]
Dyspepsia (6%)
Hepatotoxicity (2%) [12]
Nausea [8]

Respiratory
Cough (11%)
Upper respiratory tract infection (5%) [2]

Endocrine/Metabolic
ALT increased (11%) [3]
AST increased (31%) [2]
Hypercholesterolemia [2]
Hypertriglyceridemia (63%)
Hypokalemia [20]

Genitourinary
Nocturia (6%)
Urinary frequency (7%)
Urinary tract infection (12%) [2]

Hematologic
Anemia [5]
Thrombocytopenia [2]

Other
Adverse effects [6]

ACETAMINOPHEN

Synonyms: APAP; paracetamol
Trade names: Anacin-3 (Wyeth), Darvocet-N (aaiPharma), Excedrin (Bristol-Myers Squibb), Lorcet (Forest), Panadol (GSK), Percocet (Endo), Tylenol (Ortho-McNeil), Vicodin (AbbVie)
Indications: Pain, fever
Class: Analgesic, non-narcotic
Half-life: <3 hours
Clinically important, potentially hazardous interactions with: alcohol, anticonvulsants, barbiturates, busulfan, carbamazepine, cholestyramine, conivaptan, coumarins, didanosine, dong quai, exenatide, imatinib, isoniazid, liraglutide, melatonin, metoclopramide, metyrapone, PEG-interferon, pramlintide, probenecid, St John's wort
Pregnancy category: C
Important contra-indications noted in the prescribing guidelines for: nursing mothers
Note: Acetaminophen is the active metabolite of phenacetin. [IV] = intravenous. As a general point most reactions listed are those that have developed following the normal prescribing doses for acetaminophen and the overdosing, poisoning, and other toxicities that have been reported have been excluded.

Skin
AGEP [10]
Anaphylactoid reactions/Anaphylaxis [19]
Angioedema [8]
Dermatitis [3]
Erythema [3]
Erythema multiforme [3]
Exanthems [7]
Exfoliative dermatitis [2]
Fixed eruption [39]
Hyperhidrosis [2]
Hypersensitivity [12]
Neutrophilic eccrine hidradenitis [2]
Pemphigus [2]
Pruritus [5]
Purpura [6]
Rash [IV] [2]
Stevens–Johnson syndrome [10]
Toxic epidermal necrolysis [13]
Urticaria [17]
Vasculitis [4]

Mucosal
Xerostomia [3]

Cardiovascular
Hypertension [IV] [3]

Central Nervous System
Agitation [IV] (>5%)
Fever [IV] (5%)
Headache [IV] (10%) [4]
Insomnia [IV] (7%)
Somnolence (drowsiness) [6]
Vertigo (dizziness) [14]

Neuromuscular/Skeletal
Rhabdomyolysis [4]

Gastrointestinal/Hepatic
Abdominal distension [2]
Abdominal pain [IV] [3]
Constipation [IV] (>5%) [6]
Diarrhea [IV] [2]
Hepatotoxicity [69]
Nausea [IV] (34%) [16]
Pancreatitis [6]
Vomiting (15%) [15]

Respiratory
Asthma [3]
Pulmonary toxicity [IV] (>5%)

Endocrine/Metabolic
Acidosis [3]

Renal
Nephrotoxicity [8]
Renal failure [3]

Hematologic
Thrombocytopenia [2]

Other
Adverse effects [13]
Death [6]

ACETAZOLAMIDE

Trade name: Diamox (Duramed)
Indications: Epilepsy, glaucoma
Class: Carbonic anhydrase inhibitor, Diuretic
Half-life: 2–6 hours
Clinically important, potentially hazardous interactions with: arsenic, aspirin, ephedra, indacaterol, lisdexamfetamine, lithium, metformin, mivacurium, triamcinolone
Pregnancy category: C
Important contra-indications noted in the prescribing guidelines for: the elderly; nursing mothers; pediatric patients
Note: Acetazolamide is a sulfonamide and can be absorbed systemically. Sulfonamides can produce severe, possibly fatal, reactions such as toxic epidermal necrolysis and Stevens-Johnson syndrome.

Skin
AGEP [2]
Anaphylactoid reactions/Anaphylaxis [3]
Exanthems [2]
Pemphigus [2]
Stevens–Johnson syndrome [6]
Toxic epidermal necrolysis [2]

Central Nervous System
Depression [2]
Dysgeusia (taste perversion) (>10%) [8]
Paresthesias [6]

Neuromuscular/Skeletal
Asthenia (fatigue) [4]

Gastrointestinal/Hepatic
Diarrhea [2]
Dyspepsia [2]
Nausea [2]
Vomiting [2]

Endocrine/Metabolic
Acidosis [3]
Libido decreased [2]
Weight loss [2]

Renal
Nephrolithiasis [3]

Ocular
Choroidal detachment [2]
Corneal edema [2]
Glaucoma [2]
Myopia [2]

ACETYLCYSTEINE

Synonyms: N-acetylcysteine; L-Cysteine; NAC
Indications: Emphysema, bronchitis, tuberculosis, bronchiectasis, tracheostomy care, antidote for acetaminophen toxicity
Class: Antidote, Antioxidant
Half-life: N/A
Clinically important, potentially hazardous interactions with: carbamazepine, nitroglycerin
Pregnancy category: B
Note: As an antidote, it is difficult to differentiate side effects due to the drug from those due to the effects of the poison.

Skin
Anaphylactoid reactions/Anaphylaxis (8–18%) [13]
Angioedema [6]
Pruritus (<4%) [3]
Rash (2–4%) [4]
Urticaria (6–8%)

Cardiovascular
Flushing (<8%) [2]
Tachycardia (<4%)

Central Nervous System
Seizures [2]

Gastrointestinal/Hepatic
Diarrhea [2]
Nausea (<6%) [3]
Vomiting (2–10%) [2]

Other
Adverse effects [2]
Death [2]

ACITRETIN

Trade names: Neotigason (Actavis), Soriatane (Stiefel)
Indications: Psoriasis
Class: Retinoid
Half-life: 49 hours
Clinically important, potentially hazardous interactions with: alcohol, bexarotene, chloroquine, cholestyramine, corticosteroids, coumarins, danazol, demeclocycline, doxycycline, ethanolamine, isotretinoin, lithium, lymecycline, medroxyprogesterone, methotrexate, minocycline, oxytetracycline, phenytoin, progestins, St John's wort, tetracycline, tigecycline, vitamin A
Pregnancy category: X
Important contra-indications noted in the prescribing guidelines for: nursing mothers; pediatric patients
Note: Oral retinoids can cause birth defects, and women should avoid acitretin when pregnant or trying to conceive.
Black Box Warning: PREGNANCY

Skin
Atrophy (10–25%)
Bromhidrosis (<10%)
Bullous dermatitis (<10%)
Clammy skin (<10%)
Dermatitis (<10%)
Diaphoresis (<10%) [2]
Edema (<10%)
Erythema (18%)
Erythroderma [3]
Exanthems (10–25%) [2]
Exfoliative dermatitis (25–50%) [3]
Fissures (<10%)
Hot flashes (<10%)
Hyperhidrosis (<10%) [2]
Palmar–plantar desquamation (20–80%) [7]
Photosensitivity [3]
Pigmentation [3]
Pruritus (10–50%) [10]
Psoriasis (aggravated) (<10%)
Purpura (<10%)
Rash (>10%)
Seborrhea (<10%)
Stickiness (3–50%) [7]
Sunburn (<10%)
Toxicity [3]
Ulcerations (<10%)
Xerosis (25–50%) [14]

Hair
Alopecia (10–75%) [21]
Curly hair [3]
Hair changes (<10%)
Hair pigmentation [2]

Nails
Brittle nails [3]
Nail changes (25–50%)
Paronychia (10–25%) [6]
Pyogenic granuloma (<10%) [4]

Mucosal
Cheilitis (>75%) [14]
Dry mucous membranes [4]
Epistaxis (nosebleed) (10–25%) [2]
Gingival bleeding (<10%)
Gingivitis (<10%)
Mucocutaneous reactions [3]
Sialorrhea (<10%)
Stomatitis (<10%) [2]
Tongue disorder (<10%)
Ulcerative stomatitis (<10%)
Xerostomia (10–60%) [7]

Cardiovascular
Capillary leak syndrome [2]

Central Nervous System
Anorexia (<10%)
Depression (<10%) [4]
Dysgeusia (taste perversion) (<10%)
Headache (<10%) [2]
Hyperesthesia (10–25%)
Insomnia (<10%)
Neurotoxicity [3]
Pain (<10%)
Paralysis (facial) (<10%)
Paresthesias (10–25%) [2]
Pseudotumor cerebri [5]
Rigors (10–25%) [2]
Somnolence (drowsiness) (<10%)
Stroke [2]
Suicidal ideation [2]

Neuromuscular/Skeletal
Arthralgia (10–25%) [2]
Asthenia (fatigue) (<10%) [3]
Back pain (<10%)
Bone or joint pain [2]
Hyperostosis [10]
Myalgia/Myopathy [4]
Osteoporosis [2]

Gastrointestinal/Hepatic
Abdominal pain (<10%)
Diarrhea (<10%) [2]
Hepatitis [5]
Hepatotoxicity [8]
Nausea (<10%) [2]
Pancreatitis [3]
Vomiting [2]

Respiratory
Laryngitis [2]
Rhinitis (25–50%) [2]
Sinusitis (<10%)

Endocrine/Metabolic
GGT increased [2]
Hyperbilirubinemia [2]
Hypercholesterolemia (25–50%) [3]
Hyperlipidemia [5]
Hypertriglyceridemia (50–75%) [4]

Genitourinary
Vulvovaginal candidiasis [2]

Otic
Ear pain (<10%)
Tinnitus (<10%)

Ocular
Blepharitis (<10%)
Cataract (<10%)
Conjunctivitis (<10%) [2]
Diplopia (<10%)
Night blindness (<10%) [2]
Ocular adverse effects [2]
Ocular itching [2]
Ocular pain (<10%)
Photophobia (<10%) [2]
Vision blurred (<10%)
Xerophthalmia (10–25%) [3]

Other
Adverse effects [9]
Dipsia (thirst) (<10%)
Infection [2]
Side effects [4]
Teratogenicity [7]

ACYCLOVIR

Synonyms: aciclovir; ACV; acycloguanosine
Trade names: Sitavig (Cipher), Zovirax (GSK)
Indications: Herpes simplex, herpes zoster
Class: Antiviral, Antiviral, topical, Guanine nucleoside analog
Half-life: 3 hours (adults)
Clinically important, potentially hazardous interactions with: cobicistat/elvitegravir/emtricitabine/tenofovir disoproxil, meperidine, tenofovir disoproxil
Pregnancy category: B
Important contra-indications noted in the prescribing guidelines for: nursing mothers

---

Skin
Acneform eruption (<3%)
Dermatitis [12]
Exanthems (<5%) [5]
Facial edema (3–5%)
Peripheral edema [2]
Pruritus (<10%)
Radiation recall dermatitis [2]
Rash (<3%) [3]
Urticaria (<5%) [4]

Hair
Alopecia (<3%)

Central Nervous System
Headache (2%) [4]
Neurotoxicity [8]

Neuromuscular/Skeletal
Asthenia (fatigue) (12%)

Gastrointestinal/Hepatic
Diarrhea (2–3%)
Nausea (2–5%) [3]
Vomiting (3%)

Renal
Nephrotoxicity [11]
Renal failure [4]

Ocular
Hallucinations, visual [2]
Periorbital edema (3–5%)

Local
Injection-site inflammation (>10%)
Injection-site thrombophlebitis (9%)

ADALIMUMAB

Trade names: Amjevita (Amgen), Humira (AbbVie)
Indications: Rheumatoid arthritis, polyarticular juvenile idiopathic arthritis, psoriatic arthritis, ankylosing spondylitis, Crohn's disease, ulcerative colitis, psoriasis
Class: Cytokine inhibitor, Disease-modifying antirheumatic drug (DMARD), Monoclonal antibody, TNF inhibitor
Half-life: 10–20 days
Clinically important, potentially hazardous interactions with: abatacept, anakinra, live vaccines
Pregnancy category: B
Important contra-indications noted in the prescribing guidelines for: nursing mothers
Note: TNF inhibitors should be used in patients with heart failure only after consideration of other treatment options. TNF inhibitors are contraindicated in patients with a personal or family history of multiple sclerosis or demyelinating disease. TNF inhibitors should not be administered to patients with moderate to severe heart failure (New York Heart Association Functional Class III/IV).
Black Box Warning: SERIOUS INFECTIONS AND MALIGNANCY

Skin
Acneform eruption [2]
Angioedema [3]
Carcinoma [2]
Cellulitis (<5%) [2]
Dermatomyositis [5]
Eczema [2]
Erysipelas (<5%)
Granulomatous reaction [5]
Henoch–Schönlein purpura [2]
Herpes zoster [9]
Hidradenitis [2]
Hypersensitivity [3]
Lichenoid eruption [5]
Lupus erythematosus [16]
Lupus syndrome [3]
Lymphoma [8]
Malignancies [3]
Melanoma [6]
Palmoplantar pustulosis [3]
Peripheral edema (<5%)
Pruritus [5]
Psoriasis [38]
Rash (12%) [4]
Sarcoidosis [6]
Squamous cell carcinoma [5]
Stevens–Johnson syndrome [2]
Urticaria [3]
Vasculitis [8]
Vitiligo [2]

Hair
Alopecia [3]
Alopecia areata [7]
Alopecia universalis [2]

Cardiovascular
Arrhythmias (<5%)
Cardiac arrest (<5%)
Chest pain (<5%)
Congestive heart failure (<5%)
Hypertension (<5%)
Myocardial infarction (<5%)
Palpitation [2]
Pericarditis (<5%)
Tachycardia (<5%)
Thromboembolism [2]

Central Nervous System
Confusion (<5%)
Encephalitis [2]
Fever (<5%) [3]
Guillain–Barré syndrome [4]
Headache (12%) [4]
Leukoencephalopathy [3]
Multiple sclerosis (<5%) [3]
Neurotoxicity [2]
Paresthesias (<5%) [2]
Syncope (<5%)
Tremor (<5%)
Vertigo (dizziness) [2]

Neuromuscular/Skeletal
Arthralgia (<5%) [4]
Asthenia (fatigue) [2]
Back pain (6%) [2]
Tuberculous arthritis [2]

Gastrointestinal/Hepatic
Abdominal pain (7%) [2]
Cholecystitis (<5%)
Colitis [2]
Esophagitis (<5%)
Gastroenteritis (<5%)
Hepatitis [7]
Hepatotoxicity [10]
Nausea (9%) [2]
Vomiting (<5%)

Respiratory
Asthma (<5%)
Bronchitis [2]
Bronchospasm (<5%)
Dyspnea (<5%)
Flu-like syndrome (7%)
Nasopharyngitis [3]
Pleural effusion (<5%)
Pneumonia (<5%) [5]
Pneumonitis [3]
Pulmonary fibrosis [3]
Pulmonary toxicity [6]
Sinusitis (11%)
Tuberculosis [8]
Upper respiratory tract infection (17%) [6]

Endocrine/Metabolic
Creatine phosphokinase increased (<5%)
Hypercholesterolemia (6%)

Genitourinary
Cystitis (<5%)
Hematuria (5%)
Pelvic pain (<5%)
Urinary tract infection (8%)

Renal
Nephrotoxicity [2]

Hematologic
Agranulocytosis (<5%)
Eosinophilia [2]
Leukopenia (<5%)

Ocular
Cataract (<5%)
Optic neuritis [5]
Uveitis [4]

Local
Injection-site edema (15%) [2]
Injection-site erythema (15%) [2]
Injection-site pain (12%)
Injection-site reactions [23]

Other
Adverse effects [43]
Death [8]
Infection (5%) [66]
Side effects [2]

ADEFOVIR

Trade name: Hepsera (Gilead)
Indications: HIV infection, hepatitis B infection
Class: Antiretroviral, Nucleotide analog reverse transcriptase inhibitor
Half-life: 16–18 hours
Clinically important, potentially hazardous interactions with: amikacin, amphotericin B, cobicistat/elvitegravir/emtricitabine/tenofovir disoproxil, delavirdine, drugs causing kidney toxicity, foscarnet, gentamicin, hydroxyurea, pentamidine, tenofovir disoproxil, tobramycin
Pregnancy category: C
Important contra-indications noted in the prescribing guidelines for: the elderly; nursing mothers; pediatric patients
Black Box Warning: SEVERE ACUTE EXACERBATIONS OF HEPATITIS, NEPHROTOXICITY, HIV RESISTANCE, LACTIC ACIDOSIS AND SEVERE HEPATOMEGALY WITH STEATOSIS

Skin
Pruritus (<10%)
Rash (<10%)

Central Nervous System
Headache (9%) [2]
Pain [2]

Neuromuscular/Skeletal
Asthenia (fatigue) (13%) [3]
Back pain (<10%)
Osteomalacia [6]

Gastrointestinal/Hepatic
Abdominal pain (9%)
Diarrhea (3%)
Dyspepsia (3%)
Flatulence (4%)
Hepatotoxicity (<25%)
Nausea (5%)
Vomiting (<10%)

Respiratory
Cough (6–8%)
Rhinitis (<5%)

Endocrine/Metabolic
Hypophosphatemia [5]

Genitourinary
Hematuria (11%)

Renal
Fanconi syndrome [8]
Nephrotoxicity [14]

ADENOSINE

Synonym: ATP
Trade names: Adenocard (Astellas), Adenocur (Sanofi-Aventis)
Indications: Paroxysmal supraventricular tachycardia, varicose vein complications with stasis dermatitis
Class: Antiarrhythmic class IV, Neurotransmitter
Half-life: <10 seconds
Clinically important, potentially hazardous interactions with: aminophylline, antiarrhythmics, beta blockers, bupivacaine, carbamazepine, dipyridamole, levobupivacaine, nicotine, prilocaine, QT prolonging agents, ropivacaine
Pregnancy category: C
Important contra-indications noted in the prescribing guidelines for: pediatric patients

Cardiovascular
Arrhythmias [2]
Atrial fibrillation [6]
Chest pain [5]
Coronary vasospasm [2]
Flushing (18–44%)
Torsades de pointes [2]

Central Nervous System
Headache (2–18%) [2]
Vertigo (dizziness) (2–12%)

Neuromuscular/Skeletal
Jaw pain (<15%)

Gastrointestinal/Hepatic
Abdominal pain (13%)

Respiratory
Cough (6–8%)
Dyspnea [3]
Respiratory distress (11%)

Other
Adverse effects [2]

ADO-TRASTUZUMAB EMTANSINE

Synonym: T-DM1
Trade name: Kadcyla (Genentech)
Indications: HER2-positive, metastatic breast cancer in patients who previously received trastuzumab and a taxane, separately or in combination
Class: Antibody drug conjugate (ADC), HER2-targeted antibody-drug conjugate
Half-life: 4 days
Clinically important, potentially hazardous interactions with: none known
Pregnancy category: D
Important contra-indications noted in the prescribing guidelines for: nursing mothers; pediatric patients
Black Box Warning: HEPATOTOXICITY, CARDIAC TOXICITY, EMBRYO-FETAL TOXICITY

Skin
Hypersensitivity (2%)
Peripheral edema (7%)
Pruritus (6%)
Rash (12%)

Mucosal
Epistaxis (nosebleed) (23%)
Stomatitis (14%)
Xerostomia (17%)

Cardiovascular
Cardiotoxicity [2]
Hypertension (5%)

Central Nervous System
Chills (8%)
Dysgeusia (taste perversion) (8%)
Fever (19%) [2]
Headache (28%) [4]
Insomnia (12%)
Peripheral neuropathy (21%)
Vertigo (dizziness) (10%)

Neuromuscular/Skeletal
Arthralgia (19%) [3]
Asthenia (fatigue) (18–36%) [12]
Bone or joint pain (36%)
Myalgia/Myopathy (14%)

Gastrointestinal/Hepatic
Abdominal pain (19%)
Constipation (27%) [3]
Diarrhea (24%) [4]
Dyspepsia (9%)
Hepatotoxicity [12]
Nausea (40%) [8]
Vomiting (19%)

Respiratory
Cough (18%)
Dyspnea (12%)
Pneumonia [2]

Endocrine/Metabolic
ALP increased (5%)
ALT increased (82%) [3]
AST increased (98%) [5]
Hypokalemia (10%) [3]

Genitourinary
Urinary tract infection (9%)

Hematologic
Anemia (14%) [4]
Febrile neutropenia [2]
Hemorrhage (32%)
Neutropenia (7%) [3]
Thrombocytopenia (31%) [18]

Ocular
Conjunctivitis (4%)
Lacrimation (3%)
Vision blurred (5%)
Xerophthalmia (4%)

Other
Adverse effects [4]

AFATINIB

Trade name: Gilotrif (Boehringer Ingelheim)
Indications: Metastatic non-small cell lung cancer in patients whose tumors have epidermal growth factor receptor exon 19 deletions or exon 21 (L858R) substitution mutations, metastatic squamous non-small cell lung cancer progressing following platinium-based chemotherapy
Class: Tyrosine kinase inhibitor
Half-life: 37 hours
Clinically important, potentially hazardous interactions with: amiodarone, carbamazepine, cyclosporine, erythromycin, itraconazole, ketoconazole, nelfinavir, P-glycoprotein inhibitors, phenobarbital, phenytoin, quinidine, rifampin, ritonavir, saquinavir, St John's wort, tacrolimus, verapamil
Pregnancy category: D
Important contra-indications noted in the prescribing guidelines for: nursing mothers; pediatric patients

Skin
Acneform eruption [24]
Fissures [2]
Hand–foot syndrome [2]
Pruritus [2]
Rash [43]
Toxicity [2]
Xerosis [6]

Nails
Nail changes [2]
Paronychia (58%) [9]

Mucosal
Epistaxis (nosebleed) [3]
Mucosal inflammation [6]
Mucositis [10]
Rhinorrhea (11%)
Stomatitis (71%) [17]

Central Nervous System
Anorexia [3]
Fever (12%)

Neuromuscular/Skeletal
Asthenia (fatigue) [16]

Gastrointestinal/Hepatic
Diarrhea (96%) [58]
Dysphagia [2]
Hepatotoxicity (10%) [3]
Nausea [13]
Vomiting [10]

Respiratory
Dyspnea [3]
Pulmonary toxicity [3]

Endocrine/Metabolic
ALT increased [2]
Appetite decreased (29%) [4]
Dehydration [3]
Hypokalemia [2]

Hematologic
Anemia [3]
Febrile neutropenia [2]
Leukopenia [2]
Neutropenia [6]
Thrombocytopenia [2]

Other
Adverse effects [7]
Death [3]

AFLIBERCEPT

Synonym: ziv-aflibercept
Trade names: Eylea (Regeneron), Zaltrap (Sanofi-Aventis)
Indications: Neovascular (wet) age-related macular degeneration (Eylea), metastatic colorectal cancer (Zaltrap) in combination with FOLFIRI (fluorouracil, leucovorin and irinotecan)
Class: Fusion protein
Half-life: terminal 5–6 days
Clinically important, potentially hazardous interactions with: none known
Pregnancy category: C
Important contra-indications noted in the prescribing guidelines for: nursing mothers; pediatric patients
Note: Eylea: Contraindicated in patients with ocular or periocular infection or active intraocular inflammation.
Black Box Warning: Zaltrap: HEMORRHAGE, GASTROINTESTINAL PERFORATION, COMPROMISED WOUND HEALING

Mucosal
Epistaxis (nosebleed) [3]
Stomatitis [5]

Cardiovascular
Hypertension [11]
Myocardial infarction (<2%)
Venous thromboembolism [2]

Central Nervous System
Anorexia [2]
Headache [2]
Stroke (<2%)

Neuromuscular/Skeletal
Asthenia (fatigue) [6]

Gastrointestinal/Hepatic
Diarrhea [5]
Gastrointestinal perforation [4]

Respiratory
Dysphonia [5]
Dyspnea [2]
Pulmonary embolism [2]

Endocrine/Metabolic
Weight loss [2]

Renal
Proteinuria [7]

Hematologic
Hemorrhage [3]
Neutropenia [9]

Ocular
Cataract (7%) [2]
Conjunctival hemorrhage (25%) [2]
Conjunctival hyperemia (4%)
Corneal erosion (4%)
Intraocular pressure increased (5%) [2]
Lacrimation (3%)
Ocular adverse effects [3]
Ocular pain (3–9%)
Vision blurred (2%)
Vitreous detachment (6%)
Vitreous floaters (6%)

Local
Injection-site pain (3%)

Other
Adverse effects [2]
Death [2]
Infection [2]

ALBENDAZOLE

Trade name: Albenza (GSK)
Indications: Nematode infections, hydatid cyst disease
Class: Anthelmintic
Half-life: 8–12 hours
Clinically important, potentially hazardous interactions with: antimalarials, conivaptan, dexamethasone, high fat foods
Pregnancy category: C
Important contra-indications noted in the prescribing guidelines for: nursing mothers

---

Skin
Fixed eruption [2]
Pruritus [4]
Urticaria [2]

Hair
Alopecia (reversible) (<2%) [4]

Central Nervous System
Fever (<2%)
Headache (<11%) [5]
Intracranial pressure increased (<2%)
Psychosis [2]
Vertigo (dizziness) (<2%) [2]

Neuromuscular/Skeletal
Dystonia [3]

Gastrointestinal/Hepatic
Abdominal pain (<7%) [7]
Hepatitis [4]
Nausea (4–6%) [3]
Vomiting (4–6%) [2]

Other
Adverse effects [5]

ALBIGLUTIDE

Trade name: Tanzeum (GSK)
Indications: To improve glycemic control in adults with Type II diabetes mellitus
Class: Glucagon-like peptide-1 (GLP-1) receptor agonist
Half-life: 5 days
Clinically important, potentially hazardous interactions with: none known
Pregnancy category: C
Important contra-indications noted in the prescribing guidelines for: nursing mothers; pediatric patients
Note: Contraindicated in patients with a personal or family history of medullary thyroid carcinoma or in patients with multiple endocrine neoplasia syndrome Type 2.
Black Box Warning: RISK OF THYROID C-CELL TUMORS

Central Nervous System
Headache [4]
Vertigo (dizziness) [2]

Neuromuscular/Skeletal
Arthralgia (7%)
Back pain (7%) [2]

Gastrointestinal/Hepatic
Constipation [2]
Diarrhea (13%) [11]
Dyspepsia (3%)
Gastroesophageal reflux (4%)
Nausea (11%) [16]
Vomiting (4%) [12]

Respiratory
Cough (7%)
Influenza (5%)
Nasopharyngitis [3]
Pneumonia (2%)
Sinusitis (6%)
Upper respiratory tract infection (14%) [3]

Endocrine/Metabolic
GGT increased (2%)
Hypoglycemia (2%) [5]

Local
Injection-site hematoma (2%)
Injection-site reactions (11%) [12]

Other
Adverse effects [4]

ALBUTEROL

Synonym: salbutamol
Trade names: AccuNeb (Mylan Specialty), Combivent (Boehringer Ingelheim), Duoneb (Mylan Specialty), Proventil (Schering), Ventolin (GSK), Volmax (Muro)
Indications: Bronchospasm associated with asthma
Class: Beta-2 adrenergic agonist, Bronchodilator, Tocolytic
Half-life: 3–6 hours
Clinically important, potentially hazardous interactions with: atomoxetine, epinephrine, insulin degludec, insulin detemir, insulin glargine, insulin glulisine
Pregnancy category: C
Important contra-indications noted in the prescribing guidelines for: nursing mothers
Note: Combivent is albuterol and ipratropium.

Skin
Dermatitis [2]
Diaphoresis (<10%)
Erythema (palmar) (with infusion) [2]

Mucosal
Xerostomia (<10%)

Cardiovascular
Flushing (<10%)
Myocardial infarction [2]
Palpitation [2]
Tachyarrhythmia [2]
Tachycardia [2]

Central Nervous System
Dysgeusia (taste perversion) (<10%)
Tremor [2]

Endocrine/Metabolic
Acidosis [3]

Other
Adverse effects [2]

ALDESLEUKIN

Synonyms: IL-2; interleukin-2
Trade name: Proleukin (Chiron)
Indications: Metastatic renal cell carcinoma and metastatic melanoma
Class: Biologic, Immunomodulator, Interleukin-2
Half-life: 6–85 minutes
Clinically important, potentially hazardous interactions with: acebutolol, alfuzosin, altretamine, amikacin, aminoglycosides, antineoplastics, betamethasone, bleomycin, busulfan, captopril, carboplatin, carmustine, chlorambucil, ciclesonide, cilazapril, cisplatin, corticosteroids, cyclophosphamide, cytarabine, dacarbazine, dactinomycin, daunorubicin, docetaxel, doxorubicin, enalapril, estramustine, etoposide, fludarabine, fluorouracil, fosinopril, gemcitabine, gentamicin, hydroxyurea, idarubicin, ifosfamide, indomethacin, interferon alfa, irbesartan, kanamycin, levamisole, lisinopril, lomustine, mechlorethamine, melphalan, mercaptopurine, methotrexate, mitomycin, mitotane, mitoxantrone, neomycin, olmesartan, PEG-interferon, pentostatin, plicamycin, procarbazine, quinapril, ramipril, streptomycin, streptozocin, thioguanine, thiotepa, tobramycin, trandolapril, tretinoin, triamcinolone, uracil, vinblastine, vincristine, vinorelbine
Pregnancy category: C
Important contra-indications noted in the prescribing guidelines for: nursing mothers; pediatric patients
Note: Contraindicated in patients with significant cardiac, pulmonary, renal, hepatic, or CNS impairment.
Black Box Warning: CAPILLARY LEAK SYNDROME

Skin
Angioedema [2]
Dermatitis [2]
Edema (47%) [3]
Erythema (41%) [5]
Erythema nodosum [3]
Erythroderma [4]
Exanthems [5]
Exfoliative dermatitis (18%)
Linear IgA bullous dermatosis [4]
Necrosis [2]
Pemphigus [2]
Peripheral edema (28%)
Petechiae (4%)
Pruritus (24%) [7]
Psoriasis [4]
Purpura (4%)
Rash (42%) [2]
Scleroderma [2]
Toxic epidermal necrolysis [2]
Toxicity [6]
Urticaria (2%) [3]
Vitiligo [3]
Xerosis (15%)

Hair
Alopecia [2]

Mucosal
Oral mucosal eruption [2]
Stomatitis (22%)

Cardiovascular
Arrhythmias (10%)
Capillary leak syndrome [12]
Cardiotoxicity (11%) [2]
Hypotension (71%) [6]
Supraventricular tachycardia (12%)
Tachycardia (23%)
Vascular leak syndrome [6]
Vasodilation (13%)

Central Nervous System
Anorexia (20%)
Anxiety (12%)
Chills (52%)
Confusion (34%)
Depression [3]
Dysgeusia (taste perversion) (7%)
Fever (29%) [8]
Neurotoxicity [3]
Pain (12%)
Rigors [3]
Somnolence (drowsiness) (22%)
Vertigo (dizziness) (11%)

Neuromuscular/Skeletal
Asthenia (fatigue) (23–27%)
Myalgia/Myopathy (6%)
Myasthenia gravis [2]

Gastrointestinal/Hepatic
Abdominal pain (11%)
Diarrhea (67%) [3]
Hepatotoxicity [2]
Nausea (35%) [9]
Vomiting (50%) [6]

Respiratory
Cough (11%)
Dyspnea (43%)
Pulmonary toxicity (11–24%) [2]
Rhinitis (10%)

Endocrine/Metabolic
Acidosis (12%)
ALP increased (10%)
AST increased (23%)
Creatine phosphokinase increased (33%) [2]
Hypocalcemia (11%)
Hypomagnesemia [2]
Hypophosphatemia [2]
Weight gain (16%)
Weight loss [2]

Genitourinary
Oliguria (63%)

Renal
Nephrotoxicity [4]

Hematologic
Anemia (29%)
Leukopenia (16%) [2]
Sepsis [3]
Thrombocytopenia (37%) [2]

Local
Injection-site inflammation [2]
Injection-site nodules [2]
Injection-site reactions (3%) [2]

Other
Adverse effects [3]
Death [5]
Infection (13%) [2]

ALECTINIB *

Trade name: Alecensa (Genentech)
Indications: Anaplastic lymphoma kinase-positive, metastatic non-small cell lung cancer in patients who have progressed on, or are intolerant to, crizotinib
Class: Kinase inhibitor
Half-life: 33 hours
Clinically important, potentially hazardous interactions with: none known
Pregnancy category: N/A (Can cause fetal harm)
Important contra-indications noted in the prescribing guidelines for: nursing mothers; pediatric patients

---

Skin
Edema (30%)
Peripheral edema [3]
Photosensitivity (10%)
Rash (18%)

Central Nervous System
Headache (17%)

Neuromuscular/Skeletal
Asthenia (fatigue) (41%) [4]
Back pain (12%)
Myalgia/Myopathy (29%) [3]

Gastrointestinal/Hepatic
Constipation (34%) [4]
Diarrhea (16%)
Nausea (18%)
Vomiting (12%)

Respiratory
Cough (19%)
Dyspnea (16%)
Pulmonary toxicity [2]

Endocrine/Metabolic
ALP increased (47%)
ALT increased (34%)
AST increased (51%) [2]
Creatine phosphokinase increased (43%) [3]
Hyperbilirubinemia (39%)
Hyperglycemia (36%)
Hypocalcemia (32%)
Hypokalemia (29%)
Hyponatremia (20%)
Hypophosphatemia (21%)
Serum creatinine increased (28%)
Weight gain (11%)

Hematologic
Anemia (56%)
Lymphopenia (22%)
Neutropenia [3]

Ocular
Visual disturbances (10%)

ALENDRONATE

Trade names: Binosto (Mission), Fosamax (Merck)
Indications: Osteoporosis in postmenopausal women, Paget's disease
Class: Bisphosphonate
Half-life: >10 years
Clinically important, potentially hazardous interactions with: none known
Pregnancy category: C
Important contra-indications noted in the prescribing guidelines for: nursing mothers; pediatric patients

---

Skin
Angioedema [2]
Hypersensitivity [3]
Rash [5]

Mucosal
Oral ulceration [8]

Central Nervous System
Headache [2]

Neuromuscular/Skeletal
Arthralgia [6]
Bone or joint pain (<6%) [5]
Fractures [20]
Osteonecrosis [12]

Gastrointestinal/Hepatic
Abdominal pain (<7%) [8]
Dyspepsia [8]
Dysphagia [4]
Esophageal perforation [2]
Esophagitis [12]
Hepatotoxicity [7]
Nausea [7]
Vomiting [4]

Endocrine/Metabolic
Hypocalcemia (18%) [5]

Renal
Nephrotoxicity [2]
Renal failure [2]

Ocular
Conjunctivitis [2]
Ocular adverse effects [2]
Ocular inflammation [2]
Scleritis [3]
Uveitis [6]

Other
Adverse effects [5]

ALFUZOSIN

Trade names: Uroxatral (Concordia), Xatral (Sanofi-Aventis)
Indications: Benign prostatic hyperplasia
Class: Adrenergic alpha-receptor antagonist
Half-life: 10 hours
Clinically important, potentially hazardous interactions with: ACE inhibitors, adrenergic neurone blockers, alcohol, aldesleukin, alprostadil, amitriptyline, angiotensin II receptor antagonists, antipsychotics, anxiolytics and hypnotics, arsenic, atazanavir, atenolol, baclofen, beta blockers, boceprevir, calcium channel blockers, cimetidine, citalopram, clonidine, conivaptan, corticosteroids, CYP3A4 inhibitors or inducers, darunavir, dasatinib, deferasirox, degarelix, delavirdine, diazoxide, diltiazem, diuretics, estrogens, food, general anesthetics, hydralazine, indinavir, itraconazole, ketoconazole, lapatinib, levodopa, levofloxacin, lopinavir, MAO inhibitors, methyldopa, minoxidil, moxifloxacin, moxisylyte, moxonidine, nelfinavir, nitrates, nitroprusside, NSAIDs, pazopanib, phosphodiesterase 5 inhibitors, protease inhibitors, QT prolonging agents, ritonavir, sildenafil, St John's wort, tadalafil, telaprevir, telavancin, telithromycin, tipranavir, tizanidine, vardenafil, voriconazole, vorinostat, ziprasidone
Pregnancy category: B
Important contra-indications noted in the prescribing guidelines for: pediatric patients

---

Cardiovascular
Hypotension [2]
Orthostatic hypotension [3]
QT prolongation [2]

Central Nervous System
Headache (3%)
Pain (<2%)
Vertigo (dizziness) (6%) [19]

Neuromuscular/Skeletal
Asthenia (fatigue) (3%)

Gastrointestinal/Hepatic
Abdominal pain (<2%)
Hepatotoxicity [2]

Respiratory
Bronchitis (<2%)
Pharyngitis (<2%)
Sinusitis (<2%)
Upper respiratory tract infection (3%)

Genitourinary
Ejaculatory dysfunction [3]
Erectile dysfunction [2]

Ocular
Floppy iris syndrome [4]

Other
Adverse effects [2]

ALIROCUMAB

Trade name: Praluent (Regeneron)
Indications: Adjunct to diet and statin therapy in hypercholesterolemia or clinical atherosclerotic cardiovascular disease where additional lowering of low density lipoprotein cholesterol is required
Class: Monoclonal antibody, Proprotein convertase subtilisin kexin type 9 (PCSK9) inhibitor
Half-life: 17–20 days
Clinically important, potentially hazardous interactions with: none known
Pregnancy category: N/A (No data available but likely to cross the placenta in second and third trimester)
Important contra-indications noted in the prescribing guidelines for: pediatric patients

---

Skin
Hematoma (2%)

Cardiovascular
Cardiotoxicity [3]
Myocardial infarction [3]

Central Nervous System
Cognitive impairment [2]
Headache [3]
Neurotoxicity [4]
Stroke [2]
Vertigo (dizziness) [6]

Neuromuscular/Skeletal
Arthralgia [6]
Back pain [5]
Bone or joint pain (2%) [2]
Muscle spasm (3%)
Myalgia/Myopathy (4%) [5]

Gastrointestinal/Hepatic
Diarrhea (5%) [3]
Hepatotoxicity (3%)
Nausea [2]

Respiratory
Bronchitis (4%)
Cough (3%)
Influenza (6%) [4]
Nasopharyngitis (11%) [8]
Sinusitis (3%) [2]
Upper respiratory tract infection [6]

Endocrine/Metabolic
ALT increased [3]
Creatine phosphokinase increased [3]

Genitourinary
Urinary tract infection (5%)

Ocular
Ocular adverse effects [2]

Local
Injection-site pain [2]
Injection-site reactions (7%) [12]

Other
Adverse effects [3]
Allergic reactions (9%)
Death [2]

ALLOPURINOL

Trade name: Zyloprim (Prometheus)
Indications: Gouty arthritis
Class: Purine analog, Xanthine oxidase inhibitor
Half-life: <3 hours
Clinically important, potentially hazardous interactions with: acenocoumarol, amoxicillin, ampicillin, ampicillin/sulbactam, azathioprine, benazepril, capecitabine, captopril, cilazapril, cyclopenthiazide, dicumarol, enalapril, fosinopril, imidapril, lisinopril, mercaptopurine, pantoprazole, quinapril, ramipril, trandolapril, uracil/tegafur, vidarabine, zofenopril
Pregnancy category: C
Note: HLA-B*5801 confers a risk of allopurinol-induced serious skin reactions like SJS/TEN and DRESS.

Skin
AGEP [6]
DRESS syndrome [43]
Eosinophilic pustular folliculitis [2]
Erythema multiforme [7]
Exanthems (<5%) [20]

Exfoliative dermatitis (>10%) [15]
Fixed eruption [11]
Granuloma annulare (disseminated) [2]
Hypersensitivity [48]
Lupus erythematosus [3]
Pityriasis rosea [2]
Pruritus [7]
Purpura (>10%) [2]
Rash (>10%) [9]
Stevens–Johnson syndrome (>10%) [50]
Toxic epidermal necrolysis [70]
Toxic pustuloderma [3]
Toxicity [2]
Urticaria (>10%) [6]
Vasculitis [7]

Hair
Alopecia (<10%) [2]

Mucosal
Oral ulceration [2]
Stomatitis [2]

Cardiovascular
Polyarteritis nodosa [3]

Central Nervous System
Chills (<10%)
Fever [2]
Headache [3]
Vertigo (dizziness) [3]

Neuromuscular/Skeletal
Arthralgia [3]
Asthenia (fatigue) [2]
Back pain [2]
Bone or joint pain [2]
Joint disorder [2]
Myalgia/Myopathy [3]

Gastrointestinal/Hepatic
Diarrhea [5]
Hepatotoxicity [7]
Nausea [3]

Respiratory
Nasopharyngitis [2]
Upper respiratory tract infection [4]

Endocrine/Metabolic
ALT increased [2]
AST increased [3]

Renal
Nephrotoxicity [3]

Other
Adverse effects [13]
Allergic reactions (severe) [2]
Death [9]

ALMOTRIPTAN

Trade names: Almogran (Almirall), Axert (Ortho-McNeil)
Indications: Migraine headaches
Class: 5-HT1 agonist, Serotonin receptor agonist, Triptan
Half-life: 3–4 hours
Clinically important, potentially hazardous interactions with: conivaptan, darunavir, delavirdine, dihydroergotamine, ergotamine, indinavir, ketoconazole, methysergide, SNRIs, SSRIs, telithromycin, triptans, voriconazole
Pregnancy category: C
Important contra-indications noted in the prescribing guidelines for: pediatric patients
Note: Contraindicated in patients with history, symptoms, or signs of ischemic cardiac, cerebrovascular, or peripheral vascular syndromes, or with uncontrolled hypertension.

Cardiovascular
Chest pain [3]

Central Nervous System
Headache [2]
Neurotoxicity [2]
Paresthesias [4]
Somnolence (drowsiness) [5]
Vertigo (dizziness) [6]

Neuromuscular/Skeletal
Asthenia (fatigue) [4]

Gastrointestinal/Hepatic
Nausea [6]
Vomiting [3]

Respiratory
Flu-like syndrome (12%)
Upper respiratory tract infection (20%)

Other
Adverse effects [10]

ALOGLIPTIN

Trade name: Nesina (Takeda)
Indications: Type II diabetes mellitus
Class: Antidiabetic, Dipeptidyl peptidase-4 (DPP-4) inhibitor
Half-life: 21 hours
Clinically important, potentially hazardous interactions with: none known
Pregnancy category: B
Important contra-indications noted in the prescribing guidelines for: nursing mothers; pediatric patients

Skin
Hypersensitivity [2]
Pruritus [2]

Central Nervous System
Headache (4%) [8]
Vertigo (dizziness) [3]

Neuromuscular/Skeletal
Arthralgia [2]

Gastrointestinal/Hepatic
Constipation [2]
Diarrhea [2]
Pancreatitis [3]

Respiratory
Nasopharyngitis (4%) [8]
Upper respiratory tract infection (4%) [6]

Endocrine/Metabolic
Hypoglycemia [14]

Other
Adverse effects [6]
Infection [3]

ALPRAZOLAM

Trade name: Xanax (Pfizer)
Indications: Anxiety, depression, panic attacks
Class: Benzodiazepine
Half-life: 11–16 hours
Clinically important, potentially hazardous interactions with: alcohol, amprenavir, aprepitant, boceprevir, clarithromycin, CNS depressants, darunavir, delavirdine, digoxin, efavirenz, fluconazole, fluoxetine, fluvoxamine, grapefruit juice, indinavir, itraconazole, ivermectin, kava, ketoconazole, posaconazole, propoxyphene, ritonavir, saquinavir, St John's wort, telaprevir, tipranavir
Pregnancy category: D
Important contra-indications noted in the prescribing guidelines for: the elderly; nursing mothers; pediatric patients

Skin
Dermatitis (4%) [5]
Diaphoresis (16%)
Edema (5%)
Photosensitivity [4]
Pruritus (<10%) [2]
Rash (11%) [4]

Mucosal
Sialopenia (33%)
Sialorrhea (4%)
Xerostomia (15%) [6]

Cardiovascular
Hypotension (<10%)

Central Nervous System
Cognitive impairment (>10%)
Coma [2]
Depression (>10%)
Dysarthria (>10%)
Incoordination (<10%)
Memory loss [2]
Neurotoxicity [2]
Paresthesias (2%)
Restlessness [2]
Sedation [2]
Seizures (<10%) [2]
Somnolence (drowsiness) (>10%)

Neuromuscular/Skeletal
Asthenia (fatigue) (>10%) [2]

Endocrine/Metabolic
Galactorrhea [2]

Genitourinary
Micturition difficulty (>10%)

ALPROSTADIL

Synonyms: PGE; prostaglandin E_1
Trade names: Caverject (Pfizer), Edex (Schwarz), Muse (Vivus), Prostin VR (Pfizer)
Indications: Impotence, to maintain patent ductus arteriosus
Class: Prostaglandin
Half-life: 5–10 minutes
Clinically important, potentially hazardous interactions with: acebutolol, alfuzosin, captopril, cilazapril, enalapril, fosinopril, irbesartan, lisinopril, olmesartan, quinapril, ramipril
Pregnancy category: D (not indicated for use in women)
Important contra-indications noted in the prescribing guidelines for: pediatric patients
Black Box Warning: APNEA (in neonates with congenital heart defects)

Skin
Edema (<10%)
Penile rash (<10%)

Mucosal
Nasal congestion (<10%)

Cardiovascular
Bradycardia (<10%)
Flushing (>10%)
Hypertension (<10%)
Hypotension (<10%)
Tachycardia (<10%)

Central Nervous System
Fever (>10%)
Headache (>10%)
Pain (>10%)
Vertigo (dizziness) (>10%)

Neuromuscular/Skeletal
Back pain (<10%)

Gastrointestinal/Hepatic
Diarrhea (<10%)

Respiratory
Apnea (>10%)
Cough (<10%)
Flu-like syndrome (<10%)
Sinusitis (<10%)

Genitourinary
Erectile dysfunction (prolonged erection / >4 hours) (4%)
Penile pain (>10%)
Priapism (4%) [8]
Urethral burning (>10%) [2]

Local
Application-site burning [3]
Application-site erythema [2]
Application-site pain [2]
Application-site pruritus [2]
Injection-site ecchymoses (<10%)
Injection-site hematoma (3%)
Injection-site pain (2%)

ALTEPLASE

Synonym: tPA
Trade name: Activase (Genentech)
Indications: Acute myocardial infarction, acute pulmonary embolism
Class: Fibrinolytic, Plasminogen activator
Half-life: 30–45 minutes
Clinically important, potentially hazardous interactions with: nitroglycerin, ticlopidine
Pregnancy category: C
Important contra-indications noted in the prescribing guidelines for: the elderly; nursing mothers

---

Skin
Anaphylactoid reactions/Anaphylaxis [5]
Angioedema [10]
Ecchymoses (<10%)
Purpura (<10%)

Central Nervous System
Fever (<10%)
Intracranial hemorrhage [7]

Gastrointestinal/Hepatic
Hemorrhagic colitis (5%)

Hematologic
Hemorrhage (4%)

Other
Death [4]

AMBRISENTAN

Trade names: Letairis (Gilead), Volibris (GSK)
Indications: Pulmonary arterial hypertension
Class: Antihypertensive, Endothelin receptor (ETR) antagonist, Vasodilator
Half-life: 9 hours
Clinically important, potentially hazardous interactions with: conivaptan, cyclosporine, CYP2C19 inhibitors and inducers, CYP3A4 inhibitors and inducers, dasatinib, deferasirox, grapefruit juice, St John's wort
Pregnancy category: X
Important contra-indications noted in the prescribing guidelines for: nursing mothers; pediatric patients
Note: Contraindicated in pregnancy and in patients with idiopathic pulmonary fibrosis.
Black Box Warning: CONTRAINDICATED IN PREGNANCY

Skin
Edema [3]
Peripheral edema (17%) [7]

Mucosal
Nasal congestion (6%) [2]

Cardiovascular
Flushing (4%)
Palpitation (5%)

Central Nervous System
Headache (15%) [3]

Gastrointestinal/Hepatic
Abdominal pain (3%)
Constipation (4%)
Hepatotoxicity [3]

Respiratory
Dyspnea (4%)
Nasopharyngitis (3%)
Sinusitis (3%)

Hematologic
Anemia [4]

AMIKACIN

Trade name: Amikacin sulfate (Bedford)
Indications: Short-term treatment of serious infections due to gram-negative bacteria
Class: Antibiotic, aminoglycoside
Half-life: 1.5–2.5 hours (adults)
Clinically important, potentially hazardous interactions with: adefovir, aldesleukin, aminoglycosides, atracurium, bumetanide, cephalexin, doxacurium, ethacrynic acid, furosemide, succinylcholine, teicoplanin, torsemide
Pregnancy category: D
Important contra-indications noted in the prescribing guidelines for: nursing mothers; pediatric patients
Note: Aminoglycosides may cause neurotoxicity and/or nephrotoxicity.

Skin
Dermatitis [2]
Exanthems [2]

Central Nervous System
Neurotoxicity (<10%)

Renal
Nephrotoxicity (<10%) [10]

Otic
Hearing loss [5]
Ototoxicity (<10%) [8]
Tinnitus [2]

Ocular
Macular infarction [3]

AMILORIDE

Trade names: Midamor (Merck), Moduretic (Merck)
Indications: Prevention of hypokalemia associated with kaliuretic diuretics, management of edema in hypertension
Class: Diuretic, potassium-sparing
Half-life: 6–9 hours
Clinically important, potentially hazardous interactions with: ACE inhibitors, benazepril, captopril, cyclosporine, enalapril, fosinopril, lisinopril, magnesium, metformin, moexipril, potassium salts, quinapril, quinidine, ramipril, spironolactone, trandolapril, zofenopril
Pregnancy category: B
Note: Moduretic is amiloride and hydrochlorothiazide. Hydrochlorothiazide is a sulfonamide and can be absorbed systemically. Sulfonamides can produce severe, possibly fatal, reactions such as toxic epidermal necrolysis and Stevens-Johnson syndrome.

Skin
Photosensitivity [4]

Central Nervous System
Headache (<10%)
Vertigo (dizziness) (<10%)

Neuromuscular/Skeletal
Asthenia (fatigue) (<10%)
Myalgia/Myopathy (<10%)

Respiratory
Cough (<10%)
Dyspnea (<10%)

Endocrine/Metabolic
Gynecomastia (<10%)
Hyperkalemia [2]

Genitourinary
Impotence (<10%)

AMINOPHYLLINE

Synonym: theophylline ethylenediamine
Trade names: Elixophyllin (Forest), Phyllocontin (Napp), Quibron (Monarch)
Indications: Prevention or treatment of reversible bronchospasm
Class: Xanthine alkaloid
Half-life: 3–15 hours (in adult nonsmokers)
Clinically important, potentially hazardous interactions with: adenosine, anagrelide, arformoterol, azithromycin, BCG vaccine, caffeine, capsicum, carbimazole, cimetidine, ciprofloxacin, clorazepate, cocoa, erythromycin, eucalyptus, febuxostat, fluvoxamine, halothane, indacaterol, influenza vaccine, levofloxacin, mebendazole, methylprednisolone, moxifloxacin, nilutamide, norfloxacin, obeticholic acid, ofloxacin, oral contraceptives, prednisolone, prednisone, propranolol, rasagiline, raspberry leaf, roflumilast, ropivacaine, roxithromycin, St John's wort, torasemide, torsemide, triamcinolone, zafirlukast
Pregnancy category: C
Important contra-indications noted in the prescribing guidelines for: the elderly; nursing mothers

---

Skin
Dermatitis [7]
Exanthems [5]
Exfoliative dermatitis [6]
Hypersensitivity [6]
Pruritus [3]
Stevens–Johnson syndrome [3]
Urticaria [6]

Cardiovascular
Arrhythmias [2]
Palpitation [3]
Tachycardia [2]

Central Nervous System
Insomnia [2]
Seizures [11]
Tremor [2]

Neuromuscular/Skeletal
Rhabdomyolysis [5]

Gastrointestinal/Hepatic
Abdominal pain [2]
Nausea [5]
Vomiting [2]

Endocrine/Metabolic
SIADH [2]

Other
Adverse effects [3]
Allergic reactions [5]
Death [2]

AMIODARONE

Trade names: Cordarone (Wyeth), Pacerone (Upsher-Smith)
Indications: Ventricular fibrillation, ventricular tachycardia
Class: Antiarrhythmic, Antiarrhythmic class III, CYP1A2 inhibitor, CYP3A4 inhibitor
Half-life: 26–107 days
Clinically important, potentially hazardous interactions with: abarelix, acebutolol, acenocoumarol, afatinib, amisulpride, amitriptyline, amprenavir, anisindione, anticoagulants, arsenic, artemether/lumefantrine, asenapine, astemizole, atazanavir, atorvastatin, azoles, boceprevir, bosentan, carbimazole, celiprolol, cholestyramine, cimetidine, ciprofloxacin, clopidogrel, cobicistat/elvitegravir/emtricitabine/tenofovir alafenamide, cobicistat/elvitegravir/emtricitabine/tenofovir disoproxil, colchicine, cyclosporine, dabigatran, daclatasvir, darunavir, degarelix, delavirdine, dextromethorphan, dicumarol, digoxin, diltiazem, disopyramide, dronedarone, droperidol, echinacea, enoxacin, fentanyl, flecainide, fosamprenavir, gatifloxacin, grapefruit juice, indinavir, ledipasvir & sofosbuvir, lesinurad, levofloxacin, levomepromazine, lidocaine, lomefloxacin, lopinavir, loratadine, macrolide antibiotics, methotrexate, moxifloxacin, nelfinavir, nevirapine, nilotinib, norfloxacin, ofloxacin, orlistat, oxprenolol, pentamidine, phenytoin, procainamide, propranolol, quinidine, quinine, quinolones, rifabutin, rifampin, rifapentine, ritonavir, ropivacaine, rosuvastatin, simvastatin, sotalol, sparfloxacin, St John's wort, sulpiride, tacrolimus, telaprevir, tetrabenazine, thalidomide, tipranavir, trazodone, vandetanib, venetoclax, verapamil, warfarin, zuclopenthixol
Pregnancy category: D
Important contra-indications noted in the prescribing guidelines for: the elderly; nursing mothers; pediatric patients
Black Box Warning: PULMONARY TOXICITY

Skin
Anaphylactoid reactions/Anaphylaxis [2]
Angioedema [2]
Diaphoresis [2]
Edema (<10%)
Erythema nodosum [2]
Exanthems [5]
Facial erythema (3%) [2]
Iododerma [2]
Linear IgA bullous dermatosis [6]
Lupus erythematosus [5]
Myxedema [3]
Photosensitivity (10–75%) [41]
Phototoxicity [3]
Pigmentation (blue) (<10%) [68]
Pruritus (<5%) [2]
Psoriasis [2]
Purpura (2%)
Toxic epidermal necrolysis [2]
Toxicity [4]
Vasculitis [5]

Hair
Alopecia [5]

Mucosal
Sialorrhea (<10%)

Cardiovascular
Arrhythmias (<3%) [3]
Atrial fibrillation (paroxysmal) [3]
Atrioventricular block [2]
Bradycardia [17]
Cardiotoxicity [3]
Flushing (<10%)
Hypotension (16%) [4]
QT prolongation [23]
Tachycardia [2]
Thrombophlebitis [2]
Torsades de pointes [34]
Ventricular arrhythmia [2]

Central Nervous System
Anorexia (10–33%)
Coma [2]
Dysgeusia (taste perversion) (<10%)
Headache (3–40%)
Insomnia (3–40%)
Neurotoxicity [5]
Paresthesias (4–9%)
Parkinsonism [4]
Parosmia (<10%)
Peripheral neuropathy [4]
Syncope [2]
Tremor (3–40%) [4]
Vertigo (dizziness) (3–40%)

Neuromuscular/Skeletal
Ataxia [4]
Myoclonus [2]
Rhabdomyolysis [7]

Gastrointestinal/Hepatic
Abdominal pain (<10%)
Constipation (10–33%)
Hepatic failure [2]
Hepatic steatosis [2]
Hepatitis (<3%) [3]
Hepatotoxicity [26]
Nausea (10–33%)
Pancreatitis [4]
Vomiting (10–33%)

Respiratory
Cough [2]
Eosinophilic pneumonia [2]
Pneumonia [4]
Pneumonitis [5]
Pulmonary toxicity [22]

Endocrine/Metabolic
Hyperthyroidism (<3%) [8]
Hyponatremia [2]
Hypothyroidism (<3%) [16]
SIADH [10]
Thyroid dysfunction [24]
Thyrotoxicosis [17]

Genitourinary
Epididymitis [2]

Ocular
Corneal deposits (>90%) [2]
Keratopathy [6]

Ocular adverse effects [4]
Ocular toxicity [2]
Optic neuropathy [7]
Visual disturbances (2–9%)

Other
Adverse effects [5]
Death [8]
Side effects (12%) [4]

AMITRIPTYLINE

Trade names: Elavil (AstraZeneca), Limbitrol (Valeant)
Indications: Depression
Class: Antidepressant, tricyclic, Muscarinic antagonist
Half-life: 10–25 hours
Clinically important, potentially hazardous interactions with: adrenergic neurone blockers, alcohol, alfuzosin, altretamine, amiodarone, amphetamines, amprenavir, anticholinergics, antiepileptics, antihistamines, antimuscarinics, antipsychotics, apraclonidine, arsenic, artemether/lumefantrine, aspirin, atomoxetine, baclofen, barbiturates, brimonidine, bupropion, cannabis extract, carbamazepine, cimetidine, cinacalcet, ciprofloxacin, cisapride, clonidine, clozapine, cobicistat/elvitegravir/emtricitabine/tenofovir disoproxil, conivaptan, coumarins, CYP2D6 inhibitors, desmopressin, dexmethylphenidate, diltiazem, disopyramide, disulfiram, diuretics, dronedarone, droperidol, duloxetine, entacapone, ephedra, epinephrine, estrogens, eucalyptus, flecainide, gadobutrol, general anesthetics, gotu kola, grapefruit juice, guanethidine, histamine, interferon alfa, iobenguane, isocarboxazid, isoproterenol, kava, linezolid, lithium, MAO inhibitors, methylphenidate, metoclopramide, moclobemide, moxifloxacin, moxonidine, nefopam, nicorandil, nilotinib, nitrates, NSAIDs, opioid analgesics, paroxetine hydrochloride, pentamidine, phenelzine, phenothiazines, phenytoin, pimozide, pramlintide, primidone, propafenone, propoxyphene, protease inhibitors, QT interval prolonging agents, quinidine, quinine, quinolones, rasagiline, ritonavir, saquinavir, selegiline, sibutramine, sodium oxybate, sotalol, sparfloxacin, SSRIs, St John's wort, sulfonylureas, terbinafine, tetrabenazine, thioridazine, thyroid hormones, tramadol, tranylcypromine, valerian, valproic acid, verapamil, vitamin K antagonists, yohimbine, ziprasidone
Pregnancy category: C
Important contra-indications noted in the prescribing guidelines for: the elderly; nursing mothers; pediatric patients
Note: Limbitrol is amitriptyline and chlordiazepoxide.
Black Box Warning: SUICIDALITY AND ANTIDEPRESSANT DRUGS

Skin
Diaphoresis (<10%)
DRESS syndrome [2]
Photosensitivity [3]
Pigmentation [4]
Pruritus [3]
Pseudolymphoma [2]
Purpura [2]

Mucosal
Xerostomia (>10%) [15]

Cardiovascular
Brugada syndrome [4]
Myocardial infarction [2]
Postural hypotension [2]
QT prolongation [2]

Central Nervous System
Delirium [2]
Depression [2]
Dysgeusia (taste perversion) (>10%) [2]
Hallucinations [3]
Restless legs syndrome [2]
Sedation [2]
Seizures [7]
Serotonin syndrome [4]
Somnolence (drowsiness) [6]
Vertigo (dizziness) [6]

Neuromuscular/Skeletal
Asthenia (fatigue) [3]
Rhabdomyolysis [2]

Gastrointestinal/Hepatic
Cholestasis [2]
Constipation [3]
Nausea [2]

Endocrine/Metabolic
SIADH [5]
Weight gain [6]

Otic
Tinnitus [3]

Ocular
Hallucinations, visual [2]
Vision blurred [2]

Other
Adverse effects [5]
Death [3]

AMLODIPINE

Trade names: Caduet (Pfizer), Exforge (Novartis), Istin (Pfizer), Lotrel (Novartis), Norvasc (Pfizer), Prestalia (Symplmed), Tekamlo (Novartis)
Indications: Hypertension, angina
Class: Antiarrhythmic class IV, Calcium channel blocker
Half-life: 30–50 hours
Clinically important, potentially hazardous interactions with: amprenavir, carbamazepine, cobicistat/elvitegravir/emtricitabine/tenofovir disoproxil, conivaptan, delavirdine, epirubicin, imatinib, phenytoin, primidone, sildenafil, simvastatin, St John's wort, tadalafil, telaprevir
Pregnancy category: C
Important contra-indications noted in the prescribing guidelines for: the elderly; nursing mothers; pediatric patients
Note: Caduet is amlodipine and atorvastatin; Exforge is amlodipine and valsartan; Lotrel is amlodipine and benazepril; Prestalia is amlodipine and perindopril; Tekamlo is amlodipine and aliskiren.

Skin
Angioedema [6]
Dermatitis (<10%)
Edema (5–14%) [20]
Erythema multiforme [2]
Exanthems (2–4%) [2]
Peripheral edema (>10%) [44]
Pigmentation [2]
Pruritus (2–4%) [3]
Rash (<10%)
Telangiectasia (facial) [5]
Toxic epidermal necrolysis [2]
Toxicity [2]
Vasculitis [2]

Mucosal
Gingival hyperplasia/hypertrophy [28]

Cardiovascular
Flushing (<10%) [5]
Hypotension [7]

Central Nervous System
Headache [12]
Parkinsonism [2]
Syncope [2]
Vertigo (dizziness) [13]

Neuromuscular/Skeletal
Asthenia (fatigue) [5]
Rhabdomyolysis [2]

Gastrointestinal/Hepatic
Diarrhea [3]
Gastritis [2]
Hepatotoxicity [3]
Nausea [5]
Vomiting [2]

Respiratory
Bronchitis [2]
Cough [2]
Upper respiratory tract infection [4]

Other
Adverse effects [8]

AMODIAQUINE

Trade names: Camoquin (Pfizer), Flavoquin (Sanofi-Aventis)
Indications: Malaria
Class: Anti-inflammatory, Antimalarial
Half-life: 15.7–19.5 hours
Clinically important, potentially hazardous interactions with: none known
Pregnancy category: N/A
Important contra-indications noted in the prescribing guidelines for: pediatric patients

---

Skin
Pruritus [3]

Central Nervous System
Extrapyramidal symptoms [2]

Neuromuscular/Skeletal
Asthenia (fatigue) [3]

Gastrointestinal/Hepatic
Abdominal pain [3]
Diarrhea [3]
Vomiting [6]

Hematologic
Neutropenia [2]

Other
Adverse effects [2]
Death [2]

AMOXAPINE

Trade name: Amoxapine (Watson)
Indications: Depression
Class: Antidepressant, tricyclic, Muscarinic antagonist
Half-life: 11–30 hours
Clinically important, potentially hazardous interactions with: amprenavir, artemether/lumefantrine, clonidine, dronedarone, epinephrine, fluoxetine, guanethidine, iobenguane, isocarboxazid, linezolid, MAO inhibitors, nilotinib, phenelzine, pimozide, quetiapine, quinine, quinolones, sparfloxacin, tetrabenazine, thioridazine, toremifene, tranylcypromine, vandetanib, vemurafenib, ziprasidone
Pregnancy category: C
Important contra-indications noted in the prescribing guidelines for: the elderly; nursing mothers; pediatric patients
Black Box Warning: SUICIDALITY AND ANTIDEPRESSANT DRUGS

Skin
AGEP [3]
Diaphoresis (<10%)
Edema (<10%)
Exanthems [2]
Rash (<10%)
Toxic epidermal necrolysis [2]

Mucosal
Xerostomia (14%)

Central Nervous System
Dysgeusia (taste perversion) (>10%)
Headache (<10%)
Insomnia (<10%)
Neuroleptic malignant syndrome [2]
Somnolence (drowsiness) (14%)
Vertigo (dizziness) (<10%)

Neuromuscular/Skeletal
Asthenia (fatigue) (<10%)

Gastrointestinal/Hepatic
Constipation (12%)
Nausea (<10%)

Endocrine/Metabolic
Galactorrhea [2]

Ocular
Vision blurred (7%)

Other
Side effects (5%)

AMOXICILLIN

Synonym: amoxycillin
Trade names: Amoxil (GSK), Augmentin (GSK), Prevpac (TAP), Trimox (Bristol-Myers Squibb)
Indications: Infections of the respiratory tract, skin and urinary tract
Class: Antibiotic, penicillin
Half-life: 0.7–1.4 hours
Clinically important, potentially hazardous interactions with: allopurinol, bromelain, chloramphenicol, demeclocycline, doxycycline, erythromycin, imipenem/cilastatin, methotrexate, minocycline, omeprazole, oxytetracycline, sulfonamides, tetracycline
Pregnancy category: B
Note: Augmentin is amoxicillin and clavulanic acid.

Skin
AGEP [26]
Anaphylactoid reactions/Anaphylaxis [15]
Angioedema (<10%) [5]
Baboon syndrome (SDRIFE) [11]
Bullous pemphigoid [2]
Dermatitis [4]
DRESS syndrome [5]
Edema [2]
Erythema multiforme [18]
Exanthems (>5%) [33]
Fixed eruption [10]
Hypersensitivity [5]
Jarisch–Herxheimer reaction [2]
Linear IgA bullous dermatosis [3]
Pemphigus [4]
Pruritus [7]
Pustules [8]
Rash (<10%) [13]
Serum sickness (<10%) [5]
Stevens–Johnson syndrome [10]
Toxic epidermal necrolysis [13]
Toxic pustuloderma [2]
Urticaria (<5%) [16]

Mucosal
Stomatitis [2]

Central Nervous System
Anorexia [2]
Dysgeusia (taste perversion) [5]
Hallucinations [3]
Headache [5]
Somnolence (drowsiness) [3]
Vertigo (dizziness) [5]

Neuromuscular/Skeletal
Asthenia (fatigue) [3]

Gastrointestinal/Hepatic
Abdominal distension [2]
Abdominal pain [7]
Diarrhea [17]
Dyspepsia [2]
Hepatotoxicity [33]
Nausea [12]
Vomiting [9]

Genitourinary
Vaginitis [3]

Renal
Nephrotoxicity [2]

Other
Adverse effects [19]
Kounis syndrome [6]
Side effects [4]
Tooth fluorosis [2]

AMPHOTERICIN B

Trade names: Abelcet (Sigma-Tau), AmBisome (Astellas), Amphocin (Pfizer), Amphotec (Alkopharma)
Indications: Potentially life-threatening fungal infections
Class: Antifungal
Half-life: initial: 15–48 hours; terminal: 15 days
Clinically important, potentially hazardous interactions with: adefovir, aminoglycosides, arsenic, astemizole, betamethasone, cephalothin, cidofovir, cyclosporine, digoxin, ethoxzolamide, fluconazole, flucytosine, ganciclovir, griseofulvin, hydrocortisone, itraconazole, ketoconazole, micafungin, pentamidine, probenecid, sulpiride, terbinafine, triamcinolone, voriconazole
Pregnancy category: B
Important contra-indications noted in the prescribing guidelines for: nursing mothers

---

Skin
Anaphylactoid reactions/Anaphylaxis [4]
Diaphoresis (7%)
Exanthems [4]
Peripheral edema (15%)
Pruritus (11%) [2]
Purpura [3]
Rash (25%)
Toxicity [2]
Urticaria [2]

Mucosal
Epistaxis (nosebleed) (15%)

Cardiovascular
Chest pain (12%)
Flushing (<10%) [2]
Hypertension (8%) [4]
Hypotension (14%)
Tachycardia (13%)
Thrombophlebitis (<10%)

Central Nervous System
Anorexia (>10%)
Anxiety (14%)
Chills (48%) [4]
Confusion (11%)
Delirium (>10%)
Fever (>10%) [4]
Headache (20%)
Insomnia (17%)
Leukoencephalopathy [4]
Pain (14%)
Paresthesias (<10%)
Parkinsonism [2]

Neuromuscular/Skeletal
Asthenia (fatigue) (13%)
Back pain (12%)

Gastrointestinal/Hepatic
Abdominal pain (20%)
Diarrhea (30%)
Gastrointestinal bleeding (10%)
Hepatotoxicity [4]

Nausea (40%)
Vomiting (32%)

Respiratory
Cough (18%)
Dyspnea (23%)
Hypoxia (8%)
Pleural effusion (13%)
Pulmonary toxicity (18%)
Rhinitis (11%)
Tachypnea (>10%)

Endocrine/Metabolic
ALP increased (22%)
ALT increased (15%)
AST increased (13%)
Creatine phosphokinase increased (22%)
Hyperglycemia (23%)
Hypernatremia (4%)
Hypervolemia (12%)
Hypocalcemia (18%)
Hypomagnesemia (20%)

Genitourinary
Hematuria (14%)
Urinary retention (<10%)

Renal
Nephrotoxicity [47]

Hematologic
Anemia (>10%) [4]
Leukocytosis (<10%)
Sepsis (14%)

Local
Infusion-site reactions [4]
Injection-site pain (>10%)
Injection-site reactions [5]

Other
Adverse effects [5]
Death [4]
Infection (11%)

AMPICILLIN

Trade name: Totacillin (GSK)
Indications: Susceptible strains of gram-negative and gram-positive bacterial infections
Class: Antibiotic, penicillin
Half-life: 1–1.5 hours
Clinically important, potentially hazardous interactions with: allopurinol, anticoagulants, chloramphenicol, cyclosporine, demeclocycline, doxycycline, erythromycin, levodopa, methotrexate, minocycline, oxytetracycline, sulfonamides, tetracycline
Pregnancy category: B
Important contra-indications noted in the prescribing guidelines for: nursing mothers
Note: Five to 10% of people taking ampicillin develop eruptions between the 5th and 14th day following initiation of therapy. Also, there is a 95% incidence of exanthematous eruptions in patients who are treated for infectious mononucleosis with ampicillin. The allergenicity of ampicillin appears to be enhanced by allopurinol or by hyperuricemia. Ampicillin is clearly the more allergenic of the two drugs when given alone.

Skin
AGEP [9]
Anaphylactoid reactions/Anaphylaxis [10]
Angioedema [2]
Baboon syndrome (SDRIFE) [3]
Dermatitis [8]
Erythema multiforme [11]
Exanthems (>10%) [84]
Exfoliative dermatitis [3]
Fixed eruption [10]
Hypersensitivity [5]
Linear IgA bullous dermatosis [4]
Pemphigus [6]
Pruritus (<5%) [5]
Psoriasis [5]
Purpura [6]
Pustules [4]
Rash (<10%)
Stevens–Johnson syndrome [10]
Toxic epidermal necrolysis [15]
Urticaria [16]
Vasculitis [4]

Hematologic
Thrombocytopenia [2]

Local
Injection-site pain (>10%)

Other
Allergic reactions (<10%) [3]

AMPICILLIN/ SULBACTAM

Trade name: Unasyn (Pfizer)
Indications: Various infections caused by susceptible organisms
Class: Antibiotic, beta-lactam, Antibiotic, penicillin
Half-life: 1 hour
Clinically important, potentially hazardous interactions with: allopurinol, probenecid
Pregnancy category: B
Important contra-indications noted in the prescribing guidelines for: nursing mothers
Note: Serious and occasionally fatal hypersensitivity (anaphylactic) reactions have been reported in patients on penicillin therapy. Contraindicated in patients with a history of hypersensitivity reactions to any of the penicillins.

Skin
Anaphylactoid reactions/Anaphylaxis [2]
Linear IgA bullous dermatosis [3]
Rash (<10%)

Gastrointestinal/Hepatic
Diarrhea (<10%)

Local
Injection-site pain (16%)

ANAKINRA

Trade name: Kineret (Amgen)
Indications: Rheumatoid arthritis, neonatal-onset multisystem inflammatory disease
Class: Disease-modulating antirheumatoid drug, Interleukin-1 receptor antagonist (IL-IRa)
Half-life: 4–6 hours
Clinically important, potentially hazardous interactions with: abatacept, adalimumab, certolizumab, etanercept, golimumab, infliximab, lenalidomide, live vaccines
Pregnancy category: B
Important contra-indications noted in the prescribing guidelines for: nursing mothers

---

Central Nervous System
Fever (12%)
Headache (12–14%) [2]

Neuromuscular/Skeletal
Arthralgia (6–12%)

Gastrointestinal/Hepatic
Abdominal pain (5%)
Diarrhea (8%)
Nausea (8%)
Vomiting (14%)

Respiratory
Flu-like syndrome (6%)
Nasopharyngitis (12%)
Sinusitis (7%)
Upper respiratory tract infection (4%)

Local
Injection-site edema [2]
Injection-site erythema [3]
Injection-site inflammation [2]
Injection-site pain [4]
Injection-site reactions (71%) [29]

Other
Adverse effects [5]
Infection (40%) [10]

ANASTROZOLE

Trade name: Arimidex (AstraZeneca)
Indications: Breast carcinoma (localized – advanced or metastatic)
Class: Antineoplastic, Aromatase inhibitor
Half-life: 50 hours
Clinically important, potentially hazardous interactions with: estradiol, estrogens, tamoxifen
Pregnancy category: X
Important contra-indications noted in the prescribing guidelines for: nursing mothers
Note: Contraindicated in women of premenopausal endocrine status, including pregnant women. The efficacy of anastrozole in the treatment of pubertal gynecomastia in adolescent boys and in the treatment of precocious puberty in girls with McCune-Albright syndrome has not been demonstrated.

Skin
Hot flashes (12–36%) [10]
Lupus erythematosus [3]
Peripheral edema (10%)

Pruritus (2–5%)
Rash (6–11%) [2]

Hair
Alopecia (2–5%)

Cardiovascular
Angina (2%)
Flushing (>5%)
Hypertension (2–13%)
Thrombophlebitis (2–5%)

Central Nervous System
Carpal tunnel syndrome [2]
Depression (5–13%)
Headache (9–13%) [2]
Pain (14%)
Tumor pain (>5%)

Neuromuscular/Skeletal
Arthralgia (2–5%) [6]
Asthenia (fatigue) (19%) [7]
Back pain (12%) [2]
Bone or joint pain (6–11%) [2]
Joint disorder [3]
Myalgia/Myopathy (2–5%)
Osteoporosis (11%)

Gastrointestinal/Hepatic
Diarrhea [2]
Hepatotoxicity [5]
Nausea (11–19%)
Vomiting (8–13%)

Respiratory
Cough (11%)
Flu-like syndrome (7%)
Pharyngitis (6–14%)

Endocrine/Metabolic
Mastodynia (2–5%)

Genitourinary
Vaginal dryness (2%) [2]

Other
Infection (2–5%)

ANIDULAFUNGIN

Trade names: Ecalta (Pfizer), Eraxis (Pfizer)
Indications: Candidemia, candidal esophagitis
Class: Antimycobacterial, echinocandin
Half-life: 40–50 hours
Clinically important, potentially hazardous interactions with: none known
Pregnancy category: C
Important contra-indications noted in the prescribing guidelines for: nursing mothers; pediatric patients

---

Skin
Angioedema (<2%)
Erythema (<2%)
Hot flashes (<2%)
Hyperhidrosis (<2%)
Peripheral edema (11%)
Pruritus (<2%)
Ulcerations (5%)
Urticaria (<2%)

Mucosal
Oral candidiasis (5%)

Cardiovascular
Atrial fibrillation (<2%)
Bundle branch block (<2%)
Chest pain (5%)
Flushing (<2%) [2]
Hypertension (12%)
Hypotension (15%)
Phlebitis [2]
Thrombophlebitis (<2%)
Venous thromboembolism (10%)

Central Nervous System
Confusion (8%)
Depression (6%)
Fever (9–18%) [3]
Headache (8%) [5]
Insomnia (15%)
Rigors (<2%)
Seizures (<2%)
Vertigo (dizziness) (<2%)

Neuromuscular/Skeletal
Back pain (5%)

Gastrointestinal/Hepatic
Abdominal pain (6%)
Cholestasis (<2%)
Constipation (8%)
Diarrhea (9–18%)
Dyspepsia (aggravated) (7%)
Hepatotoxicity [3]
Nausea (7–24%) [4]
Vomiting (7–18%) [4]

Respiratory
Cough (7%)
Dyspnea (12%)
Pleural effusion (10%)
Pneumonia (6%)
Respiratory distress (6%)

Endocrine/Metabolic
ALP increased (12%)
ALT increased (2%)
Creatine phosphokinase increased (5%)
Dehydration (6%)
Hyperglycemia (6%)
Hyperkalemia (6%)
Hypoglycemia (7%)
Hypokalemia (5–15%)
Hypomagnesemia (12%)

Genitourinary
Urinary tract infection (15%)

Hematologic
Anemia (8–9%)
Coagulopathy (<2%)
Leukocytosis (5%)
Sepsis (7%)
Thrombocythemia (6%)
Thrombocytopenia (<2%)

Ocular
Ocular pain (<2%)
Vision blurred (<2%)
Visual disturbances (<2%)

Local
Infusion-site reactions (<2%)

Other
Adverse effects [3]
Infection (63%)

ANTHRAX VACCINE

Trade name: BioThrax (Emergent BioSolutions)
Indications: Anthrax prophylaxis
Class: Vaccine
Half-life: Requires 1 month to achieve immunity (92.5% efficient)
Clinically important, potentially hazardous interactions with: corticosteroids, immunosuppressive therapies, other vaccines
Pregnancy category: D
Important contra-indications noted in the prescribing guidelines for: the elderly; nursing mothers; pediatric patients
Note: Dr. Sue Bailey, Assistant Secretary for Health Affairs, released a statement on June 29, 1999 that 'almost one million shots given, the anthrax immunization is proving to be one of the safest vaccination programs on record.' The ADRs reported occurred for '50 service members at one installation alone.' Note that no number of military personnel was mentioned at this installation, nor did it give any percentages for the reactions reported.

Skin
Diaphoresis [2]
Edema (3%) [2]
Hypersensitivity [5]
Lupus erythematosus [2]
Pruritus (<10%) [2]
Rash [2]
Stevens–Johnson syndrome [2]
Urticaria [2]

Central Nervous System
Chills [2]
Fever [3]
Guillain–Barré syndrome [2]
Headache (4–64%) [2]

Neuromuscular/Skeletal
Arthralgia [3]
Asthenia (fatigue) (5–62%)
Myalgia/Myopathy (2–72%) [3]

Gastrointestinal/Hepatic
Diarrhea (6–8%)
Nausea (6%)

Respiratory
Flu-like syndrome [3]
Nasopharyngitis (12–15%)

Genitourinary
Dysmenorrhea (7%)

Local
Injection-site edema [4]
Injection-site nodules [2]
Injection-site pain [4]
Injection-site pruritus [2]
Injection-site reactions [6]

Other
Allergic reactions [2]

ANTIHEMOPHILIC FACTOR

Synonym: rFVIIIFc
Trade names: Afstyla (CSL Behring), Eloctate (Biogen Idec), Kovaltry (Bayer)
Indications: Control and prevention of bleeding episodes in Hemophilia A
Class: Antihemorrhagic, Recombinant fusion protein
Half-life: 20 hours (adults)
Clinically important, potentially hazardous interactions with: none known
Pregnancy category: C
Important contra-indications noted in the prescribing guidelines for: nursing mothers

Mucosal
Xerostomia (<10%)

Central Nervous System
Dysgeusia (taste perversion) (3%)

Ocular
Conjunctivitis (<5%)
Eyelid edema (<3%)
Ocular pruritus (5–15%)
Xerophthalmia (<5%)

Other
Allergic reactions [5]

APIXABAN

Trade name: Eliquis (Bristol-Myers Squibb)
Indications: Reduce the risk of stroke and systemic embolism in patients with nonvalvular atrial fibrillation
Class: Anticoagulant, Direct factor Xa inhibitor
Half-life: 5–12 hours
Clinically important, potentially hazardous interactions with: carbamazepine, darunavir, phenytoin, rifampin, St John's wort, tipranavir, voriconazole
Pregnancy category: B
Important contra-indications noted in the prescribing guidelines for: nursing mothers; pediatric patients
Note: Contraindicated in patients with active pathological bleeding.
Black Box Warning: DISCONTINUING ELIQUIS IN PATIENTS WITHOUT ADEQUATE CONTINUOUS ANTICOAGULATION INCREASES RISK OF STROKE

Gastrointestinal/Hepatic
Hepatotoxicity [2]

Hematologic
Hemorrhage [15]

Other
Adverse effects [4]

APRACLONIDINE

Trade name: Iopidine (Alcon)
Indications: Post-surgical intraocular pressure elevation
Class: Adrenergic alpha2-receptor agonist
Half-life: 8 hours
Clinically important, potentially hazardous interactions with: amitriptyline
Pregnancy category: C
Important contra-indications noted in the prescribing guidelines for: nursing mothers; pediatric patients

---

Skin
Dermatitis [3]
Pruritus (10%)

APREMILAST

Trade name: Otezla (Celgene)
Indications: Psoriatic arthritis, plaque psoriasis
Class: Phosphodiesterase inhibitor, Phosphodiesterase type 4 (PDE4) inhibitor
Half-life: 6–9 hours
Clinically important, potentially hazardous interactions with: carbamazepine, phenobarbital, phenytoin, rifampin
Pregnancy category: C
Important contra-indications noted in the prescribing guidelines for: nursing mothers; pediatric patients

---

Central Nervous System
Depression [3]
Headache (5–6%) [21]

Neuromuscular/Skeletal
Asthenia (fatigue) [5]

Gastrointestinal/Hepatic
Abdominal pain (<2%) [2]
Diarrhea (8–9%) [24]
Dyspepsia [2]
Nausea (7–9%) [26]
Vomiting (<3%) [5]

Respiratory
Nasopharyngitis (<3%) [15]
Upper respiratory tract infection (<4%) [12]

Endocrine/Metabolic
ALT increased [2]
Weight loss (10–12%) [4]

Other
Adverse effects [3]
Infection [2]

APREPITANT

Trade name: Emend (Merck)
Indications: Prevention of postoperative and chemotherapy induced nausea and vomiting
Class: Antiemetic, CYP3A4 inhibitor, Neurokinin 1 receptor antagonist
Half-life: 9–13 hours
Clinically important, potentially hazardous interactions with: alprazolam, antifungal agents, astemizole, avanafil, betamethasone, carbamazepine, cisapride, clarithromycin, colchicine, conivaptan, corticosteroids, CYP2C9 substrates, CYP3A4 inhibitors or inducers, dasatinib, deferasirox, dexamethasone, diltiazem, docetaxel, eplerenone, estrogens, everolimus, fentanyl, grapefruit juice, halofantrine, ifosfamide, imatinib, irinotecan, itraconazole, ketoconazole, methylprednisolone, midazolam, mifepristone, nefazodone, oral contraceptives, paroxetine hydrochloride, phenobarbital, phenytoin, pimecrolimus, pimozide, progestins, ranolazine, rifampin, rifamycin derivatives, rifapentine, ritonavir, salmeterol, saxagliptin, St John's wort, telithromycin, terfenadine, tolbutamide, tolvaptan, trabectedin, triamcinolone, troleandomycin, vinblastine, vincristine, voriconazole, warfarin
Pregnancy category: N/A (Insufficient evidence to inform drug-associated risk)
Important contra-indications noted in the prescribing guidelines for: nursing mothers; pediatric patients
Note: Fosaprepitant is a prodrug of aprepitant for injection. Aprepitant treatment is given along with a 5-HT3-receptor antagonist and dexamethasone.

Skin
Pruritus (8%)

Hair
Alopecia (12%)

Mucosal
Mucocutaneous reactions (3%)
Stomatitis (3%)

Cardiovascular
Hypertension (2%)
Hypotension (6%)

Central Nervous System
Anorexia (6–10%) [2]
Fever (3–6%)
Headache (5–9%) [5]
Insomnia (2–3%)
Vertigo (dizziness) (3–7%) [2]

Neuromuscular/Skeletal
Asthenia (fatigue) (5–18%) [8]

Gastrointestinal/Hepatic
Abdominal pain (5%) [3]
Constipation (9–10%) [6]
Diarrhea (<10%) [2]
Dyspepsia (5–6%)
Flatulence (4%)
Gastritis (4%)
Nausea (6–13%)
Vomiting (3–8%)

Endocrine/Metabolic
ALT increased (6%)
AST increased (3%)
Creatine phosphokinase increased (4%)
Dehydration (6%)

Genitourinary
Urinary tract infection (2%)

Renal
Proteinuria (7%)

Hematologic
Anemia (3%)
Febrile neutropenia [2]
Neutropenia (3–6%) [2]

Otic
Tinnitus (4%)

Local
Infusion-site pain [2]

Other
- Hiccups (11%) [8]
- Infection [3]

ARFORMOTEROL

Trade name: Brovana (Sunovion)
Indications: Chronic obstructive pulmonary disease including chronic bronchitis and emphysema
Class: Beta-2 adrenergic agonist, Bronchodilator
Half-life: 26 hours
Clinically important, potentially hazardous interactions with: aminophylline, beta blockers, MAO inhibitors, tricyclic antidepressants
Pregnancy category: C
Important contra-indications noted in the prescribing guidelines for: nursing mothers; pediatric patients
Note: Studies in asthma patients showed that long-acting beta$_2$-adrenergic agonists may increase the risk of asthma-related death. Contraindicated in patients with asthma without use of a long-term asthma control medication.
Black Box Warning: ASTHMA-RELATED DEATH

Skin
- Abscess (<2%)
- Edema (<2%)
- Herpes simplex (<2%)
- Herpes zoster (<2%)
- Neoplasms (<2%)
- Peripheral edema (3%)
- Pigmentation (<2%)
- Rash (4%)
- Xerosis (<2%)

Mucosal
- Oral candidiasis (<2%)

Cardiovascular
- Arteriosclerosis (<2%)
- Atrioventricular block (<2%)
- Chest pain (7%) [2]
- Digitalis intoxication (<2%)
- QT prolongation (<2%)
- Supraventricular tachycardia (<2%)

Central Nervous System
- Agitation (<2%)
- Fever (<2%)
- Headache [2]
- Hypokinesia (<2%)
- Insomnia [2]
- Nervousness [3]
- Pain (8%)
- Paresthesias (<2%)
- Somnolence (drowsiness) (<2%)
- Tremor (<2%) [3]

Neuromuscular/Skeletal
- Arthralgia (<2%)
- Back pain (6%)
- Leg cramps (4%)
- Neck rigidity (<2%)

Gastrointestinal/Hepatic
- Nausea [2]

Respiratory
- Bronchitis [3]
- COPD (exacerbation) [3]
- Dysphonia (<2%)
- Dyspnea (4%)
- Flu-like syndrome (3%)
- Nasopharyngitis [3]
- Sinusitis (4%) [2]

Genitourinary
- Cystitis (<2%)
- Nocturia (<2%)

Ocular
- Glaucoma (<2%)
- Visual disturbances (<2%)

Local
- Injection-site pain (<2%)

Other
- Adverse effects [2]
- Allergic reactions (<2%)

ARIPIPRAZOLE

Trade names: Abilify (Bristol-Myers Squibb), Aristada (Alkermes)
Indications: Schizophrenia, bipolar I disorder, major depressive disorder, irritability associated with autistic disorder
Class: Antipsychotic, Mood stabilizer
Half-life: 75–94 hours
Clinically important, potentially hazardous interactions with: alcohol, atazanavir, carbamazepine, CYP3A4 inhibitors, efavirenz, itraconazole, ketoconazole, lopinavir, nelfinavir, paroxetine hydrochloride, quinidine
Pregnancy category: C
Important contra-indications noted in the prescribing guidelines for: the elderly; pediatric patients
Black Box Warning: INCREASED MORTALITY IN ELDERLY PATIENTS WITH DEMENTIA-RELATED PSYCHOSIS
SUICIDALITY AND ANTIDEPRESSANT DRUGS

Skin
- Rash (6%)

Mucosal
- Sialorrhea (4–9%) [5]
- Xerostomia (5%) [6]

Cardiovascular
- Hypertension [2]
- QT prolongation [2]

Central Nervous System
- Agitation (19%) [3]
- Akathisia (8–13%) [26]
- Anxiety (17%) [5]
- Compulsions [2]
- Dyskinesia [3]
- Extrapyramidal symptoms [6]
- Fever (2%)
- Headache (27%) [9]
- Impulse control disorder [5]
- Insomnia (18%) [11]
- Irritability [4]
- Mania [2]
- Neuroleptic malignant syndrome [13]
- Neurotoxicity [2]
- Parkinsonism [7]
- Restlessness [7]
- Sedation [6]
- Somnolence (drowsiness) (5–11%) [5]
- Stroke [2]
- Suicidal ideation [6]
- Tardive dyskinesia [6]
- Tremor (3%) [5]

Neuromuscular/Skeletal
- Asthenia (fatigue) [3]
- Ataxia [4]
- Dystonia [11]
- Pisa syndrome [2]

Gastrointestinal/Hepatic
- Constipation (11%)
- Dyspepsia (9%)
- Nausea (15%) [7]
- Vomiting (11%) [2]

Respiratory
- Cough (3%)
- Upper respiratory tract infection [3]

Endocrine/Metabolic
- Appetite increased [3]
- Galactorrhea [2]
- Hyperprolactinemia [2]
- SIADH [2]
- Weight gain (2–30%) [21]

Genitourinary
- Priapism [3]
- Vaginitis [2]

Hematologic
- Neutropenia [2]

Ocular
- Vision blurred (3–8%)

Local
- Injection-site pain [4]

Other
- Adverse effects [4]
- Death [2]
- Hiccups [3]

ARMODAFINIL

Trade name: Nuvigil (Cephalon)
Indications: Narcolepsy, obstructive sleep apnea, shift work sleep disorder
Class: Eugeroic
Half-life: 12–15 hours
Clinically important, potentially hazardous interactions with: cyclosporine
Pregnancy category: C
Important contra-indications noted in the prescribing guidelines for: the elderly; nursing mothers; pediatric patients

---

Central Nervous System
- Anxiety [2]
- Headache (14–23%) [10]
- Insomnia (4–6%) [3]
- Vertigo (dizziness) (5%) [2]

Gastrointestinal/Hepatic
- Diarrhea [3]
- Nausea [2]

Other
- Adverse effects [2]

ARTEMETHER/ LUMEFANTRINE

Trade name: Coartem (Novartis)
Indications: Acute, uncomplicated malaria infections due to *Plasmodium falciparum* in patients of 5kg bodyweight and above
Class: Antimalarial
Half-life: ~2 hours (artemether); 3–6 days (lumefantrine)
Clinically important, potentially hazardous interactions with: amiodarone, amitriptyline, amoxapine, antimalarials, antiretrovirals, arsenic, astemizole, atazanavir, atovaquone/proguanil, azithromycin, carbamazepine, ciprofloxacin, citalopram, clomipramine, conivaptan, CYP2D6 substrates, CYP3A4 inhibitors, substrates or inducers, darunavir, dasatinib, degarelix, delavirdine, disopyramide, dolasetron, duloxetine, flecainide, halofantrine, hormonal contraceptives, imipramine, indinavir, itraconazole, lapatinib, levofloxacin, levomepromazine, lopinavir, mefloquine, moxifloxacin, nelfinavir, norfloxacin, ofloxacin, paroxetine hydrochloride, pazopanib, phenytoin, pimozide, procainamide, quinidine, quinine, rifampin, risperidone, sotalol, St John's wort, telavancin, telithromycin, terfenadine, tipranavir, venlafaxine, voriconazole, vorinostat, ziprasidone, zuclopenthixol
Pregnancy category: C
Important contra-indications noted in the prescribing guidelines for: nursing mothers; pediatric patients
Note: Artemether/Lumefantrine tablets should not be used to treat severe malaria or to prevent malaria.

Skin
Abscess (<3%)
Impetigo (<3%)
Inflammation [3]
Pruritus (4%) [2]
Rash (3%) [6]
Urticaria (<3%) [2]

Cardiovascular
Palpitation (18%) [2]

Central Nervous System
Agitation (<3%)
Anorexia (40%) [6]
Chills (23%)
Fever (25–29%) [6]
Gait instability (<3%)
Headache (56%) [8]
Hypoesthesia (<3%)
Insomnia (5%) [2]
Mood changes (<3%)
Seizures [2]
Sleep disturbances (22%)
Sleep related disorder [2]
Tremor (<3%)
Vertigo (dizziness) (39%) [8]

Neuromuscular/Skeletal
Arthralgia (34%)
Asthenia (fatigue) (38%) [8]
Ataxia (<3%)
Back pain (<3%)
Myalgia/Myopathy (32%)

Gastrointestinal/Hepatic
Abdominal pain (17%) [11]
Constipation (<3%)
Diarrhea (8%) [11]
Dyspepsia (<3%)
Dysphagia (<3%)
Gastroenteritis (<3%)
Hepatomegaly (6–9%)
Nausea [8]
Peptic ulceration (<3%)
Vomiting [16]

Respiratory
Asthma (<3%)
Bronchitis (<3%)
Cough (6–23%) [2]
Influenza (<3%)
Nasopharyngitis (4%)
Pharyngolaryngeal pain (<3%)
Pneumonia (<3%)
Rhinitis (4%)
Upper respiratory tract infection (<3%)

Endocrine/Metabolic
ALT increased (<3%)
AST increased (<3%)
Hypokalemia (<3%)

Genitourinary
Hematuria (<3%)
Urinary tract infection (<3%)

Renal
Proteinuria (<3%)

Hematologic
Anemia (4–9%) [4]
Eosinophilia (<3%)
Neutropenia [2]
Platelets decreased (<3%)

Otic
Ear infection (<3%)
Hearing impairment [2]
Tinnitus (<3%)

Ocular
Conjunctivitis (<3%)
Nystagmus (<3%)

Other
Adverse effects [3]
Infection (<3%)

ARTESUNATE

Trade name: Rtsun (Wiscon)
Indications: *Plasmodium falciparum* malaria
Class: Antimalarial
Half-life: 0.5 hours
Clinically important, potentially hazardous interactions with: efavirenz
Pregnancy category: N/A (Use carefully in first three trimesters of pregnancy)
Note: Artesunate therapy should be combined with other antimalarials (e.g. mefloquine) if given for less than 5 days.

Skin
Pruritus [3]

Cardiovascular
QT prolongation [2]

Central Nervous System
Anorexia [3]
Extrapyramidal symptoms [2]
Fever [2]
Headache [8]
Insomnia [2]
Vertigo (dizziness) [12]

Neuromuscular/Skeletal
Asthenia (fatigue) [4]
Myalgia/Myopathy [2]

Gastrointestinal/Hepatic
Abdominal pain [4]
Diarrhea [5]
Nausea [6]
Vomiting [12]

Respiratory
Cough [3]

Hematologic
Anemia [4]
Hemolysis [3]
Hemolytic anemia [2]
Neutropenia [2]

Other
Adverse effects [2]

ASENAPINE

Trade name: Saphris (Merck)
Indications: Schizophrenia, bipolar disorder
Class: Antipsychotic
Half-life: 24 hours
Clinically important, potentially hazardous interactions with: alcohol, amiodarone, chlorpromazine, CYP2D6 substrates and inhibitors, fluvoxamine, gatifloxacin, moxifloxacin, paroxetine hydrochloride, procainamide, QT prolonging drugs, quinidine, sotalol, thioridazine, ziprasidone
Pregnancy category: C
Important contra-indications noted in the prescribing guidelines for: the elderly; nursing mothers; pediatric patients
Black Box Warning: INCREASED MORTALITY IN ELDERLY PATIENTS WITH DEMENTIA-RELATED PSYCHOSIS

Skin
Peripheral edema (3%)

Mucosal
Oral numbness [4]
Salivary hypersecretion (2%)
Xerostomia (2–3%)

Cardiovascular
Hypertension (2–3%) [2]

Central Nervous System
Akathisia (4–6%) [10]
Anxiety (4%)
Depression (2%) [3]
Dysgeusia (taste perversion) (3%) [4]
Extrapyramidal symptoms (6–10%) [11]
Headache (12%) [3]
Hypersomnia [2]
Hypoesthesia (4–5%) [7]
Insomnia (6–15%) [3]
Irritability (2%)
Sedation [9]
Somnolence (drowsiness) (13–24%) [15]
Vertigo (dizziness) (4–11%) [5]

Neuromuscular/Skeletal
Arthralgia (3%)
Asthenia (fatigue) (3–4%)
Pain in extremities (2%)

Gastrointestinal/Hepatic
Abdominal pain [2]
Constipation (5%)
Dyspepsia (3–4%)
Vomiting (5%)

Endocrine/Metabolic
Appetite increased (2–4%)
Weight gain (3–5%) [12]

Other
Adverse effects [4]

ASFOTASE ALFA *

Trade name: Strensiq (Alexion)
Indications: Perinatal/infantile-and juvenile-onset hypophosphatasia
Class: Enzyme replacement
Half-life: 5 days
Clinically important, potentially hazardous interactions with: none known
Pregnancy category: N/A (No available data)
Important contra-indications noted in the prescribing guidelines for: the elderly; nursing mothers

---

Skin
Anaphylactoid reactions/Anaphylaxis (<10%)
Calcification (4%)
Erythema (<10%)

Cardiovascular
Flushing (<10%)

Central Nervous System
Chills (<10%)
Fever (<10%)
Headache (<10%)
Hypoesthesia (oral) (<10%)
Irritability (<10%)
Pain (<10%)
Rigors (<10%)

Gastrointestinal/Hepatic
Nausea (<10%)
Vomiting (5%)

Local
Injection-site bruising (8%)
Injection-site edema (13%)
Injection-site erythema (41%)
Injection-site hemorrhage (<17%)
Injection-site induration (13%)
Injection-site lipoatrophy/lipohypertrophy (5–8%)
Injection-site pain (14%)
Injection-site papules and nodules (3%)
Injection-site pigmentation (15%)
Injection-site pruritus (13%)
Injection-site reactions (9%)

Other
Adverse effects [2]

ASPARAGINASE

Synonym: L-asparaginase
Trade names: Elspar (Merck), Kidrolase (EUSA Pharma)
Indications: Acute lymphoblastic leukemia, lymphoma
Class: Antineoplastic, Enzyme
Half-life: 8–30 hours (intravenous); 34–49 hours (intramuscular)
Clinically important, potentially hazardous interactions with: none known
Pregnancy category: C
Important contra-indications noted in the prescribing guidelines for: nursing mothers

---

Skin
Anaphylactoid reactions/Anaphylaxis (3–40%) [4]
Angioedema [3]
Hypersensitivity (6–40%) [13]
Toxic epidermal necrolysis [2]
Toxicity [2]
Urticaria (<15%) [5]

Mucosal
Aphthous stomatitis (<10%)
Oral lesions (26%)
Stomatitis (<10%)

Central Nervous System
Chills (>10%)
Coma (25%)
Depression (>10%)
Encephalopathy [2]
Fever (>10%)
Leukoencephalopathy [3]
Neurotoxicity [4]
Seizures (10–60%)
Somnolence (drowsiness) (>10%)
Stroke [2]

Gastrointestinal/Hepatic
Abdominal pain (70%)
Hepatotoxicity [2]
Pancreatitis (15%) [21]
Vomiting (50–60%)

Endocrine/Metabolic
Hyperglycemia [2]
Hyperlipidemia [2]
Hypertriglyceridemia [4]

Genitourinary
Azotemia (66%)

Hematologic
Sepsis [2]
Thrombosis [9]

Other
Adverse effects [2]
Allergic reactions (15–35%) [2]

ASPIRIN

Synonyms: acetylsalicylic acid; ASA
Trade names: Aggrenox (Boehringer Ingelheim), Anacin (Wyeth), Ascriptin (Novartis) (Wallace), Darvon Compound (aaiPharma), Durlaza (New Haven), Ecotrin (GSK), Equagesic (Women First), Excedrin (Bristol-Myers Squibb), Fiorinal (Watson), Norgesic (3M), Soma Compound (MedPointe), Talwin Compound (Sanofi-Aventis), Yosprala (Aralez)
Indications: Pain, fever, inflammation
Class: Antiplatelet, Non-steroidal anti-inflammatory (NSAID), Salicylate
Half-life: 15–20 minutes
Clinically important, potentially hazardous interactions with: acemetacin, acenocoumarol, amitriptyline, anagrelide, anticoagulants, azficel-t, bismuth, calcium hydroxylapatite, capsicum, celecoxib, cholestyramine, cilazapril, citalopram, desvenlafaxine, devil's claw, dexamethasone, dexibuprofen, dichlorphenamide, diclofenac, dicumarol, duloxetine, enoxaparin, etodolac, evening primrose, flunisolide, flurbiprofen, ginkgo biloba, ginseng, heparin, ibuprofen, iloprost, indomethacin, ketoprofen, ketorolac, lumiracoxib, meloxicam, methotrexate, methyl salicylate, methylprednisolone, milnacipran, nilutamide, NSAIDs, paroxetine hydrochloride, phellodendron, piroxicam, prednisone, resveratrol, reteplase, rivaroxaban, sermorelin, sulfites, tinzaparin, tirofiban, tolmetin, triamcinolone, urokinase, valdecoxib, valproic acid, venlafaxine, verapamil, vilazodone, warfarin, zafirlukast
Pregnancy category: D
Important contra-indications noted in the prescribing guidelines for: nursing mothers; pediatric patients
Note: NSAIDs may cause an increased risk of serious cardiovascular and gastrointestinal adverse events, which can be fatal. This risk may increase with duration of use.
Aggrenox is aspirin and dipyridamole; Yosprala is aspirin and omeprazole.

Skin
Anaphylactoid reactions/Anaphylaxis (<10%) [8]
Angioedema (<5%) [32]
Bullous dermatitis [4]
Erythema multiforme [9]
Erythema nodosum [9]
Erythroderma [2]
Exanthems [11]
Fixed eruption [21]
Hypersensitivity [5]
Lichenoid eruption [2]
Pityriasis rosea [3]
Pruritus [6]
Psoriasis [3]
Purpura [8]
Rash (<10%)
Stevens–Johnson syndrome [6]
Toxic epidermal necrolysis [9]
Urticaria (<10%) [72]
Vasculitis [2]

Mucosal
Aphthous stomatitis [3]

Nasal polyp [4]
Oral mucosal eruption [3]
Oral ulceration [4]

Gastrointestinal/Hepatic
Black stools [3]
Gastritis [2]
Gastrointestinal bleeding [7]
Gastrointestinal ulceration [7]
Hepatotoxicity [4]
Pancreatitis [2]

Respiratory
Asthma [10]
Pulmonary toxicity [2]
Rhinitis [3]
Sinusitis [2]

Renal
Fanconi syndrome [2]

Hematologic
Bleeding [10]

Otic
Tinnitus [17]

Ocular
Periorbital edema [3]

Other
Adverse effects [9]
Allergic reactions [2]

ATAZANAVIR

Trade names: Evotaz (Bristol-Myers Squibb), Reyataz (Bristol-Myers Squibb)
Indications: HIV infection
Class: Antiretroviral, HIV-1 protease inhibitor
Half-life: 7 hours
Clinically important, potentially hazardous interactions with: abiraterone, alfuzosin, amiodarone, antacids, aripiprazole, artemether/lumefantrine, atorvastatin, avanafil, bepridil, bosentan, buprenorphine, cabazitaxel, cabozantinib, cisapride, clarithromycin, colchicine, crizotinib, cyclosporine, darifenacin, dasatinib, dexlansoprazole, diltiazem, dofetilide, efavirenz, ergot derivatives, erlotinib, estrogens, etravirine, everolimus, famotidine, felodipine, fentanyl, fesoterodine, flibanserin, fluticasone propionate, garlic, indinavir, irinotecan, itraconazole, ixabepilone, ketoconazole, lapatinib, lidocaine, lopinavir, lovastatin, maraviroc, marihuana, midazolam, mifepristone, nevirapine, nicardipine, nifedipine, ombitasvir/paritaprevir/ritonavir, omeprazole, oral contraceptives, paclitaxel, pantoprazole, pazopanib, pimozide, posaconazole, proton-pump inhibitors, quetiapine, quinidine, quinine, rabeprazole, raltegravir, ranolazine, rifabutin, rifampin, rilpivirine, ritonavir, rivaroxaban, romidepsin, rosuvastatin, salmeterol, saquinavir, sildenafil, simeprevir, simvastatin, sirolimus, solifenacin, St John's wort, sunitinib, tacrolimus, tadalafil, telaprevir, telithromycin, temsirolimus, tenofovir disoproxil, ticagrelor, tipranavir, trazodone, triazolam, tricyclic antidepressants, vardenafil, vemurafenib, verapamil, voriconazole, warfarin
Pregnancy category: B
Important contra-indications noted in the prescribing guidelines for: the elderly; nursing mothers; pediatric patients
Note: Evotaz is atazanavir and cobicistat.

Skin
Jaundice (5–7%) [11]
Rash (3–20%) [7]

Cardiovascular
QT prolongation [2]
Torsades de pointes [2]

Central Nervous System
Depression (2%)
Fever (2%)
Headache (<6%) [2]
Insomnia (3%)
Neurotoxicity [2]
Pain (3%)
Vertigo (dizziness) (3%)

Neuromuscular/Skeletal
Asthenia (fatigue) (2%)
Back pain (2%)
Myalgia/Myopathy (4%)

Gastrointestinal/Hepatic
Abdominal pain (4%)
Cholelithiasis (gallstones) [4]
Diarrhea (2%) [3]
Hepatotoxicity [3]
Nausea (6–14%) [3]
Vomiting (3–4%)

Respiratory
Upper respiratory tract infection [2]

Endocrine/Metabolic
ALT increased (3%)
AST increased (3%)
Creatine phosphokinase increased (8%)
Hyperbilirubinemia [5]

Genitourinary
Urolithiasis [4]

Renal
Nephrolithiasis [5]
Nephrotoxicity [6]

Hematologic
Neutropenia (5%)

Other
Adverse effects [5]
Infection (~50%)

ATENOLOL

Trade names: Beta-Adalat (Bayer), Kalten (BPC), Tenif (AstraZeneca), Tenoret 50 (AstraZeneca), Tenoretic (AstraZeneca), Tenormin (AstraZeneca)
Indications: Angina, hypertension, acute myocardial infarction
Class: Antiarrhythmic class II, Beta adrenergic blocker, Beta blocker
Half-life: 6–7 hours (adults)
Clinically important, potentially hazardous interactions with: alfuzosin, calcium channel blockers, cisplatin, clonidine, digitalis glycosides, diltiazem, disopyramide, epinephrine, indomethacin, reserpine, verapamil
Pregnancy category: D
Important contra-indications noted in the prescribing guidelines for: the elderly; nursing mothers; pediatric patients
Note: Contraindicated in patients with sinus bradycardia, heart block greater than first degree, cardiogenic shock, or overt cardiac failure. Beta-Adalat and Tenif are atenolol and nifedipine. Kalten, Tenoret 50 and Tenoretic are atenolol and chlorthalidone. Chlorthalidone is a sulfonamide and can be absorbed systemically. Sulfonamides can produce severe, possibly fatal, reactions such as toxic epidermal necrolysis and Stevens-Johnson syndrome.
Black Box Warning: CESSATION OF THERAPY

Skin
Anaphylactoid reactions/Anaphylaxis [2]
Lupus erythematosus [2]
Necrosis [3]
Pruritus (<5%)
Psoriasis [7]
Raynaud's phenomenon [2]
Urticaria [2]

Cardiovascular
Atrial fibrillation (5%) [2]
Atrial flutter (2%)
Bradycardia (3–18%) [8]
Cardiac arrest (2%)
Cardiac failure (19%)
Heart block (5%)
Hypotension (25%) [2]
Postural hypotension (12%)
Supraventricular tachycardia (12%)
Ventricular tachycardia (16%)

Central Nervous System
Depression (12%)
Somnolence (drowsiness) (2%)
Stroke [2]
Vertigo (dizziness) (15%)

Neuromuscular/Skeletal
Asthenia (fatigue) (26%)
Leg pain (3%)

Gastrointestinal/Hepatic
Diarrhea (3%)
Nausea (3%)

Respiratory
Dyspnea (6%)
Wheezing (3%)

Other
Adverse effects [5]

ATEZOLIZUMAB *

Trade name: Tecentriq (Genentech)
Indications: Locally advanced or metastatic urothelial carcinoma in patients having disease progression following platinum-containing chemotherapy
Class: Monoclonal antibody, Programmed death-ligand (PD-L1) inhibitor
Half-life: 27 days
Clinically important, potentially hazardous interactions with: none known

Pregnancy category: N/A (Can cause fetal harm)
Important contra-indications noted in the prescribing guidelines for: nursing mothers; pediatric patients

Skin
Peripheral edema (18%)
Pruritus (13%)
Rash (15%)

Cardiovascular
Venous thromboembolism (>2%)

Central Nervous System
Fever (21%)

Neuromuscular/Skeletal
Arthralgia (14%)
Asthenia (fatigue) (52%)
Back pain (15%)
Neck pain (15%)

Gastrointestinal/Hepatic
Abdominal pain (17%)
Constipation (21%)
Diarrhea (18%)
Gastric obstruction (>2%)
Nausea (25%)
Vomiting (17%)

Respiratory
Cough (14%)
Dyspnea (16%)
Pneumonia (>2%)
Pneumonitis (3%)

Endocrine/Metabolic
ALP increased (4%)
ALT increased (2%)
Appetite decreased (26%)
AST increased (2%)
Dehydration (>2%)
Hyperglycemia (5%)
Hyperthyroidism (2%)
Hyponatremia (10%)
Hypothyroidism (6%)
Serum creatinine increased (3%)

Genitourinary
Hematuria (14%)
Urinary tract infection (22%)

Renal
Nephrotoxicity (>2%)

Hematologic
Anemia (8%)
Lymphopenia (10%)
Sepsis (>2%)

Local
Infusion-related reactions (3%)

Other
Adverse effects [2]
Infection (38%)

ATOMOXETINE

Trade name: Strattera (Lilly)
Indications: Attention deficit hyperactivity disorder
Class: Norepinephrine reuptake inhibitor
Half-life: 5 hours
Clinically important, potentially hazardous interactions with: albuterol, amitriptyline, cinacalcet, citalopram, delavirdine, droperidol, duloxetine, levalbuterol, levomepromazine, linezolid, lisdexamfetamine, MAO inhibitors, moxifloxacin, paroxetine hydrochloride, sotalol, terbinafine, terbutaline, tipranavir, venlafaxine, zuclopenthixol
Pregnancy category: C
Important contra-indications noted in the prescribing guidelines for: nursing mothers; pediatric patients
Black Box Warning: SUICIDAL IDEATION IN CHILDREN AND ADOLESCENTS

Skin
Pruritus (>2%)

Mucosal
Xerostomia (>5%) [9]

Cardiovascular
Cardiotoxicity [2]
Tachycardia [2]

Central Nervous System
Aggression [3]
Anorexia [4]
Depression (>2%) [2]
Headache [8]
Hypomania [2]
Insomnia [6]
Irritability [7]
Mania [2]
Mood changes [4]
Nervousness [2]
Somnolence (drowsiness) [10]
Suicidal ideation [6]
Tic disorder [5]
Tremor (>2%) [2]
Vertigo (dizziness) (>5%) [9]

Neuromuscular/Skeletal
Asthenia (fatigue) [9]

Gastrointestinal/Hepatic
Abdominal pain [11]
Constipation [2]
Dyspepsia [3]
Hepatotoxicity [12]
Nausea [18]
Vomiting [9]

Endocrine/Metabolic
Appetite decreased [25]
Weight loss [5]

Genitourinary
Erectile dysfunction [4]
Urinary hesitancy [2]

Other
Adverse effects [10]
Bruxism [2]

ATORVASTATIN

Trade names: Caduet (Pfizer), Lipitor (Pfizer), Liptruzet (Merck Sharpe & Dohme)
Indications: Hypercholesterolemia
Class: HMG-CoA reductase inhibitor, Statin
Half-life: 14 hours
Clinically important, potentially hazardous interactions with: alcohol, aliskiren, amiodarone, amprenavir, antifungals, atazanavir, azithromycin, bexarotene, boceprevir, bosentan, ciprofibrate, clarithromycin, clopidogrel, cobicistat/elvitegravir/emtricitabine/tenofovir disoproxil, colchicine, conivaptan, cyclosporine, CYP3A4 inhibitors, dabigatran, danazol, daptomycin, darunavir, dasatinib, delavirdine, digoxin, diltiazem, dronedarone, efavirenz, eltrombopag, erythromycin, estradiol, etravirine, everolimus, fenofibrate, fenofibric acid, fibrates, fluconazole, fosamprenavir, fusidic acid, gemfibrozil, grapefruit juice, imatinib, imidazoles, indinavir, itraconazole, liraglutide, lopinavir, macrolide antibiotics, midazolam, nefazodone, nelfinavir, niacin, niacinamide, norethisterone, oral contraceptives, P-glycoprotein inhibitors, posaconazole, protease inhibitors, quinine, red rice yeast, rifampin, ritonavir, rivaroxaban, saquinavir, silodosin, St John's wort, telaprevir, telithromycin, tipranavir, topotecan, trabectedin, verapamil, voriconazole, warfarin
Pregnancy category: X
Important contra-indications noted in the prescribing guidelines for: the elderly; nursing mothers; pediatric patients
Note: Caduet is atorvastatin and amlodipine; Liptruzet is atorvastatin and ezetimibe.

Skin
Acneform eruption (<2%)
Angioedema [2]
Dermatitis (<2%)
Dermatomyositis [3]
Diaphoresis (<2%)
Ecchymoses (<2%)
Eczema (<2%)
Edema (<2%)
Facial edema (<2%)
Jaundice [2]
Lupus erythematosus [2]
Petechiae (<2%)
Photosensitivity (<2%)
Pruritus (<2%)
Rash (>3%) [2]
Seborrhea (<2%)
Toxic epidermal necrolysis [2]
Toxicity [2]
Ulcerations (<2%)
Urticaria (<2%)
Xerosis (<2%)

Hair
Alopecia (<2%)

Mucosal
Cheilitis (<2%)
Glossitis (<2%)
Oral ulceration (<2%)
Stomatitis (<2%)

Central Nervous System
Ageusia (taste loss) (<2%)
Cognitive impairment [2]

Depression [3]
Dysgeusia (taste perversion) (<2%)
Headache [4]
Neurotoxicity [2]
Paresthesias (<2%)
Parosmia (<2%)

Neuromuscular/Skeletal
Arthralgia (4–12%)
Asthenia (fatigue) [5]
Back pain [3]
Muscle spasm [2]
Myalgia/Myopathy (3–8%) [30]
Pain in extremities (6%)
Rhabdomyolysis [36]
Tendinopathy/Tendon rupture [2]

Gastrointestinal/Hepatic
Cholelithiasis (gallstones) [2]
Diarrhea (5–14%)
Hepatitis [2]
Hepatotoxicity [9]
Nausea (4–7%)
Pancreatitis [8]

Respiratory
Nasopharyngitis (4–13%)

Endocrine/Metabolic
ALT increased [3]
Creatine phosphokinase increased [5]
Diabetes mellitus [2]
Gynecomastia (<2%)

Genitourinary
Urinary tract infection (4–8%)

Renal
Nephrotoxicity [3]

Otic
Hearing loss [2]

Other
Adverse effects [9]
Allergic reactions (<2%)
Death [5]
Multiorgan failure [2]

ATOVAQUONE/ PROGUANIL

Trade name: Malarone (GSK)
Indications: Malaria prophylaxis and treatment
Class: Antimalarial
Half-life: 24 hours
Clinically important, potentially hazardous interactions with: artemether/lumefantrine, dapsone, etoposide, hypoglycemic agents, indinavir, metoclopramide, phenothiazines, rifabutin, rifampin, ritonavir, tetracycline, typhoid vaccine
Pregnancy category: C
Important contra-indications noted in the prescribing guidelines for: the elderly; nursing mothers

---

Skin
Erythema multiforme [2]
Pruritus (<10%)

Mucosal
Oral ulceration (6%) [3]

Central Nervous System
Abnormal dreams (7%)
Anorexia (5%)
Headache (10%) [4]
Insomnia (3%)
Vertigo (dizziness) (5%) [3]

Neuromuscular/Skeletal
Asthenia (fatigue) (8%)

Gastrointestinal/Hepatic
Abdominal pain (17%) [5]
Diarrhea (8%)
Dyspepsia (2%)
Gastritis (3%)
Hepatotoxicity [2]
Nausea (12%)
Vomiting (12%) [2]

Respiratory
Cough [3]

Ocular
Vision impaired (2%)

Other
Adverse effects [3]

ATROPINE SULFATE

Trade name: Lomotil (Pfizer)
Indications: Salivation, sinus bradycardia, uveitis, peptic ulcer
Class: Muscarinic antagonist
Half-life: 2–3 hours
Clinically important, potentially hazardous interactions with: anticholinergics, zuclopenthixol
Pregnancy category: C
Note: Many of the trade name drugs for atropine sulfate contain phenobarbital, scopolamine, hyoscyamine, hydrocodone, methenamine, etc.

Skin
Anaphylactoid reactions/Anaphylaxis [3]
Dermatitis [3]
Erythema multiforme [2]
Photosensitivity (<10%)

Mucosal
Xerostomia (>10%) [4]

Cardiovascular
Arrhythmias [2]
Atrial fibrillation [2]
Bradycardia [3]
Tachycardia [5]

Central Nervous System
Confusion [2]

Ocular
Amblyopia [5]
Hallucinations, visual [3]
Periocular dermatitis [3]

Local
Injection-site irritation (>10%)

Other
Allergic reactions [2]
Central anticholinergic syndrome [2]

AVANAFIL

Trade name: Stendra (Vivus)
Indications: Erectile dysfunction
Class: Phosphodiesterase type 5 (PDE5) inhibitor
Half-life: 5 hours
Clinically important, potentially hazardous interactions with: alcohol, alpha blockers, amprenavir, antihypertensives, aprepitant, atazanavir, clarithromycin, diltiazem, erythromycin, fluconazole, fosamprenavir, indinavir, itraconazole, ketoconazole, nefazodone, nelfinavir, nitrates, ritonavir, saquinavir, strong CYP3A4 inhibitors, telithromycin, verapamil
Pregnancy category: C (Not indicated for use in women)
Important contra-indications noted in the prescribing guidelines for: pediatric patients
Note: Contraindicated in patients using any form of nitrates.

Skin
Facial flushing [2]
Rash (<2%)

Mucosal
Nasal congestion (<3%) [7]

Cardiovascular
Flushing (3–10%) [10]
Hypertension (<2%)

Central Nervous System
Headache (5–12%) [9]
Vertigo (dizziness) (<2%) [2]

Neuromuscular/Skeletal
Arthralgia (<2%)
Asthenia (fatigue) [2]
Back pain (<3%) [3]

Gastrointestinal/Hepatic
Constipation (<2%)
Diarrhea (<2%)
Dyspepsia (<2%) [4]
Nausea (<2%)

Respiratory
Bronchitis (<2%)
Influenza (<2%)
Nasopharyngitis (<5%) [5]
Sinusitis (<2%) [2]
Upper respiratory tract infection (<3%)

Other
Adverse effects [4]

AXITINIB

Trade name: Inlyta (Pfizer)
Indications: Advanced renal cell carcinoma (after failure of one prior systemic therapy)
Class: Tyrosine kinase inhibitor
Half-life: 2–6 hours
Clinically important, potentially hazardous interactions with: ketoconazole, rifampin
Pregnancy category: D
Important contra-indications noted in the prescribing guidelines for: nursing mothers; pediatric patients

---

Skin
Erythema (2%)

Hand–foot syndrome (27%) [15]
Pruritus (7%)
Rash (13%) [3]
Xerosis (10%)

Hair
Alopecia (4%) [2]

Mucosal
Mucosal inflammation (15%) [2]
Stomatitis (15%)

Cardiovascular
Hypertension (40%) [32]

Central Nervous System
Anorexia [3]
Dysgeusia (taste perversion) (11%)
Headache (14%) [4]
Leukoencephalopathy [2]

Neuromuscular/Skeletal
Arthralgia (15%) [2]
Asthenia (fatigue) (39%) [24]
Pain in extremities (13%)

Gastrointestinal/Hepatic
Abdominal pain (14%)
Constipation (20%) [2]
Diarrhea (55%) [22]
Dyspepsia (10%)
Nausea (32%) [10]
Vomiting (24%) [6]

Respiratory
Cough (15%) [2]
Dysphonia (>20%) [12]
Dyspnea (15%) [4]

Endocrine/Metabolic
ALT increased (22%) [2]
Appetite decreased (34%) [7]
AST increased [2]
Dehydration [2]
Hyperthyroidism [2]
Hyponatremia [2]
Hypothyroidism (19%) [8]
Serum creatinine increased [2]
Thyroid dysfunction [2]
Weight loss (25%) [2]

Renal
Proteinuria (11%) [5]

Hematologic
Anemia [2]
Hemorrhage (16%)
Neutropenia [2]
Thrombotic complications (3%)

Other
Adverse effects [4]

AZACITIDINE

Trade name: Vidaza (Celgene)
Indications: Myelodysplastic syndromes, refractory anemia
Class: Antimetabolite, Antineoplastic, Cytosine analog
Half-life: 40–56 minutes
Clinically important, potentially hazardous interactions with: BCG vaccine, denosumab, echinacea, leflunomide, natalizumab, pimecrolimus, sipuleucel-T, tacrolimus, trastuzumab, vaccines
Pregnancy category: D
Important contra-indications noted in the prescribing guidelines for: nursing mothers; pediatric patients
Note: Contraindicated in patients with advanced malignant hepatic tumors.

Skin
Anaphylactoid reactions/Anaphylaxis (<5%)
Cellulitis (8%)
Diaphoresis (11%)
Ecchymoses (31%)
Edema (14%)
Erythema (7–17%)
Hematoma (9%)
Herpes simplex (9%)
Hypersensitivity (<5%)
Induration (<5%)
Lymphoproliferative disease [2]
Neoplasms (<5%)
Nodular eruption (5%)
Pallor (16%)
Peripheral edema (19%)
Petechiae (11–24%)
Pruritus (12%)
Pyoderma gangrenosum (<5%)
Rash (10–14%) [2]
Sweet's syndrome [4]
Toxicity [2]
Urticaria (6%)
Xerosis (5%)

Mucosal
Gingival bleeding (10%)
Oral bleeding (5%)
Stomatitis (8%)
Tongue ulceration (5%)

Cardiovascular
Arrhythmias [2]
Atrial fibrillation (<5%)
Cardiac failure (<5%)
Cardiomyopathy (<5%)
Cardiotoxicity [2]
Chest pain (5–16%) [4]
Congestive heart failure (<5%)
Hypertension (9%)
Hypotension (7%) [2]
Orthostatic hypotension (<5%)
Tachycardia [2]

Central Nervous System
Anorexia (21%)
Anxiety (5–13%)
Cerebral hemorrhage (<5%)
Depression (12%)
Fever (30–52%) [3]
Headache (22%)
Insomnia (9–11%)
Intracranial hemorrhage (<5%)
Pain (11%)
Seizures (<5%)
Syncope [2]
Vertigo (dizziness) (19%)

Neuromuscular/Skeletal
Arthralgia (22%) [2]
Asthenia (fatigue) (7–36%) [3]
Back pain (19%)
Bone or joint pain (<5%)
Myalgia/Myopathy (16%)
Neck pain (<5%)

Gastrointestinal/Hepatic
Abdominal pain (12–13%)
Black stools (<5%)
Cholecystitis (<5%)
Constipation (34–50%) [3]
Diarrhea (36%) [3]
Dyspepsia (6%)
Dysphagia (5%)
Gastrointestinal bleeding (<5%)
Loose stools (6%)
Nausea (48–71%) [5]
Vomiting (27–54%) [4]

Respiratory
Cough (30%)
Dyspnea (14–29%)
Hemoptysis (<5%)
Nasopharyngitis (15%)
Pharyngolaryngeal pain (6%)
Pneumonia (11%) [2]
Pneumonitis (<5%) [2]
Pulmonary toxicity [2]
Respiratory distress (<5%)
Rhinitis (6%)
Upper respiratory tract infection (9–13%)

Endocrine/Metabolic
Dehydration (<5%)
Hypokalemia (6%)
Weight loss (8%)

Genitourinary
Hematuria (6%)
Urinary tract infection (9%)

Renal
Renal failure (<5%)

Hematologic
Agranulocytosis (<5%)
Anemia (51–70%) [3]
Bone marrow suppression (<5%)
Cytopenia [4]
Febrile neutropenia (14–16%) [5]
Leukopenia (18–48%)
Myelosuppression [2]
Neutropenia (32–66%) [5]
Pancytopenia (<5%)
Splenomegaly (<5%)
Thrombocytopenia (66–70%) [3]

Ocular
Ocular hemorrhage (<5%)

Local
Injection-site bruising (5–14%)
Injection-site edema (5%)
Injection-site erythema (35–43%)
Injection-site hematoma (6%)
Injection-site pain (19–23%)
Injection-site pigmentation (5%)
Injection-site pruritus (7%)
Injection-site purpura (14%)
Injection-site reactions (14–29%) [6]

Other
Adverse effects [5]
Death [4]
Infection (<5%) [8]

AZATHIOPRINE

Trade names: Azasan (aaiPharma), Imuran (Prometheus)
Indications: Lupus nephritis, psoriatic arthritis, rheumatoid arthritis, autoimmune diseases, as an adjunct for the prevention of rejection in kidney transplant patients
Class: Antimetabolite, Disease-modifying antirheumatic drug (DMARD), Immunosuppressant, Purine anaolog
Half-life: 12 minutes
Clinically important, potentially hazardous interactions with: allopurinol, aminosalicylates, balsalazide, benazepril, captopril, chlorambucil, co-trimoxazole, cyclophosphamide, cyclosporine, enalapril, febuxostat, fosinopril, Hemophilus B vaccine, imidapril, lisinopril, mesalamine, mycophenolate, natalizumab, olsalazine, quinapril, ramipril, ribavirin, sulfamethoxazole, tofacitinib, trimethoprim, typhoid vaccine, vaccines, warfarin, yellow fever vaccine
Pregnancy category: D
Important contra-indications noted in the prescribing guidelines for: nursing mothers; pediatric patients
Note: Patients receiving immunosuppressants, including azathioprine, are at increased risk of developing lymphoma and other malignancies, particularly of the skin.
Black Box Warning: MALIGNANCY

Skin
Acanthosis nigricans [2]
Acneform eruption [2]
AGEP [2]
Angioedema [2]
Carcinoma [3]
Dermatitis [4]
Erythema gyratum repens [2]
Erythema multiforme [2]
Erythema nodosum [4]
Exanthems [10]
Herpes simplex [3]
Herpes zoster [8]
Hypersensitivity [27]
Kaposi's sarcoma [14]
Lymphoproliferative disease [4]
Neoplasms [2]
Neutrophilic dermatosis [4]
Nevi [3]
Porokeratosis [4]
Rash (<10%) [10]
Scabies [5]
Squamous cell carcinoma [10]
Sweet's syndrome [12]
Tinea [3]
Toxicity [3]
Tumors [8]
Urticaria [5]
Vasculitis [5]
Verrucae [3]

Hair
Alopecia [9]

Nails
Onychomycosis [2]

Mucosal
Oral ulceration [2]

Cardiovascular
Atrial fibrillation [3]

Central Nervous System
Chills (>10%)
Fever [7]
Headache [3]
Leukoencephalopathy [2]

Neuromuscular/Skeletal
Arthralgia [4]
Asthenia (fatigue) [7]

Gastrointestinal/Hepatic
Abdominal pain [2]
Hepatitis [5]
Hepatotoxicity [25]
Nausea [8]
Pancreatitis [43]
Vomiting [4]

Respiratory
Flu-like syndrome [2]
Pneumonitis [2]
Pulmonary toxicity [3]

Hematologic
Bone marrow suppression [5]
Leukopenia [11]
Myelosuppression [2]
Myelotoxicity [4]
Neutropenia [2]
Pancytopenia [3]
Thrombocytopenia [5]

Other
Adverse effects [7]
Allergic reactions [5]
Infection [9]

AZITHROMYCIN

Trade names: AzaSite (Merck), Zithromax (Pfizer)
Indications: Infections of the upper and lower respiratory tract, skin infections, sexually transmitted diseases, conjunctivitis (ophthalmic preparations only)
Class: Antibacterial, Antibiotic, macrolide
Half-life: 68 hours
Clinically important, potentially hazardous interactions with: aminophylline, antacids, artemether/lumefantrine, astemizole, atorvastatin, bromocriptine, cabergoline, colchicine, coumarins, cyclosporine, digoxin, droperidol, ergotamine, fluvastatin, lovastatin, methysergide, mizolastine, oral typhoid vaccine, pimozide, pravastatin, quetiapine, reboxetine, rifabutin, ritonavir, simvastatin, venetoclax, warfarin
Pregnancy category: B
Important contra-indications noted in the prescribing guidelines for: nursing mothers; pediatric patients
Note: AzaSite is for topical ophthalmic use only (for reactions see [Ophth] below).

Skin
AGEP [2]
Anaphylactoid reactions/Anaphylaxis [2]
Churg-Strauss syndrome [2]
DRESS syndrome [4]
Erythema [2]
Exanthems [3]
Hypersensitivity [3]
Jarisch–Herxheimer reaction [2]
Pruritus [3]
Rash [Ophth] (2–10%) [6]
Stevens–Johnson syndrome [6]
Urticaria [Ophth] [2]

Cardiovascular
Cardiotoxicity [8]
QT prolongation [11]
Torsades de pointes [4]

Central Nervous System
Anorexia (2–10%)
Headache [3]
Vertigo (dizziness) [2]

Gastrointestinal/Hepatic
Abdominal pain (2–10%) [4]
Diarrhea (4–9%) [17]
Gastrointestinal disorder [2]
Hepatotoxicity [6]
Nausea (7%) [8]
Vanishing bile duct syndrome [2]
Vomiting (2–10%) [5]

Genitourinary
Vaginitis (2–10%)

Otic
Hearing loss [3]
Tinnitus [2]

Ocular
Keratitis [2]

Local
Injection-site erythema (2–10%)
Injection-site pain (2–10%) [3]

Other
Adverse effects [14]
Death [2]
Hiccups [2]
Side effects [2]

BACLOFEN

Trade names: Baclofen (Watson), Gablofen (Mallinckrodt), Lioresal (Medtronic)
Indications: Spasticity resulting from multiple sclerosis
Class: GABA receptor agonist, Skeletal muscle relaxant
Half-life: 2.5–4 hours
Clinically important, potentially hazardous interactions with: acebutolol, alcohol, alfuzosin, amitriptyline, captopril, cilazapril, diclofenac, enalapril, fosinopril, irbesartan, levodopa, lisinopril, meloxicam, olmesartan, quinapril, ramipril, trandolapril
Pregnancy category: C
Important contra-indications noted in the prescribing guidelines for: pediatric patients
Note: Children appear to be at higher risk for complications than adults when using intrathecal baclofen (ITB). ITB therapy is a safe and effective treatment for severe spasticity in the pediatric population, but does have a 31% rate of complications requiring surgical management over a 3-year treatment period.
Black Box Warning: DO NOT DISCONTINUE ABRUPTLY

Skin
- Exanthems [2]
- Rash (<10%)
- Toxicity [2]

Cardiovascular
- Bradycardia [2]
- Hypertension [2]
- Hypotension [3]

Central Nervous System
- Coma [3]
- Confusion (<10%)
- Dyskinesia [2]
- Encephalopathy [2]
- Hallucinations [4]
- Headache (<10%)
- Insomnia (>10%)
- Seizures [9]
- Slurred speech (>10%)
- Somnolence (drowsiness) (>10%) [5]
- Vertigo (dizziness) (>10%) [5]

Neuromuscular/Skeletal
- Asthenia (fatigue) (>10%) [5]

Gastrointestinal/Hepatic
- Constipation (<10%)
- Nausea (<10%)

Genitourinary
- Polyuria (<10%)

Other
- Infection [2]
- Side effects (<2%)

BALSALAZIDE

Trade names: Colazal (Salix), Colazide (Almirall)
Indications: Mild to moderately active ulcerative colitis
Class: Aminosalicylate
Half-life: N/A
Clinically important, potentially hazardous interactions with: azathioprine, cardiac glycosides, folic acid, heparin, low molecular weight heparins, mercaptopurine, thiopurine analogs, varicella virus-containing vaccines
Pregnancy category: B
Important contra-indications noted in the prescribing guidelines for: nursing mothers; pediatric patients

---

Skin
- Hypersensitivity [2]

Mucosal
- Stomatitis (3%)

Central Nervous System
- Anorexia (2%)
- Fever (2–6%)
- Headache (15%)
- Insomnia (2%)

Neuromuscular/Skeletal
- Arthralgia (4%)
- Asthenia (fatigue) (2%)

Gastrointestinal/Hepatic
- Abdominal pain (6–13%)
- Colitis (ulcerative, exacerbation) (6%)
- Diarrhea (5–9%)
- Dyspepsia (2%)
- Flatulence (2%)
- Nausea (4%)
- Vomiting (10%)

Respiratory
- Cough (2–3%)
- Flu-like syndrome (<4%)
- Nasopharyngitis (6%)
- Pharyngitis (2%)
- Pharyngolaryngeal pain (3%)
- Rhinitis (2%)

Genitourinary
- Dysmenorrhea (3%)

BASILIXIMAB

Trade name: Simulect (Novartis)
Indications: Prophylaxis of organ rejection in renal transplantation
Class: Interleukin-2 receptor antagonist, Monoclonal antibody
Half-life: 7.2 days
Clinically important, potentially hazardous interactions with: cyclosporine, Hemophilus B vaccine, mycophenolate
Pregnancy category: B
Important contra-indications noted in the prescribing guidelines for: nursing mothers

---

Skin
- Acneform eruption (>10%)
- Candidiasis (3–10%)
- Cyst (3–10%)
- Edema (generalized) (3–10%)
- Facial edema (3–10%)
- Genital edema (3–10%)
- Hematoma (3–10%)
- Herpes simplex (3–10%)
- Herpes zoster (3–10%)
- Peripheral edema (>10%)
- Pruritus (3–10%)
- Rash (3–10%)
- Ulcerations (3–10%)
- Wound complications (>10%)

Hair
- Hypertrichosis (3–10%)

Mucosal
- Gingival hyperplasia/hypertrophy (3–10%)
- Stomatitis (3–10%)
- Ulcerative stomatitis (3–10%)

Cardiovascular
- Angina (3–10%)
- Arrhythmias (3–10%)
- Atrial fibrillation (3–10%)
- Cardiac failure (3–10%)
- Chest pain (3–10%)
- Hypertension (>10%)
- Hypotension (3–10%)
- Pulmonary edema (3–10%)
- Tachycardia (3–10%)

Central Nervous System
- Agitation (3–10%)
- Anxiety (3–10%)
- Depression (3–10%)
- Fever (>10%)
- Headache (>10%)
- Hypoesthesia (3–10%)
- Insomnia (>10%)
- Pain (>10%)
- Paresthesias (3–10%)
- Rigors (3–10%)
- Tremor (>10%)
- Vertigo (dizziness) (3–10%)

Neuromuscular/Skeletal
- Arthralgia (3–10%)
- Asthenia (fatigue) (3–10%)
- Back pain (3–10%)
- Cramps (3–10%)
- Fractures (3–10%)
- Leg pain (3–10%)
- Myalgia/Myopathy (3–10%)

Gastrointestinal/Hepatic
- Abdominal distension (3–10%)
- Abdominal pain (>10%)
- Black stools (3–10%)
- Constipation (>10%)
- Diarrhea (>10%)
- Dyspepsia (>10%)
- Esophagitis (3–10%)
- Flatulence (3–10%)
- Gastroenteritis (3–10%)
- Gastrointestinal bleeding (3–10%)
- Gastrointestinal disorder (69%)
- Hernia (3–10%)
- Nausea (>10%)
- Vomiting (>10%)

Respiratory
- Bronchitis (3–10%)
- Bronchospasm (3–10%)
- Cough (3–10%)
- Dyspnea (>10%)

Pharyngitis (3–10%)
Pneumonia (3–10%)
Rhinitis (3–10%)
Sinusitis (3–10%)
Upper respiratory tract infection (>10%)

Endocrine/Metabolic
Acidosis (3–10%)
Dehydration (3–10%)
Diabetes mellitus (3–10%)
Hypercalcemia (3–10%)
Hypercholesterolemia (>10%)
Hyperglycemia (>10%)
Hyperkalemia (>10%)
Hyperlipidemia (3–10%)
Hypertriglyceridemia (3–10%)
Hyperuricemia (>10%)
Hypocalcemia (3–10%)
Hypoglycemia (3–10%)
Hypokalemia (>10%)
Hypophosphatemia (>10%)
Weight gain (3–10%)

Genitourinary
Albuminuria (3–10%)
Dysuria (3–10%)
Hematuria (3–10%)
Impotence (3–10%)
Oliguria (3–10%)
Urinary frequency (3–10%)
Urinary retention (3–10%)
Urinary tract infection (>10%)

Renal
Renal tubular necrosis (3–10%)

Hematologic
Anemia (>10%)
Hemorrhage (3–10%)
Leukopenia (3–10%)
Polycythemia (3–10%)
Sepsis (3–10%)
Thrombocytopenia (3–10%)
Thrombosis (3–10%)

Ocular
Abnormal vision (3–10%)
Cataract (3–10%)
Conjunctivitis (3–10%)

Other
Infection (viral) (>10%)

BCG VACCINE

Synonym: Bacille Calmette-Guerin
Trade names: Mycobax (Sanofi-Aventis), TICE BCG (Organon)
Indications: Immunization against tuberculosis
Class: Vaccine
Half-life: N/A
Clinically important, potentially hazardous interactions with: alefacept, aminophylline, azacitidine, betamethasone, cabazitaxel, cefazolin, cefixime, ceftaroline fosamil, ceftobiprole, ciprofloxacin, demeclocycline, denileukin, docetaxel, doripenem, doxycycline, fingolimod, gefitinib, gemifloxacin, leflunomide, levofloxacin, monosodium glutamate, moxifloxacin, ofloxacin, oxaliplatin, pazopanib, sulfadiazine, telavancin, telithromycin, temsirolimus
Pregnancy category: C

Skin
Abscess [16]
Anaphylactoid reactions/Anaphylaxis [5]
Churg-Strauss syndrome [15]
Dermatitis [2]
Erythema [3]
Fixed eruption [2]
Hypersensitivity [2]
Keloid [4]
Lupus vulgaris [22]
Lymphadenitis [6]
Lymphadenopathy [91]
Papular lesions [6]
Sarcoidosis [4]
Scar [8]
Scrofuloderma [5]
Sweet's syndrome [2]
Ulcerations [6]
Vasculitis [2]

Mucosal
Mucocutaneous lymph node syndrome (Kawaski syndrom) [2]

Central Nervous System
Fever [6]
Neurotoxicity [2]

Neuromuscular/Skeletal
Arthralgia [7]
Asthenia (fatigue) [4]
Osteomyelitis [33]

Gastrointestinal/Hepatic
Hepatitis [3]
Hepatotoxicity [2]

Genitourinary
Balanitis [3]
Bladder disorder [2]
Hematuria [2]

Hematologic
Sepsis [3]

Ocular
Optic neuritis [2]
Uveitis [4]

Local
Injection-site abscess [2]
Injection-site ulceration [3]

Other
Adverse effects [3]
Cancer [3]
Death [14]
Infection [2]
Systemic reactions [2]

BECLOMETHASONE

Trade names: Beconase AQ (GSK), Qnasl (Teva), Qvar (3M), Vanceril (Schering)
Indications: Allergic rhinitis, asthma
Class: Corticosteroid, inhaled
Half-life: N/A
Clinically important, potentially hazardous interactions with: diuretics, estrogens, ketoconazole, live vaccines, oral contraceptives, phenytoin, rifampin, warfarin
Pregnancy category: C
Important contra-indications noted in the prescribing guidelines for: nursing mothers; pediatric patients

---

Skin
Bruising [3]
Candidiasis [2]

Mucosal
Epistaxis (nosebleed) (with nasally-inhaled formulation) (2%)
Nasal discomfort (5%)
Oral candidiasis [4]

Central Nervous System
Headache (2%) [2]

Neuromuscular/Skeletal
Osteoporosis [5]

Respiratory
Upper respiratory tract infection [2]

Ocular
Cataract [4]
Glaucoma [3]

Other
Adverse effects [10]

BEDAQUILINE

Trade name: Sirturo (Janssen)
Indications: Pulmonary multi-drug resistant tuberculosis
Class: Antimycobacterial, Diarylquinoline
Half-life: 5.5 months
Clinically important, potentially hazardous interactions with: ketoconazole, rifabutin, rifampin, rifapentine, stong CYP3A4 inhibitors and inducers
Pregnancy category: B
Important contra-indications noted in the prescribing guidelines for: nursing mothers; pediatric patients
Black Box Warning: INCREASED RISK OF DEATH / QT PROLONGATION

Skin
Rash (8%)

Cardiovascular
Chest pain (11%) [2]
QT prolongation [2]

Central Nervous System
Anorexia (9%)
Headache (28%) [2]

Neuromuscular/Skeletal
Arthralgia (33%) [2]
Pain in extremities [2]

Gastrointestinal/Hepatic
Nausea (38%) [3]

Respiratory
Hemoptysis (18%)

Endocrine/Metabolic
ALT increased (<10%)
AST increased (<10%)

Other
Infection [2]

BELATACEPT

Trade name: Nulojix (Bristol-Myers Squibb)
Indications: Prophylaxis of organ rejection in kidney transplantation
Class: Immunosuppressant, T-cell co-stimulation blocker
Half-life: 7–10 days
Clinically important, potentially hazardous interactions with: live vaccines, mycophenolate
Pregnancy category: C
Important contra-indications noted in the prescribing guidelines for: nursing mothers; pediatric patients
Note: Contraindicated in patients without immunity to Epstein-Barr virus.
Black Box Warning: POST-TRANSPLANT LYMPHOPROLIFERATIVE DISORDER, OTHER MALIGNANCIES, AND SERIOUS INFECTIONS

Skin
Acneform eruption (8%)
Hematoma (<10%)
Hyperhidrosis (<10%)
Lymphoproliferative disease (post-transplant) [7]
Malignancies [3]
Peripheral edema (34%)

Hair
Alopecia (<10%)

Mucosal
Aphthous stomatitis (<10%)
Stomatitis (<10%)

Cardiovascular
Atrial fibrillation (<10%)
Hypertension (32%)
Hypotension (18%)

Central Nervous System
Anxiety (10%)
Fever (28%)
Guillain–Barré syndrome (<10%)
Headache (21%)
Insomnia (15%)
Tremor (8%)
Vertigo (dizziness) (9%)

Neuromuscular/Skeletal
Arthralgia (17%)
Back pain (13%)
Bone or joint pain (<10%)

Gastrointestinal/Hepatic
Abdominal pain (9–19%)
Constipation (33%)
Diarrhea (39%)
Nausea (24%)
Vomiting (22%)

Respiratory
Bronchitis (10%)
Cough (24%)
Dyspnea (12%)
Influenza (11%)
Nasopharyngitis (13%)
Upper respiratory tract infection (15%)

Endocrine/Metabolic
Creatine phosphokinase increased (15%)
Hypercholesterolemia (11%)
Hyperglycemia (19%)
Hyperkalemia (20%)
Hyperuricemia (5%)
Hypocalcemia (13%)
Hypokalemia (21%)
Hypomagnesemia (7%)
Hypophosphatemia (19%)

Genitourinary
Dysuria (11%)
Hematuria (16%)
Urinary incontinence (<10%)
Urinary tract infection (37%) [2]

Renal
Proteinuria (16%)
Renal failure (<10%)
Renal tubular necrosis (9%)

Hematologic
Anemia (45%)
Dyslipidemia (19%)
Leukopenia (20%)
Neutropenia (<10%)

Other
Graft dysfunction (25%)
Infection (<10%) [7]

BELINOSTAT

Trade name: Beleodaq (Spectrum)
Indications: Peripheral T-cell lymphoma
Class: Histone deacetylase (HDAC) inhibitor
Half-life: 1 hour
Clinically important, potentially hazardous interactions with: strong UGT1A1 inhibitors
Pregnancy category: D
Important contra-indications noted in the prescribing guidelines for: nursing mothers; pediatric patients

---

Skin
Peripheral edema (20%) [2]
Pruritus (16%)
Rash (20%)

Hair
Alopecia [2]

Cardiovascular
Hypotension (10%)
Phlebitis (10%)
QT prolongation (11%) [2]

Central Nervous System
Anorexia [2]
Chills (16%)
Fever (35%) [2]
Headache (15%) [3]
Peripheral neuropathy [2]
Vertigo (dizziness) (10%) [2]

Neuromuscular/Skeletal
Asthenia (fatigue) (37%) [11]
Myalgia/Myopathy [2]

Gastrointestinal/Hepatic
Abdominal pain (11%)
Constipation (23%) [5]
Diarrhea (23%) [6]
Nausea (42%) [10]
Vomiting (29%) [10]

Respiratory
Cough (19%)
Dyspnea (22%) [4]
Pneumonia (>2%)
Pneumonitis [2]

Endocrine/Metabolic
Appetite decreased (15%)
Creatine phosphokinase increased (>2%)
Hypokalemia (12%)

Hematologic
Anemia (32%) [5]
Leukopenia [2]
Lymphopenia [2]
Neutropenia [4]
Thrombocytopenia (16%) [3]
Thrombosis [2]

Local
Infusion-site pain (14%)
Injection-site reactions [2]

Other
Allergic reactions [2]
Hiccups [2]
Multiorgan failure (>2%)

BENAZEPRIL

Trade names: Lotensin (Novartis), Lotensin HCT (Novartis), Lotrel (Novartis)
Indications: Hypertension
Class: Angiotensin-converting enzyme (ACE) inhibitor, Antihypertensive, Vasodilator
Half-life: 10–11 hours
Clinically important, potentially hazardous interactions with: allopurinol, amifostine, amiloride, angiotensin II receptor blockers, antacids, antidiabetics, antihypertensives, azathioprine, cyclosporine, diazoxide, diuretics, eplerenone, everolimus, gold & gold compounds, herbals, lithium, MAO inhibitors, methylphenidate, NSAIDs, pentoxifylline, phosphodiesterase 5 inhibitors, potassium salts, prostacyclin analogues, rituximab, sirolimus, spironolactone, temsirolimus, tizanidine, tolvaptan, triamterene, trimethoprim, yohimbine
Pregnancy category: D
Important contra-indications noted in the prescribing guidelines for: pediatric patients
Note: Lotrel is benazepril and amlodipine. Lotensin-HCT is benazepril and hydrochlorothiazide. Hydrochlorothiazide is a sulfonamide and can be absorbed systemically. Sulfonamides can produce severe, possibly fatal, reactions such as toxic epidermal necrolysis and Stevens-Johnson syndrome.
Contraindicated in patients with a history of angioedema with or without previous ACE inhibitor treatment.
Black Box Warning: FETAL TOXICITY

Skin
Angioedema [8]
Peripheral edema [3]

Central Nervous System
Headache (6%)
Vertigo (dizziness) (4%)

Respiratory
Cough [10]

BETAXOLOL

Trade names: Betoptic [Ophthalmic] (Alcon), Kerlone (Pfizer)
Indications: Open-angle glaucoma, hypertension
Class: Adrenergic beta-receptor antagonist
Half-life: 14–22 hours
Clinically important, potentially hazardous interactions with: clonidine, verapamil
Pregnancy category: C
Important contra-indications noted in the prescribing guidelines for: nursing mothers; pediatric patients
Note: Cutaneous side effects of beta-receptor blockers are clinically polymorphous. They apparently appear after several months of continuous therapy.

Skin
- Cold extremities (2%)
- Dermatitis [3]
- Diaphoresis (<2%)
- Eczema (<2%)
- Edema (<2%)
- Erythema (<2%)
- Lymphadenopathy (<2%)
- Pruritus (<2%)
- Purpura (<2%)
- Rash (<2%) [3]

Hair
- Alopecia (<2%)
- Hypertrichosis (<2%)

Mucosal
- Epistaxis (nosebleed) (<2%)
- Oral ulceration (<2%)
- Sialorrhea (<2%)
- Xerostomia (<2%)

Cardiovascular
- Angina (<2%)
- Arrhythmias (<2%)
- Atrioventricular block (<2%)
- Bradycardia (6–8%)
- Cardiac failure (<2%)
- Chest pain (2–7%)
- Flushing (<2%)
- Hypertension (<2%)
- Hypotension (<2%)
- Myocardial infarction (<2%)
- Palpitation (2%)
- Peripheral ischemia (<2%)

Central Nervous System
- Ageusia (taste loss) (<2%)
- Amnesia (<2%)
- Anorexia (<2%)
- Confusion (<2%)
- Dysgeusia (taste perversion) (<2%)
- Emotional lability (<2%)
- Fever (<2%)
- Hallucinations (<2%)
- Headache (7–15%)
- Insomnia (<5%)
- Pain (<2%)
- Paresthesias (2%)
- Rigors (<2%)
- Stupor (<2%)
- Syncope (<2%)
- Tremor (<2%)
- Twitching (<2%)
- Vertigo (dizziness) (5–15%)

Neuromuscular/Skeletal
- Arthralgia (3%)
- Asthenia (fatigue) (3–10%)
- Ataxia (<2%)
- Bone or joint pain (5%)
- Leg cramps (<2%)
- Myalgia/Myopathy (3%)
- Neck pain (<2%)
- Tendinitis (<2%)

Gastrointestinal/Hepatic
- Constipation (<2%)
- Diarrhea (2%)
- Dyspepsia (4–5%)
- Dysphagia (<2%)
- Nausea (2–6%)
- Vomiting (<2%)

Respiratory
- Bronchitis (<2%)
- Bronchospasm (<2%)
- Cough (<2%)
- Dysphonia (<2%)
- Dyspnea (2%)
- Influenza (<2%)
- Pharyngitis (2%)
- Pneumonia (<2%)
- Sinusitis (<2%)
- Upper respiratory tract infection (3%)

Endocrine/Metabolic
- Acidosis (<2%)
- ALT increased (<2%)
- Appetite increased (<2%)
- AST increased (<2%)
- Diabetes mellitus (<2%)
- Gynecomastia (<2%)
- Hypercholesterolemia (<2%)
- Hyperglycemia (<2%)
- Hyperkalemia (<2%)
- Hyperuricemia (<2%)
- Hypokalemia (<2%)
- Libido decreased (<2%)
- Mastodynia (<2%)
- Menstrual irregularities (<2%)
- Weight gain (<2%)
- Weight loss (<2%)

Genitourinary
- Cystitis (<2%)
- Dysuria (<2%)
- Oliguria (<2%)
- Peyronie's disease (<2%)
- Prostatitis (<2%)

Renal
- Proteinuria (<2%)
- Renal function abnormal (<2%)

Hematologic
- Anemia (<2%)
- Lymphocytosis (<2%)
- Thrombocytopenia (<2%)
- Thrombosis (<2%)

Otic
- Ear pain (<2%)
- Hearing loss (<2%)
- Tinnitus (<2%)

Ocular
- Abnormal vision (<2%)
- Blepharitis (<2%)
- Cataract (<2%)
- Conjunctivitis (<2%)
- Iritis (<2%)
- Lacrimation (<2%)
- Ocular hemorrhage (<2%)
- Scotoma (<2%)
- Xerophthalmia (<2%)

Other
- Allergic reactions (<2%)
- Dipsia (thirst) (<2%)

BEVACIZUMAB

Trade name: Avastin (Genentech)
Indications: Colon cancer
Class: Biologic, Monoclonal antibody, Vascular endothelial growth factor antagonist
Half-life: 20 days
Clinically important, potentially hazardous interactions with: antineoplastics, irinotecan, sorafenib, sunitinib
Pregnancy category: C
Important contra-indications noted in the prescribing guidelines for: the elderly; nursing mothers; pediatric patients
Black Box Warning: GASTROINTESTINAL PERFORATIONS, SURGERY AND WOUND HEALING COMPLICATIONS, and HEMORRHAGE

Skin
- Acneform eruption [5]
- Hand–foot syndrome [11]
- Necrosis [2]
- Rash [15]
- Toxicity [9]
- Ulcerations [3]
- Wound complications [8]

Hair
- Alopecia [5]

Mucosal
- Epistaxis (nosebleed) [5]
- Mucositis [9]
- Oral ulceration [2]
- Stomatitis [8]

Cardiovascular
- Cardiac failure [2]
- Cardiotoxicity [5]
- Hypertension (23–67%) [70]
- Hypotension (7–15%)
- Thromboembolism (<21%) [14]
- Venous thromboembolism [4]

Central Nervous System
- Anorexia [12]
- Cerebral hemorrhage [5]
- Headache [6]
- Intracranial hemorrhage [2]
- Leukoencephalopathy [19]
- Neurotoxicity [12]
- Peripheral neuropathy [9]
- Seizures [2]

Neuromuscular/Skeletal
- Arthralgia [2]
- Asthenia (fatigue) [31]
- Osteonecrosis [4]

Gastrointestinal/Hepatic
- Abdominal pain [4]
- Colitis [3]
- Diarrhea [39]

Gastrointestinal bleeding [5]
Gastrointestinal fistula [2]
Gastrointestinal perforation [23]
Hepatotoxicity [4]
Nausea [10]
Vomiting [9]

Respiratory
Hemoptysis [4]
Pulmonary embolism [4]
Pulmonary toxicity [2]

Endocrine/Metabolic
ALT increased [3]
Creatine phosphokinase increased [2]
Hyperglycemia [2]
Hypokalemia [3]
Hypomagnesemia [2]

Renal
Proteinuria [30]

Hematologic
Anemia [9]
Bleeding [9]
Febrile neutropenia [9]
Hemorrhage [13]
Leukopenia [10]
Lymphopenia [2]
Neutropenia [34]
Thrombocytopenia [20]
Thrombosis [15]
Thrombotic complications [4]

Ocular
Hallucinations, visual [2]
Intraocular pressure increased [3]
Iritis [2]
Ocular adverse effects [2]
Uveitis [2]

Other
Adverse effects [20]
Allergic reactions [2]
Death [14]
Infection [7]

BEXAROTENE

Trade name: Targretin (Eisai)
Indications: Cutaneous T-cell lymphoma, mycosis fungoides
Class: Antineoplastic, Retinoid
Half-life: 7 hours
Clinically important, potentially hazardous interactions with: acitretin, atorvastatin, beta-carotene, carboplatin, conivaptan, dexamethasone, dong quai, gemfibrozil, grapefruit juice, isotretinoin, oral contraceptives, paclitaxel, saxagliptin, St John's wort, tamoxifen, tetracyclines, tretinoin, vitamin A
Pregnancy category: X
Important contra-indications noted in the prescribing guidelines for: nursing mothers; pediatric patients
Note: Retinoids can cause birth defects, and women should avoid bexarotene when pregnant or trying to conceive.
Black Box Warning: AVOID IN PREGNANCY

Skin
Acneform eruption (<10%)
Bacterial infection (<13%)
Dermatitis [2]
Erythema [2]
Exanthems (<10%)
Exfoliative dermatitis (10–28%)
Necrosis [2]
Nodular eruption (<10%)
Peripheral edema (13%)
Pruritus (20–30%) [5]
Rash (17%) [2]
Ulcerations (<10%)
Vesiculobullous eruption (<10%)
Xerosis (11%) [2]

Hair
Alopecia (4–11%)

Mucosal
Cheilitis (<10%)
Gingivitis (<10%)
Xerostomia (<10%)

Central Nervous System
Chills (10%)
Hyperesthesia (<10%)

Neuromuscular/Skeletal
Arthralgia [2]
Asthenia (fatigue) [2]
Myalgia/Myopathy (<10%) [2]

Respiratory
Flu-like syndrome (4–13%)

Endocrine/Metabolic
Hypercholesterolemia [4]
Hyperlipidemia [4]
Hypertriglyceridemia [5]
Hypothyroidism [6]
Mastodynia (<10%)

Hematologic
Anemia [4]
Leukopenia [4]
Lymphopenia [2]
Neutropenia [6]

Other
Adverse effects [2]

BEZLOTOXUMAB *

Trade name: Zinplava (Merck)
Indications: To reduce the recurrence of *Clostridium difficile* infection (CDI) in patients who are receiving antibacterial treatment of CDI and are at high risk for CDI recurrence
Class: C. difficile toxin inhibitor, Monoclonal antibody
Half-life: ~19 days
Clinically important, potentially hazardous interactions with: none known
Pregnancy category: N/A (No data available)
Important contra-indications noted in the prescribing guidelines for: nursing mothers; pediatric patients

---

Cardiovascular
Cardiac failure (2%)

Central Nervous System
Fever (5%)
Headache (4%)

Gastrointestinal/Hepatic
Nausea (7%)

Local
Infusion-related reactions (10%)

BICALUTAMIDE

Trade name: Casodex (AstraZeneca)
Indications: Metastatic prostatic carcinoma
Class: Androgen antagonist
Half-life: up to 10 days
Clinically important, potentially hazardous interactions with: CYP3A4 substrates
Pregnancy category: X (not indicated for use in women)
Important contra-indications noted in the prescribing guidelines for: pediatric patients

---

Skin
Diaphoresis (6%)
Edema (2–5%)
Hot flashes (49%) [9]
Peripheral edema (8%)
Pruritus (2–5%)
Rash (6%)
Xerosis (2–5%)

Hair
Alopecia (2–5%)

Mucosal
Xerostomia (2–5%)

Central Nervous System
Paresthesias (6%)

Neuromuscular/Skeletal
Asthenia (fatigue) [4]
Myalgia/Myopathy (2–5%)

Gastrointestinal/Hepatic
Constipation [2]
Hepatotoxicity [4]

Endocrine/Metabolic
Gynecomastia (38%) [34]
Mastodynia (39%) [16]

Local
Injection-site reactions (2–5%)

BIMATOPROST

Trade names: Latisse (Allergan), Lumigan (Allergan)
Indications: Reduction of elevated intraocular pressure in open-angle glaucoma or ocular hypertension, hypotrichosis of the eyelashes
Class: Prostaglandin analog
Half-life: 45 minutes
Clinically important, potentially hazardous interactions with: none known
Pregnancy category: C
Important contra-indications noted in the prescribing guidelines for: nursing mothers; pediatric patients

---

Skin
Pigmentation [2]

Hair
Hirsutism (<5%)
Hypertrichosis [2]

Central Nervous System
Headache (<5%)

Neuromuscular/Skeletal
Asthenia (fatigue) (<5%)

Respiratory
Nasopharyngitis [2]
Upper respiratory tract infection (10%)

Ocular
Asthenopia (<10%)
Blepharitis (<10%)
Cataract (<10%)
Conjunctival edema (<10%)
Conjunctival hemorrhage (<10%)
Conjunctival hyperemia (25–45%) [42]
Conjunctivitis (<10%)
Deepening of upper lid sulcus [9]
Eyelashes – hypertrichosis (>10%) [13]
Eyelashes – pigmentation (<10%) [3]
Eyelid erythema (3–10%) [2]
Eyelid irritation (3–10%)
Eyelid pain (3–10%)
Eyelid pigmentation (3–10%) [6]
Eyelid xerosis (3–10%)
Eyes – adverse effects [2]
Foreign body sensation (<10%)
Iris pigmentation (<10%) [4]
Keratitis [2]
Lacrimation (<10%)
Macular edema [2]
Ocular adverse effects [10]
Ocular burning (<10%)
Ocular discharge (<10%)
Ocular hyperemia [4]
Ocular itching (<10%)
Ocular pain [2]
Ocular pigmentation (<3%) [5]
Ocular pruritus (>10%) [5]
Periorbital pigmentation (<10%) [3]
Photophobia (<10%)
Punctate keratitis (<10%) [2]
Uveitis [3]

BISMUTH

Trade names: Helidac (Prometheus), Pepto-Bismol (Procter & Gamble)
Indications: As part of 'triple therapy' (antibiotics + bismuth) for eradication of *H. pylori*. Bismuth subgallate initiates clotting via activation of factor XII, and is used for bleeding during tonsillectomy and adenoidectomy. BIPP impregnated ribbon gauze is used for packing following ear surgery. Bismuth subsalicylate is in OTC products for gastrointestinal complaints and peptic ulcer disease
Class: Disinfectant, Heavy metal
Half-life: 21–72 days
Clinically important, potentially hazardous interactions with: aspirin, ciprofloxacin, demeclocycline, doxycycline, hypoglycemics, lomefloxacin, lymecycline, methotrexate, minocycline, tetracycline, warfarin
Pregnancy category: D (category C in first and second trimesters; category D in third trimester)

Skin
Dermatitis [2]
Hypersensitivity [2]
Pigmentation [5]
Pruritus (triple therapy) [2]
Rash [4]

Mucosal
Oral pigmentation [3]
Stomatitis [4]
Tongue pigmentation (>10%) [3]
Xerostomia (triple therapy) (41%)

Central Nervous System
Dysgeusia (taste perversion) (triple therapy) (46%) [9]
Encephalopathy [4]
Pain (triple therapy) (10%)
Tremor [2]
Vertigo (dizziness) [2]

Neuromuscular/Skeletal
Arthralgia [10]
Asthenia (fatigue) [2]

Gastrointestinal/Hepatic
Diarrhea [4]
Nausea [4]
Vomiting [2]

Other
Adverse effects (triple therapy) [50]
Allergic reactions [2]
Death [10]

BISOPROLOL

Trade names: Cardicor (Merck Serono), Concor (Merck Serono), Emcor (Merck Serono), Zebeta (Barr), Ziac (Barr)
Indications: Hypertension
Class: Beta adrenergic blocker, Beta blocker
Half-life: 9–12 hours
Clinically important, potentially hazardous interactions with: diltiazem, disopyramide, guanethidine, reserpine, rifampin, verapamil
Pregnancy category: C
Important contra-indications noted in the prescribing guidelines for: nursing mothers; pediatric patients
Note: Ziac is bisoprolol and hydrochlorothiazide. Hydrochlorothiazide is a sulfonamide and can be absorbed systemically. Sulfonamides can produce severe, possibly fatal, reactions such as toxic epidermal necrolysis and Stevens-Johnson syndrome.
Contraindicated in patients with cardiogenic shock, overt cardiac failure, second or third degree AV block, and marked sinus bradycardia.

Skin
Edema (3%)
Peripheral edema (<10%)
Rash (<10%)
Raynaud's phenomenon (<10%)

Cardiovascular
Bradycardia [6]
Hypotension [3]

Central Nervous System
Headache [2]
Hyperesthesia (2%)
Vertigo (dizziness) [3]

Neuromuscular/Skeletal
Myalgia/Myopathy (<10%)

Other
Adverse effects [4]

BIVALIRUDIN

Trade name: Angiomax (The Medicines Company)
Indications: Angioplasty adjunct
Class: Thrombin inhibitor
Half-life: 25 minutes
Clinically important, potentially hazardous interactions with: anisindione, dicumarol, heparin, reteplase, streptokinase, tenecteplase, urokinase, warfarin
Pregnancy category: B

Central Nervous System
Pain (15%)

Neuromuscular/Skeletal
Back pain (42%)

Hematologic
Bleeding [5]
Thrombosis [3]

Local
Injection-site pain (8%)

BLEOMYCIN

Synonyms: bleo; BLM
Trade name: Blenoxane (Mead Johnson)
Indications: Melanomas, sarcomas, lymphomas, testicular carcinoma
Class: Antibiotic, anthracycline
Half-life: 1.3–9 hours
Clinically important, potentially hazardous interactions with: aldesleukin, brentuximab vedotin
Pregnancy category: D
Important contra-indications noted in the prescribing guidelines for: nursing mothers; pediatric patients

Skin
Acral erythema [2]
Acral necrosis [2]
Bullous dermatitis (<5%)
Calcification [2]
Erythema [6]
Exanthems [3]
Flagellate dermatitis [7]
Flagellate erythema/pigmentation [42]
Gangrene (digital) [3]
Hyperkeratosis (palms and soles) [2]
Hypersensitivity (<10%) [4]
Linear streaking [4]
Lipodystrophy [2]
Neutrophilic eccrine hidradenitis [2]
Pigmentation (~50%) [20]
Pruritus (>5%) [7]
Raynaud's phenomenon (>10%) [34]
Scleroderma [16]
Stevens-Johnson syndrome [2]

Hair
Alopecia (~50%) [7]

Nails
Nail growth reduced [2]

Nail loss [3]
Onychodystrophy [2]
Onycholysis [3]

Mucosal
Oral ulceration [2]
Stomatitis (>10%) [8]

Central Nervous System
Chills (>10%)

Neuromuscular/Skeletal
Digital necrosis [3]

Respiratory
Pneumonitis [3]
Pulmonary fibrosis [2]
Pulmonary toxicity [6]

Endocrine/Metabolic
SIADH [2]

Hematologic
Hemolytic uremic syndrome [8]

Local
Injection-site phlebitis (<10%)

Other
Adverse effects [2]
Allergic reactions [2]

BLINATUMOMAB

Trade name: Blincyto (Amgen)
Indications: Precursor B-cell acute lymphoblastic leukemia
Class: Bispecific CD19-directed CD3 T-cell engager, Monoclonal antibody
Half-life: 1.4 hours
Clinically important, potentially hazardous interactions with: none known
Pregnancy category: C
Important contra-indications noted in the prescribing guidelines for: nursing mothers
Black Box Warning: CYTOKINE RELEASE SYNDROME and NEUROLOGICAL TOXICITIES

Skin
Edema (5%) [3]
Peripheral edema (25%) [2]
Rash (21%)
Tumor lysis syndrome (4%)

Cardiovascular
Chest pain (11%)
Hypertension (8%)
Hypotension (11%)
Tachycardia (8%)

Central Nervous System
Aphasia (4%) [3]
Chills (15%)
Confusion (7%) [3]
Cytokine release syndrome (11%) [9]
Disorientation (3%) [2]
Encephalopathy (5%) [5]
Fever (62%) [7]
Headache (36%) [5]
Insomnia (15%)
Memory loss (2%)
Neurotoxicity [6]
Paresthesias (5%)
Seizures (2%) [6]
Somnolence (drowsiness) [2]
Speech disorder [2]
Tremor (20%) [6]
Vertigo (dizziness) (14%)

Neuromuscular/Skeletal
Arthralgia (10%)
Asthenia (fatigue) (17%) [3]
Back pain (14%)
Bone or joint pain (11%)
Pain in extremities (12%)

Gastrointestinal/Hepatic
Abdominal pain (15%)
Constipation (20%)
Diarrhea (20%) [2]
Nausea (25%) [3]
Vomiting (13%)

Respiratory
Cough (19%)
Dyspnea (15%)
Pneumonia (9%) [3]

Endocrine/Metabolic
ALT increased (12%) [2]
Appetite decreased (10%)
AST increased (11%)
GGT increased (6%) [2]
Hyperbilirubinemia (8%)
Hyperglycemia (11%)
Hypoalbuminemia (4%)
Hypokalemia (23%) [4]
Hypomagnesemia (12%)
Hypophosphatemia (6%)
Weight gain (11%)

Hematologic
Anemia (18%) [4]
Febrile neutropenia (25%) [6]
Leukocytosis (2%)
Leukopenia (9%) [4]
Lymphopenia [2]
Neutropenia (16%) [3]
Sepsis (7%) [2]
Thrombocytopenia (11%) [5]

Local
Catheter-related infection [2]

BOCEPREVIR

Trade name: Victrelis (Merck)
Indications: Chronic hepatitis C
Class: CYP3A4 inhibitor, Hepatitis C virus NS3/4A protease inhibitor
Half-life: 3.4 hours
Clinically important, potentially hazardous interactions with: alfuzosin, alprazolam, amiodarone, atorvastatin, bepridil, bosentan, budesonide, buprenorphine, cabozantinib, carbamazepine, cisapride, clarithromycin, colchicine, cyclosporine, dasatinib, desipramine, dexamethasone, digoxin, dihydroergotamine, drospirenone, efavirenz, ergonovine, ergotamine, estradiol, felodipine, flecainide, flibanserin, fluticasone propionate, gefitinib, itraconazole, ketoconazole, lomitapide, lovastatin, methadone, methylergonovine, midazolam, mifepristone, nicardipine, nifedipine, pazopanib, phenobarbital, phenytoin, pimozide, ponatinib, posaconazole, propafenone, quinidine, rifabutin, rifampin, ritonavir, ruxolitinib, salmeterol, sildenafil, simvastatin, sirolimus, St John's wort, tacrolimus, tadalafil, trazodone, triazolam, vardenafil, voriconazole, warfarin
Pregnancy category: X (boceprevir is pregnancy category B but must not be used in monotherapy)
Important contra-indications noted in the prescribing guidelines for: nursing mothers; pediatric patients
Note: Must be used in combination with PEG-interferon and ribavirin (see separate entries) Combination treatment is contraindicated in pregnant women and men whose female partners are pregnant because of the risks for birth defects and fetal death associated with ribavirin, or in coadministration with drugs that are highly dependent on CYP3A4/5 for clearance, or with potent CYP3A4/5 inducers.

Skin
Pruritus [3]
Rash [2]

Central Nervous System
Dysgeusia (taste perversion) [6]

Gastrointestinal/Hepatic
Hepatotoxicity [2]

Hematologic
Anemia [22]
Neutropenia [7]
Thrombocytopenia [7]

Other
Adverse effects [6]
Infection [2]

BORTEZOMIB

Trade name: Velcade (Millennium)
Indications: Multiple myeloma, mantle cell lymphoma
Class: Biologic, Proteasome inhibitor
Half-life: 9–15 hours
Clinically important, potentially hazardous interactions with: conivaptan, darunavir, delavirdine, efavirenz, indinavir, strong CYP3A4 inhibitors or inducers, telithromycin, thalidomide, voriconazole
Pregnancy category: D
Important contra-indications noted in the prescribing guidelines for: nursing mothers; pediatric patients
Note: Contraindicated in patients with hypersensitivity to boron or mannitol.

Skin
Edema (23%)
Erythema [2]
Folliculitis [2]
Herpes zoster (12%) [12]
Peripheral edema [5]
Pruritus (11%)
Purpura [2]
Rash (18%) [9]
Sweet's syndrome [7]
Toxicity [3]
Tumor lysis syndrome [2]
Vasculitis [4]

Mucosal
Mucositis [2]

Cardiovascular
Arrhythmias [2]
Cardiac failure [3]
Cardiotoxicity [3]
Hypertension [3]
Hypotension (13%) [3]

Central Nervous System
Anxiety (10%)
Dysesthesia (23%)
Dysgeusia (taste perversion) (13%)
Encephalopathy [3]
Fever (34%) [7]
Guillain–Barré syndrome [2]
Headache [3]
Insomnia (20%) [2]
Neurotoxicity [24]
Paresthesias (22%) [2]
Peripheral neuropathy (39%) [48]
Vertigo (dizziness) (17%)

Neuromuscular/Skeletal
Arthralgia (17%) [2]
Asthenia (fatigue) (64%) [33]
Back pain (13%)
Bone or joint pain (14%) [2]
Cramps (11%)
Myalgia/Myopathy (12%)

Gastrointestinal/Hepatic
Abdominal distension [2]
Abdominal pain [3]
Colitis [2]
Constipation (41%) [6]
Diarrhea (52%) [19]
Gastrointestinal disorder [2]
Hepatotoxicity [4]
Nausea (55%) [8]
Pancreatitis [2]
Vomiting (33%) [3]

Respiratory
Cough (20%) [2]
Dyspnea (21%) [6]
Nasopharyngitis (12%)
Pneumonia (12%) [7]
Pneumonitis [4]
Pulmonary toxicity [3]
Upper respiratory tract infection (12%) [3]

Endocrine/Metabolic
Appetite decreased (36%)
Dehydration (10%)
Hypocalcemia [2]
Hypokalemia [3]
Serum creatinine increased [2]
Weight loss [2]

Hematologic
Anemia (29%) [13]
Febrile neutropenia [4]
Hemotoxicity [5]
Leukopenia [6]
Lymphopenia [11]
Myelosuppression [2]
Neutropenia (17%) [30]
Sepsis [4]
Thrombocytopenia (36%) [42]

Local
Infusion-related reactions [2]
Injection-site irritation (5%)
Injection-site reactions [4]

Other
Adverse effects [12]
Death [6]
Infection [11]

BOSENTAN

Trade name: Tracleer (Actelion)
Indications: Pulmonary arterial hypertension
Class: Antihypertensive, Endothelin receptor (ETR) antagonist, Vasodilator
Half-life: ~5 hours
Clinically important, potentially hazardous interactions with: amiodarone, amprenavir, astemizole, atazanavir, atorvastatin, boceprevir, cobicistat/elvitegravir/emtricitabine/tenofovir disoproxil, cyclosporine, diltiazem, enzalutamide, erythromycin, fluconazole, fluvastatin, glibenclamide, glyburide, indinavir, itraconazole, ketoconazole, levonorgestrel, lopinavir, lovastatin, oral contraceptives, progestogens, reboxetine, rifampin, ritonavir, sildenafil, simvastatin, St John's wort, tacrolimus, tadalafil, telaprevir, tipranavir, ulipristal, vardenafil, voriconazole, warfarin
Pregnancy category: X
Important contra-indications noted in the prescribing guidelines for: nursing mothers; pediatric patients
Black Box Warning: RISKS OF HEPATOTOXICITY and TERATOGENICITY

Skin
Edema (8%) [2]
Peripheral edema (8%) [4]
Pruritus (4%)

Cardiovascular
Flushing (9%) [2]

Central Nervous System
Headache [2]
Syncope [2]

Gastrointestinal/Hepatic
Hepatotoxicity [16]

Respiratory
Bronchitis [2]

Endocrine/Metabolic
AST increased [2]

Hematologic
Anemia [3]

Other
Adverse effects [7]

BOTULINUM TOXIN (A & B)

Trade names: Azzalure (Galderma), Bocouture (Merz), Botox (Allergan), Dysport (Ipsen), Myobloc (Solstice), Neurobloc (Eisai), Vistabel (Allergan), Xeomin (Merz)
Indications: Blepharospasm, hemifacial spasm, spasmodic torticollis, sialorrhea, hyperhidrosis, strabismus, oromandibular dystonia, cervical dystonia, spasmodic dysphonia, chronic migraine, urinary incontinence in people with neurologic conditions such as spinal cord injury and multiple sclerosis who have overactivity of the bladder, cosmetic application for wrinkles
Class: Acetylcholine inhibitor, Neuromuscular blocker, Ophthalmic agent, toxin
Half-life: 3–6 months
Clinically important, potentially hazardous interactions with: aminoglycosides, anticholinergics, fesoterodine, tiotropium, trospium
Pregnancy category: C
Important contra-indications noted in the prescribing guidelines for: nursing mothers; pediatric patients
Note: Distant spread of toxin effect - postmarketing reports indicate that all botulinum toxin products may spread from the area of injection to produce symptoms consistent with botulinum toxin effects. These may include asthenia, generalized muscle weakness, diplopia, ptosis, dysphagia, dysphonia, dysarthria, urinary incontinence and breathing diffculties. These symptoms have been reported hours to weeks after injection.
An antitoxin is available in the event of overdose or misinjection.
Black Box Warning: DISTANT SPREAD OF TOXIN EFFECT

Skin
Anaphylactoid reactions/Anaphylaxis [3]
Ecchymoses [4]
Erythema [2]
Granulomas [2]
Hematoma [2]
Peripheral edema (<10%)
Pruritus (<10%)
Purpura (<10%)

Mucosal
Epistaxis (nosebleed) [2]
Stomatitis (<10%)
Xerostomia (3–34%) [11]

Central Nervous System
Dysgeusia (taste perversion) (<10%)
Headache [7]
Hyperesthesia (<10%)
Neurotoxicity [2]
Pain (6–13%) [4]
Seizures [2]
Tremor (<10%)
Vertigo (dizziness) [2]

Neuromuscular/Skeletal
Arthralgia (<7%)
Asthenia (fatigue) [15]
Myasthenia gravis [2]

Gastrointestinal/Hepatic
Constipation [2]
Dysphagia [14]

Respiratory
Dysphonia [2]
Dyspnea [2]
Flu-like syndrome (2–10%) [7]
Pulmonary toxicity [3]

Genitourinary
Hematuria [3]
Urinary incontinence [3]
Urinary retention [10]
Urinary tract infection [13]
Vulvovaginal candidiasis (<10%)

Otic
Tinnitus (<10%)

Ocular
Blepharoptosis [2]
Diplopia [10]
Eyelid edema [4]
Ocular adverse effects [2]
Ptosis (14–20%) [23]
Xerophthalmia (6%) [2]

Local
Injection-site bruising [4]
Injection-site ecchymoses [2]
Injection-site edema [7]
Injection-site erythema [3]
Injection-site pain (2–10%) [19]
Injection-site paralysis [2]
Injection-site reactions [6]

Other
Adverse effects [18]
Death [4]
Infection (13–19%)
Side effects [3]

BRENTUXIMAB VEDOTIN

Trade name: Adcetris (Seattle Genetics)
Indications: Hodgkin's lymphoma, systemic anaplastic large cell lymphoma
Class: Antibody drug conjugate (ADC), CD30-directed antibody-drug conjugate, Monoclonal antibody
Half-life: 4–6 days
Clinically important, potentially hazardous interactions with: bleomycin, efavirenz, ketoconazole, rifampin, strong CYP3A4 inhibitors
Pregnancy category: D
Important contra-indications noted in the prescribing guidelines for: the elderly; nursing mothers; pediatric patients
Black Box Warning: PROGRESSIVE MULTIFOCAL LEUKOENCEPHALOPATHY

Skin
Diaphoresis (12%)
Lymphadenopathy (11%)
Peripheral edema (4–16%)
Pruritus (19%)
Rash (31%)
Xerosis (10%)

Hair
Alopecia (14%)

Central Nervous System
Anxiety (11%)
Chills (13%)
Fever (29–38%) [3]
Headache (19%)
Insomnia (16%)
Neurotoxicity [2]
Pain (7–28%)
Peripheral neuropathy (68%) [7]
Vertigo (dizziness) (11–16%)

Neuromuscular/Skeletal
Arthralgia (9–19%)
Asthenia (fatigue) (41–49%) [4]
Back pain (14%)
Muscle spasm (10%)
Myalgia/Myopathy (17%)
Pain in extremities (10%)

Gastrointestinal/Hepatic
Abdominal pain (9–25%)
Constipation (19%)
Diarrhea (36%) [3]
Nausea (42%) [4]
Vomiting (22%)

Respiratory
Cough (17–25%)
Dyspnea (13–19%)
Pulmonary toxicity [2]
Upper respiratory tract infection (12–47%)

Endocrine/Metabolic
Appetite decreased (16%)
Weight loss (6–12%)

Hematologic
Anemia (33–52%)
Neutropenia (55%) [5]
Thrombocytopenia (16–28%)

BREXPIPRAZOLE

Trade name: Rexulti (Otsuka)
Indications: Schizophrenia, major depressive disorder (with antidepressants)
Class: Antipsychotic
Half-life: 86–91 hours
Clinically important, potentially hazardous interactions with: strong or moderate CYP2D6 inhibitors, strong or moderate CYP3A4 inducers or inhibitors
Pregnancy category: N/A (Neonatal risk in third trimester exposure)
Important contra-indications noted in the prescribing guidelines for: the elderly; nursing mothers; pediatric patients
Black Box Warning: INCREASED MORTALITY IN ELDERLY PATIENTS WITH DEMENTIA-RELATED PSYCHOSIS
SUICIDAL THOUGHTS AND BEHAVIORS

Central Nervous System
Agitation [2]
Akathisia (6–9%) [10]
Anxiety (3%)
Headache (7%) [5]
Insomnia [3]
Restlessness (3%)
Sedation (2%)
Somnolence (drowsiness) (5%) [3]
Tremor (3–4%)
Vertigo (dizziness) (3%)

Neuromuscular/Skeletal
Asthenia (fatigue) (3%)

Gastrointestinal/Hepatic
Constipation (2%)
Diarrhea (3%)
Dyspepsia (3%)
Nausea [3]

Respiratory
Nasopharyngitis (4%)

Endocrine/Metabolic
Appetite increased (3%)
Creatine phosphokinase increased (2%)
Weight gain (4–7%) [11]
Weight loss (10%)

Hematologic
Hemotoxicity (2%)

BRIMONIDINE

Trade names: Alphagan P (Allergan), Mirvaso (Galderma)
Indications: Open-angle glaucoma, ocular hypertension, topical application for rosacea
Class: Adrenergic alpha2-receptor agonist
Half-life: 12 hours
Clinically important, potentially hazardous interactions with: amitriptyline, MAO inhibitors, tricyclic antidepressants
Pregnancy category: B
Important contra-indications noted in the prescribing guidelines for: nursing mothers; pediatric patients
Note: [T] = Topical.

Skin
Burning ([T]) (2%) [3]
Erythema ([T]) (4%) [6]
Hypersensitivity [3]
Irritation [2]
Pruritus [3]
Xerosis [2]

Mucosal
Xerostomia (5–20%) [11]

Cardiovascular
Flushing ([T]) (3%) [2]
Hypertension (5–20%)

Central Nervous System
Dysgeusia (taste perversion) (<10%) [4]

Neuromuscular/Skeletal
Asthenia (fatigue) [3]

Respiratory
Upper respiratory tract infection (<10%)

Ocular
Blepharitis (<10%) [2]
Conjunctival hyperemia (5–20%) [4]
Conjunctivitis (5–20%) [7]
Eyelid crusting (<10%)
Eyelid edema (<10%)
Eyelid erythema (<10%)
Intraocular pressure increased [2]
Ocular adverse effects [4]
Ocular allergy (4%) [8]
Ocular burning (<10%) [7]
Ocular hyperemia [4]

Ocular itching [2]
Ocular pain [3]
Ocular pruritus (5–20%) [4]
Ocular stinging (<10%) [6]
Periocular dermatitis [2]
Uveitis [10]
Vision blurred ([T]) [3]
Visual disturbances (5–20%)
Xerophthalmia [3]

Other
Adverse effects [2]
Allergic reactions [2]

BRINZOLAMIDE

Trade name: Azopt (Alcon)
Indications: Open-angle glaucoma, ocular hypertension
Class: Carbonic anhydrase inhibitor, Diuretic
Half-life: 111 days
Clinically important, potentially hazardous interactions with: conivaptan, darunavir, delavirdine, indinavir, salicylates, telithromycin, voriconazole
Pregnancy category: C
Important contra-indications noted in the prescribing guidelines for: nursing mothers
Note: Brinzolamide is a sulfonamide and can be absorbed systemically. Sulfonamides can produce severe, possibly fatal, reactions such as toxic epidermal necrolysis and Stevens-Johnson syndrome.

Skin
Dermatitis (<5%)

Mucosal
Xerostomia [4]

Central Nervous System
Dysgeusia (taste perversion) (5–10%) [13]
Headache (<5%)

Neuromuscular/Skeletal
Asthenia (fatigue) [3]

Respiratory
Rhinitis (<5%)

Ocular
Blepharitis (<5%)
Conjunctival hyperemia [7]
Conjunctivitis [3]
Corneal abnormalities [2]
Foreign body sensation (<5%)
Lacrimation [2]
Ocular adverse effects [3]
Ocular allergy [2]
Ocular burning [4]
Ocular discharge (<5%)
Ocular hyperemia [5]
Ocular itching [6]
Ocular keratitis (<5%)
Ocular pain (<5%) [5]
Ocular pruritus (<5%) [3]
Ocular stinging [4]
Vision blurred (5–10%) [14]
Xerophthalmia (<5%) [4]

Other
Adverse effects [2]

BRIVARACETAM *

Trade name: Briviact (UCB)
Indications: Epilepsy adjunct therapy
Class: Anticonvulsant, Antiepileptic
Half-life: 9 hours
Clinically important, potentially hazardous interactions with: carbamazepine, phenytoin, rifampin
Pregnancy category: C
Important contra-indications noted in the prescribing guidelines for: the elderly; nursing mothers; pediatric patients

---

Central Nervous System
Balance disorder (3%)
Dysgeusia (taste perversion) (<3%)
Euphoria (<3%)
Headache [9]
Impaired concentration [2]
Insomnia [2]
Irritability (3%) [6]
Neurotoxicity (13%)
Sedation (16%)
Seizures [3]
Somnolence (drowsiness) (16%) [17]
Vertigo (dizziness) (12%) [16]

Neuromuscular/Skeletal
Asthenia (fatigue) (9%) [13]
Back pain [2]

Gastrointestinal/Hepatic
Constipation (2%)
Nausea (5%) [4]
Vomiting (5%) [2]

Respiratory
Nasopharyngitis [5]

Genitourinary
Urinary tract infection [2]

Hematologic
Leukopenia (2%)

Local
Infusion-site pain (<3%)

BROMOCRIPTINE

Trade name: Parlodel (Novartis)
Indications: Amenorrhea, Parkinsonism, infertility, acromegaly
Class: Dopamine receptor agonist
Half-life: initial: 6–8 hours; terminal: 50 hours
Clinically important, potentially hazardous interactions with: alcohol, antipsychotics, azithromycin, domperidone, erythromycin, isometheptene, lanreotide, levomepromazine, macrolides, memantine, methyldopa, metoclopramide, octreotide, pasireotide, pseudoephedrine, risperidone, sympathomimetics, zuclopenthixol
Pregnancy category: B
Important contra-indications noted in the prescribing guidelines for: nursing mothers; pediatric patients
Note: Contraindicated in women who become pregnant or in the postpartum period.

Skin
Livedo reticularis [3]
Raynaud's phenomenon (<10%) [8]
Scleroderma [2]

Hair
Alopecia [2]

Mucosal
Nasal congestion (3–4%)
Xerostomia (4–10%) [3]

Cardiovascular
Cardiotoxicity [2]
Coronary spasm [2]
Erythromelalgia [4]
Flushing [2]
Orthostatic hypotension (6%)
Postural hypotension (6%)

Central Nervous System
Anorexia (4%)
Hallucinations [4]
Headache (<19%) [3]
Seizures (in postpartum patients) [3]
Somnolence (drowsiness) (3%)
Syncope (<2%)
Vertigo (dizziness) (17%)

Neuromuscular/Skeletal
Asthenia (fatigue) (3–7%)

Gastrointestinal/Hepatic
Abdominal pain (4%)
Constipation (3–14%)
Diarrhea (3%)
Dyspepsia (4%)
Gastrointestinal bleeding (<2%)
Nausea (18–49%) [7]
Vomiting (2–5%) [4]

Respiratory
Pleural effusion [2]

Other
Adverse effects [2]

BUDESONIDE

Trade names: Pulmicort Turbuhaler (AstraZeneca), Rhinocort (AstraZeneca), Symbicort (AstraZeneca)
Indications: Asthma, rhinitis
Class: Corticosteroid, inhaled
Half-life: N/A
Clinically important, potentially hazardous interactions with: boceprevir, efavirenz, itraconazole, ketoconazole, live vaccines, oral contraceptives, telaprevir
Pregnancy category: C
Important contra-indications noted in the prescribing guidelines for: nursing mothers; pediatric patients
Note: Symbicort is budesonide and formoterol.

Skin
Acneform eruption [2]
Dermatitis [8]
Rash [2]

Respiratory
Asthma (exacerbation) [3]
Cough [2]

Endocrine/Metabolic
Adrenal insufficiency [2]

Ocular
- Cataract [2]

Other
- Adverse effects [11]
- Allergic reactions [3]
- Infection [2]
- Systemic reactions [2]

BUPRENORPHINE

Trade names: Probuphine (Braeburn), Suboxone (Reckitt Benckiser), Subutex (Reckitt Benckiser), Transtec (Napp)
Indications: Opioid dependence, moderate to severe pain
Class: Analgesic, Mixed opioid agonist/antagonist, Narcotic
Half-life: 37 hours
Clinically important, potentially hazardous interactions with: antihistamines, atazanavir, azole antifungals, benzodiazepines, boceprevir, carbamazepine, cimetidine, cobicistat/elvitegravir/emtricitabine/tenofovir disoproxil, delavirdine, diazepam, efavirenz, erythromycin, HIV protease inhibitors, hydrocodone, hydromorphone, ketoconazole, ketorolac, linezolid, macrolide antibiotics, morphine, neuroleptics, oxymorphone, phenobarbital, phenytoin, rifampin, ritonavir, tapentadol, tipranavir
Pregnancy category: C
Important contra-indications noted in the prescribing guidelines for: nursing mothers; pediatric patients
Note: Suboxone contains naloxone; Probuphine is an implant for subdermal administration.
Black Box Warning: ABUSE POTENTIAL, LIFE-THREATENING RESPIRATORY DEPRESSION, and ACCIDENTAL EXPOSURE Probuphine: IMPLANT MIGRATION, PROTRUSION, EXPULSION, and NERVE DAMAGE ASSOCIATED WITH INSERTION and REMOVAL

Skin
- Abscess (2%)
- Dermatitis [2]
- Diaphoresis (12–14%)
- Erythema [4]
- Hyperhidrosis [3]
- Pruritus [9]

Mucosal
- Xerostomia [2]

Cardiovascular
- Bradycardia [3]
- Hypotension [4]
- Pulmonary edema [2]
- QT prolongation [2]
- Vasodilation (9%)

Central Nervous System
- Anxiety (12%)
- Chills (6–8%)
- Depression (11%)
- Fever (3%)
- Headache (30–36%) [2]
- Insomnia (14–25%)
- Nervousness (6%)
- Neurotoxicity [2]
- Pain (22–24%)
- Seizures [3]
- Somnolence (drowsiness) (5%) [2]
- Vertigo (dizziness) (4%) [12]

Neuromuscular/Skeletal
- Asthenia (fatigue) (7–14%) [3]
- Back pain (4–14%)
- Myalgia/Myopathy [2]

Gastrointestinal/Hepatic
- Abdominal pain (11%) [2]
- Constipation (11–12%) [7]
- Diarrhea (4–5%)
- Dyspepsia (3%)
- Hepatotoxicity [6]
- Nausea (10–15%) [11]
- Vomiting (5–8%) [9]

Respiratory
- Cough (4%)
- Flu-like syndrome (6%)
- Pharyngitis (4%)
- Respiratory depression [2]
- Rhinitis (5–11%)

Ocular
- Lacrimation (5%)

Local
- Application-site reactions [2]

Other
- Adverse effects [4]
- Death [9]
- Infection (6–20%)

BUPROPION

Trade names: Wellbutrin (GSK), Zyban (GSK)
Indications: Depression, aid to smoking cessation
Class: Antidepressant, Dopamine reuptake inhibitor
Half-life: 14 hours
Clinically important, potentially hazardous interactions with: amitriptyline, citalopram, cobicistat/elvitegravir/emtricitabine/tenofovir disoproxil, cyclosporine, efavirenz, erythromycin, escitalopram, isocarboxazid, levodopa, linezolid, lopinavir, lorcaserin, methylphenidate, mifepristone, phenelzine, ritonavir, tranylcypromine, trimipramine, vortioxetine
Pregnancy category: C
Important contra-indications noted in the prescribing guidelines for: nursing mothers; pediatric patients
Black Box Warning: NEUROPSYCHIATRIC REACTIONS; AND SUICIDAL THOUGHTS AND BEHAVIORS

Skin
- Acneform eruption (<10%)
- AGEP [2]
- Anaphylactoid reactions/Anaphylaxis [2]
- Angioedema [3]
- Diaphoresis (5%) [4]
- Erythema multiforme [4]
- Exanthems [2]
- Hypersensitivity [6]
- Lupus erythematosus [2]
- Peripheral edema [2]
- Pruritus (4%) [3]
- Psoriasis [2]
- Rash (4%) [3]
- Serum sickness [11]
- Stevens–Johnson syndrome [2]
- Thrombocytopenic purpura [2]
- Urticaria [9]
- Xerosis (<10%)

Hair
- Hirsutism (<10%)

Mucosal
- Tongue edema [2]
- Xerostomia (<64%) [17]

Cardiovascular
- Arrhythmias [2]
- Flushing (4%)
- Hypertension [2]
- Myocardial ischemia [2]
- Tachycardia [3]

Central Nervous System
- Agitation [4]
- Anxiety [3]
- Delirium [2]
- Depression [3]
- Dysgeusia (taste perversion) (4%)
- Hallucinations [6]
- Headache [4]
- Insomnia [6]
- Nightmares [2]
- Paresthesias (2%)
- Parkinsonism [2]
- Psychosis [6]
- Seizures [40]
- Serotonin syndrome [2]
- Sleep related disorder [2]
- Somnolence (drowsiness) [4]
- Suicidal ideation [5]
- Tremor (>10%) [6]
- Twitching (2%)
- Vertigo (dizziness) [4]

Neuromuscular/Skeletal
- Arthralgia [3]
- Asthenia (fatigue) [3]
- Dystonia [2]
- Myalgia/Myopathy (6%) [2]
- Rhabdomyolysis [3]

Gastrointestinal/Hepatic
- Constipation [3]
- Hepatotoxicity [2]
- Nausea [12]
- Vomiting [5]

Respiratory
- Upper respiratory tract infection [2]

Genitourinary
- Priapism [2]

Ocular
- Hallucinations, visual [3]

Other
- Adverse effects [2]
- Congenital malformations [2]
- Death [5]

BUSPIRONE

Trade name: BuSpar (Bristol-Myers Squibb)
Indications: Anxiety
Class: Anxiolytic, Serotonin antagonist
Half-life: 2–3 hours
Clinically important, potentially hazardous interactions with: citalopram, cobicistat/elvitegravir/emtricitabine/tenofovir disoproxil, grapefruit juice, itraconazole, linezolid, nefazodone, paclitaxel, rifapentine, ritonavir, St John's wort, telithromycin, vilazodone, voriconazole
Pregnancy category: B

Hair
Alopecia [2]

Mucosal
Xerostomia (3%)

Central Nervous System
Serotonin syndrome [4]

BUSULFAN

Trade name: Myleran (GSK)
Indications: Chronic myelogenous leukemia, bone marrow disorders
Class: Alkylating agent
Half-life: 3.4 hours (after first dose)
Clinically important, potentially hazardous interactions with: acetaminophen, aldesleukin, itraconazole, metronidazole, voriconazole
Pregnancy category: D
Black Box Warning: LEUKEMOGENESIS and PANCYTOPENIA

Skin
Erythema (macular) (>10%)
Erythema multiforme [5]
Erythema nodosum [3]
Exanthems [2]
Pigmentation ('busulfan tan') (<10%) [13]
Urticaria (>10%) [5]
Vasculitis [3]

Hair
Alopecia (>10%) [7]

Mucosal
Mucositis [3]
Oral mucositis [2]
Stomatitis [2]

Central Nervous System
Neurotoxicity [3]
Seizures [3]

Gastrointestinal/Hepatic
Hepatotoxicity [3]

Respiratory
Pulmonary toxicity [2]

Endocrine/Metabolic
Gynecomastia [3]
Porphyria cutanea tarda [2]

Hematologic
Febrile neutropenia [3]

Other
Death [2]
Infection [3]

CABERGOLINE

Trade name: Dostinex (Pfizer)
Indications: Hyperprolactinemia, Parkinsonism
Class: Dopamine receptor agonist
Half-life: 63–69 hours
Clinically important, potentially hazardous interactions with: azithromycin, levomepromazine, risperidone, zuclopenthixol
Pregnancy category: B
Important contra-indications noted in the prescribing guidelines for: the elderly; nursing mothers; pediatric patients

---

Skin
- Edema [2]
- Hot flashes (3%)

Mucosal
- Xerostomia (2%)

Cardiovascular
- Cardiac failure [2]
- Hypotension [5]
- Myocardial toxicity [3]
- Pericarditis [4]
- Valve regurgitation [2]
- Valvulopathy [9]

Central Nervous System
- Dyskinesia [2]
- Headache (26%) [6]
- Mania [2]
- Neurotoxicity [3]
- Paresthesias (5%) [2]
- Psychosis [3]
- Somnolence (drowsiness) (<5%)
- Vertigo (dizziness) (15–17%) [6]

Neuromuscular/Skeletal
- Asthenia (fatigue) (6%) [4]

Gastrointestinal/Hepatic
- Abdominal pain (5%)
- Constipation (7–10%)
- Nausea (28%) [2]

Endocrine/Metabolic
- Mastodynia (2%)

CABOZANTINIB

Trade names: Carbometyx (Exelixis), Cometriq (Exelixis)
Indications: Metastatic medullary thyroid cancer (Cometriq), advanced renal cell carcinoma (Cabometyx)
Class: Tyrosine kinase inhibitor
Half-life: 55 hours (Cometriq); 99 hours (Cabometyx)
Clinically important, potentially hazardous interactions with: atazanavir, boceprevir, carbamazepine, clarithromycin, conivaptan, grapefruit juice, indinavir, itraconazole, ketoconazole, lopinavir, nefazodone, nelfinavir, phenobarbital, phenytoin, posaconazole, rifabutin, rifampin, rifapentine, ritonavir, saquinavir, St John's wort, telithromycin, voriconazole
Pregnancy category: D
Important contra-indications noted in the prescribing guidelines for: the elderly; nursing mothers; pediatric patients
Black Box Warning: PERFORATIONS AND FISTULAS, and HEMORRHAGE

Skin
- Erythema (11%)
- Hand–foot syndrome (50%) [14]
- Hyperkeratosis (7%)
- Jaundice (25%)
- Rash (19%)
- Toxicity [2]
- Xerosis (19%)

Hair
- Alopecia (16%)
- Hair changes (34%)
- Hair pigmentation (34%) [2]

Mucosal
- Mucosal inflammation [2]
- Stomatitis (51%)

Cardiovascular
- Chest pain (9%)
- Hypertension (33%) [10]
- Hypotension (7%)

Central Nervous System
- Anorexia [2]
- Anxiety (9%)
- Dysgeusia (taste perversion) (34%)
- Headache (18%)
- Paresthesias (7%)
- Peripheral neuropathy (5%)
- Vertigo (dizziness) (14%)

Neuromuscular/Skeletal
- Arthralgia (14%)
- Asthenia (fatigue) (21–41%) [14]
- Muscle spasm (12%)
- Pain in extremities (14%)

Gastrointestinal/Hepatic
- Abdominal pain (27%)
- Constipation (27%) [2]
- Diarrhea (63%) [13]
- Dyspepsia (11%)
- Dysphagia (13%)
- Gastrointestinal perforation (3%)
- Hemorrhoids (9%)
- Nausea (43%) [7]
- Vomiting (24%) [4]

Respiratory
- Cough (18%)
- Dysphonia (20%)
- Dyspnea (19%)
- Pulmonary embolism [2]

Endocrine/Metabolic
- ALP increased (52%)
- ALT increased (86%) [2]
- Appetite decreased (46%) [4]
- AST increased (86%) [2]
- Dehydration (7%)
- GGT increased (27%)
- Hypoalbuminemia (36%)
- Hypocalcemia (52%)
- Hypokalemia (18%)
- Hypomagnesemia (19%)
- Hyponatremia (10%)
- Hypophosphatemia (28%)
- Serum creatinine increased (58%)
- Weight loss (48%) [6]

Renal
- Proteinuria (2%)

Hematologic
- Anemia [2]
- Lymphopenia (53%)
- Neutropenia (35%)
- Thrombocytopenia (35%) [2]
- Thrombosis [2]

Other
- Adverse effects [4]
- Death (6%) [3]

CALCIFEDIOL *

Synonym: calcidiol
Trade name: Rayaldee (Opko)
Indications: Hyperparathyroidism in stage 3 or 4 chronic kidney disease
Class: Vitamin D analog
Half-life: 11 days
Clinically important, potentially hazardous interactions with: anticonvulsants, atazanavir, cholestyramine, clarithromycin, indinavir, itraconazole, ketoconazole, nefazodone, nelfinavir, phenobarbital, ritonavir, saquinavir, telithromycin, thiazides, voriconazole
Pregnancy category: C
Important contra-indications noted in the prescribing guidelines for: nursing mothers; pediatric patients

---

Skin
- Hematoma (2%)

Cardiovascular
- Congestive heart failure (4%)

Neuromuscular/Skeletal
- Arthralgia (2%)

Gastrointestinal/Hepatic
- Constipation (3%)

Respiratory
- Bronchitis (3%)
- Cough (4%)
- Dyspnea (4%)
- Nasopharyngitis (5%)

Endocrine/Metabolic
- Hyperkalemia (3%)
- Hyperuricemia (2%)
- Serum creatinine increased (5%)

Hematologic
- Anemia (5%)

CALCIPOTRIOL

Synonym: calcipotriene
Trade name: Dovonex (Leo Pharma)
Indications: Psoriasis
Class: Antipsoriatic agent, Vitamin D analog
Half-life: ~30 minutes
Clinically important, potentially hazardous interactions with: none known

Pregnancy category: C
Important contra-indications noted in the prescribing guidelines for: nursing mothers; pediatric patients
Note: Contraindicated in patients with acute psoriatic eruptions, hypercalcemia or vitamin D toxicity.

Skin
- Burning (23%)
- Contact dermatitis [8]
- Erythema (<10%)
- Pigmentation [3]
- Pruritus (>10%) [6]
- Psoriasis (<10%) [3]
- Rash (11%)
- Xerosis (<5%)

Respiratory
- Nasopharyngitis [2]

Endocrine/Metabolic
- Hypercalcemia [3]

Local
- Application-site pain [2]
- Application-site pruritus [2]
- Application-site reactions [2]

Other
- Adverse effects [3]

CALCITONIN

Trade names: Calcimar (Sanofi-Aventis), Miacalcin (Novartis)
Indications: Paget's disease of bone
Class: Parathyroid hormone antagonist
Half-life: 70–90 minutes
Clinically important, potentially hazardous interactions with: none known
Pregnancy category: C

Cardiovascular
- Flushing (>10%) [5]

Gastrointestinal/Hepatic
- Diarrhea [2]
- Nausea [2]

Respiratory
- Rhinitis (12%)

Local
- Injection-site edema (>10%)
- Injection-site inflammation (>10%) [2]
- Injection-site reactions (10%)

CALCIUM HYDROXYLAPATITE

Trade name: Radiesse (Merz)
Indications: Correction of facial wrinkles and folds
Class: Dermal filler
Half-life: N/A
Clinically important, potentially hazardous interactions with: anticoagulants, antiplatelet drugs, aspirin

---

Skin
- Ecchymoses [2]
- Granulomas [5]
- Necrosis [2]
- Nodular eruption [3]

Mucosal
- Oral lesions [3]

CANAGLIFLOZIN

Trade names: Invokamet (Janssen), Invokana (Janssen)
Indications: Type II diabetes mellitus
Class: Sodium-glucose co-transporter 2 (SGLT2) inhibitor
Half-life: 11–13 hours
Clinically important, potentially hazardous interactions with: digoxin, rifampin
Pregnancy category: C
Important contra-indications noted in the prescribing guidelines for: nursing mothers; pediatric patients
Note: Contraindicated in patients with severe renal impairment, end stage renal disease, or on dialysis. Invokamet is canagliflozin and metformin.

Central Nervous System
- Headache [3]

Neuromuscular/Skeletal
- Arthralgia [2]
- Asthenia (fatigue) (2%)
- Back pain [2]

Gastrointestinal/Hepatic
- Abdominal pain (2%) [3]
- Constipation (2%) [2]
- Diarrhea [2]
- Nausea (2%) [4]

Respiratory
- Nasopharyngitis [2]
- Upper respiratory tract infection [2]

Endocrine/Metabolic
- Hypoglycemia [6]

Genitourinary
- Genital mycotic infections (4–11%) [25]
- Pollakiuria [6]
- Polyuria [2]
- Urinary frequency (5%) [6]
- Urinary tract infection (4–6%) [18]
- Vulvovaginal pruritus (2–3%) [2]

Renal
- Nephrotoxicity [2]

Other
- Adverse effects [3]
- Dipsia (thirst) (2–3%) [3]

CANAKINUMAB

Trade name: Ilaris (Novartis)
Indications: Periodic fever syndromes, systemic juvenile idiopathic arthritis
Class: Interleukin-1 inhibitor, Monoclonal antibody
Half-life: 26 days
Clinically important, potentially hazardous interactions with: cytochrome P450, IL-1 blockers, lenalidomide, TNF-blockers
Pregnancy category: C
Important contra-indications noted in the prescribing guidelines for: nursing mothers; pediatric patients
Note: Interleukin-1 blockade may interfere with immune response to infections. Treatment with medications that work through inhibition of IL-1 has been associated with an increased risk of serious infections.

Cardiovascular
- Hypertension [2]

Central Nervous System
- Headache [2]
- Vertigo (dizziness) (11%) [2]

Neuromuscular/Skeletal
- Myalgia/Myopathy (11%)

Gastrointestinal/Hepatic
- Gastroenteritis (11%) [2]
- Nausea (14%)

Respiratory
- Bronchitis (11%)
- Flu-like syndrome (20%)
- Nasopharyngitis (34%) [3]
- Pharyngitis (11%)
- Rhinitis (17%)
- Upper respiratory tract infection [5]

Endocrine/Metabolic
- Weight gain (11%)

Hematologic
- Macrophage activation syndrome [2]
- Neutropenia [2]

Local
- Injection-site reactions [4]

Other
- Adverse effects [5]
- Infection [9]

CANDESARTAN

Trade name: Atacand (AstraZeneca)
Indications: Hypertension and heart failure
Class: Angiotensin II receptor antagonist (blocker), Antihypertensive
Half-life: 9 hours
Clinically important, potentially hazardous interactions with: aliskiren
Pregnancy category: D
Important contra-indications noted in the prescribing guidelines for: nursing mothers; pediatric patients
Black Box Warning: FETAL TOXICITY

Skin
Angioedema [3]

Cardiovascular
Hypotension [5]

Central Nervous System
Dysgeusia (taste perversion) [2]
Headache [5]
Vertigo (dizziness) (4%) [6]

Neuromuscular/Skeletal
Back pain (3%) [3]

Gastrointestinal/Hepatic
Gastroenteritis [2]

Respiratory
Pharyngitis (2%)
Rhinitis (2%)
Upper respiratory tract infection (6%) [3]

Endocrine/Metabolic
Hyperkalemia (2%)

Renal
Renal failure [3]

Hematologic
Neutropenia [2]

Other
Adverse effects [4]
Fetotoxicity [2]

CANGRELOR

Trade name: Kengreal (Medicines Co)
Indications: Adjunct to percutaneous coronary intervention for reducing the risk of periprocedural myocardial infarction, repeat coronary revascularization and stent thrombosis
Class: Antiplatelet, Antiplatelet, cyclopentyl triazolo-pyrimidine (CPTP)
Half-life: 3–6 minutes
Clinically important, potentially hazardous interactions with: clopidogrel, prasugrel
Pregnancy category: C
Important contra-indications noted in the prescribing guidelines for: nursing mothers; pediatric patients
Note: Contraindicated in patients with significant active bleeding.

Respiratory
Dyspnea [5]

Renal
Nephrotoxicity (3%)

Hematologic
Bleeding (<15%) [7]

CAPECITABINE

Trade name: Xeloda (Roche)
Indications: Metastatic breast or colorectal cancer, adjuvant colon cancer
Class: Antimetabolite, Antineoplastic
Half-life: 0.5–1 hour
Clinically important, potentially hazardous interactions with: allopurinol, anticoagulants, CYP2C9 substrates, erlotinib, leucovorin, phenprocoumon, phenytoin, warfarin
Pregnancy category: D
Important contra-indications noted in the prescribing guidelines for: nursing mothers
Note: Patients receiving concomitant capecitabine and oral coumarin-derivative anticoagulants such as warfarin and phenprocoumon should have their anticoagulant response (INR or prothrombin time) monitored frequently in order to adjust the anticoagulant dose accordingly. Altered coagulation parameters and/or bleeding, including death, have been reported during concomitant use.
Contraindicated in patients with severe renal impairment or with known hypersensitivity to fluorouracil.
Black Box Warning: XELODA - WARFARIN INTERACTION

Skin
Acneform eruption [3]
Actinic keratoses [3]
Dermatitis (37%) [10]
Edema (9%) [3]
Exfoliative dermatitis (31–37%)
Hand–foot syndrome (7–58%) [158]
Jaundice [3]
Lupus erythematosus [4]
Photosensitivity [2]
Pigmentation [9]
Pruritus [2]
Radiation recall dermatitis [6]
Rash [13]
Toxicity [3]
Vitiligo [2]
Xerosis [2]

Hair
Alopecia [10]

Nails
Nail changes (7%)
Onycholysis [3]
Onychomadesis [2]
Paronychia [2]
Pyogenic granuloma [2]

Mucosal
Mucosal inflammation [2]
Mucositis [15]
Stomatitis (24%) [19]

Cardiovascular
Angina [4]
Cardiotoxicity [4]
Chest pain [3]
Hypertension [6]
Myocardial infarction [3]
QT prolongation [2]
Thromboembolism [2]

Central Nervous System
Anorexia [11]
Fever [2]
Headache [2]
Leukoencephalopathy [4]
Neurotoxicity [13]
Pain [4]
Paresthesias (21%)
Peripheral neuropathy [8]
Vertigo (dizziness) [3]

Neuromuscular/Skeletal
Asthenia (fatigue) [47]
Ataxia [2]
Myalgia/Myopathy (9%) [3]
Pain in extremities [2]

Gastrointestinal/Hepatic
Abdominal pain [8]
Constipation [2]
Diarrhea [65]
Hepatotoxicity [6]
Ileus [2]
Nausea [32]
Vomiting [27]

Endocrine/Metabolic
ALT increased [5]
Appetite decreased [2]
AST increased [4]
Hyperbilirubinemia [3]
Hyperglycemia [2]
Hypertriglyceridemia [2]

Hematologic
Anemia [22]
Febrile neutropenia [3]
Hemotoxicity [2]
Leukocytopenia [3]
Leukopenia [12]
Neutropenia [38]
Thrombocytopenia [18]

Other
Adverse effects [5]
Allergic reactions [2]
Death [6]
Infection [2]

CAPTOPRIL

Trade names: Capoten (Par), Capozide (Par)
Indications: Hypertension, congestive heart failure, to improve survival following myocardial infarction in clinically stable patients with left ventricular dysfunction, diabetic nephropathy in patients with Type I insulin-dependent diabetes mellitus and retinopathy
Class: Angiotensin-converting enzyme (ACE) inhibitor, Antihypertensive, Vasodilator
Half-life: <3 hours
Clinically important, potentially hazardous interactions with: alcohol, aldesleukin, allopurinol, alpha blockers, alprostadil, amifostine, amiloride, angiotensin II receptor antagonists, antacids, antidiabetics, antihypertensives, antipsychotics, anxiolytics and hypnotics, aprotinin, azathioprine, baclofen, beta blockers, calcium channel blockers, clonidine, cyclosporine, CYP2D6 inhibitors, darunavir, diazoxide, digoxin, diuretics, eplerenone, estrogens, everolimus, general anesthetics, gold & gold compounds, heparins, herbals, hydralazine, hypotensives, insulin, interferon alfa, levodopa, lithium, MAO inhibitors, metformin, methyldopa, methylphenidate, minoxidil, moxisylyte, moxonidine, nitrates, nitroprusside, NSAIDs, pentoxifylline, phosphodiesterase 5 inhibitors, potassium salts, probenecid, prostacyclin analogues, rituximab, salicylates, sirolimus, spironolactone, sulfonylureas, temsirolimus, tizanidine, tolvaptan, triamterene, trimethoprim, venetoclax, yohimbine

Pregnancy category: D (category C in first trimester; category D in second and third trimesters)
Important contra-indications noted in the prescribing guidelines for: nursing mothers; pediatric patients
Note: Capozide is captopril and hydrochlorothiazide. Hydrochlorothiazide is a sulfonamide and can be absorbed systemically. Sulfonamides can produce severe, possibly fatal, reactions such as toxic epidermal necrolysis and Stevens-Johnson syndrome.
Black Box Warning: FETAL TOXICITY

Skin
Angioedema (<15%) [45]
Bullous pemphigoid [2]
Dermatitis [3]
DRESS syndrome [2]
Erythroderma [2]
Exanthems (4–7%) [19]
Exfoliative dermatitis (<2%) [4]
Kaposi's sarcoma [2]
Lichen planus pemphigoides [2]
Lichenoid eruption [12]
Linear IgA bullous dermatosis [5]
Lupus erythematosus [8]
Mycosis fungoides [2]
Pemphigus (<2%) [23]
Pemphigus foliaceus [2]
Penile ulcers [2]
Photosensitivity [3]
Phototoxicity (<2%)
Pigmentation [2]
Pityriasis rosea (<2%) [6]
Pruritus (<7%) [8]
Pseudolymphoma [2]
Psoriasis [8]
Rash (4–7%) [11]
Toxic epidermal necrolysis [3]
Urticaria [9]
Vasculitis [7]

Hair
Alopecia (<2%) [4]

Nails
Nail dystrophy [2]
Onycholysis [2]

Mucosal
Aphthous stomatitis (<2%) [5]
Glossitis [3]
Oral mucosal eruption [3]
Oral ulceration [4]
Sialadenitis [2]
Tongue ulceration [3]
Xerostomia (<2%)

Cardiovascular
Flushing [2]

Central Nervous System
Ageusia (taste loss) (2–4%) [11]
Dysgeusia (taste perversion) (metallic or salty taste) (2–4%) [14]
Hallucinations [2]
Paresthesias (<2%)

Gastrointestinal/Hepatic
Hepatotoxicity [4]

Respiratory
Cough [18]

Endocrine/Metabolic
Gynecomastia [3]

Other
Adverse effects [3]
Allergic reactions [2]

CARBAMAZEPINE

Trade names: Epitol (Teva), Tegretol (Novartis)
Indications: Epilepsy, pain or trigeminal neuralgia
Class: Anticonvulsant, Antipsychotic, CYP1A2 inducer, CYP3A4 inducer, Mood stabilizer
Half-life: 18–55 hours
Clinically important, potentially hazardous interactions with: abiraterone, acetaminophen, acetylcysteine, adenosine, afatinib, amitriptyline, amlodipine, amprenavir, apixaban, apremilast, aprepitant, aripiprazole, artemether/lumefantrine, boceprevir, buprenorphine, cabazitaxel, cabozantinib, caffeine, caspofungin, cefixime, charcoal, citalopram, clarithromycin, clobazam, clopidogrel, clorazepate, clozapine, cobicistat/elvitegravir/emtricitabine/tenofovir disoproxil, cobimetinib, crizotinib, dabigatran, daclatasvir, darunavir, dasatinib, delavirdine, dexamethasone, diltiazem, doxacurium, doxycycline, dronedarone, efavirenz, emtricitabine/rilpivirine/tenofovir alafenamide, enzalutamide, erythromycin, eslicarbazepine, estradiol, ethosuximide, etravirine, ezogabine, felodipine, fesoterodine, flibanserin, fosamprenavir, gefitinib, imatinib, indinavir, influenza vaccine, isotretinoin, itraconazole, ixabepilone, lacosamide, lapatinib, ledipasvir & sofosbuvir, lesinurad, levetiracetam, levomepromazine, levonorgestrel, linezolid, lopinavir, methylprednisolone, midazolam, mifepristone, nelfinavir, nevirapine, nifedipine, nilotinib, olanzapine, ombitasvir/paritaprevir/ritonavir, ondansetron, osimertinib, oxcarbazepine, oxtriphylline, paclitaxel, paliperidone, perampanel, piracetam, ponatinib, prednisolone, propoxyphene, regorafenib, rilpivirine, riociguat, risperidone, ritonavir, rivaroxaban, roflumilast, romidepsin, rufinamide, simeprevir, simvastatin, sodium picosulfate, sofosbuvir, solifenacin, sorafenib, St John's wort, sunitinib, telaprevir, telithromycin, temsirolimus, terbinafine, thalidomide, tiagabine, ticagrelor, tipranavir, tolvaptan, tramadol, triamcinolone, troleandomycin, ulipristal, vandetanib, vemurafenib, verapamil, voriconazole, vortioxetine, ziprasidone, zuclopenthixol
Pregnancy category: D
Note: Carbamazepine is the main cause of Stevens-Johnson syndrome (SJS), toxic epidermal necrolysis (TEN), and the hypersensitivity syndrome in Han Chinese, and in peoples of other Southeast Asian countries, as a result of a strong pharmacogenetic association that has been reported in these patients between the human leukocyte antigen (HLA)-B*1502 and carbamazepine.
Black Box Warning: SERIOUS DERMATOLOGIC REACTIONS AND HLA-B*1502 ALLELE
APLASTIC ANEMIA AND AGRANULOCYTOSIS

Skin
AGEP [5]
Angioedema [5]
Anticonvulsant hypersensitivity syndrome [19]
Bullous dermatitis [4]
Dermatitis [7]
Diaphoresis (<10%)
DRESS syndrome [46]
Eczema [2]
Erythema multiforme [16]
Erythroderma [12]
Exanthems (>5%) [35]
Exfoliative dermatitis [24]
Facial edema [2]
Fixed eruption [10]
Hypersensitivity [69]
Lichen planus [2]
Lichenoid eruption [7]
Lupus erythematosus [35]
Lymphoma [2]
Lymphoproliferative disease [5]
Mycosis fungoides [3]
Pemphigus [3]
Photosensitivity [9]
Pruritus [7]
Pseudolymphoma [17]
Purpura [8]
Pustules [5]
Rash (>10%) [29]
Stevens–Johnson syndrome (<10%) [95]
Toxic epidermal necrolysis (<10%) [86]
Toxic pustuloderma [3]
Toxicity [2]
Urticaria [14]
Vasculitis [7]

Hair
Alopecia [7]

Mucosal
Mucocutaneous eruption [4]
Mucocutaneous lymph node syndrome (Kawasaki syndrome) [2]
Oral ulceration [2]
Tongue ulceration [2]

Cardiovascular
Bradycardia [3]
Myocarditis [2]

Central Nervous System
Ageusia (taste loss) [3]
Coma [2]
Dysgeusia (taste perversion) [2]
Headache [4]
Memory loss [2]
Seizures [12]
Somnolence (drowsiness) [7]
Tic disorder [4]
Vertigo (dizziness) [7]

Neuromuscular/Skeletal
Asthenia (fatigue) [2]
Ataxia [5]
Myasthenia gravis [2]
Osteoporosis [2]

Gastrointestinal/Hepatic
Diarrhea [2]
Hepatotoxicity [11]
Nausea [5]
Pancreatitis [3]
Vanishing bile duct syndrome [4]
Vomiting [3]

Endocrine/Metabolic
Acute intermittent porphyria [5]
Hyponatremia [4]
SIADH [16]
Weight gain [5]

Renal
Nephrotoxicity [2]

Hematologic
Agranulocytosis [2]
Leukopenia [3]
Thrombocytopenia [3]

Ocular
Diplopia [2]

Other
Adverse effects [6]
Allergic reactions [8]
Death [6]
Side effects [3]
Teratogenicity [12]

CARBOPLATIN

Trade name: Paraplatin (Bristol-Myers Squibb)
Indications: Various carcinomas and sarcomas
Class: Alkylating agent, Antineoplastic
Half-life: terminal: 22–40 hours
Clinically important, potentially hazardous interactions with: aldesleukin, bexarotene
Pregnancy category: D
Important contra-indications noted in the prescribing guidelines for: the elderly; nursing mothers; pediatric patients

---

Skin
Anaphylactoid reactions/Anaphylaxis [5]
Erythema (2%) [2]
Exanthems [3]
Hand–foot syndrome [4]
Hypersensitivity (2%) [26]
Pigmentation [2]
Pruritus (2%) [2]
Radiation recall dermatitis [2]
Rash (2%) [9]
Scleroderma [2]
Toxicity [4]
Urticaria (2%) [4]

Hair
Alopecia (3%) [15]
Alopecia areata [2]

Mucosal
Epistaxis (nosebleed) [2]
Mucositis [4]
Stomatitis (>10%) [2]

Cardiovascular
Flushing [3]
Hypertension [5]

Central Nervous System
Anorexia [7]
Headache [2]
Leukoencephalopathy [2]
Neurotoxicity [15]
Paresthesias [2]
Peripheral neuropathy [7]
Vertigo (dizziness) [2]

Neuromuscular/Skeletal
Asthenia (fatigue) [21]
Myalgia/Myopathy [2]

Gastrointestinal/Hepatic
Constipation [3]
Diarrhea [13]
Dyspepsia [2]
Gastrointestinal perforation [2]
Hepatotoxicity [4]
Nausea [15]
Pancreatitis [2]
Vomiting [16]

Respiratory
Cough [2]
Hemoptysis [2]
Pneumonia [2]
Pulmonary toxicity [3]

Endocrine/Metabolic
ALT increased [3]
AST increased [2]
Hyperglycemia [5]
Hyponatremia [3]
SIADH [3]

Renal
Nephrotoxicity [9]

Hematologic
Anemia [22]
Febrile neutropenia [15]
Hemorrhage [2]
Hemotoxicity [3]
Leukopenia [11]
Lymphopenia [2]
Myelotoxicity [2]
Neutropenia [43]
Pancytopenia [2]
Thrombocytopenia [33]

Otic
Ototoxicity [7]
Tinnitus [3]

Local
Injection-site pain (>10%)

Other
Allergic reactions [3]
Death [3]
Infection [4]

CARFILZOMIB

Trade name: Kyprolis (Onyx)
Indications: Multiple myeloma
Class: Proteasome inhibitor
Half-life: ~1 hour
Clinically important, potentially hazardous interactions with: none known
Pregnancy category: D
Important contra-indications noted in the prescribing guidelines for: nursing mothers; pediatric patients

---

Skin
Herpes zoster (reactivation) (2%)
Peripheral edema (24%) [2]
Tumor lysis syndrome [2]

Cardiovascular
Cardiac failure (7%) [2]
Cardiotoxicity [4]
Chest pain (11%)
Hypertension (14%) [5]

Central Nervous System
Anorexia (12%)
Chills (16%)
Fever (30%) [5]
Headache (28%)
Hypoesthesia (12%)
Insomnia (18%) [2]
Pain (12%)
Peripheral neuropathy (14%) [14]
Vertigo (dizziness) (13%)

Neuromuscular/Skeletal
Arthralgia (16%)
Asthenia (fatigue) (13–56%) [14]
Back pain (20%)
Muscle spasm (14%) [2]
Pain in extremities (13%)

Gastrointestinal/Hepatic
Constipation (21%) [2]
Diarrhea (33%) [4]
Nausea (45%) [12]
Vomiting (22%) [3]

Respiratory
Cough (26%) [4]
Dyspnea (35%) [8]
Pneumonia (13%) [5]
Pulmonary hypertension (2%)
Upper respiratory tract infection (28%) [3]

Endocrine/Metabolic
AST increased (13%)
Hypercalcemia (11%)
Hyperglycemia (12%) [3]
Hypokalemia (14%) [3]
Hypomagnesemia (14%)
Hyponatremia (10%) [2]
Hypophosphatemia (11%) [3]
Serum creatinine increased [4]

Renal
Nephrotoxicity [2]

Hematologic
Anemia (47%) [17]
Leukopenia (14%) [3]
Lymphopenia (24%) [7]
Neutropenia (21%) [9]
Thrombocytopenia (36%) [16]

Other
Adverse effects [3]

CARIPRAZINE

Trade name: Vraylar (Forest)
Indications: Schizophrenia, manic or mixed episodes associated with bipolar I disorder
Class: Antipsychotic
Half-life: 2–4 days
Clinically important, potentially hazardous interactions with: CYP3A4 inducers
Pregnancy category: N/A (Neonatal risk in third trimester exposure)
Important contra-indications noted in the prescribing guidelines for: the elderly; nursing mothers; pediatric patients
Black Box Warning: INCREASED MORTALITY IN ELDERLY PATIENTS WITH DEMENTIA-RELATED PSYCHOSIS

Skin
Rash (<2%)

Mucosal
Oropharyngeal pain (<3%)
Xerostomia (<3%)

Cardiovascular
Hypertension (2–6%)
Tachycardia (<3%)

Central Nervous System
Agitation (3–5%)
Akathisia (20–21%) [17]
Anxiety (3–6%) [2]
Extrapyramidal symptoms (15–29%) [14]
Fever (<4%) [3]
Headache (9–18%) [6]
Insomnia (8–13%) [9]
Parkinsonism (13–26%) [3]
Restlessness (4–7%) [5]
Sedation [6]
Somnolence (drowsiness) (5–10%) [2]
Tremor [9]
Vertigo (dizziness) (3–7%) [7]

Neuromuscular/Skeletal
Arthralgia (<2%)
Asthenia (fatigue) (<5%)
Back pain (<3%)
Dystonia (2–5%)
Pain in extremities [2]

Gastrointestinal/Hepatic
Abdominal pain (3–8%)
Constipation (6–11%) [9]
Diarrhea (<5%) [4]
Dyspepsia (4–9%) [5]
Hepatotoxicity (<3%)
Nausea (5–13%) [9]
Vomiting (4–10%) [7]

Respiratory
Cough (<4%)
Nasopharyngitis (<2%)

Endocrine/Metabolic
Appetite decreased (<4%)
Creatine phosphokinase increased (<3%)
Weight gain (2–3%) [3]

Genitourinary
Urinary tract infection (<2%)

Ocular
Vision blurred (4%) [2]

Other
Toothache (3–6%)

CARISOPRODOL

Trade name: Soma (MedPointe)
Indications: Painful musculoskeletal disorders
Class: Central muscle relaxant
Half-life: 4–6 hours
Clinically important, potentially hazardous interactions with: CNS depressants, eucalyptus, meprobamate
Pregnancy category: C
Important contra-indications noted in the prescribing guidelines for: the elderly; nursing mothers; pediatric patients
Note: Contraindicated in patients with acute intermittent porphyria.

Skin
Angioedema (<10%)
Fixed eruption [2]
Urticaria [2]

Cardiovascular
Flushing (<10%)

Central Nervous System
Amnesia [2]
Trembling (<10%)

Other
Death [2]

CARMUSTINE

Trade names: BiCNU (Bristol-Myers Squibb), Gliadel Wafer (Guilford)
Indications: Brain tumors, Hodgkin's disease, multiple myeloma
Class: Alkylating agent, Nitrosourea
Half-life: initial: 1.4 minutes; secondary: 20 minutes
Clinically important, potentially hazardous interactions with: aldesleukin, cimetidine, clorazepate
Pregnancy category: D
Important contra-indications noted in the prescribing guidelines for: nursing mothers; pediatric patients

---

Skin
Dermatitis [3]
Pigmentation (on accidental contact) [2]
Telangiectasia [2]

Hair
Alopecia (<10%)

Mucosal
Stomatitis (<10%)

Cardiovascular
Flushing (<10%) [2]

Central Nervous System
Intracranial hemorrhage [2]
Meningococcal infection [2]
Seizures [2]

Neuromuscular/Skeletal
Asthenia (fatigue) [2]

Gastrointestinal/Hepatic
Nausea [2]
Vomiting [2]

Hematologic
Leukopenia [2]
Thrombocytopenia [2]

Local
Injection-site burning (>10%)

CARVEDILOL

Trade name: Coreg (GSK)
Indications: Hypertension
Class: Adrenergic beta-receptor antagonist
Half-life: 7–10 hours
Clinically important, potentially hazardous interactions with: cinacalcet, delavirdine, efavirenz, irbesartan, leflunomide, propafenone, trimethoprim, venetoclax, voriconazole, zafirlukast
Pregnancy category: C
Important contra-indications noted in the prescribing guidelines for: nursing mothers; pediatric patients

---

Skin
Diaphoresis (3%)
Edema (generalized) (5–6%) [2]
Peripheral edema (<7%)
Purpura (<3%)

Cardiovascular
Angina (2–6%)
Atrioventricular block (<3%)
Bradycardia (2–10%) [6]
Cardiac failure [2]
Congestive heart failure [2]
Extrasystoles [2]
Hypertension (<3%)
Hypotension (9–14%) [7]
Palpitation (<3%)
Postural hypotension (<3%)

Central Nervous System
Fever (<3%)
Headache (5–8%) [2]
Pain (9%)
Paresthesias (2%)
Somnolence (drowsiness) (<3%)
Syncope (3–8%)
Vertigo (dizziness) (24–32%) [5]

Neuromuscular/Skeletal
Arthralgia (<6%)
Asthenia (fatigue) (7–24%) [2]
Muscle spasm (<3%)
Myalgia/Myopathy (3%)

Gastrointestinal/Hepatic
Black stools (<3%)
Diarrhea (2–12%)
Nausea (4–9%)
Vomiting (<6%)

Respiratory
Cough (5–8%)
Dyspnea [4]
Stridor [2]

Endocrine/Metabolic
ALP increased (<3%) [2]
Creatine phosphokinase increased (<3%) [3]
Diabetes mellitus (<3%)
GGT increased (<3%)
Hypercholesterolemia (<4%)
Hyperglycemia (5–12%)
Hyperkalemia (<3%) [2]
Hyperuricemia (<3%)
Hypervolemia (<3%)
Hypoglycemia (<3%)
Hyponatremia (<3%)
Hypovolemia (<3%)
Weight gain (10–12%)
Weight loss (<3%)

Genitourinary
Albuminuria (<3%)
Hematuria (<3%)
Impotence (<3%)

Hematologic
Anemia [2]
Prothrombin time decreased (<3%)
Thrombocytopenia (<3%)

Ocular
- Abnormal vision (5%)
- Vision blurred (<3%)

Other
- Adverse effects [8]
- Infection (2%)

CASPOFUNGIN

Trade name: Cancidas (Merck)
Indications: Invasive *Aspergillus* and *Candida* infections
Class: Antifungal
Half-life: beta phase: 9–11 hours; terminal: 40–50 hours
Clinically important, potentially hazardous interactions with: carbamazepine, cyclosporine, dexamethasone, efavirenz, nevirapine, phenytoin, rifampin, tacrolimus
Pregnancy category: C
Important contra-indications noted in the prescribing guidelines for: nursing mothers; pediatric patients

---

Skin
- Anaphylactoid reactions/Anaphylaxis (<2%)
- Edema (~3%)
- Erythema (<4%)
- Facial edema (3%)
- Jaundice (<5%)
- Peripheral edema (11%)
- Petechiae (<5%)
- Pruritus (2–7%)
- Rash (4–16%) [5]
- Septic–toxic shock (11–13%)
- Ulcerations (3%)
- Urticaria (<5%)
- Vasculitis (2%)

Mucosal
- Epistaxis (nosebleed) (<5%)
- Mucosal inflammation (6–10%)

Cardiovascular
- Arrhythmias (<5%)
- Atrial fibrillation (<5%)
- Bradycardia (<5%)
- Cardiac arrest (<5%)
- Flushing (3%)
- Hypertension (5–10%)
- Hypotension (6–12%)
- Myocardial infarction (<5%)
- Phlebitis (18%) [3]
- Tachycardia (4–7%)
- Thrombophlebitis [2]

Central Nervous System
- Anxiety (<5%)
- Chills (9–23%)
- Confusion (<5%)
- Depression (<5%)
- Fever (6–29%) [8]
- Headache (5–15%) [3]
- Insomnia (<5%)
- Pain (<5%)
- Paresthesias (<3%)
- Seizures (<5%)
- Tremor (<2%)
- Vertigo (dizziness) (<5%)

Neuromuscular/Skeletal
- Arthralgia (<5%)
- Asthenia (fatigue) (<5%)
- Back pain (<5%)
- Myalgia/Myopathy (~3%)
- Pain in extremities (<5%)

Gastrointestinal/Hepatic
- Abdominal distension (<5%)
- Abdominal pain (7–9%)
- Constipation (<5%)
- Diarrhea (6–27%)
- Dyspepsia (<5%)
- Hepatic failure (<5%)
- Hepatotoxicity (<5%) [5]
- Nausea (5–15%) [2]
- Vomiting (9–17%) [2]

Respiratory
- Cough (6–11%)
- Dyspnea (9%)
- Flu-like syndrome (3%)
- Hypoxia (<5%)
- Pleural effusion (9%)
- Pneumonia (4–11%)
- Respiratory distress (8%)
- Respiratory failure (6–11%)
- Tachypnea (8%)

Endocrine/Metabolic
- ALP increased (12–23%) [4]
- ALT increased (4–18%) [4]
- Appetite decreased (<5%)
- AST increased (6–16%) [5]
- Hypercalcemia (<5%)
- Hyperglycemia (<5%)
- Hypokalemia (6–8%) [3]
- Hypomagnesemia (<5%)

Genitourinary
- Hematuria (<5%)
- Urinary tract infection (<5%)

Renal
- Nephrotoxicity [5]
- Renal failure (<5%)

Hematologic
- Anemia (2–11%)
- Coagulopathy (<5%)
- Eosinophilia [2]
- Febrile neutropenia (<5%)
- Neutropenia (<5%)
- Sepsis (5%)
- Thrombocytopenia (<5%) [2]

Local
- Infusion-site pain (<5%)
- Infusion-site reactions (<5%) [5]
- Injection-site induration (~3%)
- Injection-site reactions (2–12%) [4]

Other
- Adverse effects [8]

CEFACLOR

Trade name: Ceclor (Lilly)
Indications: Various infections caused by susceptible organisms
Class: Cephalosporin, 2nd generation
Half-life: 0.6–0.9 hours
Clinically important, potentially hazardous interactions with: none known
Pregnancy category: B
Important contra-indications noted in the prescribing guidelines for: the elderly; nursing mothers; pediatric patients
Note: Penicillin and cephalosporins share a common beta-lactam structure. People who are allergic to penicillin are approximately 4 times more likely to develop an allergic reaction to a cephalosporin than those people who have no penicillin allergy (from 5–16% of patients allergic to penicillin develop reactions to cephalosporins).

Skin
- AGEP [2]
- Anaphylactoid reactions/Anaphylaxis [4]
- Erythema multiforme [6]
- Exanthems [9]
- Fixed eruption [2]
- Pruritus [4]
- Purpura [2]
- Rash (<2%)
- Serum sickness [31]
- Urticaria [5]

Gastrointestinal/Hepatic
- Diarrhea [2]

Other
- Adverse effects [3]

CEFADROXIL

Trade name: Duricef (Warner Chilcott)
Indications: Various infections caused by susceptible organisms
Class: Cephalosporin, 1st generation
Half-life: 1.2–1.5 hours
Clinically important, potentially hazardous interactions with: none known
Pregnancy category: B
Important contra-indications noted in the prescribing guidelines for: nursing mothers
Note: Penicillin and cephalosporins share a common beta-lactam structure. People who are allergic to penicillin are approximately 4 times more likely to develop an allergic reaction to a cephalosporin than those people who have no penicillin allergy (from 5–16% of patients allergic to penicillin develop reactions to cephalosporins).

Skin
- Urticaria [2]

Gastrointestinal/Hepatic
- Diarrhea [2]
- Nausea [2]

Other
- Adverse effects [3]

CEFDINIR

Trade name: Omnicef (Medicis)
Indications: Community-acquired pneumonia and various infections caused by susceptible organisms
Class: Cephalosporin, 3rd generation
Half-life: 1–2 hours
Clinically important, potentially hazardous interactions with: none known

Pregnancy category: B
Important contra-indications noted in the prescribing guidelines for: pediatric patients
Note: Penicillin and cephalosporins share a common beta-lactam structure. People who are allergic to penicillin are approximately 4 times more likely to develop an allergic reaction to a cephalosporin than those people who have no penicillin allergy (from 5–16% of patients allergic to penicillin develop reactions to cephalosporins).

Skin
Rash (3%)

Gastrointestinal/Hepatic
Red stools [2]

Genitourinary
Vulvovaginal candidiasis (5%)

Other
Adverse effects [2]

CEFEPIME

Trade name: Maxipime (Elan)
Indications: Various infections caused by susceptible organisms
Class: Cephalosporin, 4th generation
Half-life: 2–2.3 hours
Clinically important, potentially hazardous interactions with: none known
Pregnancy category: B
Important contra-indications noted in the prescribing guidelines for: the elderly; nursing mothers
Note: Penicillin and cephalosporins share a common beta-lactam structure. People who are allergic to penicillin are approximately 4 times more likely to develop an allergic reaction to a cephalosporin than those people who have no penicillin allergy (from 5–16% of patients allergic to penicillin develop reactions to cephalosporins).

Skin
Exanthems (2%)
Hypersensitivity [2]
Lupus erythematosus [2]
Pruritus [3]
Rash (51%) [12]

Central Nervous System
Encephalopathy [9]
Headache [3]
Neurotoxicity [14]
Seizures [16]
Status epilepticus [4]

Neuromuscular/Skeletal
Myoclonus [2]

Local
Injection-site reactions (3%) [2]

Other
Adverse effects [2]

CEFIXIME

Trade name: Suprax (Lupin)
Indications: Various infections caused by susceptible organisms
Class: Cephalosporin, 3rd generation
Half-life: 3–4 hours
Clinically important, potentially hazardous interactions with: aminoglycosides, anticoagulants, BCG vaccine, carbamazepine, probenecid, typhoid vaccine, warfarin
Pregnancy category: B
Important contra-indications noted in the prescribing guidelines for: nursing mothers; pediatric patients
Note: Penicillin and cephalosporins share a common beta-lactam structure. People who are allergic to penicillin are approximately 4 times more likely to develop an allergic reaction to a cephalosporin than those people who have no penicillin allergy (from 5–16% of patients allergic to penicillin develop reactions to cephalosporins).

Skin
Anaphylactoid reactions/Anaphylaxis (<2%)
Angioedema (<2%)
Erythema multiforme (<2%)
Facial edema (<2%)
Jaundice (<2%)
Pruritus (<2%)
Pruritus ani et vulvae (<2%)
Rash (<2%) [2]
Serum sickness (<2%)
Stevens–Johnson syndrome (<2%)
Toxic epidermal necrolysis (<2%)
Urticaria (<2%) [2]

Central Nervous System
Fever (<2%)

Gastrointestinal/Hepatic
Abdominal pain (3%)
Diarrhea (16%)
Dyspepsia (3%)
Flatulence (4%)
Hepatitis (<2%)
Loose stools (6%)
Nausea (7%)
Pseudomembranous colitis (<2%)

Endocrine/Metabolic
ALP increased (<2%)
Creatine phosphokinase increased (<2%)

Genitourinary
Vaginitis (<2%)
Vulvovaginal candidiasis (<2%)

Renal
Renal failure (<2%)

CEFOTAXIME

Trade name: Claforan (Sanofi-Aventis)
Indications: Various infections caused by susceptible organisms
Class: Cephalosporin, 3rd generation
Half-life: 1 hour (adults)
Clinically important, potentially hazardous interactions with: none known
Pregnancy category: B
Important contra-indications noted in the prescribing guidelines for: nursing mothers
Note: Penicillin and cephalosporins share a common beta-lactam structure. People who are allergic to penicillin are approximately 4 times more likely to develop an allergic reaction to a cephalosporin than those people who have no penicillin allergy (from 5–16% of patients allergic to penicillin develop reactions to cephalosporins).

Skin
Anaphylactoid reactions/Anaphylaxis (2%)
DRESS syndrome [4]
Erythema multiforme [2]
Exanthems [3]
Hypersensitivity [2]
Pruritus (2%) [3]
Rash (2%) [3]
Urticaria (2%)

Local
Injection-site inflammation (4%)
Injection-site pain (<10%)

Other
Adverse effects [2]

CEFOTETAN

Indications: Various infections caused by susceptible organisms
Class: Cephalosporin, 2nd generation
Half-life: 3–5 hours
Clinically important, potentially hazardous interactions with: none known
Pregnancy category: B
Important contra-indications noted in the prescribing guidelines for: nursing mothers; pediatric patients
Note: Penicillin and cephalosporins share a common beta-lactam structure. People who are allergic to penicillin are approximately 4 times more likely to develop an allergic reaction to a cephalosporin than those people who have no penicillin allergy (from 5–16% of patients allergic to penicillin develop reactions to cephalosporins).

Skin
Anaphylactoid reactions/Anaphylaxis [3]
Rash [2]

Hematologic
Hemolytic anemia [12]

Other
Death [5]

CEFTAROLINE FOSAMIL

Trade name: Teflaro (Forest)
Indications: Acute bacterial skin and skin structure infections, community-acquired bacterial pneumonia
Class: Antibacterial, Cephalosporin, 5th generation
Half-life: 3 hours
Clinically important, potentially hazardous interactions with: BCG vaccine, probenecid, typhoid vaccine
Pregnancy category: B
Important contra-indications noted in the prescribing guidelines for: the elderly; nursing mothers; pediatric patients
Note: Penicillin and cephalosporins share a common beta-lactam structure. People who are allergic to penicillin are approximately 4 times more likely to develop an allergic reaction to a cephalosporin than those people who have no penicillin allergy (from 5–16% of patients allergic to penicillin develop reactions to cephalosporins).

Skin
Anaphylactoid reactions/Anaphylaxis (<2%)
Hypersensitivity (<2%) [2]
Pruritus [7]
Rash (3%) [7]
Urticaria (<2%)

Cardiovascular
Bradycardia (<2%)
Hypertension [2]
Palpitation (<2%)
Phlebitis (2%) [3]

Central Nervous System
Fever (<2%)
Headache [9]
Insomnia [5]
Seizures (<2%)
Vertigo (dizziness) (<2%)

Gastrointestinal/Hepatic
Abdominal pain (<2%)
Colitis (<2%)
Constipation (2%)
Diarrhea (5%) [10]
Hepatotoxicity (<2%)
Nausea (4%) [9]
Vomiting (2%)

Respiratory
Eosinophilic pneumonia [3]

Endocrine/Metabolic
ALT increased (2%)
Hyperglycemia (<2%)
Hyperkalemia (<2%)
Hypokalemia (2%) [2]

Renal
Renal failure (<2%)

Hematologic
Anemia (<2%)
Eosinophilia (<2%)
Neutropenia (<2%)
Thrombocytopenia (<2%)

Other
Adverse effects [3]

CEFTAZIDIME

Trade names: Ceptaz (GSK), Fortaz (Concordia), Tazicef (Hospira)
Indications: Various infections caused by susceptible organisms
Class: Cephalosporin, 3rd generation
Half-life: 1–2 hours
Clinically important, potentially hazardous interactions with: none known
Pregnancy category: B
Important contra-indications noted in the prescribing guidelines for: the elderly; nursing mothers
Note: Penicillin and cephalosporins share a common beta-lactam structure. People who are allergic to penicillin are approximately 4 times more likely to develop an allergic reaction to a cephalosporin than those people who have no penicillin allergy (from 5–16% of patients allergic to penicillin develop reactions to cephalosporins). See also separate profile for Ceftazidime & Avibactam.

Skin
Anaphylactoid reactions/Anaphylaxis (2%) [3]
Angioedema (2%)
Erythema multiforme (2%)
Hypersensitivity (2%)
Pemphigus erythematodes [2]
Pruritus (2%) [3]
Rash (2%) [4]
Stevens–Johnson syndrome (2%)
Toxic epidermal necrolysis (2%)

Central Nervous System
Encephalopathy [2]
Seizures [3]

Local
Injection-site inflammation (2%)
Injection-site reactions [2]
Injection-site thrombophlebitis (2%)

Other
Adverse effects [3]
Death [2]

CEFTAZIDIME & AVIBACTAM *

Trade name: Avycaz (Cerexa)
Indications: Various infections caused by susceptible organisms
Class: Antibiotic, beta-lactam (avibactam), Cephalosporin, 3rd generation (ceftazidime)
Half-life: <3 hours
Clinically important, potentially hazardous interactions with: probenecid
Pregnancy category: B
Important contra-indications noted in the prescribing guidelines for: the elderly; nursing mothers; pediatric patients
Note: See also separate entry for ceftazidime.

Skin
Rash (<5%)

Central Nervous System
Anxiety (10%) [3]
Fever [4]
Headache [3]
Vertigo (dizziness) (6%)

Gastrointestinal/Hepatic
Abdominal pain (7%) [5]
Constipation (10%) [2]
Diarrhea [5]
Hepatotoxicity [4]
Nausea (2%) [5]
Vomiting [5]

Endocrine/Metabolic
ALP increased (3%)
ALT increased (3%) [3]
AST increased [3]
GGT increased (<5%)

Renal
Nephrotoxicity (<5%)
Renal failure (<5%) [4]

Hematologic
Eosinophilia (<5%)
Prothrombin time increased (<5%)
Thrombocytopenia (<5%)

Local
Injection-site reactions [4]

Other
Adverse effects [2]

CEFTOBIPROLE

Trade names: BAL5788 (Basilea) (Cilag AG), Zeftera (Janssen)
Indications: Bacterial infections, MRSA
Class: Cephalosporin, 5th generation
Half-life: 3 hours
Clinically important, potentially hazardous interactions with: alcohol, anticoagulants, BCG vaccine, carbenicillin, dipyridamole, heparin, pentoxifylline, plicamycin, sulfinpyrazone, ticarcillin, typhoid vaccine, valproic acid
Pregnancy category: N/A (not recommended in pregnancy)
Important contra-indications noted in the prescribing guidelines for: nursing mothers; pediatric patients
Note: Penicillin and cephalosporins share a common beta-lactam structure. People who are allergic to penicillin are approximately 4 times more likely to develop an allergic reaction to a cephalosporin than those people who have no penicillin allergy (from 5–16% of patients allergic to penicillin develop reactions to cephalosporins).

Skin
Erythema (9%)
Pruritus (9%)

Central Nervous System
Dysgeusia (taste perversion) (8%) [3]
Headache [2]

Gastrointestinal/Hepatic
Abdominal pain [2]
Diarrhea [4]
Nausea [6]
Vomiting [4]

Endocrine/Metabolic
Hyponatremia [2]

Local
Infusion-site reactions [2]

Other
Adverse effects [3]

CEFTOLOZANE & TAZOBACTAM *

Trade name: Zerbaxa (Cubist)
Indications: Various infections caused by susceptible organisms
Class: Antibacterial, Antibiotic, beta-lactam, Cephalosporin, 5th generation
Half-life: <3 hours
Clinically important, potentially hazardous interactions with: none known
Pregnancy category: B
Important contra-indications noted in the prescribing guidelines for: the elderly; nursing mothers; pediatric patients

---

Cardiovascular
Hypertension [3]

Central Nervous System
Fever (2%) [5]
Headache (3%) [8]
Insomnia [2]
Somnolence (drowsiness) [2]

Neuromuscular/Skeletal
Myalgia/Myopathy [2]

Gastrointestinal/Hepatic
Constipation (4%) [4]
Diarrhea (2%) [10]
Nausea (3%) [11]
Vomiting [3]

Endocrine/Metabolic
ALT increased (2%)
AST increased (2%)

Hematologic
Anemia [2]

Local
Infusion-site reactions [2]

CEFTRIAXONE

Trade name: Rocephin (Roche)
Indications: Various infections caused by susceptible organisms
Class: Antibiotic, Cephalosporin, 3rd generation
Half-life: 5–9 hours
Clinically important, potentially hazardous interactions with: aminoglycosides, coumarins, histamine H_2 antagonists, oral typhoid vaccine, probenecid
Pregnancy category: B
Important contra-indications noted in the prescribing guidelines for: nursing mothers; pediatric patients
Note: Penicillin and cephalosporins share a common beta-lactam structure. People who are allergic to penicillin are approximately 4 times more likely to develop an allergic reaction to a cephalosporin than those people who have no penicillin allergy (from 5–16% of patients allergic to penicillin develop reactions to cephalosporins).

Skin
AGEP [4]
Anaphylactoid reactions/Anaphylaxis [14]
Angioedema [3]
Candidiasis (5%) [3]
Dermatitis [2]
DRESS syndrome [2]
Erythroderma [2]
Exanthems [7]
Hypersensitivity [4]
Linear IgA bullous dermatosis [2]
Pruritus [2]
Rash (2%) [5]
Serum sickness [2]
Urticaria [4]

Mucosal
Glossitis [2]

Cardiovascular
Flushing [2]
Hypotension [2]
Phlebitis [2]

Central Nervous System
Fever [2]

Gastrointestinal/Hepatic
Cholelithiasis (gallstones) [4]
Diarrhea [6]
Hepatotoxicity [7]
Nausea [4]
Vomiting [2]

Respiratory
Dyspnea [2]

Renal
Biliary pseudolithiasis [7]
Nephrolithiasis [2]
Nephrotoxicity [6]
Renal failure [3]

Hematologic
Eosinophilia [2]
Hemolysis [9]
Hemolytic anemia [14]
Thrombocytopenia [4]

Local
Injection-site pain (<10%) [3]
Injection-site phlebitis [2]

Other
Adverse effects [6]
Death [9]
Side effects (3%) [2]

CEFUROXIME

Trade names: Ceftin (GSK), Zinacef (Concordia)
Indications: Various infections caused by susceptible organisms
Class: Cephalosporin, 2nd generation
Half-life: 1–2 hours
Clinically important, potentially hazardous interactions with: none known
Pregnancy category: B
Important contra-indications noted in the prescribing guidelines for: nursing mothers
Note: Penicillin and cephalosporins share a common beta-lactam structure. People who are allergic to penicillin are approximately 4 times more likely to develop an allergic reaction to a cephalosporin than those people who have no penicillin allergy (from 5–16% of patients allergic to penicillin develop reactions to cephalosporins).

Skin
AGEP [2]
Anaphylactoid reactions/Anaphylaxis [7]
Exanthems [2]
Hypersensitivity [4]
Serum sickness [2]
Toxic epidermal necrolysis [2]
Urticaria [2]

Cardiovascular
Thrombophlebitis (<10%)

Gastrointestinal/Hepatic
Nausea [2]

Ocular
Ocular toxicity [2]

Other
Kounis syndrome [3]

CELECOXIB

Trade name: Celebrex (Pfizer)
Indications: Osteoarthritis, rheumatoid arthritis (adults and juveniles aged 2 years and over), ankylosing spondylitis, acute pain, primary dysmenorrhea
Class: COX-2 inhibitor, Non-steroidal anti-inflammatory (NSAID), Sulfonamide
Half-life: 11 hours
Clinically important, potentially hazardous interactions with: ACE inhibitors, aliskiren, angiotensin II receptor antagonists, aspirin, dexibuprofen, fluconazole, furosemide, lithium, NSAIDs, warfarin
Pregnancy category: D (pregnancy category C prior to 30 weeks gestation; category D starting at 30 weeks gestation)
Important contra-indications noted in the prescribing guidelines for: the elderly; nursing mothers; pediatric patients
Note: Celecoxib is a sulfonamide and can be absorbed systemically. Sulfonamides can produce severe, possibly fatal, reactions such as toxic epidermal necrolysis and Stevens-Johnson syndrome. NSAIDs may cause an increased risk of serious cardiovascular and gastrointestinal adverse events, which can be fatal. This risk may increase with duration of use.
Contraindicated in patients with known hypersensitivity to celecoxib, aspirin, or other NSAIDs; in patients who have demonstrated allergic-type reactions to sulfonamides; in patients who have experienced asthma, urticaria, or allergic-type reactions after taking aspirin or other NSAIDs; and for the treatment of peri-operative pain in the setting of coronary artery bypass graft surgery.

Black Box Warning: CARDIOVASCULAR AND GASTROINTESTINAL RISKS

Skin
AGEP [7]
Anaphylactoid reactions/Anaphylaxis [8]
Angioedema [9]
Bacterial infection (<2%)
Candidiasis (<2%)
Dermatitis (<2%) [2]
Diaphoresis (<2%)
Edema (<2%) [5]
Erythema [2]
Erythema multiforme [3]
Exanthems (<2%) [7]
Facial edema (<2%)
Fixed eruption [2]
Herpes simplex (<2%)
Herpes zoster (<2%)
Hot flashes (<2%)
Hypersensitivity [8]
Nodular eruption (<2%)
Peripheral edema (2%) [2]
Photosensitivity (<2%)
Pruritus (<2%) [6]
Rash (2%) [11]
Stevens–Johnson syndrome [2]
Sweet's syndrome [3]
Toxic epidermal necrolysis [5]
Urticaria (<2%) [11]
Vasculitis [4]
Xerosis (<2%)

Hair
Alopecia (<2%) [3]

Nails
Nail changes (<2%)

Mucosal
Stomatitis (<2%) [4]
Xerostomia (<2%)

Cardiovascular
Cardiotoxicity [2]
Hypertension [2]
Myocardial infarction [4]

Central Nervous System
Anorexia [3]
Depression [2]
Dysgeusia (taste perversion) (<2%)
Headache [3]
Paresthesias (<2%)
Stroke [3]
Vertigo (dizziness) [3]

Neuromuscular/Skeletal
Asthenia (fatigue) [6]
Myalgia/Myopathy (<2%)
Tendinopathy/Tendon rupture (<2%)

Gastrointestinal/Hepatic
Abdominal pain [10]
Constipation [5]
Diarrhea [11]
Dyspepsia [10]
Flatulence [2]
Gastrointestinal bleeding [4]
Nausea [14]
Vomiting [9]

Endocrine/Metabolic
Dehydration [2]
Mastodynia (<2%)

Genitourinary
Vaginitis (<2%)
Vulvovaginal candidiasis (<2%)

Renal
Nephrotoxicity [4]

Hematologic
Anemia [2]
Neutropenia [4]

Ocular
Visual disturbances [3]

Local
Application-site cellulitis (<2%)
Application-site reactions (<2%)

Other
Adverse effects [16]
Allergic reactions (<2%) [2]
Death [4]
Infection (<2%)
Tooth disorder (<2%)

CELIPROLOL

Trade names: Celectol (Winthrop), Celol (Pacific), Selectol (Sanofi-Aventis)
Indications: Hypertension, angina pectoris
Class: Beta blocker
Half-life: 5–6 hours
Clinically important, potentially hazardous interactions with: amiodarone, bepridil, diltiazem, disopyramide, floctafenine, quinidine, theophylline, verapamil
Pregnancy category: N/A
Important contra-indications noted in the prescribing guidelines for: nursing mothers

---

Central Nervous System
Headache [2]
Vertigo (dizziness) [2]

Neuromuscular/Skeletal
Asthenia (fatigue) [3]

CEPHALEXIN

Synonym: cefalexin
Trade names: Keflex (Advancis), Keftab (Biovail)
Indications: Various infections caused by susceptible organisms
Class: Cephalosporin, 1st generation
Half-life: 0.9–1.2 hours
Clinically important, potentially hazardous interactions with: amikacin, gentamicin, metformin
Pregnancy category: B
Important contra-indications noted in the prescribing guidelines for: the elderly; nursing mothers
Note: Penicillin and cephalosporins share a common beta-lactam structure. People who are allergic to penicillin are approximately 4 times more likely to develop an allergic reaction to a cephalosporin than those people who have no penicillin allergy (from 5–16% of patients allergic to penicillin develop reactions to cephalosporins).

Skin
AGEP [4]
Anaphylactoid reactions/Anaphylaxis [4]
Angioedema [2]
Bullous pemphigoid [2]
Erythema multiforme [3]
Exanthems [3]
Pemphigus [2]
Pruritus [3]
Pustules [2]
Stevens–Johnson syndrome [3]
Toxic epidermal necrolysis [4]
Urticaria [2]

Other
Adverse effects [2]
Side effects (2%) [2]

CERTOLIZUMAB

Trade name: Cimzia (Celltech) (UCB)
Indications: Crohn's disease, rheumatoid arthritis
Class: Disease-modifying antirheumatic drug (DMARD), Monoclonal antibody, TNF inhibitor
Half-life: 14 days
Clinically important, potentially hazardous interactions with: abatacept, anakinra, lenalidomide, live vaccines, natalizumab, rituximab
Pregnancy category: B
Important contra-indications noted in the prescribing guidelines for: nursing mothers; pediatric patients
Note: TNF inhibitors should be used in patients with heart failure only after consideration of other treatment options. TNF inhibitors are contraindicated in patients with a personal or family history of multiple sclerosis or demyelinating disease. TNF inhibitors should not be administered to patients with moderate to severe heart failure (New York Heart Association Functional Class III/IV).
Black Box Warning: SERIOUS INFECTIONS AND MALIGNANCY

Skin
Herpes zoster [2]
Lupus syndrome [2]
Neoplasms [2]
Psoriasis [6]
Rash [2]

Cardiovascular
Hypertension [2]

Central Nervous System
Fever (5%) [2]
Headache (7–18%) [5]
Vertigo (dizziness) (~6%)

Neuromuscular/Skeletal
Arthralgia (6–7%) [4]
Back pain [3]

Gastrointestinal/Hepatic
Nausea [2]

Respiratory
Nasopharyngitis (4–13%) [8]
Pulmonary toxicity [2]
Sinusitis [2]
Upper respiratory tract infection (20%) [11]

Endocrine/Metabolic
Creatine phosphokinase increased [2]

Genitourinary
Urinary tract infection (~8%) [8]

Local
Injection-site pain [3]
Injection-site reactions (~7%) [3]

Other
Adverse effects [14]
Death [2]
Infection (14–38%) [14]

CETIRIZINE

Trade name: Zyrtec (Pfizer)
Indications: Allergic rhinitis, urticaria
Class: Histamine H1 receptor antagonist
Half-life: 8–11 hours
Clinically important, potentially hazardous interactions with: alcohol, CNS depressants, pilsicainide
Pregnancy category: B
Important contra-indications noted in the prescribing guidelines for: nursing mothers

---

Skin
Acneform eruption (<2%)
Anaphylactoid reactions/Anaphylaxis (<2%) [2]
Angioedema (<2%)
Bullous dermatitis (<2%)
Dermatitis (<2%)
Diaphoresis (<2%)
Exanthems (<2%)
Fixed eruption [6]
Furunculosis (<2%)
Hyperkeratosis (<2%)
Photosensitivity (<2%)
Phototoxicity (<2%)
Pruritus (<2%)
Purpura (<2%)
Rash (<2%)
Seborrhea (<2%)
Urticaria (<2%) [9]
Xerosis (<2%)

Hair
Alopecia (<2%)
Hypertrichosis (<2%)

Mucosal
Sialorrhea (<2%)
Stomatitis (<2%)
Tongue edema (<2%)
Tongue pigmentation (<2%)
Xerostomia (6%) [2]

Cardiovascular
Flushing (<2%)
QT prolongation [2]

Central Nervous System
Ageusia (taste loss) (<2%)
Dysgeusia (taste perversion) (<2%)
Hyperesthesia (<2%)
Insomnia [2]
Paresthesias (<2%)
Parosmia (<2%)
Somnolence (drowsiness) [4]

Neuromuscular/Skeletal
Asthenia (fatigue) [3]
Dystonia [5]
Myalgia/Myopathy (<2%)

Endocrine/Metabolic
Mastodynia (<2%)

Genitourinary
Vaginitis (<2%)

Other
Adverse effects [4]

CETRORELIX

Trade name: Cetrotide (Merck)
Indications: Inhibition of premature luteinizing hormone surges in women undergoing controlled ovarian stimulation
Class: Gonadotropin-releasing hormone (GnRH) antagonist
Half-life: 5 hours
Clinically important, potentially hazardous interactions with: none known
Pregnancy category: X
Important contra-indications noted in the prescribing guidelines for: nursing mothers

---

Skin
Hot flashes [2]

Central Nervous System
Headache [2]

CETUXIMAB

Trade name: Erbitux (Bristol-Myers Squibb)
Indications: Metastatic colorectal cancer, squamous cell carcinoma of the head and neck
Class: Antineoplastic, Biologic, Epidermal growth factor receptor (EGFR) inhibitor, Monoclonal antibody
Half-life: 75–188 hours
Clinically important, potentially hazardous interactions with: none known
Pregnancy category: C
Important contra-indications noted in the prescribing guidelines for: nursing mothers; pediatric patients
Black Box Warning: SERIOUS INFUSION REACTIONS and CARDIOPULMONARY ARREST

Skin
Acneform eruption (88%) [61]
Anaphylactoid reactions/Anaphylaxis [5]
Dermatitis [4]
Desquamation (89%) [3]
Erythema [3]
Exanthems [5]
Fissures [4]
Folliculitis [12]
Hand–foot syndrome [5]
Hypersensitivity [8]
Papulopustular eruption [6]
Peripheral edema (10%)
Pruritus (40%) [9]
Rash (89%) [46]
Toxic epidermal necrolysis [2]
Toxicity [18]
Xerosis (49%) [14]

Hair
Abnormal hair growth [2]
Alopecia (5%)
Hair changes [3]
Hypertrichosis [3]

Nails
Nail changes (21%)
Nail disorder [2]
Paronychia [14]

Mucosal
Mucositis [10]
Stomatitis (25%) [3]
Xerostomia (11%)

Cardiovascular
Cardiotoxicity [2]
Flushing [2]
Thromboembolism [2]

Central Nervous System
Anorexia [2]
Anxiety (14%)
Aseptic meningitis [6]
Chills (13%) [2]
Confusion (15%)
Depression (13%)
Fever (30%) [4]
Headache (33%)
Insomnia (30%)
Pain (51%)
Peripheral neuropathy [3]
Rigors (13%)
Seizures [2]

Neuromuscular/Skeletal
Asthenia (fatigue) (89%) [23]
Back pain (11%)
Bone or joint pain (15%)

Gastrointestinal/Hepatic
Abdominal pain (59%)
Constipation (46%)
Diarrhea (39%) [18]
Dysphagia [2]
Hepatotoxicity [4]
Nausea [10]
Vomiting (37%) [7]

Respiratory
Cough (29%)
Dyspnea (48%) [5]
Pneumonia [2]
Pneumonitis [3]
Pulmonary toxicity [5]

Endocrine/Metabolic
Hypokalemia [6]
Hypomagnesemia [15]
Hyponatremia [4]

Hematologic
Anemia [6]
Febrile neutropenia [4]
Leukopenia [7]
Neutropenia [21]
Sepsis (<4%)
Thrombocytopenia [5]
Thrombosis [3]

Ocular
Blepharitis [3]
Conjunctivitis (7%) [2]
Ectropion [2]

Eyelashes – hypertrichosis [3]
Trichomegaly [11]

Local
Application-site reactions (~3%)
Infusion-related reactions [6]
Infusion-site reactions (15–21%) [10]

Other
Adverse effects [6]
Allergic reactions [3]
Death [6]
Infection (13–35%) [3]

CEVIMELINE

Trade name: Evoxac (Daiichi Sankyo)
Indications: Sicca syndrome in patients with Sjøgren's syndrome
Class: Muscarinic cholinergic agonist
Half-life: 3–4 hours
Clinically important, potentially hazardous interactions with: none known
Pregnancy category: C
Important contra-indications noted in the prescribing guidelines for: nursing mothers; pediatric patients
Note: Contraindicated in patients with uncontrolled asthma, acute iritis or narrow-angle glaucoma.

Skin
Abscess (<3%)
Candidiasis (<3%)
Diaphoresis (20%)
Edema (<3%)
Erythema (<3%)
Exanthems (<10%)
Fungal dermatitis (<10%)
Hot flashes (2%)
Hyperhidrosis (19%) [5]
Peripheral edema (<3%)
Pruritus (<3%)
Rash (4%)

Mucosal
Epistaxis (nosebleed) (<3%)
Sialadenitis (<3%)
Sialorrhea (2%)
Ulcerative stomatitis (<3%)
Xerostomia (<3%)

Cardiovascular
Chest pain (<3%)
Palpitation (<3%)

Central Nervous System
Anorexia (<3%)
Depression (<3%)
Fever (<3%)
Headache (14%)
Hypoesthesia (<3%)
Hyporeflexia (<3%)
Insomnia (2%)
Migraine (<3%)
Pain (3%)
Tremor (<3%)
Vertigo (dizziness) (4%)

Neuromuscular/Skeletal
Arthralgia (4%)
Back pain (5%)
Bone or joint pain (3%)
Hypertonia (<3%)
Leg cramps (<3%)
Myalgia/Myopathy (<3%)

Gastrointestinal/Hepatic
Abdominal pain (8%)
Constipation (<3%)
Diarrhea (10%)
Dyspepsia (8%)
Eructation (belching) (<3%)
Gastroesophageal reflux (<3%)
Nausea (14%) [3]
Vomiting (5%)

Respiratory
Bronchitis (4%)
Cough (6%)
Flu-like syndrome (<3%)
Pharyngitis (5%)
Pneumonia (<3%)
Rhinitis (11%)
Sinusitis (12%)
Upper respiratory tract infection (11%)

Genitourinary
Urinary tract infection (6%)
Vaginitis (<3%)

Hematologic
Anemia (<3%)

Otic
Ear pain (<3%)
Otitis media (<3%)

Ocular
Abnormal vision (<3%)
Conjunctivitis (4%)
Ocular pain (<3%)
Xerophthalmia (<3%)

Other
Allergic reactions (<3%)
Infection (<3%)
Tooth disorder (<3%)

CHLORAL HYDRATE

Indications: Insomnia, sedation
Class: Anesthetic, general, Hypnotic
Half-life: 8–11 hours
Clinically important, potentially hazardous interactions with: antihistamines, azatadine, brompheniramine, buclizine, chlorpheniramine, clemastine, dexchlorpheniramine, diphenhydramine, meclizine, tripelennamine
Pregnancy category: C
Important contra-indications noted in the prescribing guidelines for: nursing mothers

---

Skin
Acneform eruption [2]
Angioedema [2]
Dermatitis [2]
Erythema multiforme [2]
Exanthems [3]
Fixed eruption [5]
Pruritus [2]
Purpura [2]
Rash (<10%)
Urticaria (<10%) [2]

Mucosal
Oral lesions [2]

Cardiovascular
Hypotension [2]

Central Nervous System
Agitation [2]
Sedation (prolonged) [2]

Gastrointestinal/Hepatic
Vomiting [4]

Respiratory
Apnea [2]

Other
Adverse effects [3]
Death [3]

CHLORAMPHENICOL

Indications: Various infections caused by susceptible organisms
Class: Antibiotic, CYP3A4 inhibitor
Half-life: 1.5–3.5 hours
Clinically important, potentially hazardous interactions with: amoxicillin, ampicillin, clopidogrel, clozapine, ethotoin, fosphenytoin, gliclazide, levodopa, mephenytoin, phenytoin, propyphenazone, voriconazole
Pregnancy category: C
Important contra-indications noted in the prescribing guidelines for: nursing mothers

---

Skin
AGEP [2]
Dermatitis [18]
Erythema multiforme [6]
Exanthems (<5%) [5]
Hypersensitivity [2]
Purpura [2]
Pustules [2]
Sensitization [2]
Toxic epidermal necrolysis [2]
Urticaria [3]

Nails
Photo-onycholysis [2]

CHLORDIAZEPOXIDE

Trade names: Libritabs (Valeant), Librium (Valeant), Limbitrol (Valeant)
Indications: Anxiety
Class: Benzodiazepine
Half-life: 6–25 hours
Clinically important, potentially hazardous interactions with: chlorpheniramine, clarithromycin, efavirenz, esomeprazole, imatinib, indinavir, ketoconazole, nelfinavir, nilutamide, ritonavir
Pregnancy category: D
Important contra-indications noted in the prescribing guidelines for: the elderly; nursing mothers; pediatric patients
Note: Limbitrol is chlordiazepoxide and amitriptyline.

Skin
Angioedema [3]
Dermatitis (<10%)
Diaphoresis (>10%)
Edema (<10%)

Erythema multiforme [5]
Erythema nodosum [2]
Exanthems [3]
Fixed eruption [7]
Lupus erythematosus [3]
Photosensitivity [6]
Purpura [5]
Rash (>10%)
Urticaria [4]
Vasculitis [2]

Hair
Alopecia [3]

Mucosal
Sialopenia (>10%)
Sialorrhea (<10%)
Xerostomia (>10%)

Endocrine/Metabolic
Galactorrhea [3]

CHLORHEXIDINE

Trade name: Hibiclens (SSL)
Indications: Skin antisepsis, gingivitis
Class: Antiseptic
Half-life: N/A
Clinically important, potentially hazardous interactions with: none known
Pregnancy category: B
Important contra-indications noted in the prescribing guidelines for: nursing mothers; pediatric patients

---

Skin
Anaphylactoid reactions/Anaphylaxis [28]
Dermatitis [16]
Hypersensitivity [9]
Rash [2]
Urticaria [4]

Mucosal
Gingival pigmentation [2]
Gingivitis [3]
Glossitis (<10%)
Stomatitis (<10%)
Tongue irritation (<10%)
Tongue pigmentation (>10%)

Central Nervous System
Dysgeusia (taste perversion) (>10%) [5]

Other
Allergic reactions [6]
Tooth pigmentation [3]

CHLOROQUINE

Trade name: Aralen (Sanofi-Aventis)
Indications: Malaria, rheumatoid arthritis, lupus erythematosus
Class: Antimalarial, Antiprotozoal, Disease-modifying antirheumatic drug (DMARD)
Half-life: 3–5 days
Clinically important, potentially hazardous interactions with: acitretin, antacids, arsenic, cholestyramine, citalopram, dapsone, dasatinib, degarelix, droperidol, ethosuximide, furazolidone, halofantrine, hydroxychloroquine, lacosamide, lanthanum, lapatinib, levofloxacin, methotrexate, methoxsalen, mivacurium, moxifloxacin, neostigmine, nilotinib, oxcarbazepine, pazopanib, penicillamine, sulfonamides, telavancin, telithromycin, tiagabine, typhoid vaccine, vandetanib, vigabatrin, voriconazole, vorinostat, ziprasidone
Pregnancy category: D
Important contra-indications noted in the prescribing guidelines for: nursing mothers

---

Skin
Dermatitis [2]
Erythema annulare centrifugum [2]
Erythroderma [3]
Exanthems (<5%) [3]
Exfoliative dermatitis [4]
Lichenoid eruption [6]
Photosensitivity [8]
Pigmentation [15]
Pruritus [36]
Psoriasis [18]
Stevens–Johnson syndrome [4]
Toxic epidermal necrolysis [5]
Toxicity [2]
Urticaria [4]
Vitiligo [7]

Hair
Hair pigmentation [10]
Poliosis [3]

Nails
Nail pigmentation [2]

Mucosal
Mucosal membrane pigmentation [2]
Oral pigmentation [12]

Cardiovascular
Atrioventricular block [2]
Cardiac failure [2]
Cardiomyopathy [8]
Cardiotoxicity [3]
Congestive heart failure [2]
Myocardial toxicity [2]
QT prolongation [3]
Torsades de pointes [2]

Central Nervous System
Headache [4]
Psychosis [4]
Seizures [2]
Vertigo (dizziness) [4]

Neuromuscular/Skeletal
Myalgia/Myopathy [8]
Myasthenia gravis [7]

Gastrointestinal/Hepatic
Diarrhea [2]
Nausea [3]
Vomiting [5]

Endocrine/Metabolic
Porphyria [7]

Ocular
Corneal deposits [2]
Keratopathy [2]
Maculopathy [3]
Ocular adverse effects [2]
Ocular toxicity [4]
Retinopathy [10]
Vision blurred [2]

Other
Adverse effects [2]
Death [3]

CHLORPHENIRAMINE

Synonym: chlorphenamine
Trade names: Chlor-Trimeton (Schering), Triaminic (Novartis)
Indications: Allergic rhinitis, urticaria
Class: Histamine H1 receptor antagonist, Muscarinic antagonist
Half-life: 20–40 hours
Clinically important, potentially hazardous interactions with: alcohol, anticholinergics, barbiturates, benzodiazepines, butabarbital, chloral hydrate, chlordiazepoxide, chlorpromazine, clonazepam, clorazepate, diazepam, ethchlorvynol, fluphenazine, flurazepam, hypnotics, lopinavir, lorazepam, MAO inhibitors, mephobarbital, mesoridazine, midazolam, narcotics, oxazepam, pentobarbital, phenobarbital, phenothiazines, phenylbutazone, primidone, prochlorperazine, promethazine, quazepam, secobarbital, sedatives, temazepam, thioridazine, tranquilizers, trifluoperazine, zolpidem
Pregnancy category: B
Important contra-indications noted in the prescribing guidelines for: the elderly; nursing mothers; pediatric patients

---

Skin
Angioedema (<10%)
Dermatitis (<10%) [4]
Photosensitivity (<10%)

Mucosal
Xerostomia (<10%)

Central Nervous System
Seizures [2]

CHLORPROMAZINE

Trade name: Thorazine (GSK)
Indications: Psychosis, manic-depressive disorders
Class: Antiemetic, Antipsychotic, Muscarinic antagonist, Phenothiazine
Half-life: initial: 2 hours; terminal: 30 hours
Clinically important, potentially hazardous interactions with: alcohol, antihistamines, arsenic, asenapine, chlorpheniramine, dofetilide, epinephrine, evening primrose, guanethidine, lisdexamfetamine, mivacurium, propranolol, quinolones, sodium picosulfate, sparfloxacin, tetrabenazine, zolpidem
Pregnancy category: N/A
Important contra-indications noted in the prescribing guidelines for: the elderly; nursing mothers; pediatric patients
Note: The prolonged use of chlorpromazine can produce a gray-blue or purplish pigmentation over light-exposed areas. This is a result of either dermal deposits of melanin, a chlorpromazine metabolite, or to a combination of both. Chlorpromazine melanosis is seen more often in women.
Black Box Warning: INCREASED MORTALITY IN ELDERLY PATIENTS WITH DEMENTIA-RELATED PSYCHOSIS

Skin
Exanthems (>5%) [8]
Lupus erythematosus [12]
Photosensitivity (<10%) [22]
Phototoxicity [6]
Pigmentation [16]
Pruritus (<10%) [2]
Purpura [6]
Rash (<10%)
Seborrheic dermatitis [4]
Toxic epidermal necrolysis [2]
Urticaria [4]
Vasculitis [3]

Nails
Nail pigmentation [4]

Mucosal
Xerostomia (<10%)

Cardiovascular
Hypotension [3]
QT prolongation [4]
Tachycardia [2]
Torsades de pointes [2]

Central Nervous System
Neuroleptic malignant syndrome [5]
Sedation [2]

Endocrine/Metabolic
Galactorrhea (<10%)
Gynecomastia (<10%)
Mastodynia (<10%)

Genitourinary
Priapism [7]

Otic
Tinnitus [2]

Ocular
Cataract [2]
Corneal opacity [2]
Eyelid edema [2]
Retinopathy [2]

Other
Adverse effects [3]

CHOLERA VACCINE *

Trade name: Vaxchora (PaxVax)
Indications: Immunization against cholera for adults traveling to cholera-affected areas
Class: Vaccine
Half-life: N/A
Clinically important, potentially hazardous interactions with: antibiotics, chloroquine
Pregnancy category: N/A (Not expected to cause fetal risk)
Important contra-indications noted in the prescribing guidelines for: the elderly; pediatric patients

---

Central Nervous System
Headache (29%)

Neuromuscular/Skeletal
Asthenia (fatigue) (31%)

Gastrointestinal/Hepatic
Abdominal pain (19%)
Diarrhea (4%)
Nausea (18%)
Vomiting (18%)

Endocrine/Metabolic
Appetite decreased (17%)

CHOLESTYRAMINE

Trade name: Questran (Par)
Indications: Pruritus associated with biliary obstruction, primary hypercholesterolemia
Class: Bile acid sequestrant
Half-life: N/A
Clinically important, potentially hazardous interactions with: acarbose, acetaminophen, acitretin, amiodarone, aspirin, bezafibrate, chloroquine, cyclopenthiazide, cyclosporine, deferasirox, digoxin, doxepin, doxercalciferol, ergocalciferol, hydroxychloroquine, isotretinoin, leflunomide, levodopa, lovastatin, meloxicam, mycophenolate, phytonadione, propranolol, raloxifene, sulfasalazine, sulfonylureas, tetracycline, tricyclic antidepressants, troglitazone, ursodiol, valproic acid, vitamin A, vitamin E
Pregnancy category: C
Important contra-indications noted in the prescribing guidelines for: nursing mothers; pediatric patients
Note: Contraindicated in patients with complete biliary obstruction.

Skin
Pruritus [2]

Neuromuscular/Skeletal
Osteomalacia [2]

Hematologic
Hemorrhage [2]

CHOLIC ACID

Trade name: Cholbam (Asklepion Pharmaceuticals)
Indications: Bile acid synthesis disorders, adjunctive treatment of peroxisomal disorders
Class: Bile acid
Half-life: N/A
Clinically important, potentially hazardous interactions with: cyclosporine
Pregnancy category: N/A
Important contra-indications noted in the prescribing guidelines for: the elderly; nursing mothers

---

Gastrointestinal/Hepatic
Diarrhea (2%)

CIDOFOVIR

Trade name: Vistide (Gilead)
Indications: Cytomegalovirus (CMV) retinitis in patients with acquired immunodeficiency syndrome (AIDS)
Class: Antiviral, nucleotide analog
Half-life: ~2.6 hours
Clinically important, potentially hazardous interactions with: amphotericin B, cobicistat/elvitegravir/emtricitabine/tenofovir disoproxil, tenofovir disoproxil
Pregnancy category: C
Important contra-indications noted in the prescribing guidelines for: the elderly; nursing mothers; pediatric patients
Black Box Warning: RENAL TOXICITY and NEUTROPENIA

Skin
Acneform eruption (>10%)
Diaphoresis (<10%)
DRESS syndrome [2]
Pallor (<10%)
Pigmentation (>10%)
Pruritus (<10%) [2]
Rash (27%) [2]
Toxicity [3]
Ulcerations [2]
Urticaria (<10%)

Hair
Alopecia (22%) [2]

Mucosal
Stomatitis (<10%)

Central Nervous System
Chills (24%)
Dysgeusia (taste perversion) (<10%)
Headache [4]
Paresthesias (>10%)

Neuromuscular/Skeletal
Asthenia (fatigue) [2]
Myalgia/Myopathy [2]

Renal
Fanconi syndrome [2]
Nephrotoxicity [5]

Ocular
Intraocular inflammation [2]
Iritis [6]
Ocular hypotension [2]
Retinal detachment [3]
Uveitis [18]
Vision impaired [3]
Vision loss [3]

Local
Application-site reactions (39%) [3]

Other
Allergic reactions (<10%)

CILOSTAZOL

Trade name: Pletal (Otsuka)
Indications: Peripheral vascular disease, intermittent claudication
Class: Antiplatelet, Phosphodiesterase inhibitor, Vasodilator, peripheral
Half-life: 11–13 hours
Clinically important, potentially hazardous interactions with: anagrelide, anticoagulants, antifungals, antiplatelet agents, clarithromycin, collagenase, conivaptan, CYP2C19 inhibitors, CYP3A4 inhibitors and inducers, dasatinib, deferasirox, diltiazem, drotrecogin alfa, erythromycin, esomeprazole, fondaparinux, glucosamine, grapefruit juice, high-fat foods, ibritumomab, itraconazole, ketoconazole, macrolide antibiotics, NSAIDs, omeprazole, PEG-interferon, pentosan, pentoxifylline, prostacyclin analogues, salicylates, St John's wort, telithromycin, thrombolytic agents, tositumomab & iodine^{131}, voriconazole
Pregnancy category: C
Important contra-indications noted in the prescribing guidelines for: nursing mothers; pediatric patients
Note: Contraindicated in patients with congestive heart failure or active pathological bleeding.
Black Box Warning: CONTRAINDICATED IN HEART FAILURE PATIENTS

Skin
Ecchymoses (<2%)
Edema (<2%)
Facial edema (<2%)
Furunculosis (<2%)
Hypertrophy (<2%)
Peripheral edema (7–9%)
Purpura (<2%)
Rash (2%) [2]
Urticaria (<2%)
Varicosities (<2%)
Xerosis (<2%)

Mucosal
Epistaxis (nosebleed) (<2%)
Gingival bleeding (<2%)
Perioral abscess (<2%)
Rectal hemorrhage (<2%)
Tongue edema (<2%)

Cardiovascular
Arrhythmias (<2%)
Atrial fibrillation (<2%)
Atrial flutter (<2%)
Cardiac arrest (<2%)
Cardiotoxicity [4]
Congestive heart failure (<2%)
Extrasystoles (<2%)
Hypotension (<2%)
Myocardial infarction (<2%) [4]
Myocardial ischemia (<2%)
Palpitation (5–10%) [6]
Postural hypotension (<2%)
Supraventricular tachycardia (<2%)
Tachycardia (4%) [3]
Vasodilation (<2%)
Ventricular tachycardia (<2%)

Central Nervous System
Anorexia (<2%)
Anxiety (<2%)
Cerebral ischemia (<2%)
Chills (<2%)
Headache (27–34%) [18]
Hyperesthesia (2%)
Insomnia (<2%)
Neurotoxicity (<2%)
Paresthesias (2%)
Syncope (<2%)
Vertigo (dizziness) (<10%) [3]

Neuromuscular/Skeletal
Arthralgia (<2%)
Asthenia (fatigue) (<2%)
Back pain (6–7%)
Bone or joint pain (<2%)
Gouty tophi (<2%)
Myalgia/Myopathy (2–3%)

Gastrointestinal/Hepatic
Abdominal pain (4–5%)
Black stools (<2%)
Cholelithiasis (gallstones) (<2%)
Colitis (<2%)
Diarrhea (12–19%) [6]
Dyspepsia (6%)
Esophagitis (<2%)
Flatulence (2–3%)
Gastritis (<2%)
Gastroenteritis (<2%)
Gastrointestinal ulceration (<2%)
Hematemesis (<2%)
Nausea (6–7%) [4]
Peptic ulceration (<2%)
Vomiting (>2%)

Respiratory
Asthma (<2%)
Cough (3–4%) [2]
Hemoptysis (<2%)
Pharyngitis (7–10%)
Pneumonia (<2%)
Rhinitis (7–12%)
Sinusitis (<2%)

Endocrine/Metabolic
Creatine phosphokinase increased (<2%)
Diabetes mellitus (<2%)
GGT increased (<2%)
Hyperlipidemia (<2%)
Hyperuricemia (<2%)

Genitourinary
Albuminuria (<2%)
Cystitis (<2%)
Urinary frequency (<2%)
Vaginal bleeding (<2%)
Vaginitis (<2%)

Renal
Retroperitoneal bleeding (<2%)

Hematologic
Anemia (<2%)
Hemorrhage (<2%)
Polycythemia (<2%)
Thrombosis [3]

Otic
Ear pain (<2%)
Tinnitus (<2%)

Ocular
Amblyopia (<2%)
Blindness (<2%)
Conjunctivitis (<2%)
Diplopia (<2%)
Ocular hemorrhage (<2%)

Other
Adverse effects [4]
Death [3]
Infection (10–14%)

CIMETIDINE

Trade name: Tagamet (GSK)
Indications: Duodenal ulcer
Class: CYP1A2 inhibitor, CYP3A4 inhibitor, Histamine H2 receptor antagonist
Half-life: 2 hours
Clinically important, potentially hazardous interactions with: acenocoumarol, alfuzosin, aminophylline, amiodarone, amitriptyline, anisindione, anticoagulants, buprenorphine, butorphanol, caffeine, carmustine, citalopram, clobazam, clopidogrel, clozapine, cocoa, delavirdine, dicumarol, dofetilide, duloxetine, dutasteride, epirubicin, eszopiclone, fentanyl, ferrous sulfate, floxuridine, fluorouracil, galantamine, gliclazide, hydromorphone, itraconazole, ketoconazole, labetalol, levomepromazine, lidocaine, lomustine, meptazinol, metformin, metronidazole, midazolam, mizolastine, moclobemide, morphine, narcotic analgesics, oxprenolol, oxtriphylline, oxycodone, oxymorphone, pentazocine, phenytoin, pimecrolimus, posaconazole, prednisone, propranolol, quinine, rilpivirine, risperidone, roflumilast, sertindole, sildenafil, sufentanil, tamsulosin, terbinafine, thalidomide, tolazoline, warfarin, xanthines, zaleplon, zofenopril, zolmitriptan, zolpidem
Pregnancy category: B
Important contra-indications noted in the prescribing guidelines for: nursing mothers; pediatric patients

---

Skin
Angioedema [3]
Erythema annulare centrifugum [2]
Erythema multiforme [5]
Exanthems [3]
Exfoliative dermatitis [2]
Fixed eruption [2]
Hypersensitivity [4]
Lupus erythematosus [3]
Pruritus [6]
Pseudolymphoma [2]
Psoriasis [6]
Rash (<2%)
Stevens-Johnson syndrome [3]
Toxic epidermal necrolysis [2]
Urticaria [6]
Vasculitis [3]

Hair
Alopecia [4]

Central Nervous System
Hallucinations [3]

Neuromuscular/Skeletal
Myalgia/Myopathy [2]

Endocrine/Metabolic
Gynecomastia [12]

Renal
Nephrotoxicity [3]

CIPROFLOXACIN

Trade names: Ciloxan Ophthalmic (Alcon), Cipro (Bayer), Ciproxin (Bayer)
Indications: Various infections caused by susceptible organisms, inhalational anthrax (post exposure)
Class: Antibiotic, fluoroquinolone, CYP1A2 inhibitor, CYP3A4 inhibitor
Half-life: 4 hours
Clinically important, potentially hazardous interactions with: agomelatine, aminophylline, amiodarone, amitriptyline, antacids, antineoplastics, arsenic, artemether/lumefantrine, BCG vaccine, bendamustine, bepridil, bismuth, bismuth subsalicylate, bretylium, calcium salts, citalopram, clopidogrel, clozapine, corticosteroids, cyclosporine, dairy products, dasatinib, degarelix, didanosine, disopyramide, dolasetron, duloxetine, dutasteride, erlotinib, erythromycin, flibanserin, insulin, lanthanum, lapatinib, levofloxacin, magnesium salts, meptazinol, methotrexate, methylxanthines, mifepristone, moxifloxacin, mycophenolate, NSAIDs, olanzapine, opiod analgesics, oral iron, oxtriphylline, P-glycoprotein inhibitors, pazopanib, pentoxifylline, phenothiazines, phenytoin, pirfenidone, probenecid, procainamide, propranolol, QT prolonging agents, quinapril, quinidine, rasagiline, ropinirole, ropivacaine, sevelamer, sotalol, St John's wort, strontium ranelate, sucralfate, sulfonylureas, telavancin, telithromycin, tizanidine, tricyclic antidepressants, typhoid vaccine, venetoclax, vitamin K antagonists, voriconazole, vorinostat, warfarin, zinc, ziprasidone, zolmitriptan
Pregnancy category: C
Important contra-indications noted in the prescribing guidelines for: the elderly; nursing mothers
Note: Fluoroquinolones are associated with an increased risk of tendinitis and tendon rupture in all ages. This risk is further increased in older patients usually over 60 years of age, in patients taking corticosteroid drugs, and in patients with kidney, heart or lung transplants.
Fluoroquinolones may exacerbate muscle weakness in persons with myasthenia gravis.
Ciprofloxacin is chemically related to nalidixic acid.
Black Box Warning: SERIOUS ADVERSE REACTIONS INCLUDING TENDINITIS, TENDON RUPTURE, PERIPHERAL NEUROPATHY, CENTRIAL NERVOUS SYSTEM EFFECTS and EXACERBATION OF MYASTHENIA GRAVIS

Skin
- Acneform eruption [3]
- AGEP [3]
- Anaphylactoid reactions/Anaphylaxis [15]
- Angioedema [7]
- Candidiasis [2]
- Diaphoresis [4]
- Erythema multiforme [5]
- Exanthems [4]
- Fixed eruption [12]
- Hypersensitivity [5]
- Linear IgA bullous dermatosis [2]
- Photosensitivity [18]
- Phototoxicity [5]
- Pruritus [10]
- Purpura [4]
- Rash (<10%) [12]
- Serum sickness [2]
- Stevens–Johnson syndrome [8]
- Toxic epidermal necrolysis [10]
- Toxicity [2]
- Urticaria [8]
- Vasculitis [11]

Mucosal
- Stomatitis [3]
- Xerostomia [3]

Cardiovascular
- QT prolongation [11]
- Torsades de pointes [8]

Central Nervous System
- Dysgeusia (taste perversion) [2]
- Fever [2]
- Headache [5]
- Mania [3]
- Psychosis [5]
- Seizures [5]

Neuromuscular/Skeletal
- Arthralgia [2]
- Asthenia (fatigue) [2]
- Myasthenia gravis (exacerbation) [2]
- Myoclonus [3]
- Rhabdomyolysis [3]
- Tendinitis [3]
- Tendinopathy/Tendon rupture [31]

Gastrointestinal/Hepatic
- Flatulence [2]
- Hepatitis [4]
- Hepatotoxicity [5]
- Nausea (3%) [3]
- Pancreatitis [2]

Genitourinary
- Vaginitis [2]

Renal
- Nephrotoxicity [9]
- Renal failure [3]

Hematologic
- Bone marrow suppression [2]
- Hemolytic anemia [2]
- Thrombocytopenia [3]

Ocular
- Hallucinations, visual [6]

Local
- Injection-site pain [2]

Other
- Adverse effects [7]
- Death [3]

CISPLATIN

Synonym: CDDP
Trade name: Platinol (Bristol-Myers Squibb)
Indications: Carcinomas, lymphomas
Class: Alkylating agent, Antineoplastic
Half-life: alpha phase: 25–49 minutes; beta phase: 58–73 hours
Clinically important, potentially hazardous interactions with: aldesleukin, atenolol, chlorothiazide, gadobenate, methotrexate, paclitaxel, pentamidine, rituximab, selenium, thalidomide, zinc
Pregnancy category: D
Important contra-indications noted in the prescribing guidelines for: the elderly; nursing mothers

---

Skin
- Acneform eruption [6]
- Anaphylactoid reactions/Anaphylaxis [10]
- Angioedema [4]
- Edema [3]
- Erythema [3]
- Exanthems [4]
- Hand–foot syndrome [9]
- Hypersensitivity [5]
- Necrosis [2]
- Peripheral edema [2]
- Pigmentation [5]
- Pruritus [7]
- Rash [19]
- Raynaud's phenomenon [14]
- Thrombocytopenic purpura [2]
- Toxic epidermal necrolysis [2]
- Toxicity [6]
- Urticaria [7]

Hair
- Alopecia (>10%) [23]

Mucosal
- Epistaxis (nosebleed) [3]
- Mucositis [14]
- Oral lesions [2]
- Stomatitis [16]

Cardiovascular
- Cardiotoxicity [2]
- Flushing [5]
- Hypertension [7]
- Thromboembolism [4]
- Venous thromboembolism [3]

Central Nervous System
- Anorexia [20]
- Dysgeusia (taste perversion) [3]
- Fever [5]
- Headache [4]
- Insomnia [4]
- Leukoencephalopathy [10]
- Neurotoxicity [12]
- Pain [3]
- Peripheral neuropathy [8]
- Seizures [3]
- Vertigo (dizziness) [2]

Neuromuscular/Skeletal
- Asthenia (fatigue) [31]
- Ataxia [2]
- Myalgia/Myopathy [3]

Gastrointestinal/Hepatic
- Abdominal pain [3]

Constipation [4]
Diarrhea [32]
Esophagitis [2]
Gastrointestinal bleeding [2]
Hepatotoxicity [6]
Nausea [40]
Pancreatitis [2]
Vomiting [30]

Respiratory
Cough [4]
Dysphonia [4]
Dyspnea [4]
Pneumonia [4]
Pneumonitis [3]
Pulmonary toxicity [4]

Endocrine/Metabolic
ALP increased [2]
ALT increased [5]
Appetite decreased [6]
AST increased [5]
Dehydration [3]
Hyperglycemia [3]
Hyperkalemia [2]
Hypocalcemia [2]
Hypokalemia [5]
Hypomagnesemia [11]
Hyponatremia [16]
Serum creatinine increased [5]
SIADH [18]
Weight loss [4]

Renal
Nephrotoxicity [54]
Proteinuria [2]
Renal failure [3]
Renal function abnormal [2]

Hematologic
Anemia [41]
Febrile neutropenia [29]
Hemolytic uremic syndrome [12]
Hemotoxicity [3]
Leukopenia [26]
Lymphopenia [4]
Myelosuppression [6]
Myelotoxicity [3]
Neutropenia [79]
Thrombocytopenia [44]
Thrombosis [2]

Otic
Hearing loss [12]
Ototoxicity [38]
Tinnitus [26]

Local
Injection-site cellulitis [4]

Other
Adverse effects [15]
Death [15]
Hiccups [5]
Infection [9]

CITALOPRAM

Trade names: Celexa (Forest), Cipramil (Lundbeck)
Indications: Depression, obsessive-compulsive disorder, panic disorder
Class: Antidepressant, Selective serotonin reuptake inhibitor (SSRI)
Half-life: ~35 hours
Clinically important, potentially hazardous interactions with: alcohol, alfuzosin, alpha or beta blockers, antidepressants, antiepileptics, antiplatelet agents, artemether/lumefantrine, aspirin, atomoxetine, barbiturates, bupropion, buspirone, carbamazepine, chloroquine, cimetidine, ciprofloxacin, clozapine, CNS depressants, collagenase, conivaptan, coumarins/anticoagulants, CYP2C19 inhibitors, CYP3A4 inhibitors, cyproheptadine, desmopressin, dexibuprofen, dextromethorphan, dronedarone, drotrecogin alfa, duloxetine, efavirenz, fluconazole, gadobutrol, glucosamine, haloperidol, ibritumomab, iobenguane, isocarboxazid, lithium, macrolide antibiotics, MAO inhibitors, methadone, methylphenidate, metoclopramide, mexiletine, moclobemide, nilotinib, NSAIDs, opioid anagesics, pentoxifylline, phenelzine, phenytoin, pimozide, QT prolonging agents, quinine, rasagiline, risperidone, ritonavir, salicylates, selegiline, serotonin modulators, sibutramine, SSRIs, St John's wort, sumatriptan, tetrabenazine, thioridazine, thrombolytic agents, tositumomab & iodine^{131}, tramadol, tranylcypromine, trazodone, tricyclic antidepressants, tryptophan, vitamin K antagonists, ziprasidone
Pregnancy category: C
Important contra-indications noted in the prescribing guidelines for: nursing mothers; pediatric patients
Black Box Warning: SUICIDALITY AND ANTIDEPRESSANT DRUGS

Skin
Diaphoresis (11%) [3]
Hyperhidrosis (11%) [2]
Pigmentation [2]
Pruritus (<10%) [2]
Rash (<10%)

Mucosal
Xerostomia (20%) [4]

Cardiovascular
Bradycardia [2]
Cardiotoxicity [4]
Chest pain [2]
Palpitation [2]
QT prolongation [21]
Tachycardia [3]
Torsades de pointes [8]

Central Nervous System
Agitation (3%)
Akathisia [2]
Anorexia (4%)
Anxiety (4%) [2]
Fever (2%)
Headache [5]
Incoordination [2]
Insomnia (15%) [3]
Nightmares [2]
Restless legs syndrome [4]
Seizures (overdose) [5]
Serotonin syndrome [19]
Somnolence (drowsiness) (18%) [6]
Suicidal ideation [3]
Tremor (8%) [5]
Vertigo (dizziness) [5]
Yawning (2%)

Neuromuscular/Skeletal
Arthralgia (2%)
Asthenia (fatigue) (5%) [4]
Dystonia [2]
Myalgia/Myopathy (2%)

Gastrointestinal/Hepatic
Abdominal pain (3%)
Constipation [2]
Diarrhea (8%) [2]
Dyspepsia (5%)
Nausea (21%) [3]
Vomiting (4%) [2]

Respiratory
Rhinitis (5%)
Sinusitis (3%)
Upper respiratory tract infection (5%)

Endocrine/Metabolic
Galactorrhea [4]
Hyponatremia [2]
Libido decreased (2%)
SIADH [18]
Weight gain [2]

Genitourinary
Dysmenorrhea (3%)
Ejaculatory dysfunction (6%) [2]
Impotence (3%)
Priapism [4]
Sexual dysfunction [4]
Urinary frequency [2]

Otic
Hallucinations, auditory [2]

Ocular
Diplopia [2]
Glaucoma [2]
Hallucinations, visual [3]

Other
Adverse effects [2]
Death [8]

CLADRIBINE

Trade name: Leustatin (Janssen Biotech)
Indications: Leukemias
Class: Antimetabolite, Antineoplastic
Half-life: alpha phase: 25 minutes; beta phase: 7 hours
Clinically important, potentially hazardous interactions with: none known
Pregnancy category: D
Important contra-indications noted in the prescribing guidelines for: the elderly; nursing mothers

---

Skin
Diaphoresis (<10%)
Edema (6%)
Erythema (6%)
Exanthems (27–50%) [2]

Herpes zoster [5]
Petechiae (8%)
Pruritus (6%)
Purpura (10%)
Rash (27%) [2]

Neuromuscular/Skeletal
Myalgia/Myopathy (7%)

Hematologic
Lymphocytopenia [4]
Lymphopenia [2]
Neutropenia [7]
Thrombocytopenia [2]

Local
Injection-site edema (9%)
Injection-site erythema (9%)
Injection-site pain (9%)
Injection-site phlebitis (2%)
Injection-site thrombosis (2%)

Other
Adverse effects [2]
Death [3]
Infection [7]

CLARITHROMYCIN

Trade name: Biaxin (AbbVie)
Indications: Various infections caused by susceptible organisms
Class: Antibiotic, macrolide, CYP3A4 inhibitor
Half-life: 5–7 hours
Clinically important, potentially hazardous interactions with: abiraterone, alprazolam, aprepitant, astemizole, atazanavir, atorvastatin, avanafil, benzodiazepines, boceprevir, cabazitaxel, cabozantinib, carbamazepine, chlordiazepoxide, cilostazol, clonazepam, clorazepate, cobicistat/elvitegravir/emtricitabine/tenofovir disoproxil, colchicine, conivaptan, crizotinib, cyclosporine, dabigatran, darunavir, dasatinib, delavirdine, diazepam, digoxin, dihydroergotamine, disopyramide, dronedarone, efavirenz, eletriptan, ergot alkaloids, estradiol, etravirine, everolimus, fesoterodine, flibanserin, fluoxetine, flurazepam, fluticasone propionate, fluvastatin, HMG-CoA reductase inhibitors, imatinib, indinavir, itraconazole, ixabepilone, lapatinib, lomitapide, lopinavir, lorazepam, lovastatin, maraviroc, methylergonovine, methylprednisolone, methysergide, midazolam, mifepristone, nevirapine, nilotinib, omeprazole, oxazepam, oxtriphylline, paclitaxel, paroxetine hydrochloride, pazopanib, pimozide, ponatinib, pravastatin, prednisone, quazepam, ranolazine, regorafenib, repaglinide, rilpivirine, rimonabant, rivaroxaban, romidepsin, ruxolitinib, sertraline, sildenafil, silodosin, simeprevir, simvastatin, solifenacin, sunitinib, tadalafil, temazepam, temsirolimus, ticagrelor, tipranavir, tolvaptan, trabectedin, triazolam, ulipristal, vandetanib, vemurafenib, venetoclax, warfarin, zidovudine
Pregnancy category: C
Important contra-indications noted in the prescribing guidelines for: the elderly; nursing mothers; pediatric patients

---

Skin
Anaphylactoid reactions/Anaphylaxis [2]
Fixed eruption [3]
Hypersensitivity [3]
Psoriasis [2]
Purpura [3]
Rash (3%) [2]
Toxic epidermal necrolysis [4]
Vasculitis [3]

Mucosal
Stomatitis [2]

Cardiovascular
QT prolongation [7]
Torsades de pointes [9]

Central Nervous System
Anorexia [2]
Dysgeusia (taste perversion) (3%) [8]
Mania [3]
Neurotoxicity [4]
Psychosis [3]

Neuromuscular/Skeletal
Arthralgia [2]
Rhabdomyolysis [14]

Gastrointestinal/Hepatic
Abdominal distension [2]
Abdominal pain [5]
Diarrhea [9]
Dyspepsia [2]
Hepatotoxicity [3]
Nausea [4]
Vomiting [3]

Endocrine/Metabolic
Hypoglycemia [3]

Renal
Nephrotoxicity [2]

Ocular
Hallucinations, visual [4]

Local
Injection-site pain [2]

Other
Adverse effects [11]

CLINDAMYCIN

Trade names: Benzaclin (Dermik), Cleocin (Pfizer), Cleocin-T (Pfizer), Clindagel (Galderma), Clindets (Stiefel)
Indications: Various serious infections caused by susceptible organisms
Class: Antibiotic, lincosamide
Half-life: 2–3 hours
Clinically important, potentially hazardous interactions with: cisatracurium, erythromycin, kaolin, mivacurium, neostigmine, pyridostigmine, rocuronium, saquinavir
Pregnancy category: B

Skin
AGEP [6]
Anaphylactoid reactions/Anaphylaxis [5]
Dermatitis (from topical preparations) [7]
DRESS syndrome [2]
Erythema multiforme [2]
Erythroderma [2]
Exanthems [5]
Hypersensitivity [4]
Rash (<10%) [3]
Stevens–Johnson syndrome [3]
Sweet's syndrome [2]
Toxic epidermal necrolysis [3]
Urticaria [3]
Vasculitis [2]

Mucosal
Burning mouth syndrome [2]
Xerostomia [2]

Central Nervous System
Ageusia (taste loss) [2]

Gastrointestinal/Hepatic
Colitis [2]
Diarrhea [4]
Esophagitis [2]
Hepatotoxicity [2]
Pseudomembranous colitis [5]

Hematologic
Neutropenia [2]

Otic
Tinnitus [2]

Local
Application-site erythema [3]

Other
Adverse effects [5]
Death [3]

CLOMIPRAMINE

Trade name: Anafranil (Mallinckrodt)
Indications: Obsessive-compulsive disorder
Class: Antidepressant, tricyclic, Muscarinic antagonist
Half-life: 21–31 hours
Clinically important, potentially hazardous interactions with: amprenavir, arbutamine, arsenic, artemether/lumefantrine, clonidine, duloxetine, epinephrine, formoterol, guanethidine, isocarboxazid, linezolid, MAO inhibitors, milnacipran, moclobemide, phenelzine, quinolones, sparfloxacin, tranylcypromine
Pregnancy category: C
Important contra-indications noted in the prescribing guidelines for: the elderly; nursing mothers; pediatric patients
Black Box Warning: SUICIDALITY AND ANTIDEPRESSANT DRUGS

Skin
Acneform eruption (2%)
Cellulitis (2%)
Dermatitis (2%)
Diaphoresis (29%) [2]
Edema (2%)
Hypersensitivity [2]
Photosensitivity [3]
Pruritus (6%)
Purpura (3%)
Rash (8%)
Xerosis (2%)

Mucosal
Xerostomia (84%) [6]

Cardiovascular
Flushing (8%)
QT prolongation [4]
Torsades de pointes [2]

Central Nervous System
Dysgeusia (taste perversion) (8%)
Seizures [4]

Serotonin syndrome [3]

Neuromuscular/Skeletal

Myalgia/Myopathy (13%)

Endocrine/Metabolic

Gynecomastia (2%)
SIADH [3]

Genitourinary

Vaginitis (2%)

Other

Adverse effects [3]
Allergic reactions (<3%)

CLONAZEPAM

Trade name: Klonopin (Roche)
Indications: Petit mal and myoclonic seizures
Class: Benzodiazepine
Half-life: 18–50 hours
Clinically important, potentially hazardous interactions with: amprenavir, chlorpheniramine, clarithromycin, cobicistat/ elvitegravir/emtricitabine/tenofovir disoproxil, efavirenz, esomeprazole, imatinib, indinavir, nelfinavir, nevirapine, oxycodone, piracetam
Pregnancy category: D
Important contra-indications noted in the prescribing guidelines for: the elderly; nursing mothers; pediatric patients

---

Skin

Bullous dermatitis [2]
Dermatitis (<10%)
Diaphoresis (>10%)
Pseudolymphoma [2]
Rash (>10%)

Hair

Alopecia [2]

Mucosal

Sialopenia (>10%)
Sialorrhea (<10%)
Xerostomia (>10%)

Central Nervous System

Psychosis [2]
Seizures [2]

Other

Adverse effects [2]
Allergic reactions (<10%)

CLONIDINE

Trade name: Catapres (Boehringer Ingelheim)
Indications: Hypertension
Class: Adrenergic alpha-receptor agonist
Half-life: 6–24 hours
Clinically important, potentially hazardous interactions with: acebutolol, alfuzosin, amitriptyline, amoxapine, atenolol, betaxolol, captopril, carteolol, cilazapril, clomipramine, desipramine, dexmethylphenidate, diclofenac, doxepin, enalapril, esmolol, fosinopril, imipramine, insulin aspart, insulin degludec, insulin detemir, insulin glargine, insulin glulisine, irbesartan, levodopa, levomepromazine, lisinopril, meloxicam, metoprolol, milnacipran, nadolol, nebivolol, nortriptyline, olmesartan, oxprenolol, penbutolol, pericyazine, pindolol, propranolol, protriptyline, quinapril, ramipril, sotalol, sulpiride, timolol, trandolapril, triamcinolone, tricyclic antidepressants, trimipramine, verapamil
Pregnancy category: C
Important contra-indications noted in the prescribing guidelines for: nursing mothers; pediatric patients

---

Skin

Depigmentation [2]
Dermatitis (from patch) (20%) [23]
Eczema [2]
Erythema [2]
Lupus erythematosus [5]
Pigmentation [2]
Pityriasis rosea [2]
Pruritus (>5%) [6]
Psoriasis [2]
Rash (<10%)
Ulcerations (<10%)

Mucosal

Xerostomia (40%) [11]

Cardiovascular

Bradycardia [8]
Hypotension [18]

Central Nervous System

Hallucinations [3]
Headache [2]
Hyperesthesia (<10%)
Seizures [2]
Somnolence (drowsiness) [2]
Vertigo (dizziness) [2]

Other

Adverse effects [2]

CLOPIDOGREL

Trade name: Plavix (Bristol-Myers Squibb) (Sanofi-Aventis)
Indications: Acute coronary syndrome, recent myocardial infarction, recent stroke, or established peripheral arterial disease
Class: Antiplatelet, Antiplatelet, thienopyridine
Half-life: 6 hours
Clinically important, potentially hazardous interactions with: amiodarone, anisindione, anticoagulants, atorvastatin, calcium channel blockers, carbamazepine, chloramphenicol, cimetidine, ciprofloxacin, collagenase, dabigatran, dasatinib, delavirdine, dexlansoprazole, diclofenac, dicumarol, dipyridamole, drotrecogin alfa, efavirenz, enoxaparin, erythromycin, esomeprazole, etravirine, fluconazole, fluoxetine, fluvoxamine, fondaparinux, glucosamine, herbals with anticoagulant properties, ibritumomab, iloprost, itraconazole, ketoconazole, lansoprazole, lepirudin, macrolide antibiotics, meloxicam, miconazole, moclobemide, NSAIDs, omega-3 fatty acids, omeprazole, oxcarbazepine, pantoprazole, pentosan, pentoxifylline, polysulfate sodium, prasugrel, rabeprazole, rifapentine, rivaroxaban, salicylates, simvastatin, telithromycin, thrombolytic agents, tinzaparin, tositumomab & iodine[131], voriconazole, warfarin
Pregnancy category: B
Important contra-indications noted in the prescribing guidelines for: nursing mothers; pediatric patients
Note: Contraindicated in patients with active pathological bleeding.
Black Box Warning: DIMINISHED EFFECTIVENESS IN POOR METABOLIZERS

Skin

AGEP [2]
Angioedema [4]
Bullous dermatitis (<3%)
Eczema (<3%)
Edema (3–5%)
Exanthems (<3%) [2]
Hypersensitivity [9]
Pruritus (3%) [2]
Psoriasis [2]
Purpura [18]
Rash (4%) [5]
Stevens–Johnson syndrome [2]
Thrombocytopenic purpura [9]
Ulcerations (<3%)
Urticaria (<3%) [2]

Cardiovascular

Acute coronary syndrome [2]
Myocardial infarction [2]

Central Nervous System

Ageusia (taste loss) [3]
Fever [3]
Hyperesthesia (<3%)
Intracranial hemorrhage [2]
Paresthesias (<3%)

Neuromuscular/Skeletal

Arthralgia [5]
Rhabdomyolysis [3]

Gastrointestinal/Hepatic

Gastrointestinal bleeding [3]
Hepatotoxicity [6]

Respiratory

Dyspnea [3]
Flu-like syndrome (8%)

Hematologic

Bleeding [16]
Hemolytic uremic syndrome [2]
Neutropenia [4]
Thrombocytopenia [3]
Thrombosis [2]

Other

Adverse effects [2]
Allergic reactions (<3%) [2]

CLORAZEPATE

Trade name: Tranxene (Recordati)
Indications: Anxiety and panic disorders
Class: Benzodiazepine
Half-life: 48–96 hours
Clinically important, potentially hazardous interactions with: aminophylline, amprenavir, antacids, carbamazepine, carmustine, chlorpheniramine, clarithromycin, cobicistat/ elvitegravir/emtricitabine/tenofovir disoproxil, efavirenz, esomeprazole, imatinib, indinavir,

itraconazole, ketoconazole, MAO inhibitors, midazolam, moclobemide, nelfinavir, phenytoin, sucralfate, warfarin
Pregnancy category: D
Important contra-indications noted in the prescribing guidelines for: nursing mothers; pediatric patients

---

Skin
- Dermatitis (<10%)
- Diaphoresis (>10%)
- Rash (>10%)

Mucosal
- Sialopenia (>10%)
- Sialorrhea (<10%)
- Xerostomia (>10%)

CLOZAPINE

Trade names: Clozaril (Novartis), Denzapine (Merz), Leponex (Novartis), Zaponex (Teva)
Indications: Treatment-resistant schizophrenia
Class: Antipsychotic
Half-life: 4–12 hours
Clinically important, potentially hazardous interactions with: alcohol, amitriptyline, antimuscarinics, arsenic, benzodiazepines, cabazitaxel, caffeine, carbamazepine, chloramphenicol, cimetidine, ciprofloxacin, citalopram, cocoa, cyclophosphamide, cytotoxics, darifenacin, dasatinib, encainide, epinephrine, erythromycin, everolimus, flecainide, fluoxetine, flupentixol, fluphenazine, fluvoxamine, gefitinib, guarana, haloperidol, insulin degludec, insulin detemir, insulin glargine, insulin glulisine, lapatinib, lithium, lomustine, lorazepam, MAO inhibitors, nilotinib, norfloxacin, ofloxacin, omeprazole, oxaliplatin, oxybutynin, paroxetine hydrochloride, pazopanib, pemetrexed, penicillamine, pipotiazine, propafenone, quinidine, rifampin, risperidone, ritonavir, saquinavir, selenium, sertraline, sorafenib, sulfonamides, sunitinib, telithromycin, temozolomide, temsirolimus, tetrazepam, tricyclic antidepressants, trospium, uracil/tegafur, valproic acid, venlafaxine, zuclopenthixol
Pregnancy category: B
Important contra-indications noted in the prescribing guidelines for: the elderly; nursing mothers; pediatric patients
Note: Contraindicated in patients with myeloproliferative disorders, uncontrolled epilepsy, paralytic ileus, or a history of clozapine-induced agranulocytosis or severe granulocytopenia.
Black Box Warning: AGRANULOCYTOSIS / SEIZURES / MYOCARDITIS / OTHER ADVERSE CARDIOVASCULAR AND RESPIRATORY EFFECTS
INCREASED MORTALITY IN ELDERLY PATIENTS WITH DEMENTIA-RELATED PSYCHOSIS

Skin
- Angioedema [2]
- Diaphoresis (6%) [4]
- Exanthems [2]
- Lupus erythematosus [4]
- Pityriasis rosea [2]
- Rash (2%) [2]
- Toxicity [3]

Mucosal
- Parotitis [3]
- Sialorrhea (31%) [71]
- Xerostomia [3]

Cardiovascular
- Atrial fibrillation [2]
- Cardiomyopathy [12]
- Hypertension (4%) [4]
- Hypotension (9%) [3]
- Myocarditis [35]
- Orthostatic hypotension [2]
- Pericardial effusion [3]
- Pericarditis [7]
- QT prolongation [5]
- Tachycardia (25%) [8]
- Venous thromboembolism [5]

Central Nervous System
- Akathisia [3]
- Anxiety [2]
- Compulsions [8]
- Fever [5]
- Headache (7%)
- Neuroleptic malignant syndrome [28]
- Neurotoxicity [2]
- Pain [2]
- Sedation (39%) [7]
- Seizures [23]
- Somnolence (drowsiness) [9]
- Syncope [2]
- Tardive dyskinesia [5]
- Tic disorder [2]
- Tremor (<10%) [2]
- Vertigo (dizziness) (19%)

Neuromuscular/Skeletal
- Myoclonus [2]
- Rhabdomyolysis [7]

Gastrointestinal/Hepatic
- Colitis [2]
- Constipation (14%) [6]
- Gastric obstruction [3]
- Gastrointestinal hypomotitlity [2]
- Hepatotoxicity [5]
- Ileus [6]
- Pancreatitis [6]

Respiratory
- Pleural effusion [4]
- Pneumonia [2]
- Pulmonary embolism [2]

Endocrine/Metabolic
- Diabetes mellitus [7]
- Diabetic ketoacidosis [2]
- Galactorrhea [2]
- Hyperglycemia [5]
- Hyperlipidemia [3]
- Metabolic syndrome [12]
- Weight gain [26]

Genitourinary
- Priapism [14]

Renal
- Enuresis [4]

Hematologic
- Agranulocytosis [25]
- Dyslipidemia [3]
- Eosinophilia [9]
- Hemotoxicity [2]
- Leukopenia [8]
- Neutropenia [12]
- Pancytopenia [2]
- Thrombosis [2]

Other
- Adverse effects [10]
- Death [11]
- Serositis [6]

CO-TRIMOXAZOLE

Synonyms: sulfamethoxazole-trimethoprim; SMX-TMP; SMZ-TMP; TMP-SMX; TMP-SMZ
Trade names: Bactrim (GSK), Septra (Monarch)
Indications: Various infections caused by susceptible organisms
Class: Antibiotic, sulfonamide
Half-life: 6–10 hours
Clinically important, potentially hazardous interactions with: anticoagulants, azathioprine, cyclosporine, dofetilide, isotretinoin, methotrexate, prilocaine, repaglinide, warfarin
Pregnancy category: C
Important contra-indications noted in the prescribing guidelines for: the elderly; nursing mothers; pediatric patients
Note: Co-trimoxazole is a sulfonamide and can be absorbed systemically. Sulfonamides can produce severe, possibly fatal, reactions such as toxic epidermal necrolysis and Stevens-Johnson syndrome.
Co-trimoxazole is sulfamethoxazole and trimethoprim.

Skin
- AGEP [4]
- Anaphylactoid reactions/Anaphylaxis [6]
- Angioedema [3]
- Bullous dermatitis [2]
- Dermatitis [4]
- DRESS syndrome [9]
- Erythema multiforme [19]
- Erythema nodosum [2]
- Exanthems [35]
- Exfoliative dermatitis [5]
- Fixed eruption [49]
- Hypersensitivity [17]
- Jarisch–Herxheimer reaction [2]
- Linear IgA bullous dermatosis [4]
- Lupus erythematosus [4]
- Photosensitivity [4]
- Pruritus [10]
- Purpura [3]
- Pustules [6]
- Radiation recall dermatitis [3]
- Rash (>10%) [14]
- Serum sickness [2]
- Stevens–Johnson syndrome (<10%) [39]
- Sweet's syndrome [9]
- Toxic epidermal necrolysis (<10%) [51]
- Toxicity [2]
- Urticaria [12]
- Vasculitis [11]

Mucosal
- Oral mucosal eruption [2]
- Oral ulceration [2]

Cardiovascular
QT prolongation [2]
Torsades de pointes [3]

Central Nervous System
Aseptic meningitis [4]
Fever [4]
Psychosis [4]
Tremor [4]
Vertigo (dizziness) [2]

Neuromuscular/Skeletal
Asthenia (fatigue) [2]
Myalgia/Myopathy [2]
Rhabdomyolysis [7]

Gastrointestinal/Hepatic
Hepatotoxicity [7]
Nausea [2]
Pancreatitis [4]
Vomiting [4]

Endocrine/Metabolic
ALT increased [2]
Hyperkalemia [4]
Hypoglycemia [4]
Hyponatremia [2]
Serum creatinine increased [4]

Hematologic
Anemia [3]
Neutropenia [4]
Thrombocytopenia [9]

Ocular
Glaucoma [2]
Myopia [2]

Other
Adverse effects [11]
Allergic reactions [2]
Death [4]
Side effects [2]

COBICISTAT/ ELVITEGRAVIR/ EMTRICITABINE/ TENOFOVIR ALAFENAMIDE *

Trade name: Genvoya (Gilead)
Indications: HIV-1 infection
Class: Antiretroviral, CYP3A inhibitor (cobicistat), Hepatitis B virus necleoside analog reverse transcriptase inhibitor (tenofovir alafenamide), Integrase strand transfer inhibitor (elvitegravir), Nucleoside analog reverse transcriptase inhibitor (emtricitabine)
Half-life: 3.5 hours (cobicistat); 13 hours (elvitegravir); 10 hours (emtricitabine); <1 hour (tenofovir alafenamide)
Clinically important, potentially hazardous interactions with: acyclovir, aminoglycosides, amiodarone, amitriptyline, amlodipine, antacids, antiarrhythmics, atorvastatin, benzodiazepines, bepridil, beta blockers, bosentan, buprenorphine, bupropion, buspirone, calcium channel blockers, cidofovir, clarithromycin, clorazepate, colchicine, desipramine, dexamethasone, diazepam, digoxin, diltiazem, disopyramide, drugs affecting renal function, estazolam, ethosuximide, felodipine, flecainide, flurazepam, fluticasone furoate, fluticasone propionate, ganciclovir, gentamicin, hormonal contraceptives, imipramine, immunosuppressants, itraconazole, ketoconazole, lidocaine, lorazepam, metoprolol, mexiletine, midazolam, naloxone, neuroleptics, nicardipine, nifedipine, nortriptyline, oxcarbazepine, paroxetine hydrochloride, perphenazine, propafenone, quinidine, rifabutin, rifapentine, risperidone, salmeterol, sildenafil, SSRIs, tadalafil, telithromycin, thioridazine, timolol, trazodone, tricyclic antidepressants, valacyclovir, valganciclovir, vardenafil, verapamil, voriconazole, warfarin, zolpidem
Pregnancy category: B
Important contra-indications noted in the prescribing guidelines for: nursing mothers
Note: See also separate profiles for emtricitabine and tenofovir alafenamide.
Black Box Warning: LACTIC ACIDOSIS/ SEVERE HEPATOMEGALY WITH STEATOSIS and POST TREATMENT ACUTE EXACERBATION OF HEPATITIS B

Central Nervous System
Headache (6%)

Neuromuscular/Skeletal
Asthenia (fatigue) (5%)

Gastrointestinal/Hepatic
Diarrhea (7%)
Nausea (5%) [2]

Other
Adverse effects [2]

COBICISTAT/ ELVITEGRAVIR/ EMTRICITABINE/ TENOFOVIR DISOPROXIL

Trade name: Stribild (Gilead)
Indications: HIV-1 infection
Class: Antiretroviral, CYP3A inhibitor (cobicistat), Integrase strand transfer inhibitor (elvitegravir), Nucleoside analog reverse transcriptase inhibitor (emtricitabine and tenofovir disoproxil)
Half-life: 3.5 hours (cobicistat); 13 hours (elvitegravir); 10 hours (emtricitabine); 12–18 hours (tenofovir disoproxil)
Clinically important, potentially hazardous interactions with: acyclovir, adefovir, amiodarone, amitriptyline, amlodipine, antacids, antiarrhythmics, antiretrovirals, atorvastatin, benzodiazepines, bepridil, beta blockers, bosentan, buprenorphine, bupropion, buspirone, calcium channel blockers, carbamazepine, cidofovir, clarithromycin, clonazepam, clorazepate, colchicine, cyclosporine, desipramine, dexamethasone, diazepam, digoxin, diltiazem, disopyramide, drugs affecting renal function, elbasvir & grazoprevir, emtricitabine, estazolam, ethosuximide, felodipine, flecainide, flurazepam, fluticasone propionate, ganciclovir, hormonal contraceptives, imipramine, immunosuppressants, itraconazole, ketoconazole, lamivudine, ledipasvir & sofosbuvir, lidocaine, metoprolol, mexiletine, midazolam, naloxone, neuroleptics, nicardipine, nifedipine, non-nucleoside reverse transcriptase inhibitors, nortriptyline, oxcarbazepine, paroxetine hydrochloride, perphenazine, phenobarbital, phenytoin, propafenone, protease inhibitors, quinidine, rifabutin, rifapentine, risperidone, ritonavir, salmeterol, sedatives / hypnotics, sildenafil, simeprevir, sirolimus, SSRIs, tacrolimus, tadalafil, telithromycin, tenofovir disoproxil, thioridazine, timolol, trazodone, tricyclic antidepressants, valacyclovir, valganciclovir, vardenafil, verapamil, voriconazole, warfarin, zolpidem
Pregnancy category: B
Important contra-indications noted in the prescribing guidelines for: the elderly; nursing mothers; pediatric patients
Note: See also separate profiles for emtricitabine and tenofovir disoproxil.
Black Box Warning: LACTIC ACIDOSIS/ SEVERE HEPATOMEGALY WITH STEATOSIS and POST TREATMENT ACUTE EXACERBATION OF HEPATITIS B

Skin
Rash (3%) [3]

Central Nervous System
Abnormal dreams (9%) [3]
Headache (7%) [5]
Insomnia (3%) [2]
Vertigo (dizziness) (3%) [3]

Neuromuscular/Skeletal
Asthenia (fatigue) (5%) [2]

Gastrointestinal/Hepatic
Diarrhea (12%) [6]
Flatulence (2%)
Gastrointestinal disorder [2]
Nausea (16%) [8]

Respiratory
Upper respiratory tract infection [2]

Endocrine/Metabolic
AST increased (2%)
Serum creatinine increased [2]

Genitourinary
Hematuria (3%)

Renal
Nephrotoxicity [2]
Proteinuria (39%)

Other
Adverse effects [5]

COBIMETINIB *

Trade name: Cotellic (Genentech)
Indications: Melanoma (unresectable or metastatic) in patients with BRAF V600E or V600K mutations, in combination with vemurafenib
Class: MEK inhibitor
Half-life: 23–70 hours
Clinically important, potentially hazardous interactions with: carbamazepine, efavirenz, itraconazole, phenytoin, rifampin, St John's wort,

strong or moderate CYP3A inhibitors or inducers
Pregnancy category: N/A (Can cause fetal harm)
Important contra-indications noted in the prescribing guidelines for: nursing mothers; pediatric patients

Skin
- Acneform eruption (16%) [2]
- Basal cell carcinoma (5%)
- Erythema (10%)
- Hyperkeratosis (11%) [2]
- Keratoacanthoma [2]
- Photosensitivity (46%) [7]
- Rash [6]
- Squamous cell carcinoma (6%) [5]

Hair
- Alopecia (15%) [2]

Mucosal
- Stomatitis (14%)

Cardiovascular
- Hypertension (15%)

Central Nervous System
- Chills (10%)
- Fever (28%) [2]

Neuromuscular/Skeletal
- Arthralgia [2]
- Asthenia (fatigue) [5]

Gastrointestinal/Hepatic
- Diarrhea (60%) [6]
- Gastrointestinal bleeding (4%)
- Hepatotoxicity [5]
- Nausea (41%) [5]
- Vomiting (24%) [2]

Respiratory
- Pneumonitis (<10%)

Endocrine/Metabolic
- ALP increased (71%) [2]
- ALT increased (68%) [2]
- AST increased (73%) [2]
- Creatine phosphokinase increased (79%) [3]
- GGT increased (65%)
- Hyperkalemia (26%)
- Hypoalbuminemia (42%)
- Hypocalcemia (24%)
- Hypokalemia (25%)
- Hyponatremia (38%)
- Hypophosphatemia (68%)
- Serum creatinine increased (100%)

Genitourinary
- Hematuria (2%)

Hematologic
- Anemia (69%) [2]
- Hemorrhage (13%)
- Lymphopenia (73%)
- Thrombocytopenia (18%)

Ocular
- Chorioretinopathy (13%)
- Retinal detachment (12%) [2]
- Vision impaired (15%)

COCAINE

Indications: Topical anesthesia
Class: Anesthetic, local, CNS stimulant
Half-life: 75 minutes
Clinically important, potentially hazardous interactions with: epinephrine, iobenguane
Pregnancy category: C (the pregnancy category is X for non-medicinal use)

Skin
- Angioedema [3]
- Diaphoresis [3]
- Hyperkeratosis (fingers and palms) [2]
- Necrosis [6]
- Purpura [4]
- Raynaud's phenomenon [2]
- Scleroderma (reversible) [3]
- Vasculitis [14]

Mucosal
- Nasal septal perforation [4]
- Palatal perforation [7]

Cardiovascular
- Angina [2]
- Brugada syndrome [3]
- Chest pain [5]
- Myocardial infarction [6]
- Myocardial ischemia [2]

Central Nervous System
- Ageusia (taste loss) (>10%)
- Anosmia (>10%)
- Compulsions [2]
- Hallucinations [4]
- Leukoencephalopathy [3]
- Psychosis [2]
- Seizures [6]
- Suicidal ideation [2]
- Tic disorder [2]
- Tremor (<10%)

Neuromuscular/Skeletal
- Arthralgia [2]
- Rhabdomyolysis [19]

Genitourinary
- Priapism [5]

Renal
- Glomerulonephritis [2]
- Nephrotoxicity [2]

Hematologic
- Agranulocytosis [2]
- Hemolytic uremic syndrome [2]
- Neutropenia [6]

Otic
- Hallucinations, auditory [2]

Ocular
- Hallucinations, visual [3]

Other
- Death [3]

CODEINE

Synonym: methylmorphine
Trade names: Halotussin (Watson), Nucofed (Monarch), Robitussin AC (Wyeth), Tussi-Organidin (MedPointe)
Indications: Pain, cough suppressant
Class: Opiate agonist
Half-life: 2.5–4 hours
Clinically important, potentially hazardous interactions with: alcohol, cinacalcet, CNS depressants, delavirdine, MAO inhibitors, mianserin, terbinafine, tipranavir
Pregnancy category: C
Important contra-indications noted in the prescribing guidelines for: the elderly; nursing mothers; pediatric patients
Black Box Warning: DEATH RELATED TO ULTRA-RAPID METABOLISM OF CODEINE TO MORPHINE

Skin
- Angioedema [2]
- Dermatitis [5]
- Erythema multiforme [4]
- Exanthems [6]
- Fixed eruption [6]
- Pruritus [3]
- Rash (<10%)
- Toxic epidermal necrolysis [2]
- Urticaria (<10%) [9]

Mucosal
- Xerostomia (<10%)

Central Nervous System
- Vertigo (dizziness) [2]

Gastrointestinal/Hepatic
- Constipation [2]
- Pancreatitis [5]
- Vomiting [2]

Respiratory
- Respiratory depression [3]

Local
- Injection-site pain (<10%)

Other
- Death [5]

COLCHICINE

Indications: Gouty arthritis (in adults), gout, familial Mediterranean fever
Class: Alkaloid, Anti-inflammatory
Half-life: 27–31 hours (following multiple doses)
Clinically important, potentially hazardous interactions with: amiodarone, aprepitant, atazanavir, atorvastatin, azithromycin, boceprevir, clarithromycin, cobicistat/elvitegravir/emtricitabine/tenofovir disoproxil, conivaptan, cyanocobalamin, cyclosporine, darunavir, dasatinib, delavirdine, digoxin, diltiazem, efavirenz, erythromycin, fenofibrate, fibrates, fluvastatin, gemfibrozil, grapefruit juice, HMG-CoA reductase inhibitors, indinavir, itraconazole, ketoconazole, lapatinib, lopinavir, ombitasvir/paritaprevir/ritonavir, P-glycoprotein inhibitors or inducers, pravastatin, protease inhibitors, ritonavir, rosuvastatin, saxagliptin, simvastatin,

strong CYP3A4 inhibitors, telithromycin, troleandomycin, verapamil, voriconazole
Pregnancy category: C
Important contra-indications noted in the prescribing guidelines for: the elderly
Note: Contraindicated in patients with renal or hepatic impairment where P-glycoprotein or strong CYP3A4 inhibitors are also prescribed.

Skin
Pruritus [2]
Staphylococcal scalded skin syndrome [2]
Toxic epidermal necrolysis [3]
Vasculitis [2]

Hair
Alopecia (<10%) [6]

Central Nervous System
Headache (2%)
Neurotoxicity [3]

Neuromuscular/Skeletal
Asthenia (fatigue) (<4%)
Gouty tophi (4%)
Myalgia/Myopathy [18]
Rhabdomyolysis [17]

Gastrointestinal/Hepatic
Abdominal pain (<20%) [2]
Diarrhea (23%) [5]
Gastrointestinal disorder [2]
Hepatotoxicity [3]
Nausea (<20%) [2]
Vomiting (<20%) [3]

Respiratory
Pharyngolaryngeal pain (3%)

Other
Adverse effects [6]
Death [3]
Side effects (14%)

COLESEVELAM

Trade names: Cholestagel (Genzyme), Welchol (Sankyo)
Indications: Hypercholesterolemia, hyperlipidemia, Type II diabetes mellitus
Class: Bile acid sequestrant
Half-life: N/A
Clinically important, potentially hazardous interactions with: cyclosporine, deferasirox, estradiol, glyburide, levothyroxine, olmesartan, phenytoin, warfarin
Pregnancy category: B
Important contra-indications noted in the prescribing guidelines for: pediatric patients
Note: Contraindicated in patients with a history of bowel obstruction, with serum triglyceride concentrations >500 mg/dL or with a history of hypertriglyceridemia-induced pancreatitis.

Cardiovascular
Hypertension (3%)

Central Nervous System
Headache [2]

Neuromuscular/Skeletal
Myalgia/Myopathy (2%)

Gastrointestinal/Hepatic
Abdominal pain (4%)
Constipation (9–10%) [3]
Diarrhea (3%)
Dyspepsia (4–6%) [3]
Flatulence (11%)
Gastrointestinal disorder [4]
Nausea (3%)

Respiratory
Nasopharyngitis (4%)

Endocrine/Metabolic
Hypoglycemia (3%) [3]

Other
Adverse effects [4]

COLLAGEN (BOVINE)

Trade names: Bellafill (Suneva), Zyderm (Inamed), Zyplast (Inamed)
Indications: Cataract surgery (collagen shields), depressed cutaneous scars, facial lines, wrinkles, glottic insufficiency, phonosurgey, urinary incontinence
Class: Protein
Half-life: Several months to years
Clinically important, potentially hazardous interactions with: argatroban, avitene
Pregnancy category: N/A
Important contra-indications noted in the prescribing guidelines for: nursing mothers
Note: A reaction to the anesthetic, lidocaine, in liquid collagen injections may occur. Artecoll and Bellafill contain polymethyl-methacrylate microspheres.

Skin
Abscess [2]
Churg-Strauss syndrome [7]
Dermatomyositis [3]
Edema [2]
Erythema [3]
Granulomatous reaction [2]
Hypersensitivity [10]
Induration [3]
Panniculitis [2]

Neuromuscular/Skeletal
Arthralgia [2]
Polymyositis [3]

Other
Adverse effects [12]
Allergic reactions [7]

CONIVAPTAN

Trade name: Vaprisol (Astellas)
Indications: Hyponatremia, SIADH
Class: CYP3A4 inhibitor, Vasopressin receptor antagonist
Half-life: 5 hours
Clinically important, potentially hazardous interactions with: acetaminophen, albendazole, alfuzosin, almotriptan, alosetron, ambrisentan, amitriptyline, amlodipine, antifungals, aprepitant, artemether/lumefantrine, atorvastatin, bexarotene, bortezomib, brinzolamide, bupivacaine, cabazitaxel, cabozantinib, ciclesonide, cilostazol, cinacalcet, citalopram, clarithromycin, colchicine, cyclobenzaprine, CYP3A4 inhibitors or substrates, darunavir, dasatinib, deferasirox, delavirdine, dienogest, digoxin, docetaxel, dronedarone, dutasteride, efavirenz, enalapril, eplerenone, estradiol, eszopiclone, everolimus, fentanyl, fesoterodine, fingolimod, flibanserin, gefitinib, guanfacine, halofantrine, indinavir, itraconazole, ixabepilone, ketoconazole, lapatinib, lomitapide, maraviroc, meloxicam, metaxalone, methylprednisolone, micafungin, midazolam, mifepristone, mometasone, nilotinib, nisoldipine, oxybutynin, pantoprazole, paricalcitol, pazopanib, pimecrolimus, pioglitazone, ponatinib, prasugrel, ramelteon, ranolazine, ritonavir, rivaroxaban, romidepsin, rosuvastatin, ruxolitinib, salmeterol, saxagliptin, sildenafil, silodosin, simvastatin, sorafenib, St John's wort, tadalafil, tamsulosin, telithromycin, temsirolimus, terbinafine, tiagabine, tiotropium, tipranavir, tolvaptan, trimethoprim, ulipristal, vardenafil, venetoclax, voriconazole, ziprasidone
Pregnancy category: C
Important contra-indications noted in the prescribing guidelines for: nursing mothers; pediatric patients

---

Skin
Erythema (3%)
Peripheral edema (3–8%)
Pruritus (<5%)

Mucosal
Oral candidiasis (2%)
Xerostomia (4%)

Cardiovascular
Atrial fibrillation (2–5%)
Hypertension (6–8%)
Hypotension (5–8%) [4]
Orthostatic hypotension (6–14%)
Phlebitis (32–51%)

Central Nervous System
Confusion (<5%)
Fever (5–11%) [2]
Headache (8–10%)
Insomnia (4–5%)

Gastrointestinal/Hepatic
Constipation (6–8%)
Diarrhea (<7%)
Nausea (3–5%)
Vomiting (5–7%)

Respiratory
Pharyngolaryngeal pain (<5%)
Pneumonia (2–5%)

Endocrine/Metabolic
Hypokalemia (10–22%)
Hypomagnesemia (2–5%)
Hyponatremia (6–8%)

Genitourinary
Urinary tract infection (4–5%)

Hematologic
Anemia (5–6%)

Local
Infusion-site erythema (<6%)
Infusion-site pain (<5%)
Infusion-site reactions (63–73%) [5]

Other
Dipsia (thirst) (3–6%) [2]

CORTISONE

Trade name: Cortone (Merck)
Indications: Arthralgia, dermatoses
Class: Corticosteroid
Half-life: N/A
Clinically important, potentially hazardous interactions with: chlorpropamide, diuretics, ethambutol, live vaccines, pancuronium, rifampin
Pregnancy category: C
Important contra-indications noted in the prescribing guidelines for: nursing mothers

---

Neuromuscular/Skeletal
Osteonecrosis [15]
Osteoporosis [10]
Tendinopathy/Tendon rupture [2]

Ocular
Cataract [5]
Glaucoma [8]

Other
Adverse effects [2]

CRIZOTINIB

Trade name: Xalkori (Pfizer)
Indications: Advanced or metastatic non-small cell lung cancer in ALK-positive patients
Class: Tyrosine kinase inhibitor
Half-life: 42 hours
Clinically important, potentially hazardous interactions with: alfentanil, atazanavir, carbamazepine, clarithromycin, cyclosporine, CYP3A inhibitors or inducers, CYP3A substrates, dihydroergotamine, efavirenz, ergotamine, fentanyl, grapefruit juice, indinavir, itraconazole, ketoconazole, nefazodone, nelfinavir, phenobarbital, phenytoin, pimozide, quinidine, rifabutin, rifampin, ritonavir, saquinavir, sirolimus, St John's wort, tacrolimus, telithromycin, troleandomycin, voriconazole
Pregnancy category: D
Important contra-indications noted in the prescribing guidelines for: nursing mothers; pediatric patients

---

Skin
Edema (38%) [9]
Peripheral edema [5]
Photosensitivity [2]
Rash (16%) [4]

Mucosal
Stomatitis (11%)

Cardiovascular
Bradycardia (5%) [6]
Cardiotoxicity [2]
Chest pain (12%)
QT prolongation [6]

Central Nervous System
Dysgeusia (taste perversion) (13%) [4]
Fever (12%)
Headache (13%)
Insomnia (12%)
Neurotoxicity (23%)
Vertigo (dizziness) (24%) [4]

Neuromuscular/Skeletal
Arthralgia (11%)
Asthenia (fatigue) (31%) [7]
Back pain (11%)

Gastrointestinal/Hepatic
Abdominal pain (16%)
Constipation (38%) [10]
Diarrhea (49%) [19]
Dyspepsia [3]
Dysphagia [3]
Esophagitis [7]
Gastroesophageal reflux [2]
Hepatitis [2]
Hepatotoxicity [8]
Nausea (57%) [18]
Vomiting (45%) [18]

Respiratory
Cough (21%)
Dyspnea (22%)
Pneumonitis [6]
Pulmonary toxicity [8]
Upper respiratory tract infection (20%)

Endocrine/Metabolic
ALT increased (15%) [10]
Appetite decreased (27%) [4]
AST increased (11%) [8]
Dehydration [2]
Hypocalcemia [2]
Hypogonadism [6]
Hypophosphatemia [5]

Renal
Nephrotoxicity [8]

Hematologic
Anemia [2]
Lymphopenia (11%) [5]
Neutropenia (5%) [8]

Ocular
Diplopia [2]
Ocular adverse effects (64%) [13]
Photophobia [2]
Photopsia [2]
Reduced visual acuity [2]
Vision blurred [2]
Vision impaired [2]
Visual disturbances [12]
Vitreous floaters [2]

Other
Adverse effects [5]
Death [2]

CROFELEMER

Trade name: Fulyzaq (Salix)
Indications: Non-infectious diarrhea in adult patients with HIV/AIDS on anti-retroviral therapy
Class: Proanthocyanidin oligomer
Half-life: N/A
Clinically important, potentially hazardous interactions with: none known
Pregnancy category: C
Important contra-indications noted in the prescribing guidelines for: the elderly; nursing mothers; pediatric patients
Note: Derived from the red latex of *Croton lechleri* which is also known as Sangre de Drago or dragon's blood.

Skin
Acneform eruption (<2%)
Dermatitis (<2%)
Herpes zoster (<2%)

Mucosal
Xerostomia (<2%)

Central Nervous System
Anxiety (2%)
Depression (<2%)
Vertigo (dizziness) (<2%)

Neuromuscular/Skeletal
Arthralgia (3%)
Back pain (3%)
Bone or joint pain (2%)
Pain in extremities (<2%)

Gastrointestinal/Hepatic
Abdominal distension (2%)
Abdominal pain (<2%)
Constipation (<2%)
Dyspepsia (<2%)
Flatulence (3%)
Gastroenteritis (<2%)
Nausea (3%)

Respiratory
Bronchitis (4%)
Cough (4%)
Nasopharyngitis (2%)
Sinusitis (<2%)
Upper respiratory tract infection (6%)

Endocrine/Metabolic
ALT increased (2%)
AST increased (<2%)

Genitourinary
Pollakiuria (<2%)

Renal
Nephrolithiasis (<2%)

Hematologic
Leukopenia (<2%)

Other
Infection (giardiasis) (2%)

CYANOCOBALAMIN

Synonym: Vitamin B_{12}
Trade name: Nascobal (Nastech)
Indications: Vitamin B_{12} deficiency, pernicious anemia
Class: Vitamin
Half-life: 6 days
Clinically important, potentially hazardous interactions with: colchicine
Pregnancy category: C

Skin
Acneform eruption [8]
Anaphylactoid reactions/Anaphylaxis [6]
Dermatitis [2]
Exanthems [3]
Hypersensitivity [2]
Nicolau syndrome [2]
Pruritus (<10%)
Urticaria [7]

Other
Allergic reactions [3]

CYCLOBENZAPRINE

Trade name: Flexeril (McNeil)
Indications: Muscle spasms
Class: Central muscle relaxant
Half-life: 8–37 hours
Clinically important, potentially hazardous interactions with: acetylcholinesterase inhibitors, anticholinergics, barbiturates, cisapride, CNS depressants, conivaptan, CYP1A2 inhibitors, droperidol, levomepromazine, linezolid, MAO inhibitors, phendimetrazine, pramlintide
Pregnancy category: B
Important contra-indications noted in the prescribing guidelines for: the elderly; nursing mothers; pediatric patients

---

Mucosal
Xerostomia (7–32%) [7]

Central Nervous System
Confusion (<3%)
Dysgeusia (taste perversion) (<3%)
Headache (5%) [3]
Irritability (<3%)
Nervousness (<3%)
Serotonin syndrome [3]
Somnolence (drowsiness) (29–39%) [8]
Vertigo (dizziness) (<11%) [8]

Neuromuscular/Skeletal
Asthenia (fatigue) (6%) [3]

Gastrointestinal/Hepatic
Abdominal pain (<3%)
Constipation (<3%) [3]
Diarrhea (<3%)
Nausea (<3%)

Respiratory
Pharyngitis (<3%)
Upper respiratory tract infection (<3%)

Ocular
Vision blurred (<3%)

Other
Adverse effects [2]

CYCLOPHOSPHAMIDE

Synonyms: CPM; CTX; CYT
Trade names: Cytoxan (Mead Johnson), Neosar (Gensia)
Indications: Lymphomas, minimal change nephrotic syndrome in pediatric patients
Class: Alkylating agent
Half-life: 3–12 hours
Clinically important, potentially hazardous interactions with: aldesleukin, azathioprine, belimumab, clozapine, cyclopenthiazide, cyclosporine, dexamethasone, etanercept, itraconazole, mycophenolate, pentostatin, prednisone, vaccines
Pregnancy category: D
Important contra-indications noted in the prescribing guidelines for: nursing mothers
Note: Contraindicated in patients with urinary outflow obstruction.

Skin
Acral erythema [3]
Anaphylactoid reactions/Anaphylaxis [3]
Edema [5]
Exanthems [4]
Graft-versus-host reaction [2]
Hand–foot syndrome [9]
Herpes zoster [4]
Hypersensitivity [6]
Kaposi's sarcoma [2]
Lupus erythematosus [2]
Lymphoma [4]
Malignancies [2]
Pemphigus [2]
Pigmentation [15]
Radiation recall dermatitis [6]
Rash (<10%) [6]
Scleroderma [2]
Squamous cell carcinoma [2]
Stevens–Johnson syndrome [2]
Toxicity [5]
Urticaria [8]
Vasculitis [2]

Hair
Alopecia [28]

Nails
Leukonychia (Mees' lines) (Muehrcke's lines) [3]
Nail pigmentation [16]

Mucosal
Gingival pigmentation [2]
Mucositis [3]
Oral ulceration [2]
Stomatitis (10%) [6]

Cardiovascular
Cardiotoxicity [6]
Flushing (<10%)
Hypotension [2]

Central Nervous System
Anorexia [2]
Dysgeusia (taste perversion) [2]
Fever [2]
Headache [3]
Leukoencephalopathy [6]
Neurotoxicity [7]
Peripheral neuropathy [6]

Neuromuscular/Skeletal
Arthralgia [2]
Asthenia (fatigue) [11]
Myalgia/Myopathy [7]

Gastrointestinal/Hepatic
Abdominal pain [2]
Diarrhea [7]
Hepatotoxicity [10]
Nausea [9]
Vomiting [10]

Respiratory
Pneumonia [2]

Endocrine/Metabolic
Amenorrhea [16]
Hyperglycemia [2]
Hyponatremia [3]
Menstrual irregularities [2]
SIADH [9]

Genitourinary
Cystitis [9]
Urinary tract infection [2]

Hematologic
Anemia [8]
Cytopenia [2]
Febrile neutropenia [13]
Hemotoxicity [8]
Leukopenia [7]
Lymphopenia [2]
Myelosuppression [4]
Neutropenia [28]
Sepsis [2]
Thrombocytopenia [13]

Local
Infusion-related reactions [2]

Other
Adverse effects [14]
Allergic reactions [2]
Death [7]
Hiccups [4]
Infection [19]

CYCLOSERINE

Trade name: Seromycin (Lilly)
Indications: Tuberculosis
Class: Antibiotic
Half-life: 10 hours
Clinically important, potentially hazardous interactions with: none known
Pregnancy category: C
Important contra-indications noted in the prescribing guidelines for: nursing mothers; pediatric patients

---

Skin
Dermatitis [2]
Exanthems [4]

Mucosal
Gingival hyperplasia/hypertrophy [3]

Central Nervous System
Depression [2]
Neurotoxicity [2]
Psychosis [7]
Seizures [4]

Renal
Nephrotoxicity [2]

Other
Adverse effects [4]

CYCLOSPORINE

Synonyms: CsA; CyA
Trade names: Neoral (Novartis), Restasis (Allergan), Sandimmune (Novartis)
Indications: Rheumatoid arthritis, prophylaxis of organ rejection in transplants, psoriasis, Restasis is indicated for patients with moderate-to-severe dry eye syndrome
Class: Calcineurin inhibitor, Disease-modifying antirheumatic drug (DMARD), Immunosuppressant
Half-life: 10–27 hours (adults)
Clinically important, potentially hazardous interactions with: afatinib, aliskiren, ambrisentan, amiloride, aminoglycosides, amiodarone, amphotericin B, ampicillin, amprenavir, anisindione, anticoagulants,

armodafinil, atazanavir, atorvastatin, azathioprine, azithromycin, bacampicillin, basiliximab, benazepril, bezafibrate, boceprevir, bosentan, bupropion, captopril, carbenicillin, caspofungin, cholestyramine, choline fenofibrate, cilazapril, ciprofloxacin, clarithromycin, cloxacillin, co-trimoxazole, cobicistat/elvitegravir/emtricitabine/tenofovir disoproxil, colchicine, colesevelam, corticosteroids, crizotinib, cyclophosphamide, dabigatran, daclizumab, danazol, daptomycin, darifenacin, darunavir, dasatinib, delavirdine, dichlorphenamide, diclofenac, dicloxacillin, dicumarol, digoxin, diltiazem, disulfiram, docetaxel, doxycycline, dronedarone, echinacea, efavirenz, enalapril, enzalutamide, erythromycin, ethotoin, etoposide, etoricoxib, everolimus, ezetimibe, flunisolide, fluoxymesterone, fluvastatin, foscarnet, fosinopril, fosphenytoin, gemfibrozil, grapefruit juice, Hemophilus B vaccine, HMG-CoA reductase inhibitors, imatinib, imipenem/cilastatin, indinavir, influenza vaccine, irbesartan, itraconazole, ketoconazole, lanreotide, levofloxacin, lisinopril, lopinavir, lovastatin, meloxicam, mephenytoin, methicillin, methoxsalen, methylphenidate, methylprednisolone, methyltestosterone, mezlocillin, micafungin, mifepristone, mizolastine, moxifloxacin, mycophenolate, nafcillin, natalizumab, nelfinavir, nevirapine, nifedipine, nisoldipine, norfloxacin, NSAIDs, ofloxacin, olmesartan, omeprazole, orlistat, osimertinib, oxacillin, oxcarbazepine, pasireotide, penicillins, phenytoin, pitavastatin, posaconazole, pravastatin, prednisolone, prednisone, pristinamycin, quinapril, rabeprazole, ramipril, ranolazine, rifabutin, rifampin, rifapentine, ritonavir, rosuvastatin, sevelamer, silodosin, simvastatin, sirolimus, spironolactone, St John's wort, sulfacetamide, sulfadiazine, sulfamethoxazole, sulfisoxazole, sulfonamides, tacrolimus, telithromycin, temsirolimus, tenoxicam, terbinafine, testosterone, ticarcillin, tinidazole, tipranavir, tofacitinib, tolvaptan, trabectedin, trandolapril, triamterene, trimethoprim, troleandomycin, ursodiol, vaccines, vecuronium, venetoclax, voriconazole, warfarin, zofenopril

Pregnancy category: C

Important contra-indications noted in the prescribing guidelines for: nursing mothers; pediatric patients

Note: Restasis is an ophthalmic emulsion.

Skin

Acne keloid [2]
Acneform eruption [7]
Anaphylactoid reactions/Anaphylaxis [8]
Basal cell carcinoma [4]
Candidiasis [2]
Cyst [5]
Edema (5–14%)
Fibroadenoma [2]
Folliculitis [8]
Herpes simplex [4]
Herpes zoster [2]
Hot flashes [2]
Hypersensitivity [2]
Kaposi's sarcoma [5]
Keratoses [3]
Keratosis pilaris [2]
Linear IgA bullous dermatosis [2]
Lymphocytic infiltration [5]
Lymphoma [12]
Lymphoproliferative disease [2]
Malignancies [2]
Mycosis fungoides [2]
Peripheral edema [3]
Pruritus (<2%) [2]
Pseudolymphoma [6]
Psoriasis [2]
Purpura (3%) [4]
Rash (7–12%)
Raynaud's phenomenon [2]
Sebaceous hyperplasia [9]
Squamous cell carcinoma [12]
Thrombocytopenic purpura [5]
Toxicity [2]
Urticaria [2]
Vasculitis [3]

Hair

Alopecia (3–4%) [2]
Alopecia areata [6]
Hirsutism [10]
Hypertrichosis (5–19%) [33]
Pseudofolliculitis barbae [2]

Nails

Brittle nails (<2%)
Leukonychia (Mees' lines) [2]

Mucosal

Aphthous stomatitis [2]
Gingival hyperplasia/hypertrophy (2–6%) [156]
Gingivitis (3–4%)
Oral ulceration [2]
Rectal hemorrhage (<3%)
Stomatitis (5–7%)

Cardiovascular

Arrhythmias (2–5%)
Capillary leak syndrome [2]
Chest pain (4–6%)
Flushing (2–5%) [5]
Hypertension (8–28%) [26]

Central Nervous System

Anorexia (3%)
Depression (<6%)
Dysesthesia [2]
Encephalopathy [4]
Fever (3–6%)
Headache (14–25%) [4]
Insomnia (<4%)
Leukoencephalopathy [17]
Migraine (2–3%)
Neurotoxicity [10]
Pain (3–13%)
Paresthesias (5–11%) [8]
Parkinsonism [6]
Pseudotumor cerebri [3]
Rigors (<3%)
Seizures [4]
Tremor (7–13%) [4]
Vertigo (dizziness) (6–8%)

Neuromuscular/Skeletal

Arthralgia (<6%)
Asthenia (fatigue) (3–6%) [4]
Myalgia/Myopathy [10]
Rhabdomyolysis [13]

Gastrointestinal/Hepatic

Abdominal pain (15%) [3]
Diarrhea (5–13%) [3]
Dyspepsia (2–12%)
Flatulence (4–5%)
Gastrointestinal disorder (2–4%) [2]
Hepatotoxicity [9]
Nausea (6–23%)
Vomiting (6–9%)

Respiratory

Bronchitis (<3%)
Bronchospasm (5%)
Cough (3–5%)
Dyspnea (<5%)
Influenza (<10%)
Pharyngitis (3–4%)
Pneumonia (<4%)
Rhinitis (<5%)
Sinusitis (3–4%)
Upper respiratory tract infection (8–15%)

Endocrine/Metabolic

Diabetes mellitus [2]
Gynecomastia (>3%) [3]
Hypertriglyceridemia [2]
Hypomagnesemia (4–6%)
Menstrual irregularities (<3%)
Serum creatinine increased (16–43%) [4]

Genitourinary

Urinary frequency (2–4%)
Urinary tract infection (3%)

Renal

Nephrotoxicity [94]
Renal function abnormal [2]

Hematologic

Anemia [3]
Dyslipidemia [4]
Hemolytic uremic syndrome [17]
Leukopenia [2]
Neutropenia [2]

Ocular

Hallucinations, visual [2]
Ocular burning (Restasis) (17%)
Papilledema [2]

Other

Adverse effects [18]
Infection [6]

CYPROTERONE

Trade name: Androcur (Bayer)

Indications: Control of libido in severe hypersexuality and/or sexual deviation in the adult male

Class: Androgen antagonist, Progesterone agonist

Half-life: 1.7 days

Clinically important, potentially hazardous interactions with: alcohol, clotrimazole, fingolimod, itraconazole, ketoconazole, pazopanib, phenytoin, rifampin, ritonavir, St John's wort

Pregnancy category: X (not indicated for use in women)

Important contra-indications noted in the prescribing guidelines for: pediatric patients

---

Skin

Tumors [3]

Cardiovascular

Venous thromboembolism [2]

Neuromuscular/Skeletal
Osteoporosis [2]

Gastrointestinal/Hepatic
Hepatotoxicity [23]

Respiratory
Dyspnea [4]

CYTARABINE

Synonym: ara-C
Trade names: Cytosar-U (Sicor), DepoCyt (Pacira)
Indications: Leukemias
Class: Antimetabolite, Antineoplastic, Antiviral
Half-life: initial: 10–15 minutes
Clinically important, potentially hazardous interactions with: aldesleukin
Pregnancy category: D
Important contra-indications noted in the prescribing guidelines for: nursing mothers; pediatric patients
Note: DepoCyt is a liposomal formulation. Vasculitis, a part of the cytarabine syndrome, consists of fever, malaise, myalgia, conjunctivitis, arthralgia and a diffuse erythematous maculopapular eruption that occurs from 6–12 hours following the administration of the drug.
Black Box Warning: DepoCyt: CHEMICAL ARACHNOIDITIS ADVERSE REACTIONS

Skin
Acral erythema [16]
Anaphylactoid reactions/Anaphylaxis [3]
Ephelides (<10%)
Erythema [5]
Exanthems [7]
Hand–foot syndrome [20]
Herpes zoster [2]
Neutrophilic eccrine hidradenitis [11]
Pruritus (<10%)
Rash (>10%) [2]
Seborrheic keratoses (inflammation of) (Leser–Trélat syndrome) [2]
Toxic epidermal necrolysis [2]
Toxicity [5]
Vasculitis [3]

Hair
Alopecia (<10%) [5]

Nails
Leukonychia (Mees' lines) [2]

Mucosal
Mucositis [2]
Oral lesions [5]
Oral ulceration (>10%)
Perianal ulcerations (>10%)
Stomatitis [2]

Cardiovascular
Thrombophlebitis (>10%)

Central Nervous System
Fever [3]
Headache [4]
Leukoencephalopathy [8]
Neurotoxicity [11]
Peripheral neuropathy [2]

Neuromuscular/Skeletal
Myalgia/Myopathy (<10%)
Rhabdomyolysis [3]

Gastrointestinal/Hepatic
Diarrhea [4]
Hepatotoxicity [4]
Nausea [3]
Pancreatitis [5]
Vomiting [3]

Respiratory
Pneumonia [3]

Endocrine/Metabolic
Hypokalemia [2]

Hematologic
Anemia [2]
Bleeding [2]
Febrile neutropenia [8]
Hemotoxicity [3]
Leukopenia [2]
Myelosuppression [3]
Neutropenia [5]
Sepsis [2]
Thrombocytopenia [4]

Ocular
Ocular adverse effects [2]

Local
Injection-site cellulitis (<10%)

Other
Adverse effects [5]
Death [4]
Infection [6]

DABIGATRAN

Trade name: Pradaxa (Boehringer Ingelheim)
Indications: Prevention of venous thromboembolic events, reduce stroke risk
Class: Anticoagulant, Thrombin inhibitor
Half-life: 2.5 days
Clinically important, potentially hazardous interactions with: amiodarone, antacids, anticoagulants, atorvastatin, carbamazepine, clarithromycin, clopidogrel, collagenase, cyclosporine, darunavir, dasatinib, deferasirox, desirudin, dextran, diclofenac, dronedarone, fondaparinux, heparin, ibritumomab, itraconazole, ketoconazole, ketorolac, lapatinib, meloxicam, nandrolone, NSAIDs, P-glycoprotein inducers and inhibitors, pantoprazole, pentosan, phenytoin, polysulfate sodium, prostacyclin analogues, proton pump inhibitors, quinidine, rifampin, rivaroxaban, salicylates, St John's wort, sulfinpyrazone, tacrolimus, telaprevir, thrombolytic agents, ticlopidine, tipranavir, tositumomab & iodine^{131}, ulipristal, verapamil, vitamin K antagonists
Pregnancy category: C
Important contra-indications noted in the prescribing guidelines for: the elderly; nursing mothers; pediatric patients
Note: Contraindicated in patients with active pathological bleeding or with a mechanical prosthetic heart valve.
Black Box Warning: DISCONTINUING PRADAXA IN PATIENTS WITHOUT ADEQUATE CONTINUOUS ANTICOAGULATION INCREASES RISK OF STROKE

Skin
Bruising (<10%)
Exanthems [2]
Rash [2]

Mucosal
Epistaxis (nosebleed) [2]

Cardiovascular
Myocardial infarction [5]

Central Nervous System
Headache [2]
Intracranial hemorrhage [4]
Subarachnoid hemorrhage [2]

Gastrointestinal/Hepatic
Abdominal pain [2]
Dyspepsia (11%) [6]
Esophagitis [3]
Gastritis [2]
Gastrointestinal bleeding (6%) [10]

Renal
Renal failure [3]

Hematologic
Anemia (<4%)
Anticoagulation [2]
Hemorrhage [9]
Thrombosis [3]

Other
Adverse effects [5]
Death [6]

DABRAFENIB

Trade name: Tafinlar (Novartis)
Indications: Melanoma (unresectable or metastatic) in patients with BRAF V600E mutation
Class: BRAF inhibitor, Kinase inhibitor
Half-life: 8 hours
Clinically important, potentially hazardous interactions with: strong CYP3A4 or CYP2C8 inducers or inhibitors
Pregnancy category: D
Important contra-indications noted in the prescribing guidelines for: nursing mothers; pediatric patients

---

Skin
Acneform eruption [3]
Actinic keratoses [3]
Basal cell carcinoma [4]
Bullae (<10%)
Grover's disease [4]
Hand–foot syndrome (20%) [6]
Hyperkeratosis (37%) [9]
Hypersensitivity (<10%)
Keratoacanthoma (7%) [5]
Keratosis pilaris [3]
Lesions [2]
Malignant melanoma (2%)
Panniculitis [5]
Papillomas (27%) [3]
Photosensitivity [5]
Pruritus [2]
Rash (17%) [4]
Seborrheic keratoses [2]
Squamous cell carcinoma (7%) [15]
Toxicity [3]
Xerosis [2]

Hair
Alopecia (22%) [4]
Hair changes [2]

Cardiovascular
Chest pain [2]

Central Nervous System
Chills [3]
Fever (28%) [14]
Headache (32%) [5]
Intracranial hemorrhage [3]

Neuromuscular/Skeletal
Arthralgia (27%) [7]
Asthenia (fatigue) [10]
Back pain (12%)
Myalgia/Myopathy (11%)

Gastrointestinal/Hepatic
Constipation (11%)
Diarrhea [2]
Nausea [6]
Pancreatitis (<10%)
Vomiting [4]

Respiratory
Cough (12%)
Nasopharyngitis (10%)

Endocrine/Metabolic
ALP increased (19%)
Appetite decreased [2]
Hyperglycemia (50%)
Hyponatremia (8%) [2]
Hypophosphatemia (37%)

Renal
Nephrotoxicity (<10%)

Hematologic
Anemia [4]
Neutropenia [4]

Other
Adverse effects [5]

DACARBAZINE

Synonym: DIC
Trade name: DTIC-Dome (Bayer)
Indications: Malignant melanoma, carcinomas
Class: Alkylating agent, Antineoplastic
Half-life: 5 hours
Clinically important, potentially hazardous interactions with: aldesleukin
Pregnancy category: C
Important contra-indications noted in the prescribing guidelines for: nursing mothers

---

Skin
Anaphylactoid reactions/Anaphylaxis (<10%)
Hypersensitivity [2]
Photosensitivity [10]
Rash (<10%) [2]
Urticaria [2]

Hair
Alopecia (<10%) [3]

Mucosal
Stomatitis (48%)

Cardiovascular
Flushing (<10%) [2]

Central Nervous System
Dysgeusia (taste perversion) (<10%)

Neuromuscular/Skeletal
Asthenia (fatigue) (75%) [4]
Myalgia/Myopathy (<10%)

Gastrointestinal/Hepatic
Hepatotoxicity [4]
Nausea [3]
Vomiting [2]

Respiratory
Flu-like syndrome [2]

Endocrine/Metabolic
ALT increased [2]
AST increased [2]

Hematologic
Neutropenia [4]
Thrombocytopenia [2]

Local
Injection-site burning (>10%)
Injection-site necrosis (>10%)
Injection-site pain (>10%)

Other
Adverse effects [7]

DACLATASVIR

Trade name: Daklinza (Bristol-Myers Squibb)
Indications: Hepatitis C (in combination with sofosbuvir)
Class: Hepatitis C virus NS5A inhibitor
Half-life: 12–15 hours
Clinically important, potentially hazardous interactions with: amiodarone, carbamazepine, dabigatran, phenytoin, rifampin, St John's wort
Pregnancy category: N/A (No data available)
Important contra-indications noted in the prescribing guidelines for: nursing mothers; pediatric patients
Note: See also separate entry for sofosbuvir.

Skin
Pruritus [2]

Central Nervous System
Fever [3]
Headache (14%) [15]
Insomnia [4]

Neuromuscular/Skeletal
Asthenia (fatigue) (14%) [12]

Gastrointestinal/Hepatic
Abdominal pain [2]
Diarrhea (5%) [8]
Nausea (8%) [11]

Endocrine/Metabolic
ALT increased [8]
AST increased [3]

Hematologic
Anemia [5]
Lymphopenia [2]
Neutropenia [2]

Other
Adverse effects [7]

DACLIZUMAB

Trade names: Zenapax (Roche), Zinbryta (Biogen)
Indications: Transplant rejection (Zenapax), relapsing forms of multiple sclerosis (Zinbryta)
Class: Immunosuppressant, Monoclonal antibody
Half-life: 11–38 days
Clinically important, potentially hazardous interactions with: corticosteroids, cyclosporine, Hemophilus B vaccine, methylprednisolone, mycophenolate, prednisolone
Pregnancy category: C
Important contra-indications noted in the prescribing guidelines for: the elderly; nursing mothers; pediatric patients
Black Box Warning: Zinbryta: HEPATIC INJURY INCLUDING AUTOIMMUNE HEPATITIS and OTHER IMMUNE-MEDIATED DISORDERS

Skin
Acneform eruption (>5%)
Dermatitis [2]
Eczema [5]
Edema (>5%)
Hypersensitivity [2]
Hypohidrosis (2–5%)
Lymphadenopathy [4]
Peripheral edema (>5%)
Pruritus (2–5%)
Psoriasis [2]
Rash (2–5%) [7]
Toxicity [2]
Wound complications (>5%)

Hair
Hirsutism (2–5%)

Cardiovascular
Chest pain (>5%)
Hypertension (>5%)
Hypotension (>5%)
Pulmonary edema (>5%)
Tachycardia (>5%)

Central Nervous System
Anxiety (2–5%)
Depression (2–5%)
Fever (>5%)
Headache (>5%) [2]
Insomnia (>5%)
Pain (>5%)
Tremor (>5%)
Vertigo (dizziness) (>5%)

Neuromuscular/Skeletal
Arthralgia (2–5%)
Asthenia (fatigue) (>5%)
Back pain (>5%)
Bone or joint pain (>5%)
Myalgia/Myopathy (2–5%)

Gastrointestinal/Hepatic
Abdominal distension (>5%)
Abdominal pain (>5%)
Colitis [2]
Constipation (>5%)
Diarrhea (>5%)
Flatulence (2–5%)
Gastritis (2–5%)
Hemorrhoids (2–5%)
Hepatotoxicity [3]
Nausea (>5%)
Vomiting (>5%)

Respiratory
Cough (>5%)
Dyspnea (>5%)
Hypoxia (2–5%)
Nasopharyngitis [2]
Pharyngitis (2–5%)
Pleural effusion (2–5%)
Pneumonia [2]
Rhinitis (2–5%)
Upper respiratory tract infection [3]

Endocrine/Metabolic
ALT increased [2]
AST increased [2]
Dehydration (2–5%)
Diabetes mellitus (2–5%)

Genitourinary
Urinary retention (2–5%)
Urinary tract infection [2]

Renal
Nephrotoxicity (2–5%)

Hematologic
Hemorrhage (>5%)
Thrombosis (>5%)

Ocular
Vision blurred (2–5%)

Local
Application-site reactions (2–5%)

Other
Adverse effects [3]
Infection [5]

DACTINOMYCIN

Synonyms: ACT; actinomycin-D
Trade name: Cosmegen (Merck)
Indications: Melanomas, sarcomas
Class: Antibiotic, anthracycline
Half-life: 36 hours
Clinically important, potentially hazardous interactions with: aldesleukin
Pregnancy category: D
Important contra-indications noted in the prescribing guidelines for: the elderly; nursing mothers; pediatric patients
Note: Contraindicated in patients with chickenpox or herpes zoster infection.

Skin
Acneform eruption (>10%) [6]
Erythema [2]
Folliculitis [2]
Pigmentation [4]
Pruritus [2]
Pustules [2]
Radiation recall dermatitis (>10%) [4]

Hair
Alopecia (>10%)

Mucosal
Oral lesions [3]
Stomatitis (ulcerative) (>5%)

Hematologic
Febrile neutropenia [2]
Neutropenia [2]
Thrombocytopenia [2]

Local
Injection-site extravasation (>10%)
Injection-site necrosis (>10%)
Injection-site phlebitis (>10%)

DALFAMPRIDINE

Synonym: 4-aminopyridine
Trade name: Ampyra (Acorda)
Indications: Multiple sclerosis (to improve walking)
Class: Potassium channel blocker
Half-life: 5–6.5 hours
Clinically important, potentially hazardous interactions with: none known
Pregnancy category: C
Important contra-indications noted in the prescribing guidelines for: nursing mothers; pediatric patients
Note: Contraindicated in patients with a history of seizure, or with moderate or severe renal impairment.

Central Nervous System
Balance disorder (5%)
Gait instability [2]
Headache (7%) [5]

Insomnia (9%) [5]
Multiple sclerosis (relapse) (4%)
Paresthesias (4%) [2]
Seizures [5]
Vertigo (dizziness) (7%) [9]

Neuromuscular/Skeletal
Asthenia (fatigue) (7%) [3]
Back pain (5%)

Gastrointestinal/Hepatic
Constipation (3%)
Dyspepsia (2%)
Nausea (7%) [4]

Respiratory
Nasopharyngitis (4%)
Pharyngolaryngeal pain (2%)

Genitourinary
Urinary tract infection (12%) [2]

Other
Adverse effects [4]

DALTEPARIN

Trade name: Fragmin (Pfizer)
Indications: Prophylaxis of deep vein thrombosis
Class: Heparin, low molecular weight
Half-life: 4–8 hours
Clinically important, potentially hazardous interactions with: butabarbital, danaparoid
Pregnancy category: B
Important contra-indications noted in the prescribing guidelines for: nursing mothers; pediatric patients
Black Box Warning: SPINAL/EPIDURAL HEMATOMA

Skin
Anaphylactoid reactions/Anaphylaxis (<10%) [2]
Bullous dermatitis (<10%)
Pruritus (<10%)
Rash (<10%)

Hair
Alopecia [2]

Local
Injection-site hematoma (<10%)
Injection-site pain (<10%)

Other
Allergic reactions (<10%) [3]

DANAZOL

Indications: Endometriosis, fibrocystic breast disease
Class: Pituitary hormone inhibitor
Half-life: ~4.5 hours
Clinically important, potentially hazardous interactions with: acenocoumarol, acitretin, atorvastatin, cyclosporine, insulin aspart, insulin degludec, insulin detemir, insulin glargine, insulin glulisine, oral contraceptives, paricalcitol, simvastatin, tacrolimus, warfarin
Pregnancy category: X
Important contra-indications noted in the prescribing guidelines for: nursing mothers; pediatric patients

Skin
Acneform eruption (>10%) [6]
Diaphoresis (3%)
Edema (>10%)
Erythema multiforme [2]
Exanthems [2]
Lupus erythematosus [4]
Rash (3%)
Seborrhea [4]

Hair
Alopecia [3]
Hirsutism (<10%) [5]

Cardiovascular
Flushing [3]

Neuromuscular/Skeletal
Rhabdomyolysis [5]

Gastrointestinal/Hepatic
Hepatotoxicity [4]

Endocrine/Metabolic
Pseudomenopause [2]
Weight gain [2]

Other
Adverse effects [2]
Death [2]

DANTROLENE

Trade names: Dantrium (Par), Ryanodex (Eagle)
Indications: Spasticity, malignant hyperthermia
Class: Skeletal muscle relaxant, hydantoin
Half-life: 8.7 hours
Clinically important, potentially hazardous interactions with: verapamil
Pregnancy category: C
Important contra-indications noted in the prescribing guidelines for: the elderly; nursing mothers; pediatric patients
Black Box Warning: HEPATOTOXICITY

Skin
Acneform eruption [3]
Rash (>10%)

Cardiovascular
Pericarditis [3]

Central Nervous System
Chills (<10%)
Vertigo (dizziness) [2]

Neuromuscular/Skeletal
Asthenia (fatigue) [2]
Myalgia/Myopathy [2]

Gastrointestinal/Hepatic
Hepatotoxicity [2]

Respiratory
Eosinophillic pleural effusion [3]
Pleural effusion [5]

Other
Adverse effects [2]
Death [4]

DAPAGLIFLOZIN

Trade names: Farxiga (AstraZeneca), Xigduo XR (AstraZeneca)
Indications: Type II diabetes mellitus
Class: Sodium-glucose co-transporter 2 (SGLT2) inhibitor
Half-life: 13 hours
Clinically important, potentially hazardous interactions with: pioglitazone
Pregnancy category: C
Important contra-indications noted in the prescribing guidelines for: the elderly; nursing mothers; pediatric patients
Note: Contraindicated in patients with severe renal impairment, end-stage renal disease, or undergoing dialysis. Xigduo XR is dapagliflozin and metformin.

Skin
Eczema [2]

Cardiovascular
Hypertension [2]
Hypotension [3]

Central Nervous System
Headache [2]

Neuromuscular/Skeletal
Arthralgia [2]
Back pain (3–4%) [3]
Pain in extremities (2%)

Gastrointestinal/Hepatic
Constipation (2%)
Diarrhea [3]
Nausea (3%) [2]

Respiratory
Bronchitis [2]
Cough [2]
Influenza (2–3%) [2]
Nasopharyngitis (6–7%) [6]
Upper respiratory tract infection [4]

Endocrine/Metabolic
Dehydration [2]
Hypoglycemia (>10%) [13]
Hypovolemia [2]

Genitourinary
Genital mycotic infections (particularly in women) (3–8%) [30]
Pollakiuria [2]
Urinary frequency (3–4%)
Urinary tract infection (4–6%) [32]

Hematologic
Dyslipidemia (2–3%)

Other
Adverse effects [8]
Dipsia (thirst) [2]
Infection (<10%)

DAPSONE

Trade name: Aczone (Allergan)
Indications: Leprosy, dermatitis herpetiformis, acne
Class: Antibiotic, Antimycobacterial
Half-life: 10–50 hours
Clinically important, potentially hazardous interactions with: atovaquone/proguanil, chloroquine, didanosine, furazolidone, ganciclovir, hydroxychloroquine, methotrexate, pyrimethamine, rifabutin, rifampin, rifapentine, sulfonamides, trimethoprim, ursodiol
Pregnancy category: C
Important contra-indications noted in the prescribing guidelines for: nursing mothers
Note: A hypersensitivity reaction – termed the 'sulfone syndrome' or 'dapsone syndrome' – may infrequently develop during the first six weeks of treatment. This syndrome consists of exfoliative dermatitis, fever, malaise, nausea, anorexia, hepatitis, jaundice, lymphadenopathy and hemolytic anemia.

Skin
AGEP [2]
Cyanosis [2]
Dapsone syndrome [38]
DRESS syndrome [12]
Erythema multiforme [8]
Erythema nodosum [4]
Exanthems (<5%) [11]
Exfoliative dermatitis [9]
Fixed eruption [3]
Hypersensitivity [20]
Lupus erythematosus [5]
Photosensitivity [9]
Pigmentation [6]
Rash [6]
Stevens–Johnson syndrome [3]
Toxic epidermal necrolysis [7]

Nails
Beau's lines (transverse nail bands) [3]

Central Nervous System
Headache (4%) [2]
Peripheral neuropathy [2]

Gastrointestinal/Hepatic
Hepatitis [3]
Hepatotoxicity [2]
Pancreatitis [2]

Respiratory
Cough (2%)
Eosinophilic pneumonia [2]
Nasopharyngitis (5%)
Pharyngitis (2%)
Sinusitis (2%)
Upper respiratory tract infection (3%)

Hematologic
Agranulocytosis [6]
Anemia [2]
Hemolysis [5]
Hemolytic anemia [6]
Methemoglobinemia [17]

Local
Application-site erythema (13%) [2]
Application-site reactions (18%)

Other
Adverse effects [4]
Death [5]

DAPTOMYCIN

Trade name: Cubicin (Cubist)
Indications: Complicated skin and skin structure infections, *Staphylococcus aureus* bloodstream infections
Class: Antibiotic, glycopeptide
Half-life: ~8 hours
Clinically important, potentially hazardous interactions with: atorvastatin, cyclosporine, fibrates, HMG-CoA reductase inhibitors, rosuvastatin, statins, tobramycin, typhoid vaccine, warfarin
Pregnancy category: B
Important contra-indications noted in the prescribing guidelines for: the elderly; nursing mothers; pediatric patients

---

Skin
AGEP [2]
Cellulitis (<2%)
Edema (<7%)
Fungal dermatitis (3%)
Hyperhidrosis (5%)
Pruritus (3–6%)
Rash (4%)

Cardiovascular
Chest pain (7%)
Hypertension (6%)
Hypotension (2%)

Central Nervous System
Fever (2%)
Headache (5%)
Insomnia (9%)
Vertigo (dizziness) (2%)

Neuromuscular/Skeletal
Back pain (<2%)
Myalgia/Myopathy [7]
Rhabdomyolysis [6]

Gastrointestinal/Hepatic
Abdominal pain (<6%)
Constipation (6%)
Diarrhea (5%) [2]
Hepatotoxicity [3]
Nausea (6%) [2]
Vomiting (3%)

Respiratory
Cough (<2%)
Dyspnea (2%)
Eosinophilic pneumonia [14]
Pharyngolaryngeal pain (8%)
Pneumonia [2]

Endocrine/Metabolic
Creatine phosphokinase increased (7%) [5]

Genitourinary
Urinary tract infection (2%)

Renal
Nephrotoxicity [2]
Renal failure [2]

Hematologic
Eosinophilia [2]
Neutropenia [2]
Thrombocytopenia [2]

Local
Injection-site reactions (6%)

Other
Adverse effects [3]

DARATUMUMAB *

Trade name: Darzalex (Janssen Biotech)
Indications: Multiple myeloma in patients who have received at least three prior lines of therapy including a proteasome inhibitor (PI) and an immunomodulatory agent or who are double-refractory to a PI and an immunomodulatory agent
Class: Monoclonal antibody
Half-life: 18 days
Clinically important, potentially hazardous interactions with: none known
Pregnancy category: N/A (No data available)
Important contra-indications noted in the prescribing guidelines for: pediatric patients

---

Skin
Herpes zoster (3%)

Mucosal
Nasal congestion (17%)

Cardiovascular
Chest pain (12%)
Hypertension (10%)

Central Nervous System
Chills (10%)
Cytokine release syndrome [2]
Fever (21%) [2]
Headache (12%)

Neuromuscular/Skeletal
Arthralgia (17%)
Asthenia (fatigue) (39%) [2]
Back pain (23%)
Pain in extremities (15%)

Gastrointestinal/Hepatic
Constipation (15%)
Diarrhea (16%)
Nausea (27%)
Vomiting (14%)

Respiratory
Bronchospasm (<2%) [2]
Cough (21%)
Dyspnea (15%) [2]
Hypoxia (<2%)
Nasopharyngitis (15%)
Pneumonia (11%)
Rhinitis (>5%)
Upper respiratory tract infection (20%)

Endocrine/Metabolic
Appetite decreased (15%)

Hematologic
Anemia (45%) [5]
Lymphopenia (72%)
Neutropenia (60%) [2]
Thrombocytopenia (48%) [5]

Local
Infusion-related reactions (48%) [5]

DARBEPOETIN ALFA

Synonym: erythropoiesis stimulating protein
Trade name: Aranesp (Amgen)
Indications: Anemia associated with renal failure and chemotherapy
Class: Colony stimulating factor, Erythropoiesis-stimulating agent (ESA), Erythropoietin
Half-life: 21 hours
Clinically important, potentially hazardous interactions with: none known
Pregnancy category: C
Important contra-indications noted in the prescribing guidelines for: nursing mothers; pediatric patients
Note: There is an increased risk of death for patients suffering from chronic renal failure with this drug (6%).
Black Box Warning: ERYTHROPOIESIS-STIMULATING AGENTS (ESAs) INCREASE THE RISK OF DEATH, MYOCARDIAL INFARCTION, STROKE, VENOUS THROMBOEMBOLISM, THROMBOSIS OF VASCULAR ACCESS AND TUMOR PROGRESSION OR RECURRENCE

Skin
Edema (21%)
Peripheral edema (11%)
Pruritus (8%)
Rash (7%) [2]

Central Nervous System
Fever (9–19%)
Vertigo (dizziness) (8–14%)

Neuromuscular/Skeletal
Arthralgia (11–13%)
Asthenia (fatigue) (9–33%)
Back pain (8%)
Myalgia/Myopathy (21%)

Gastrointestinal/Hepatic
Abdominal pain (12%)

Respiratory
Cough (10%)
Flu-like syndrome (6%)
Upper respiratory tract infection (14%)

Hematologic
Thrombosis [2]

Local
Injection-site pain (7%)

Other
Adverse effects [3]

DARIFENACIN

Trade names: Emselex (Novartis), Enablex (Novartis)
Indications: Overactive bladder
Class: Anticholinergic, Antimuscarinic, Muscarinic antagonist
Half-life: 13–19 hours
Clinically important, potentially hazardous interactions with: anticholinergics, antihistamines, atazanavir, clozapine, cyclosporine, digoxin, disopyramide, domperidone, erythromycin, flecainide, fosamprenavir, haloperidol, imipramine, indinavir, itraconazole, ketoconazole, levodopa, lopinavir, MAO inhibitors, memantine, metoclopramide, nefopam, nelfinavir, nitrates (sublingual), parasympathomimetics, paroxetine hydrochloride, phenothiazines, potent CYP3A4 inhibitors, ritonavir, saquinavir, thioridazine, tipranavir, tricyclic antidepressants, verapamil
Pregnancy category: C
Important contra-indications noted in the prescribing guidelines for: nursing mothers; pediatric patients
Note: Contraindicated in patients with, or at risk for, urinary retention, gastric retention or uncontrolled narrow-angle glaucoma.

Mucosal
Xerostomia (20%) [12]

Gastrointestinal/Hepatic
Abdominal pain (2%)
Constipation [3]

DARUNAVIR

Trade names: Prezcobix (Janssen), Prezista (Janssen)
Indications: HIV infection (must be co-administered with ritonavir and with other antiretroviral agents)
Class: Antiretroviral, HIV-1 protease inhibitor
Half-life: 15 hours
Clinically important, potentially hazardous interactions with: abacavir, alfuzosin, almotriptan, alosetron, alprazolam, amiodarone, antifungals, apixaban, artemether/lumefantrine, astemizole, atorvastatin, bortezomib, brinzolamide, calcium channel blockers, captopril, carbamazepine, ciclesonide, cisapride, clarithromycin, colchicine, conivaptan, cyclosporine, CYP2D6 substrates, CYP3A4 inhibitors, inducers and substrates, dabigatran, dasatinib, deferasirox, delavirdine, didanosine, dienogest, digoxin, dihydroergotamine, dronedarone, duloxetine, dutasteride, efavirenz, enfuvirtide, eplerenone, ergotamine, estrogens, etravirine, everolimus, fentanyl, fesoterodine, food, fusidic acid, guanfacine, halofantrine, HMG-CoA reductase inhibitors, indinavir, inhaled corticosteroids, ixabepilone, ketoconazole, lidocaine, lopinavir, lovastatin, maraviroc, meperidine, methadone, methylprednisolone, midazolam, mifepristone, mometasone, nefazodone, nilotinib, nisoldipine, P-glycoprotein substrates, paricalcitol, paroxetine hydrochloride, pazopanib, phenobarbital, phenytoin, pimecrolimus, pimozide, prasugrel, pravastatin, protease inhibitors, quetiapine, quinidine, quinine, ranolazine, rifabutin, rifampin, rilpivirine, rivaroxaban, romidepsin, rosuvastatin, salmeterol, saquinavir, saxagliptin, sertraline, sildenafil, silodosin, simeprevir, simvastatin, sirolimus, sorafenib, St John's wort, tacrolimus, tadalafil, tamsulosin, telaprevir, temsirolimus, tenofovir disoproxil, terfenadine, theophylline, tolvaptan, topotecan, trazodone, triazolam, tricyclic antidepressants, vardenafil, voriconazole, warfarin, zidovudine
Pregnancy category: C
Important contra-indications noted in the prescribing guidelines for: nursing mothers; pediatric patients
Note: Darunavir is a sulfonamide and can be absorbed systemically. Sulfonamides can produce severe, possibly fatal, reactions such as toxic epidermal necrolysis and Stevens-Johnson syndrome.
Prezcobix is darunavir and cobicistat.

Skin
Angioedema (<2%)
Hypersensitivity (<2%)
Pruritus (<2%)
Rash (6–10%) [9]
Stevens–Johnson syndrome (<2%)
Urticaria (<2%)

Central Nervous System
Abnormal dreams (<2%)
Anorexia (2%)
Headache (7%) [6]

Neuromuscular/Skeletal
Asthenia (fatigue) (2–3%)
Osteonecrosis (<2%)

Gastrointestinal/Hepatic
Abdominal distension (2%)
Abdominal pain (6%)
Diarrhea (9–14%) [10]
Dyspepsia (<3%)
Flatulence (<2%)
Gastrointestinal disorder [3]
Hepatotoxicity (<2%) [6]
Nausea (4–7%) [6]
Pancreatitis (<2%)
Vomiting (2–5%)

Endocrine/Metabolic
Diabetes mellitus (new onset or exacebated) (2%)

Other
Adverse effects [6]

DASABUVIR/ OMBITASVIR/PARITA-PREVIR/RITONAVIR *

Trade name: Viekira XR (AbbVie)
Indications: Genotype 1a chronic hepatitis C virus with or without cirrhosis, genotype 1b chronic hepatitis C virus with or without cirrhosis in combination with ribavirin
Class: CYP3A4 inhibitor (ritonavir), Hepatitis C virus non-nucleoside NS5B palm polymerase inhibitor (dasabuvir), Hepatitis C virus NS3/4A protease inhibitor (paritaprevir), Hepatitis C virus NS5A inhibitor (ombitasvir)
Half-life: 6 hours (dasabuvir); 21–25 hours (ombitasvir); 6 hours (paritaprevir); 4 hours (ritonavir)
Clinically important, potentially hazardous interactions with: alfuzosin, carbamazepine, cisapride, dihydroergotamine, dronedarone, efavirenz, ergotamine, ethinyl estradiol-containing medications, gemfibrozil, lovastatin, lurasidone, methylergonovine, midazolam, phenobarbital, phenytoin, pimozide, ranolazine, rifampin,

sildenafil, simvastatin, St John's wort, triazolam
Pregnancy category: N/A (Insufficient evidence to inform drug-associated risk; contraindicated in pregnancy when given with ribavirin)
Important contra-indications noted in the prescribing guidelines for: nursing mothers; pediatric patients
Note: Contraindicated in patients with moderate to severe hepatic impairment. See also separate entries for Ombitasvir/Paritaprevir/Ritonavir (co-packaged with Dasabuvir as Viekira Pak) and Ribavirin.

Skin
Pruritus (7%) [2]
Rash (7%)

Central Nervous System
Insomnia (5%) [2]

Neuromuscular/Skeletal
Asthenia (fatigue) (4%) [2]

Gastrointestinal/Hepatic
Nausea (8%)

Endocrine/Metabolic
Hyperbilirubinemia (2%)

DASATINIB

Trade name: Sprycel (Bristol-Myers Squibb)
Indications: Leukemia (chronic myeloid), acute lymphoblastic leukemia
Class: Antineoplastic, Biologic, Tyrosine kinase inhibitor
Half-life: 3–5 hours
Clinically important, potentially hazardous interactions with: abciximab, alfentanil, alfuzosin, ambrisentan, antacids, anticoagulants, antiplatelet agents, aprepitant, argatroban, artemether/lumefantrine, astemizole, atazanavir, atorvastatin, boceprevir, cabazitaxel, carbamazepine, chloroquine, ciclesonide, cilostazol, cinacalcet, ciprofloxacin, cisapride, clarithromycin, clopidogrel, clozapine, colchicine, conivaptan, cyclosporine, CYP3A4 inhibitors, inducers and substrates, dabigatran, darunavir, deferasirox, dexamethasone, dihydroergotamine, docetaxel, dronedarone, efavirenz, eptifibatide, ergotamine, erythromycin, eszopiclone, famotidine, fentanyl, fesoterodine, gadobutrol, gefitinib, H_2 antagonists, indinavir, itraconazole, ixabepilone, ketoconazole, lopinavir, lurasidone, maraviroc, meloxicam, nefazodone, nelfinavir, nilotinib, omeprazole, pantoprazole, phenobarbital, phenytoin, pimozide, proton pump inhibitors, QT prolonging agents, quinidine, quinine, rifampin, ritonavir, saquinavir, saxagliptin, sildenafil, simvastatin, sirolimus, St John's wort, tacrolimus, tadalafil, temsirolimus, terfenadine, tetrabenazine, thioridazine, tiagabine, tinzaparin, vardenafil, ziprasidone
Pregnancy category: D
Important contra-indications noted in the prescribing guidelines for: nursing mothers; pediatric patients

---

Skin
Acneform eruption (<10%)
Dermatitis (<10%)
Eczema (<10%)
Edema (13–18%) [5]
Herpes (<10%)
Hyperhidrosis (<10%)
Panniculitis [3]
Peripheral edema [3]
Pruritus (<10%) [3]
Rash (11–21%) [9]
Toxicity [6]
Urticaria (<10%)
Xerosis (<10%)

Hair
Alopecia (<10%)
Hair pigmentation [2]

Mucosal
Mucositis (16%)

Cardiovascular
Arrhythmias (<10%)
Cardiac failure (3%)
Congestive heart failure (2%)
Flushing (<10%)
Hypertension (<10%)
Palpitation (<10%)
Pericardial effusion (2–3%) [6]
QT prolongation [3]
Tachycardia (<10%)

Central Nervous System
Anorexia (<10%) [6]
Anxiety [2]
Depression (<10%)
Dysgeusia (taste perversion) (<10%)
Fever (5–39%)
Headache (12–33%) [7]
Insomnia (<10%)
Neurotoxicity (13%)
Pain (26%) [2]
Peripheral neuropathy (<10%)
Somnolence (drowsiness) (<10%)
Subdural hemorrhage [4]
Vertigo (dizziness) (<10%)

Neuromuscular/Skeletal
Arthralgia (<19%)
Asthenia (fatigue) (8%) [14]
Bone or joint pain (12–19%) [2]
Myalgia/Myopathy (6–13%) [2]

Gastrointestinal/Hepatic
Abdominal distension (<10%)
Abdominal pain (<25%)
Colitis (<10%) [3]
Constipation (<10%)
Diarrhea (18–31%) [18]
Dyspepsia (<10%)
Enterocolitis (<10%)
Gastritis (<10%)
Gastrointestinal bleeding (2–8%) [3]
Hemorrhagic colitis [2]
Hepatitis [2]
Hepatotoxicity [2]
Nausea (9–23%) [10]
Vomiting (7–15%) [6]

Respiratory
Cough (<10%)
Dyspnea (20%) [5]
Pleural effusion (12–21%) [35]
Pneumonia (<10%) [3]
Pneumonitis (<10%)
Pulmonary hypertension (<10%) [9]
Pulmonary toxicity [3]
Upper respiratory tract infection (<10%)

Endocrine/Metabolic
Weight gain (<10%)
Weight loss (<10%)

Renal
Proteinuria [2]
Renal failure [3]

Hematologic
Anemia [3]
Bleeding (6–26%)
Cytopenia [3]
Febrile neutropenia (<12%)
Hemorrhage [2]
Hemotoxicity [4]
Myelosuppression [9]
Neutropenia [7]
Pancytopenia (<10%)
Thrombocytopenia [13]

Otic
Tinnitus (<10%)

Ocular
Reduced visual acuity (<10%)
Vision blurred (<10%)
Visual disturbances (<10%)
Xerophthalmia (<10%)

Other
Adverse effects [4]
Death [2]
Infection (<14%) [2]
Side effects [2]

DAUNORUBICIN

Synonyms: daunomycin; DNR; rubidomycin
Trade name: DaunoXome (Gilead)
Indications: Acute leukemias
Class: Antibiotic, anthracycline
Half-life: 14–20 hours; 4 hours (intramuscular)
Clinically important, potentially hazardous interactions with: aldesleukin, gadobenate
Pregnancy category: D
Important contra-indications noted in the prescribing guidelines for: the elderly; nursing mothers; pediatric patients
Black Box Warning: MYOCARDIAL TOXICITY / MYELOSUPPRESSION

Skin
Angioedema [4]
Dermatitis [2]
Edema (11%)
Exanthems [2]
Folliculitis (<5%)
Hot flashes (<5%)
Hyperhidrosis (14%)
Lymphadenopathy (<5%)
Neutrophilic eccrine hidradenitis [2]
Pigmentation [3]
Pruritus (7%)
Seborrhea (<5%)
Urticaria [3]
Xerosis (<5%)

Hair
Alopecia (8%) [4]

Nails
Nail pigmentation [5]

Mucosal
Gingival bleeding (<5%)
Oral lesions [2]
Sialorrhea (<5%)
Stomatitis (10%)
Xerostomia (<5%)

Cardiovascular
Chest pain (9–14%)
Flushing (14%)
Hypertension (<5%)
Myocardial toxicity [5]
Palpitation (<5%)
Tachycardia (<5%)

Central Nervous System
Amnesia (<5%)
Anorexia (23%)
Anxiety (<5%)
Cognitive impairment (<5%)
Depression (10%)
Dysgeusia (taste perversion) (<5%)
Gait instability (<5%)
Hallucinations (<5%)
Headache (25%)
Insomnia (6%)
Meningococcal infection (<5%)
Neurotoxicity (13%)
Rigors (19%)
Seizures (<5%)
Somnolence (drowsiness) (<5%)
Syncope (<5%)
Tremor (<5%)
Vertigo (dizziness) (8%)

Neuromuscular/Skeletal
Arthralgia (7%)
Asthenia (fatigue) (10%)
Ataxia (<5%)
Back pain (16%)
Hyperkinesia (<5%)
Hypertonia (<5%)
Myalgia/Myopathy (7%)

Gastrointestinal/Hepatic
Abdominal pain (23%)
Black stools (<5%)
Constipation (7%)
Diarrhea (38%)
Dysphagia (<5%)
Gastritis (<5%)
Gastrointestinal bleeding (<5%)
Hemorrhoids (<5%)
Hepatomegaly (<5%)
Nausea (54%)
Tenesmus (5%)
Vomiting (23%)

Respiratory
Cough (28%)
Dyspnea (26%)
Flu-like syndrome (5%)
Hemoptysis (<5%)
PIE syndrome (<5%)
Rhinitis (12%)
Sinusitis (8%)

Endocrine/Metabolic
Appetite increased (<5%)
Dehydration (<5%)

Genitourinary
Dysuria (<5%)
Nocturia (<5%)
Polyuria (<5%)

Hematologic
Neutropenia (15–36%)
Splenomegaly (<5%)

Otic
Ear pain (<5%)
Hearing loss (<5%)
Tinnitus (<5%)

Ocular
Abnormal vision (5%)
Conjunctivitis (<5%)
Ocular pain (<5%)

Local
Injection-site inflammation (<5%)
Injection-site necrosis (<10%) [2]
Injection-site ulceration (<10%)

Other
Dipsia (thirst) (<5%)
Hiccups (<5%)
Infection (40%)
Tooth decay (<5%)

DECITABINE

Synonym: 5-aza-2'-deoxycytidine
Trade name: Dacogen (MGI Pharma)
Indications: Myelodysplastic syndromes, leukemia
Class: Antineoplastic
Half-life: ~30 minutes
Clinically important, potentially hazardous interactions with: none known
Pregnancy category: D
Important contra-indications noted in the prescribing guidelines for: nursing mothers; pediatric patients

---

Skin
Bacterial infection (5%)
Candidiasis (10%)
Cellulitis (12%)
Ecchymoses (22%)
Edema (18%)
Erythema (14%)
Facial edema (6%)
Hematoma (5%)
Lymphadenopathy (12%)
Pallor (23%)
Peripheral edema (25%)
Petechiae (39%)
Pruritus (11%)
Rash (19%) [2]
Urticaria (6%)

Mucosal
Gingival bleeding (8%)
Glossodynia (5%)
Lip ulceration (5%)
Mucositis [2]
Oral candidiasis (6%)
Stomatitis (12%)
Tongue ulceration (7%)

Cardiovascular
Chest pain (7%)
Hypotension (6%)
Pulmonary edema (6%)

Central Nervous System
Anorexia (16%)
Anxiety (11%)
Confusion (12%)
Fever (53%)
Headache (28%)
Hypoesthesia (11%)
Insomnia (28%)
Pain (13%)
Rigors (22%)
Vertigo (dizziness) (18%)

Neuromuscular/Skeletal
Arthralgia (20%)
Asthenia (fatigue) (5–12%) [5]
Back pain (17%)
Bone or joint pain (6–19%)
Myalgia/Myopathy (5%)

Gastrointestinal/Hepatic
Abdominal distension (5%)
Abdominal pain (14%)
Ascites (10%)
Constipation (35%)
Diarrhea (34%) [2]
Dyspepsia (12%)
Dysphagia (6%)
Gastroesophageal reflux (5%)
Hemorrhoids (8%)
Hepatotoxicity [2]
Loose stools (7%)
Nausea (42%) [6]
Vomiting (25%) [3]

Respiratory
Cough (40%)
Hypoxia (10%)
Pharyngitis (16%)
Pneumonia (22%) [2]
Sinusitis (5%)

Endocrine/Metabolic
ALP increased (11%)
Appetite decreased (16%)
AST increased (10%)
Dehydration (6%)
Hyperglycemia (33%)
Hyperkalemia (13%)
Hypoalbuminemia (24%)
Hypokalemia (22%)
Hypomagnesemia (24%)
Hyponatremia (19%)

Genitourinary
Dysuria (6%)
Urinary frequency (5%)
Urinary tract infection (7%)

Hematologic
Anemia (82%) [4]
Bacteremia (5%)
Febrile neutropenia (29%) [6]
Hemotoxicity [2]
Leukopenia (28%)
Lymphopenia [2]
Myelosuppression [11]
Neutropenia (90%) [11]
Thrombocytopenia (89%) [6]

Ocular
Vision blurred (6%)

Local
Injection-site edema (5%)
Injection-site erythema (5%)

Other
Adverse effects [2]
Infection [3]

DEFERASIROX

Trade names: Exjade (Novartis), Jadenu (Novartis)
Indications: Chronic iron overload due to blood transfusions and in non-transfuson dependent thalassemia syndromes
Class: Chelator, iron
Half-life: 8–16 hours
Clinically important, potentially hazardous interactions with: alfuzosin, aluminum-containing antacids, ambrisentan, aprepitant, cabazitaxel, cholestyramine, cilostazol, colesevelam, colestipol, conivaptan, dabigatran, darunavir, dasatinib, delavirdine, docetaxel, efavirenz, enalapril, estradiol, eszopiclone, fesoterodine, gefitinib, indinavir, ixabepilone, lapatinib, lurasidone, maraviroc, pazopanib, phenobarbital, phenytoin, pioglitazone, repaglinide, rifampin, ritonavir, sildenafil, telithromycin, theophylline, tiagabine, tipranavir, trimethoprim, ulipristal
Pregnancy category: C
Important contra-indications noted in the prescribing guidelines for: the elderly; nursing mothers
Black Box Warning: RENAL FAILURE, HEPATIC FAILURE, AND GASTROINTESTINAL HEMORRHAGE

Skin
Rash (2–11%) [24]
Urticaria (4%)

Central Nervous System
Headache (16%) [2]

Neuromuscular/Skeletal
Arthralgia (7%)
Asthenia (fatigue) [2]
Back pain (6%)

Gastrointestinal/Hepatic
Abdominal pain (21–28%) [11]
Diarrhea (5–20%) [18]
Gastrointestinal bleeding [3]
Gastrointestinal disorder [3]
Hepatotoxicity [8]
Nausea (2–6%) [19]
Vomiting (10–21%) [6]

Respiratory
Cough (14%)
Flu-like syndrome (11%)
Upper respiratory tract infection (9%)

Endocrine/Metabolic
ALT increased [8]
AST increased [3]
Serum creatinine increased [21]

Renal
Fanconi syndrome [10]
Nephrotoxicity [7]
Proteinuria [4]
Renal failure [3]
Renal function abnormal [2]

Other
Adverse effects [15]

DEFERIPRONE

Trade name: Ferriprox (ApoPharma)
Indications: Treatment of patients with transfusional iron overload due to thalassemia syndromes when current chelation therapy is inadequate
Class: Chelator, iron
Half-life: 1.9 hours
Clinically important, potentially hazardous interactions with: antacids containing iron, aluminum, zinc, diclofenac, mineral supplements, probenecid
Pregnancy category: D
Important contra-indications noted in the prescribing guidelines for: the elderly; nursing mothers; pediatric patients
Black Box Warning: AGRANULOCYTOSIS / NEUTROPENIA

Central Nervous System
Headache (3%)

Neuromuscular/Skeletal
Arthralgia (10%) [8]
Arthropathy [5]
Back pain (2%)
Bone or joint pain [2]
Pain in extremities (2%)

Gastrointestinal/Hepatic
Abdominal pain (10%) [2]
Diarrhea (3%) [2]
Dyspepsia (2%)
Gastrointestinal disorder [5]
Hepatotoxicity [3]
Nausea (13%) [4]
Vomiting (10%)

Endocrine/Metabolic
ALT increased (8%) [5]
Appetite increased (4%)
AST increased [2]
Weight gain (2%)

Renal
Chromaturia (15%)

Hematologic
Agranulocytosis (2%) [14]
Neutropenia [11]
Thrombocytopenia [2]

Other
Adverse effects [2]
Death [2]

DEFEROXAMINE

Trade name: Desferal (Novartis)
Indications: Hemochromatosis, acute iron overload
Class: Chelator, iron
Half-life: 6.1 hours
Clinically important, potentially hazardous interactions with: ascorbic acid, ferrous sulfate, zinc
Pregnancy category: C

Skin
Anaphylactoid reactions/Anaphylaxis [3]
Hypersensitivity [2]

Central Nervous System
Neurotoxicity [2]

Neuromuscular/Skeletal
Arthralgia [6]

Endocrine/Metabolic
Serum creatinine increased [2]

Otic
Hearing loss [2]
Ototoxicity [7]

Ocular
Night blindness [2]
Retinopathy [12]

Local
Injection-site inflammation (<10%)
Injection-site pain (<10%)

Other
Death [3]

DEFIBROTIDE *

Trade name: Defitelio (Jazz)
Indications: Hepatic veno-occlusive disease in patients with renal or pulmonary dysfunction following hematopoietic stem-cell transplantation
Class: Oligonucleotide
Half-life: <2 hours
Clinically important, potentially hazardous interactions with: alteplase, heparin
Pregnancy category: N/A (No data available)
Important contra-indications noted in the prescribing guidelines for: nursing mothers
Note: Contraindicated for concomitant administration with systemic anticoagulant or fibrinolytic therapy.

Skin
Graft-versus-host reaction (6%)

Mucosal
Epistaxis (nosebleed) (14%)

Cardiovascular
Hypotension (37%) [3]

Central Nervous System
Cerebral hemorrhage (2%)
Intracranial hemorrhage (3%)

Gastrointestinal/Hepatic
Diarrhea (24%)
Gastrointestinal bleeding (9%) [3]
Nausea (16%)
Vomiting (18%)

Respiratory
Alveolar hemorrhage (pulmonary) (9%)
Pneumonia (5%)
Pulmonary hemorrhage (4%)
Pulmonary toxicity (6%)

Endocrine/Metabolic
Hyperuricemia (2%)

Hematologic
Hemorrhage [2]
Sepsis (7%)

Other
Adverse effects [3]
Infection (3%)

DENOSUMAB

Trade names: Prolia (Amgen), Xgeva (Amgen)
Indications: Osteoporosis (postmenopausal women), prevention of skeletal-related events in patients with bone metastases from solid tumors
Class: Bone resorption inhibitor, Monoclonal antibody, RANK ligand (RANKL) inhibitor
Half-life: 25–28 days
Clinically important, potentially hazardous interactions with: abatacept, alcohol, azacitidine, betamethasone, cabazitaxel, denileukin, docetaxel, fingolimod, gefitinib, immuosuppressants, leflunomide, lenalidomide, oxaliplatin, pazopanib, temsirolimus, triamcinolone
Pregnancy category: X
Important contra-indications noted in the prescribing guidelines for: nursing mothers; pediatric patients
Note: Contraindicated in patients with hypocalcemia.

Skin
Cellulitis [9]
Dermatitis [2]
Eczema [10]
Herpes zoster (2%)
Hypersensitivity [2]
Peripheral edema (5%)
Pruritus (2%)
Rash (3%) [4]

Cardiovascular
Angina (3%)
Atrial fibrillation (2%)
Cardiotoxicity [2]

Central Nervous System
Headache [3]
Insomnia (3%)
Pain [2]
Vertigo (dizziness) (5%)

Neuromuscular/Skeletal
Arthralgia [3]
Asthenia (fatigue) (2%) [2]
Back pain (35%) [6]
Bone or joint pain (4–8%) [3]
Fractures [8]
Myalgia/Myopathy (3%)
Osteonecrosis (jaw) [24]
Pain in extremities (12%) [6]

Gastrointestinal/Hepatic
Abdominal pain (3%)
Flatulence (2%)
Gastroesophageal reflux (2%)
Pancreatitis [2]

Respiratory
Pharyngitis (2%)
Pneumonia (4%)
Upper respiratory tract infection (5%)

Endocrine/Metabolic
Hypercholesterolemia (7%) [2]
Hypocalcemia (2%) [30]
Hypophosphatemia [2]

Genitourinary
Cystitis (6%)

Hematologic
Anemia (3%) [2]

Other
Adverse effects [11]
Infection [12]

DEOXYCHOLIC ACID

Trade name: Kybella (Kythera)
Indications: Improvement in the appearance of moderate to severe convexity or fullness associated with submental fat
Class: Cytolytic
Half-life: N/A
Clinically important, potentially hazardous interactions with: none known
Pregnancy category: N/A
Important contra-indications noted in the prescribing guidelines for: the elderly; pediatric patients
Note: Contraindicated in the presence of infection at the injection sites.

Skin
Lymphadenopathy (<2%)

Mucosal
Oropharyngeal pain (3%)

Cardiovascular
Hypertension (3%)

Central Nervous System
Headache (8%)
Syncope (<2%)

Neuromuscular/Skeletal
Neck pain (<2%)

Gastrointestinal/Hepatic
Dysphagia (2%)
Nausea (2%)

Local
Injection-site bruising (72%) [2]
Injection-site edema [2]
Injection-site erythema (27%)
Injection-site hemorrhage (<2%)
Injection-site induration (23%) [2]
Injection-site nodules (13%)
Injection-site numbness (66%) [2]
Injection-site pain (70%) [2]
Injection-site pigmentation (<2%)
Injection-site pruritus (12%)
Injection-site urticaria (<2%)

Other
Adverse effects [2]

DESLORATADINE

Trade name: Clarinex (Schering)
Indications: Allergic rhinitis, urticaria
Class: Histamine H1 receptor antagonist
Half-life: 27 hours
Clinically important, potentially hazardous interactions with: none known
Pregnancy category: C
Important contra-indications noted in the prescribing guidelines for: nursing mothers; pediatric patients

---

Skin
Urticaria [2]

Mucosal
Xerostomia [5]

Central Nervous System
Headache [7]
Somnolence (drowsiness) [6]

Neuromuscular/Skeletal
Asthenia (fatigue) [7]

Gastrointestinal/Hepatic
Diarrhea [2]
Nausea [2]

Other
Adverse effects [6]

DESMOPRESSIN

Trade names: DDAVP (Sanofi-Aventis), Minirin (Ferring), Stimate (CSL Behring)
Indications: Primary nocturnal enuresis
Class: Antidiuretic hormone analog
Half-life: 75 minutes
Clinically important, potentially hazardous interactions with: amitriptyline, citalopram, demeclocycline, hydromorphone, meloxicam, tapentadol
Pregnancy category: B
Important contra-indications noted in the prescribing guidelines for: the elderly; nursing mothers

---

Cardiovascular
Flushing (<10%)
Myocardial infarction [2]

Central Nervous System
Headache [6]
Seizures [5]

Endocrine/Metabolic
Hyponatremia [11]
SIADH [2]

Local
Injection-site pain (<10%)

DESOXIMETASONE

Trade name: Topicort (Taro)
Indications: Dermatoses
Class: Corticosteroid, topical
Half-life: N/A
Clinically important, potentially hazardous interactions with: live vaccines
Pregnancy category: C
Important contra-indications noted in the prescribing guidelines for: nursing mothers; pediatric patients

---

Local
Application-site irritation (3%)
Application-site pruritus (2%) [2]

Other
Adverse effects [3]

DESVENLAFAXINE

Trade name: Pristiq (Wyeth)
Indications: Major depressive disorder
Class: Antidepressant, Serotonin-norepinephrine reuptake inhibitor
Half-life: 11 hours
Clinically important, potentially hazardous interactions with: alcohol, aspirin, CNS-active agents, heparin, ketoconazole, linezolid, lithium, MAO inhibitors, NSAIDs, sibutramine, tramadol, venlafaxine, warfarin
Pregnancy category: C
Important contra-indications noted in the prescribing guidelines for: the elderly; nursing mothers; pediatric patients
Black Box Warning: SUICIDAL THOUGHTS AND BEHAVIORS

Skin
- Hot flashes (<2%)
- Hyperhidrosis (10–21%)
- Hypersensitivity (2%)
- Rash (<2%)

Mucosal
- Epistaxis (nosebleed) (<2%)
- Xerostomia (11–25%) [3]

Cardiovascular
- Hypertension (<2%)
- Hypotension (~2%)
- Orthostatic hypotension (<2%)
- Palpitation (<3%)
- Tachycardia (<2%)

Central Nervous System
- Abnormal dreams (2–4%)
- Anorexia (5–8%) [2]
- Anorgasmia (3–8%)
- Anxiety (3–5%)
- Chills (<4%)
- Dysgeusia (taste perversion) (<2%)
- Extrapyramidal symptoms (<2%)
- Headache (20–29%) [3]
- Impaired concentration (<2%)
- Insomnia (9–12%) [3]
- Irritability (2%)
- Nervousness (<2%) [2]
- Paresthesias (<3%)
- Seizures (~2%)
- Somnolence (drowsiness) (4–12%) [4]
- Suicidal ideation [2]
- Syncope (<2%)
- Tremor (~3%)
- Vertigo (dizziness) (10–16%) [5]
- Yawning (<4%)

Neuromuscular/Skeletal
- Asthenia (fatigue) (7–11%) [2]

Gastrointestinal/Hepatic
- Constipation (9–14%)
- Diarrhea (5–11%)
- Nausea (22–41%) [6]
- Vomiting (3–9%)

Endocrine/Metabolic
- Appetite decreased (5–10%)
- Libido decreased (3–6%)
- Weight gain (<2%)
- Weight loss (<2%)

Genitourinary
- Ejaculatory dysfunction (<5%)
- Erectile dysfunction (3–11%)
- Sexual dysfunction (<2%)

Otic
- Tinnitus (<2%)

Ocular
- Mydriasis (2–6%)
- Vision blurred (3–4%)

DEXAMETHASONE

Trade names: Decadron (Merck), Dexone (Solvay), Ozurdex (Allergan)
Indications: Antiemetic, arthralgias, dermatoses, diagnostic aid, macular edema following branch retinal vein occlusion (BRVO) or central retinal vein occlusion (CRVO), non-infectious uveitis affecting the posterior segment of the eye
Class: Antiemetic, Corticosteroid, systemic, Corticosteroid, topical
Half-life: N/A
Clinically important, potentially hazardous interactions with: albendazole, aminoglutethimide, amprenavir, aprepitant, aspirin, bexarotene, boceprevir, carbamazepine, caspofungin, cobicistat/elvitegravir/emtricitabine/tenofovir disoproxil, cyclophosphamide, dasatinib, delavirdine, diuretics, ephedrine, imatinib, itraconazole, ixabepilone, lapatinib, lenalidomide, live vaccines, lopinavir, methotrexate, midazolam, phenobarbital, phenytoin, praziquantel, primidone, rifampin, rilpivirine, romidepsin, simeprevir, sorafenib, sunitinib, telaprevir, temsirolimus, ticagrelor, vandetanib, warfarin
Pregnancy category: C
Important contra-indications noted in the prescribing guidelines for: nursing mothers; pediatric patients

---

Skin
- Acneform eruption [6]
- AGEP [2]
- Anaphylactoid reactions/Anaphylaxis [3]
- Dermatitis [5]
- Edema [3]
- Erythema multiforme [3]
- Exanthems [4]
- Herpes zoster [2]
- Hyperhidrosis [2]
- Hypersensitivity [5]
- Peripheral edema [7]
- Pigmentation [2]
- Pruritus [7]
- Pruritus ani et vulvae [2]
- Rash [9]
- Striae [4]
- Toxicity [5]
- Tumor lysis syndrome [2]
- Xerosis [2]

Mucosal
- Oral candidiasis [2]

Cardiovascular
- Bradycardia [8]
- Flushing [5]
- Hypertension [16]
- Myocardial toxicity [11]
- Tachycardia [2]
- Thromboembolism [2]
- Venous thromboembolism [5]

Central Nervous System
- Anorexia [2]
- Catatonia [2]
- Dysgeusia (taste perversion) [3]
- Fever [6]
- Headache (<5%) [8]
- Insomnia [9]
- Leukoencephalopathy [2]
- Neurotoxicity [11]
- Paresthesias [2]
- Peripheral neuropathy [19]
- Vertigo (dizziness) [3]

Neuromuscular/Skeletal
- Arthralgia [5]
- Asthenia (fatigue) [37]
- Back pain [4]
- Bone or joint pain [4]
- Muscle spasm [4]
- Myalgia/Myopathy [6]
- Osteonecrosis [15]
- Osteoporosis [3]

Gastrointestinal/Hepatic
- Abdominal distension [2]
- Abdominal pain [5]
- Constipation [7]
- Diarrhea [15]
- Dyspepsia [2]
- Gastrointestinal disorder [3]
- Hepatotoxicity [4]
- Nausea [10]
- Pancreatitis [2]
- Vomiting [6]

Respiratory
- Cough [3]
- Dyspnea [5]
- Pneumonia [12]
- Upper respiratory tract infection [3]

Endocrine/Metabolic
- ALT increased [2]
- AST increased [2]
- Dehydration [2]
- Hyperglycemia [6]
- Hypokalemia [5]
- Hypophosphatemia [4]
- Serum creatinine increased [2]

Hematologic
- Anemia [30]
- Febrile neutropenia [6]
- Hemoglobin decreased [2]
- Hemotoxicity [5]
- Leukopenia [8]
- Lymphopenia [11]
- Myelosuppression [5]
- Neutropenia [39]
- Sepsis [3]
- Thrombocytopenia [39]
- Thrombosis [2]

Otic
- Ototoxicity [4]

Ocular
- Cataract (<10%) [7]
- Conjunctival hemorrhage (>10%)
- Glaucoma [9]
- Intraocular pressure increased (>10%) [10]
- Ocular hypertension (<10%) [6]

Ocular pain (<10%) [6]
Vision blurred [3]

Local
Infusion-related reactions [2]
Infusion-site reactions [2]

Other
Adverse effects [18]
Allergic reactions [2]
Death [10]
Hiccups [16]
Infection [26]
Side effects [3]

DEXLANSOPRAZOLE

Trade name: Dexilant (Takeda)
Indications: Erosive esophagitis, heartburn associated with gastroesophageal reflux disease
Class: Proton pump inhibitor (PPI)
Half-life: <2 hours
Clinically important, potentially hazardous interactions with: atazanavir, clopidogrel, digoxin, emtricitabine/rilpivirine/tenofovir alafenamide, ketoconazole, tacrolimus, warfarin
Pregnancy category: B
Important contra-indications noted in the prescribing guidelines for: nursing mothers

Skin
Acneform eruption (<2%)
Dermatitis (<2%)
Erythema (<2%)
Hot flashes (<2%)
Lesions (<2%)
Lymphadenopathy (<2%)
Pruritus (<2%)
Rash (<2%)
Urticaria (<2%)

Mucosal
Mucosal inflammation (<2%)
Oral candidiasis (<2%)
Xerostomia (<2%)

Cardiovascular
Cardiac disorder (<2%)

Central Nervous System
Headache [2]

Gastrointestinal/Hepatic
Abdominal pain (4%) [4]
Constipation [2]
Diarrhea (5%) [4]
Flatulence (<3%) [3]
Gastrointestinal disorder (<2%)
Nausea (3%) [4]
Vomiting (<2%) [2]

Respiratory
Upper respiratory tract infection (2–3%) [3]

Hematologic
Anemia (<2%)

Otic
Ear pain (<2%)
Tinnitus (<2%)

Ocular
Ocular edema (<2%)
Ocular pruritus (<2%)

Other
Adverse effects [2]

DEXMETHYLPHENIDATE

Trade name: Focalin (Novartis)
Indications: Attention deficit disorder
Class: CNS stimulant
Half-life: 2–4.5 hours
Clinically important, potentially hazardous interactions with: amitriptyline, clonidine, linezolid, MAO inhibitors, pantoprazole
Pregnancy category: C
Important contra-indications noted in the prescribing guidelines for: nursing mothers; pediatric patients
Note: Contraindicated in patients with marked anxiety, tension and agitation, with glaucoma, or with motor tics or history/diagnosis of Tourette's syndrome.

Central Nervous System
Fever (5%)
Headache [4]

Gastrointestinal/Hepatic
Abdominal pain (15%) [2]

Endocrine/Metabolic
Appetite decreased [2]

DEXTROAMPHETAMINE

Trade names: Adderall (Shire), Dexedrine (Alliant)
Indications: Narcolepsy, attention deficit disorder (ADD)
Class: Amphetamine, CNS stimulant
Half-life: 10–12 hours
Clinically important, potentially hazardous interactions with: fluoxetine, fluvoxamine, MAO inhibitors, paroxetine hydrochloride, phenelzine, sertraline, tranylcypromine
Pregnancy category: C
Important contra-indications noted in the prescribing guidelines for: nursing mothers; pediatric patients
Black Box Warning: POTENTIAL FOR ABUSE

Skin
Diaphoresis (<10%)

Mucosal
Xerostomia (<10%)

Central Nervous System
Insomnia [2]

Neuromuscular/Skeletal
Rhabdomyolysis [10]

DEXTROMETHORPHAN

Trade names: Robitussin (Wyeth), Vicks Formula 44 (Procter & Gamble)
Indications: Nonproductive cough
Class: Analgesic, narcotic, NMDA receptor antagonist
Half-life: N/A
Clinically important, potentially hazardous interactions with: amiodarone, citalopram, iloperidone, linezolid, lorcaserin, memantine, moclobemide, phenelzine, rasagiline, sibutramine, tranylcypromine, valdecoxib
Pregnancy category: C
Important contra-indications noted in the prescribing guidelines for: nursing mothers; pediatric patients

Skin
Bullous dermatitis [2]
Fixed eruption [2]

Central Nervous System
Serotonin syndrome [4]
Vertigo (dizziness) [2]

Gastrointestinal/Hepatic
Diarrhea [2]

Genitourinary
Urinary tract infection [2]

Other
Adverse effects [2]

DIAZEPAM

Trade names: Diastat (Xcel), Valium (Roche)
Indications: Anxiety
Class: Benzodiazepine, Skeletal muscle relaxant
Half-life: 20–70 hours
Clinically important, potentially hazardous interactions with: alcohol, amprenavir, barbiturates, buprenorphine, chlorpheniramine, clarithromycin, CNS depressants, cobicistat/elvitegravir/emtricitabine/tenofovir disoproxil, efavirenz, esomeprazole, eucalyptus, fluoroquinolones, imatinib, indinavir, itraconazole, ivermectin, macrolide antibiotics, MAO inhibitors, methadone, mianserin, nalbuphine, narcotics, nelfinavir, nilutamide, olanzapine, omeprazole, phenothiazines, propranolol, ritonavir, SSRIs, voriconazole
Pregnancy category: D
Important contra-indications noted in the prescribing guidelines for: nursing mothers

Skin
Dermatitis (<10%) [3]
Diaphoresis (>10%)
Exanthems [6]
Exfoliative dermatitis [2]
Fixed eruption [2]
Pigmentation [2]
Purpura [4]
Rash (>10%) [2]

Mucosal
Xerostomia (>10%)

Central Nervous System
Amnesia [17]
Hallucinations [2]
Sedation [3]
Somnolence (drowsiness) [6]
Vertigo (dizziness) [2]

Neuromuscular/Skeletal
Ataxia [2]

Endocrine/Metabolic
Gynecomastia [4]
Porphyria [2]

Local
Injection-site pain [2]
Injection-site phlebitis (>10%) [2]

Other
Adverse effects [3]
Allergic reactions [2]

DICLOFENAC

Trade names: Arthrotec (Pfizer), Cataflam (Novartis), Dicolmax (Galen), Motifene (Daiichi Sankyo), Pennsaid (Mallinckrodt), Solaraze Gel (Nycomed), Voltaren (Novartis), Voltarol (Novartis), Zipsor (Depomed)
Indications: Rheumatoid and osteoarthritis, topical treatment of actinic keratosis, postoperative inflammation in patients who have undergone cataract extraction and for the temporary relief of pain and photophobia in patients undergoing corneal refractive surgery
Class: Non-steroidal anti-inflammatory (NSAID)
Half-life: 1–2 hours
Clinically important, potentially hazardous interactions with: ACE inhibitors, adrenergic neurone blockers, aldosterone antagonists, aliskiren, alpha blockers, angiotensin II receptor antagonists, anticoagulants, aspirin, baclofen, beta blockers, calcium channel blockers, cardiac glycosides, clonidine, clopidogrel, corticosteroids, coumarins, cyclosporine, dabigatran, deferiprone, diazoxide, diuretics, enoxaparin, erlotinib, furosemide, heparins, hydralazine, iloprost, ketorolac, lithium, methotrexate, methyldopa, mifamurtide, minoxidil, moxonidine, nitrates, nitroprusside, penicillamine, pentoxifylline, phenindione, potassium canrenoate, prasugrel, rifampin, ritonavir, rivaroxaban, SSRIs, sulfonylureas, tacrolimus, thiazides, tinzaparin, venlafaxine, voriconazole, warfarin, zidovudine
Pregnancy category: D (category B for topical use; category C for oral and ophthalmic use; category D in third trimester.)
Important contra-indications noted in the prescribing guidelines for: nursing mothers; pediatric patients
Note: NSAIDs may cause an increased risk of serious cardiovascular and gastrointestinal adverse events, which can be fatal. This risk may increase with duration of use.
Contraindicated in patients who have experienced asthma, urticaria, or allergic-type reactions after taking aspirin or other NSAIDs. Severe, rarely fatal, anaphylactic-like reactions to NSAIDs have been reported in such patients.
Arthrotec is diclofenac and misoprostol.
Black Box Warning: RISK OF SERIOUS CARDIOVASCULAR AND GASTROINTESTINAL EVENTS

Skin
Anaphylactoid reactions/Anaphylaxis (<3%) [16]
Angioedema (<3%) [2]
Bullous dermatitis (<3%) [2]
Dermatitis (<3%) [9]
Dermatitis herpetiformis [2]
Eczema (<3%)
Erythema [4]
Erythema multiforme [6]
Exanthems (<5%) [6]
Fixed eruption [4]
Hypersensitivity [4]
Linear IgA bullous dermatosis [6]
Nicolau syndrome [16]
Photosensitivity (<3%) [4]
Pruritus (<10%) [6]
Purpura (<3%) [2]
Purpura fulminans [2]
Rash (>10%) [4]
Stevens–Johnson syndrome [5]
Toxic epidermal necrolysis [4]
Urticaria (<3%) [7]
Vasculitis [3]
Xerosis [3]

Hair
Alopecia (<3%)

Mucosal
Tongue edema (<3%)
Xerostomia (<3%) [2]

Cardiovascular
Cardiotoxicity [2]
Myocardial infarction [4]

Central Nervous System
Dysgeusia (taste perversion) (<3%)
Headache [2]
Stroke [3]
Vertigo (dizziness) [3]

Neuromuscular/Skeletal
Rhabdomyolysis [3]

Gastrointestinal/Hepatic
Abdominal pain [6]
Constipation [3]
Diarrhea [3]
Dyspepsia [5]
Gastritis [3]
Gastrointestinal bleeding [4]
Gastrointestinal ulceration [4]
Hepatotoxicity [9]
Nausea [7]
Vomiting [3]

Renal
Nephrotoxicity [4]
Renal failure [2]

Hematologic
Agranulocytosis [3]
Bleeding [2]

Local
Application-site reactions [3]

Other
Adverse effects [11]
Allergic reactions [2]
Death [6]

DICUMAROL

Indications: Atrial fibrillation, pulmonary embolism, venous thrombosis
Class: Coumarin
Half-life: 1–4 days
Clinically important, potentially hazardous interactions with: allopurinol, amiodarone, amobarbital, anabolic steroids, anti-thyroid agents, aprobarbital, aspirin, barbiturates, bivalirudin, butabarbital, butalbital, cimetidine, clofibrate, clopidogrel, cyclosporine, delavirdine, disulfiram, fenofibrate, fluconazole, gemfibrozil, glutethimide, imatinib, itraconazole, ketoconazole, levothyroxine, liothyronine, mephobarbital, methimazole, metronidazole, miconazole, penicillins, pentobarbital, phenobarbital, phenylbutazones, piperacillin, prednisone, primidone, propylthiouracil, quinidine, quinine, rifabutin, rifampin, rifapentine, rofecoxib, salicylates, secobarbital, sulfinpyrazone, sulfonamides, testosterone, zileuton
Pregnancy category: D
Important contra-indications noted in the prescribing guidelines for: nursing mothers

---

Skin
Dermatitis [2]
Exanthems [5]
Necrosis [10]
Purplish erythema (feet and toes) [2]
Purpura [2]
Urticaria [3]

Hair
Alopecia (<10%) [5]

Hematologic
Hemorrhage [3]

DIDANOSINE

Trade name: Videx (Bristol-Myers Squibb)
Indications: Advanced HIV infection
Class: Antiretroviral, Nucleoside analog reverse transcriptase inhibitor
Half-life: 1.5 hours
Clinically important, potentially hazardous interactions with: acetaminophen, amprenavir, ciprofloxacin, corticosteroids, dapsone, darunavir, febuxostat, gemifloxacin, indinavir, itraconazole, ketoconazole, levofloxacin, lomefloxacin, lopinavir, moxifloxacin, norfloxacin, ofloxacin, sulfones, tenofovir disoproxil, tetracycline, tipranavir, voriconazole
Pregnancy category: B
Important contra-indications noted in the prescribing guidelines for: the elderly; nursing mothers
Black Box Warning: PANCREATITIS, LACTIC ACIDOSIS and HEPATOMEGALY with STEATOSIS

Skin
Erythema multiforme [2]
Lipodystrophy [2]
Pruritus (9%)
Rash (9%)

Stevens–Johnson syndrome [3]

Mucosal
Xerostomia [4]

Cardiovascular
Myocardial infarction [2]

Central Nervous System
Neurotoxicity [4]

Gastrointestinal/Hepatic
Hepatotoxicity [2]
Non-cirrhotic portal hypertension [5]
Pancreatitis [23]

Endocrine/Metabolic
Acidosis [6]
Diabetes mellitus [2]
Gynecomastia [3]

Renal
Fanconi syndrome [5]

Ocular
Retinopathy [3]

Other
Death [3]

DIGOXIN

Trade name: Lanoxin (Concordia)
Indications: Congestive heart failure, atrial fibrillation
Class: Antiarrhythmic class IV, Cardiac glycoside, Inotrope
Half-life: 36–48 hours
Clinically important, potentially hazardous interactions with: acarbose, alprazolam, amiodarone, amphotericin B, arbutamine, atorvastatin, azithromycin, bendroflumethiazide, benzthiazide, bisacodyl, boceprevir, bosutinib, bumetanide, canagliflozin, captopril, carbimazole, chlorothiazide, chlorthalidone, cholestyramine, clarithromycin, cobicistat/elvitegravir/emtricitabine/tenofovir alafenamide, cobicistat/elvitegravir/emtricitabine/tenofovir disoproxil, colchicine, conivaptan, cyclopenthiazide, cyclosporine, cyclothiazide, darifenacin, darunavir, demeclocycline, dexlansoprazole, dexmedetomidine, doxycycline, dronedarone, erythromycin, eslicarbazepine, esomeprazole, ethacrynic acid, etravirine, everolimus, ezogabine, fingolimod, flibanserin, flunisolide, furosemide, glycopyrrolate, glycopyrronium, hydrochlorothiazide, hydroflumethiazide, indapamide, indinavir, itraconazole, lapatinib, lenalidomide, liraglutide, lomustine, lopinavir, meloxicam, mepenzolate, metformin, methyclothiazide, metolazone, milnacipran, minocycline, mirabegron, nifedipine, nilotinib, omeprazole, oxprenolol, oxytetracycline, pantoprazole, paricalcitol, paroxetine hydrochloride, pemetrexed, phenylbutazone, polythiazide, posaconazole, propafenone, propantheline, quinethazone, quinidine, quinine, rabeprazole, rifampin, roxithromycin, sitagliptin, sodium picosulfate, sorafenib, St John's wort, sunitinib, telaprevir, telithromycin, temozolomide, temsirolimus, teriparatide, tetracycline, thalidomide, thiazide diuretics, ticagrelor, tipranavir, tolvaptan, trichlormethiazide, trimethoprim, troglitazone, ulipristal, verapamil, zuclopenthixol
Pregnancy category: C
Important contra-indications noted in the prescribing guidelines for: the elderly; nursing mothers; pediatric patients
Note: This is the pure form of Digitalis. Contraindicated in ventricular fibrillation.

Skin
Exanthems (2%) [2]
Psoriasis [2]
Toxicity [4]

Cardiovascular
Arrhythmias [7]
Atrial fibrillation [4]
Bradycardia [3]
Tachycardia [2]

Central Nervous System
Anorexia [2]

Gastrointestinal/Hepatic
Nausea [3]
Vomiting [2]

Endocrine/Metabolic
Gynecomastia [2]

Ocular
Dyschromatopsia (green) [6]
Hallucinations, visual [2]

Other
Death [5]

DIHYDROCODEINE

Trade name: DHC-Continus (Napp)
Indications: Severe pain in cancer and other chronic conditions
Class: Analgesic, opioid
Half-life: 12 hours
Clinically important, potentially hazardous interactions with: CNS depressants, MAO inhibitors, phenothiazines, tranquilizers
Pregnancy category: C
Important contra-indications noted in the prescribing guidelines for: nursing mothers

---

Skin
AGEP [2]

Mucosal
Xerostomia [2]

Central Nervous System
Narcosis [2]
Seizures [3]
Somnolence (drowsiness) [2]

Gastrointestinal/Hepatic
Abdominal pain [2]
Constipation [2]
Nausea [2]
Vomiting [2]

Respiratory
Respiratory depression [2]

Genitourinary
Priapism [2]

Renal
Renal failure [5]

DILTIAZEM

Trade names: Cardizem (Biovail), Dilacor XR (Watson), Teczem (Sanofi-Aventis), Tiazac (Forest)
Indications: Angina, essential hypertension
Class: Antiarrhythmic class IV, Calcium channel blocker, CYP3A4 inhibitor
Half-life: 5–8 hours (for extended-release capsules)
Clinically important, potentially hazardous interactions with: acebutolol, alfuzosin, amiodarone, amitriptyline, amprenavir, aprepitant, atazanavir, atenolol, atorvastatin, avanafil, bisoprolol, bosentan, carbamazepine, celiprolol, cilostazol, cobicistat/elvitegravir/emtricitabine/tenofovir disoproxil, colchicine, corticosteroids, cyclosporine, delavirdine, dronedarone, dutasteride, efavirenz, epirubicin, erythromycin, fingolimod, flibanserin, lurasidone, mifepristone, moricizine, nevirapine, nifedipine, oxprenolol, posaconazole, ranolazine, silodosin, simvastatin, sulpiride, telaprevir, venetoclax
Pregnancy category: C
Important contra-indications noted in the prescribing guidelines for: the elderly; nursing mothers; pediatric patients
Note: Teczem is diltiazem and enalapril.

Skin
AGEP [21]
Angioedema [3]
Diaphoresis [2]
Edema (<10%) [4]
Erythema [2]
Erythema multiforme (<31%) [11]
Exanthems [17]
Exfoliative dermatitis [6]
Hypersensitivity [2]
Leg ulceration [2]
Lupus erythematosus [5]
Palmar–plantar desquamation [2]
Peripheral edema (5–8%)
Photosensitivity [11]
Phototoxicity [2]
Pigmentation [10]
Pruritus [6]
Psoriasis [3]
Purpura [3]
Pustules [2]
Rash [4]
Stevens–Johnson syndrome [4]
Thickening [2]
Toxic epidermal necrolysis [4]
Toxic erythema [2]
Toxicity [2]
Urticaria [5]
Vasculitis [6]

Hair
Alopecia [2]

Mucosal
Gingival hyperplasia/hypertrophy (21%) [10]
Xerostomia [2]

Cardiovascular
Bradycardia [6]
Cardiogenic shock [2]
Flushing (<10%) [6]

Central Nervous System
- Dysgeusia (taste perversion) [2]
- Parkinsonism [3]
- Somnolence (drowsiness) [2]

Neuromuscular/Skeletal
- Rhabdomyolysis [3]

Other
- Side effects [2]

DIMENHYDRINATE

Trade name: Dramamine (Pfizer)
Indications: Motion sickness, dizziness, nausea, vomiting
Class: Antiemetic, Cholinesterase absorption inhibitor
Half-life: N/A
Clinically important, potentially hazardous interactions with: none known
Pregnancy category: B
Important contra-indications noted in the prescribing guidelines for: nursing mothers

---

Skin
- Fixed eruption [12]

Mucosal
- Xerostomia (<10%)

Central Nervous System
- Somnolence (drowsiness) [5]

DIMETHYL FUMARATE

Synonyms: dimethyl (E) butenedioate; BG-12
Trade names: Fumaderm (Biogen Idec), Tecfidera (Biogen Idec)
Indications: Relapsing forms of multiple sclerosis, psoriasis
Class: Fumaric acid ester
Half-life: 1 hour
Clinically important, potentially hazardous interactions with: none known
Pregnancy category: C
Important contra-indications noted in the prescribing guidelines for: the elderly; nursing mothers; pediatric patients
Note: Fumaderm is mixed dimethyl fumarate and monoethylfumarate salts.

Skin
- Contact dermatitis (from topical contact) [14]
- Erythema (5%) [2]
- Pruritus (8%) [3]
- Rash (8%)

Cardiovascular
- Flushing (40%) [24]

Central Nervous System
- Leukoencephalopathy [4]

Neuromuscular/Skeletal
- Asthenia (fatigue) [3]

Gastrointestinal/Hepatic
- Abdominal pain (18%) [11]
- Diarrhea (14%) [10]
- Dyspepsia (5%) [2]
- Nausea [7]
- Vomiting (9%) [3]

Endocrine/Metabolic
- AST increased (4%) [2]

Genitourinary
- Albuminuria (6%)

Hematologic
- Hemotoxicity [2]
- Lymphopenia (2%) [6]

Other
- Adverse effects (gastrointestinal) [17]

DINOPROSTONE

Trade names: Cervidel (Forest), Prepidil (Pfizer)
Indications: Pregnancy termination, uterine content evacuation, cervical ripening
Class: Prostaglandin
Half-life: 2.5–5 minutes
Clinically important, potentially hazardous interactions with: none known
Pregnancy category: C
Note: Dinoprostone is the naturally occurring form of Prostaglandin E2 (PGE2).

DINUTUXIMAB

Trade name: Unituxin (United Therapeutics)
Indications: High-risk neuroblastoma in combination with granulocyte-macrophage colony-stimulating factor (GM-CSF), interleukin-2 (IL-2), and isotretinoin (13-*cis*-retinoic acid), in pediatric patients who achieve at least a partial response to prior first-line multiagent, multimodality therapy
Class: Monoclonal antibody
Half-life: 10 days
Clinically important, potentially hazardous interactions with: none known
Pregnancy category: N/A (may cause fetal harm)
Important contra-indications noted in the prescribing guidelines for: the elderly; nursing mothers
Black Box Warning: SERIOUS INFUSION REACTIONS AND NEUROPATHY

Skin
- Edema (17%)
- Urticaria (25–37%)

Mucosal
- Nasal congestion (20%)

Cardiovascular
- Capillary leak syndrome (22–40%)
- Hypertension (14%)
- Hypotension (60%)
- Tachycardia (19%)

Central Nervous System
- Fever (55–72%)
- Pain (61–85%)
- Peripheral neuropathy (13%)

Gastrointestinal/Hepatic
- Diarrhea (31–43%)
- Nausea (10%)
- Vomiting (33–46%)

Respiratory
- Hypoxia (24%)
- Wheezing (15%)

Endocrine/Metabolic
- ALT increased (43–56%)
- AST increased (16–28%)
- Creatine phosphokinase increased (15%)
- Hyperglycemia (18%)
- Hypertriglyceridemia (16%)
- Hypoalbuminemia (29–33%)
- Hypocalcemia (20–27%)
- Hypokalemia (26–43%)
- Hypomagnesemia (12%)
- Hyponatremia (36–58%)
- Hypophosphatemia (20%)
- Weight gain (10%)

Renal
- Proteinuria (16%)

Hematologic
- Anemia (42–51%)
- Hemorrhage (17%)
- Lymphopenia (54–62%)
- Neutropenia (25–39%)
- Sepsis (18%)
- Thrombocytopenia (61–66%)

Local
- Infusion-related reactions (47–60%)

DIPHENHYDRAMINE

Trade name: Benadryl (Pfizer)
Indications: Allergic rhinitis, urticaria
Class: Antiemetic, Histamine H1 receptor antagonist, Muscarinic antagonist
Half-life: 2–8 hours
Clinically important, potentially hazardous interactions with: alcohol, anticholinergics, chloral hydrate, CNS depressants, glutethimide, MAO inhibitors
Pregnancy category: B
Important contra-indications noted in the prescribing guidelines for: nursing mothers

---

Skin
- Anaphylactoid reactions/Anaphylaxis [4]
- Contact dermatitis [2]
- Dermatitis [4]
- Eczema [2]
- Fixed eruption [4]
- Photosensitivity [3]
- Pruritus [2]
- Toxic epidermal necrolysis [3]
- Toxicity [2]

Mucosal
- Xerostomia (<10%)

Cardiovascular
- QT prolongation [5]
- Torsades de pointes [3]

Central Nervous System
- Delirium [2]
- Sedation [2]
- Seizures [2]
- Somnolence (drowsiness) [7]

Neuromuscular/Skeletal
- Rhabdomyolysis [5]

Ocular
Hallucinations, visual [2]

Other
Death [4]

DIPHENOXYLATE

Trade name: Lomotil (Pfizer)
Indications: Diarrhea
Class: Antimotility, Opioid agonist
Half-life: 2.5 hours
Clinically important, potentially hazardous interactions with: oxybutynin
Pregnancy category: C
Important contra-indications noted in the prescribing guidelines for: nursing mothers; pediatric patients
Note: Diphenoxylate is almost always prescribed with atropine sulfate.

Mucosal
Xerostomia (3%)

DIPYRIDAMOLE

Trade names: Aggrenox (Boehringer Ingelheim), Persantine (Boehringer Ingelheim)
Indications: Thromboembolic complications following cardiac valve replacement
Class: Adenosine reuptake inhibitor, Antiplatelet
Half-life: 10–12 hours
Clinically important, potentially hazardous interactions with: adenosine, ceftobiprole, clopidogrel, enoxaparin, fondaparinux, regadenoson, reteplase, riociguat, tinzaparin
Pregnancy category: B
Important contra-indications noted in the prescribing guidelines for: nursing mothers; pediatric patients
Note: Aggrenox is dipyridamole and aspirin.

Skin
Rash (2%)
Stevens–Johnson syndrome [2]

Cardiovascular
Flushing (3%)

Central Nervous System
Headache [2]

Other
Adverse effects [2]

DISOPYRAMIDE

Trade name: Norpace (Pfizer)
Indications: Ventricular arrhythmias
Class: Antiarrhythmic, Antiarrhythmic class Ia, Muscarinic antagonist
Half-life: 4–10 hours
Clinically important, potentially hazardous interactions with: acebutolol, amiodarone, amisulpride, amitriptyline, arsenic, artemether/lumefantrine, astemizole, atenolol, bisoprolol, celiprolol, ciprofloxacin, clarithromycin, cobicistat/elvitegravir/emtricitabine/tenofovir alafenamide, cobicistat/elvitegravir/emtricitabine/tenofovir disoproxil, darifenacin, degarelix, dronedarone, droperidol, enoxacin, erythromycin, gatifloxacin, gliclazide, glycopyrrolate, glycopyrronium, insulin aspart, insulin degludec, insulin glargine, insulin glulisine, itraconazole, ketoconazole, levomepromazine, lomefloxacin, lurasidone, metformin, moxifloxacin, nevirapine, nilotinib, norfloxacin, ofloxacin, oxprenolol, oxybutynin, quinine, quinolones, rifapentine, roxithromycin, sildenafil, sotalol, sparfloxacin, sulpiride, tadalafil, telithromycin, tiotropium, trospium, vandetanib, vardenafil, zuclopenthixol
Pregnancy category: C
Important contra-indications noted in the prescribing guidelines for: nursing mothers; pediatric patients

---

Skin
Dermatitis (<3%)
Edema (<3%)
Exanthems (<5%)
Lupus erythematosus [3]
Pruritus (<3%)
Rash (generalized) (<3%)

Mucosal
Oral lesions (40%)
Xerostomia (32%) [2]

Cardiovascular
Chest pain (<3%)
Hypotension (<3%)
QT prolongation [8]
Torsades de pointes [13]

Central Nervous System
Anorexia (<3%)
Headache (3–9%)
Nervousness (<3%)
Syncope (<3%)
Vertigo (dizziness) (3–9%)

Neuromuscular/Skeletal
Asthenia (fatigue) (3–9%)

Gastrointestinal/Hepatic
Abdominal pain (3–9%)
Constipation (11%) [2]
Diarrhea (<3%)
Nausea (3–9%)
Vomiting (<3%)

Respiratory
Dyspnea (<3%)

Endocrine/Metabolic
Hypocalcemia [3]
Hypoglycemia [4]
Hypokalemia (<3%)
Weight gain (<3%)

Genitourinary
Impotence (<3%)
Urinary hesitancy (14%)
Urinary retention (3–9%)

Ocular
Vision blurred (3–9%)
Xerophthalmia (3–9%)

DISULFIRAM

Trade name: Antabuse (Odyssey)
Indications: Alcoholism
Class: Antialcoholism, Antioxidant
Half-life: N/A
Clinically important, potentially hazardous interactions with: acenocoumarol, alcohol, amitriptyline, anisindione, anticoagulants, clobazam, cyclosporine, dicumarol, dronabinol, ethanolamine, ethotoin, fosphenytoin, lopinavir, mephenytoin, metronidazole, omeprazole, oxtriphylline, phenytoin, thalidomide, tipranavir, warfarin
Pregnancy category: C
Important contra-indications noted in the prescribing guidelines for: nursing mothers; pediatric patients

---

Skin
Acneform eruption [3]
Bullous dermatitis [2]
Dermatitis [17]
Eczema [2]
Exanthems [2]
Fixed eruption [2]
Rash (<10%)
Recall reaction (nickel) [4]
Urticaria [3]

Cardiovascular
Flushing (with alcohol) [5]
Hypertension [2]
Hypotension [2]
Polyarteritis nodosa [2]
Tachycardia [2]

Central Nervous System
Dysgeusia (taste perversion) (metallic or garlic aftertaste) (<10%)
Neurotoxicity [6]
Psychosis [4]
Seizures [2]
Somnolence (drowsiness) [2]
Vertigo (dizziness) [2]

Neuromuscular/Skeletal
Asthenia (fatigue) [2]

Ocular
Optic neuropathy [2]

Other
Adverse effects [2]

DOCETAXEL

Trade name: Taxotere (Sanofi-Aventis)
Indications: Metastatic breast cancer, non-small cell lung cancer, with prednisone in hormone refractory prostate cancer, with cisplatin and fluorouracil for gastric adenocarcinoma and squamous cell carcinoma of the head and neck
Class: Antineoplastic, Taxane
Half-life: 11–18 hours
Clinically important, potentially hazardous interactions with: alcohol, aldesleukin, anthracyclines, antifungals, aprepitant, BCG vaccine, conivaptan, cyclosporine, CYP3A4 inhibitors or inducers, dasatinib, deferasirox, denosumab, echinacea, erythromycin, itraconazole, ketoconazole, lapatinib,

leflunomide, natalizumab, P-glycoprotein inhibitors or inducers, pimecrolimus, prednisone, ritonavir, sipuleucel-T, sorafenib, St John's wort, tacrolimus, thalidomide, trastuzumab, vaccines, voriconazole
Pregnancy category: D
Important contra-indications noted in the prescribing guidelines for: the elderly; nursing mothers; pediatric patients
Note: Contraindicated in patients with hypersensitivity to docetaxel or polysorbate 80, or with neutrophil counts of <1500 cells/mm^3.
Black Box Warning: TOXIC DEATHS, HEPATOTOXICITY, NEUTROPENIA, HYPERSENSITIVITY REACTIONS, and FLUID RETENTION

Skin
AGEP [2]
Anaphylactoid reactions/Anaphylaxis [2]
Edema (34%) [22]
Erythema [4]
Exanthems [3]
Facial erythema [2]
Flagellate erythema/pigmentation [2]
Hand–foot syndrome [39]
Hypersensitivity (6%) [14]
Peripheral edema [8]
Photosensitivity [6]
Pigmentation [2]
Psoriasis [3]
Radiation recall dermatitis [17]
Rash [12]
Recall reaction [2]
Scleroderma [8]
Thrombocytopenic purpura [2]
Toxicity (20–48%) [8]
Xerosis [2]

Hair
Alopecia (56–76%) [29]

Nails
Beau's lines (transverse nail bands) [2]
Discoloration [2]
Melanonychia [2]
Nail changes [17]
Nail disorder (11–41%)
Nail loss [3]
Nail pigmentation [6]
Onycholysis [15]
Paronychia [4]
Pyogenic granuloma [2]
Subungual abscess [2]
Subungual hemorrhage [2]
Transverse superficial loss of nail plate [2]

Mucosal
Aphthous stomatitis [2]
Mucositis [13]
Oral mucositis [2]
Stomatitis (19–53%) [19]

Cardiovascular
Capillary leak syndrome [2]
Cardiotoxicity [2]
Flushing [2]
Hypertension [8]
Hypotension (3%)
Thromboembolism [2]

Central Nervous System
Anorexia [10]
Dysesthesia (4%)
Dysgeusia (taste perversion) (6%) [7]
Fever (31–35%) [4]
Headache [2]
Mood changes [2]
Neurotoxicity [18]
Pain [4]
Paresthesias (4%) [2]
Peripheral neuropathy [8]
Vertigo (dizziness) [2]

Neuromuscular/Skeletal
Arthralgia (3–9%) [2]
Asthenia (fatigue) (53–66%) [54]
Bone or joint pain [2]
Myalgia/Myopathy (3–23%) [9]

Gastrointestinal/Hepatic
Abdominal pain [3]
Constipation [3]
Diarrhea (23–43%) [44]
Dysphagia [2]
Hepatotoxicity [2]
Nausea (34–42%) [21]
Vomiting (22–23%) [16]

Respiratory
Cough [2]
Dyspnea [5]
Pneumonitis [8]
Pulmonary embolism [2]
Pulmonary toxicity (41%) [3]
Upper respiratory tract infection [2]

Endocrine/Metabolic
ALP increased (4–7%)
ALT increased [5]
Amenorrhea [4]
Appetite decreased [3]
AST increased [4]
Dehydration [2]
Hyperglycemia [3]
Hyponatremia [2]
Hypophosphatemia [2]

Hematologic
Anemia (65–94%) [21]
Febrile neutropenia (6%) [36]
Hemolytic uremic syndrome [3]
Hemotoxicity [3]
Leukocytopenia [3]
Leukopenia (84–99%) [20]
Lymphopenia [3]
Neutropenia (84–99%) [70]
Thrombocytopenia (8–14%) [9]

Ocular
Epiphora [8]

Local
Injection-site erythema [2]
Injection-site extravasation [3]
Injection-site pigmentation [3]

Other
Adverse effects [2]
Allergic reactions [2]
Death [13]
Infection (<34%) [9]

DOLUTEGRAVIR

Trade names: Tivicay (ViiV), Triumeq (ViiV)
Indications: HIV-1 infection
Class: Antiretroviral, Integrase strand transfer inhibitor
Half-life: ~14 hours
Clinically important, potentially hazardous interactions with: dofetilide
Pregnancy category: B
Important contra-indications noted in the prescribing guidelines for: nursing mothers; pediatric patients
Note: Triumeq is abacavir, dolutegravir and lamivudine.

Skin
Hypersensitivity [5]
Pruritus (<2%)
Rash [3]

Central Nervous System
Abnormal dreams [2]
Headache (<2%) [15]
Insomnia (<3%) [4]

Neuromuscular/Skeletal
Asthenia (fatigue) (<2%) [2]
Myalgia/Myopathy (<2%)

Gastrointestinal/Hepatic
Abdominal pain (<2%)
Diarrhea [15]
Flatulence (<2%)
Hepatitis (<2%)
Nausea [12]
Vomiting (<2%)

Respiratory
Nasopharyngitis [3]
Upper respiratory tract infection [2]

Endocrine/Metabolic
ALT increased (<2%) [2]
AST increased (<3%)
Creatine phosphokinase increased (<4%)
Hyperglycemia (5–7%)

Renal
Nephrotoxicity (<2%)

Other
Adverse effects [3]

DONEPEZIL

Trade names: Aricept (Eisai), Aricept Evess (Eisai)
Indications: Mild, moderate and severe dementia of the Alzheimer's type
Class: Acetylcholinesterase inhibitor, Cholinesterase inhibitor, Parasympathomimetic
Half-life: 50–70 hours
Clinically important, potentially hazardous interactions with: anticholinergics, cholinergic agonists, galantamine, non-depolarising muscle relaxants, ramelteon, succinylcholine

Pregnancy category: C
Important contra-indications noted in the prescribing guidelines for: nursing mothers; pediatric patients
Note: Contraindicated in patients with known hypersensitivity to donepezil hydrochloride or to piperidine derivatives.

Skin
Diaphoresis [2]
Ecchymoses (4–5%)
Eczema (3%)
Purpura (<10%)

Cardiovascular
Atrioventricular block [2]
Bradycardia [7]
Chest pain (2%)
Hypertension [2]
Hypotension (3%)
QT prolongation [4]
Torsades de pointes [2]

Central Nervous System
Abnormal dreams (3%) [2]
Agitation [2]
Anorexia (4–8%) [5]
Confusion (2%) [3]
Delirium [2]
Depression (2–3%) [3]
Emotional lability (2%)
Fever (3%)
Gait instability [2]
Hallucinations (3%)
Headache (4–10%) [6]
Hostility (3%)
Insomnia (5–9%) [4]
Mania [2]
Nervousness (3%)
Neuroleptic malignant syndrome [2]
Pain (3–9%)
Parkinsonism [2]
Somnolence (drowsiness) (2%) [2]
Syncope (2%) [5]
Tremor [3]
Vertigo (dizziness) (2–8%) [6]

Neuromuscular/Skeletal
Arthralgia (2%)
Asthenia (fatigue) (5%) [3]
Back pain (3%)
Dystonia [2]
Muscle spasm [2]
Myoclonus [2]

Gastrointestinal/Hepatic
Constipation [3]
Diarrhea (10%) [10]
Hepatotoxicity [3]
Nausea (6–11%) [12]
Vomiting (5–8%) [7]

Endocrine/Metabolic
Appetite decreased [4]
Creatine phosphokinase increased (3%)
Dehydration (2%)
Hyperlipidemia (2%)
Weight loss (3%)

Genitourinary
Urinary frequency (2%) [2]
Urinary incontinence (2%)
Urinary tract infection [3]

Hematologic
Hemorrhage (2%)

Other
Adverse effects [9]
Infection (11%)

DOPAMINE

Trade name: Intropin (Hospira)
Indications: Hemodynamic imbalances present in shock
Class: Adrenergic alpha-receptor agonist, Catecholamine, Inotropic sympathomimetic
Half-life: 2 minutes
Clinically important, potentially hazardous interactions with: ethotoin, fosphenytoin, furazolidone, lurasidone, MAO inhibitors, mephenytoin, phenelzine, phenytoin, quetiapine, tranylcypromine
Pregnancy category: C
Important contra-indications noted in the prescribing guidelines for: nursing mothers; pediatric patients

---

Cardiovascular
QT prolongation [2]

Local
Injection-site extravasation [2]
Injection-site necrosis [3]

DORZOLAMIDE

Trade names: Cosopt (Merck), Trusopt (Banyu)
Indications: Glaucoma, ocular hypertension
Class: Carbonic anhydrase inhibitor, Diuretic
Half-life: ~4 months
Clinically important, potentially hazardous interactions with: none known
Pregnancy category: C
Important contra-indications noted in the prescribing guidelines for: nursing mothers
Note: Dorzolamide is a sulfonamide and can be absorbed systemically. Sulfonamides can produce severe, possibly fatal, reactions such as toxic epidermal necrolysis and Stevens-Johnson syndrome.
Cosopt is dorzolamide and timolol.

Skin
Contact dermatitis [4]

Central Nervous System
Dysgeusia (taste perversion) (25%) [8]

Ocular
Ocular burning (33%) [5]
Ocular pain [2]
Ocular pruritus [4]
Ocular stinging [10]
Vision blurred [3]

Other
Adverse effects [2]

DOXAZOSIN

Trade name: Cardura (Pfizer)
Indications: Hypertension
Class: Adrenergic alpha-receptor antagonist
Half-life: 19–22 hours
Clinically important, potentially hazardous interactions with: tadalafil, vardenafil, zuclopenthixol
Pregnancy category: C
Important contra-indications noted in the prescribing guidelines for: the elderly; nursing mothers; pediatric patients

---

Skin
Edema (4%)
Exanthems (2%)

Mucosal
Xerostomia (2%) [2]

Cardiovascular
Hypotension [3]
Orthostatic hypotension [2]
Postural hypotension [2]

Central Nervous System
Headache [2]
Vertigo (dizziness) [9]

Neuromuscular/Skeletal
Asthenia (fatigue) [4]

Gastrointestinal/Hepatic
Abdominal pain [2]

Genitourinary
Erectile dysfunction [3]

Ocular
Floppy iris syndrome [3]

DOXEPIN

Trade names: Adapin (LGM Pharma), Silenor (Somaxon), Sinquan (Pfizer)
Indications: Mental depression, anxiety, insomnia
Class: Antidepressant, tricyclic, Muscarinic antagonist
Half-life: 6–8 hours
Clinically important, potentially hazardous interactions with: alcohol, amprenavir, arbutamine, cholestyramine, clonidine, CNS depressants, epinephrine, formoterol, guanethidine, isocarboxazid, linezolid, MAO inhibitors, phenelzine, QT prolonging agents, quinolones, ramelteon, selegiline, sparfloxacin, sympathomimetics, tranylcypromine
Pregnancy category: C (pregnancy category is B for topical use)
Important contra-indications noted in the prescribing guidelines for: nursing mothers
Black Box Warning: SUICIDALITY AND ANTIDEPRESSANT DRUGS

Skin
Dermatitis (from topical) [9]
Diaphoresis (<10%)
Pseudolymphoma [2]

Mucosal
Xerostomia (>10%) [6]

Cardiovascular
QT prolongation [2]

Central Nervous System
Dysgeusia (taste perversion) (>10%)
Headache [4]
Somnolence (drowsiness) [7]

DOXORUBICIN

Synonym: hydroxydaunomycin
Trade names: Adriamycin (Bedford), Doxil (Tibotec), Rubex (Mead Johnson)
Indications: Carcinomas, leukemias, sarcomas
Class: Antibiotic, anthracycline
Half-life: 20–48 hours
Clinically important, potentially hazardous interactions with: aldesleukin, cabazitaxel, CYP2D6 inhibitors or inducers, CYP3A4 inhibitors or inducers, gadobenate, P-glycoprotein inhibitors or inducers, paclitaxel, sorafenib, stavudine, trastuzumab, zidovudine
Pregnancy category: D
Important contra-indications noted in the prescribing guidelines for: nursing mothers
Black Box Warning: CARDIOMYOPATHY, SECONDARY MALIGNANCIES, EXTRAVASATION AND TISSUE NECROSIS, and SEVERE MYELOSUPPRESSION

Skin
Anaphylactoid reactions/Anaphylaxis [2]
Angioedema [5]
Erythema [2]
Exanthems [3]
Exfoliative dermatitis [2]
Hand–foot syndrome [58]
Intertrigo [3]
Lupus erythematosus [3]
Necrosis (local) [5]
Palmar–plantar erythema (painful) [4]
Pigmentation [15]
Pruritus [2]
Purpura [2]
Radiation recall dermatitis [8]
Rash [6]
Toxicity [11]
Urticaria [10]

Hair
Alopecia (>10%) [38]

Nails
Beau's lines [2]
Nail changes [2]
Nail pigmentation [16]
Onycholysis [5]

Mucosal
Aphthous stomatitis [2]
Mucositis [16]
Oral lesions [7]
Stomatitis (>10%) [19]
Tongue pigmentation [3]

Cardiovascular
Atrial fibrillation [2]
Cardiomyopathy [4]
Cardiotoxicity [17]
Chest pain [2]
Congestive heart failure [4]
Flushing (<10%) [2]
Myocardial toxicity [4]

Central Nervous System
Anorexia [3]
Dysgeusia (taste perversion) [2]
Fever [4]
Headache [3]
Leukoencephalopathy [4]
Neurotoxicity [4]
Peripheral neuropathy [5]

Neuromuscular/Skeletal
Asthenia (fatigue) [15]
Bone or joint pain [2]
Myalgia/Myopathy [2]

Gastrointestinal/Hepatic
Constipation [3]
Diarrhea [4]
Gastrointestinal perforation [2]
Hepatotoxicity [6]
Nausea [8]
Pancreatitis [2]
Vomiting [7]

Respiratory
Dyspnea [3]
Pneumonia [3]
Pneumonitis [2]

Endocrine/Metabolic
ALT increased [3]
Amenorrhea [2]

Renal
Nephrotoxicity [2]

Hematologic
Anemia [11]
Febrile neutropenia [14]
Hemorrhage [2]
Hemotoxicity [2]
Leukopenia [3]
Neutropenia [27]
Thrombocytopenia [18]

Local
Injection-site erythema [7]
Injection-site extravasation (>10%) [12]
Injection-site necrosis (>10%) [5]
Injection-site reactions [2]
Injection-site ulceration (>10%) [4]

Other
Adverse effects [5]
Allergic reactions [3]
Death [10]
Infection [4]

DOXYCYCLINE

Trade names: Adoxa (Bioglan), Doryx (Warner Chilcott), Oracea (Galderma), Vibra-Tabs (Pfizer), Vibramycin-D (Pfizer)
Indications: Various infections caused by susceptible organisms
Class: Antibiotic, tetracycline
Half-life: 12–22 hours
Clinically important, potentially hazardous interactions with: acitretin, amoxicillin, ampicillin, antacids, bacampicillin, barbiturates, BCG vaccine, bismuth, calcium salts, carbamazepine, carbenicillin, cloxacillin, corticosteroids, coumarins, cyclosporine, dairy products, digoxin, ergotamine, kaolin, methotrexate, methoxyflurane, methysergide, mezlocillin, nafcillin, oral contraceptives, oral iron, oral typhoid vaccine, oxacillin, penicillins, phenindione, phenytoin, piperacillin, primidone, quinapril, retinoids, rifampin, St John's wort, strontium ranelate, sucralfate, sulfonylureas, ticarcillin, tripotassium dicitratobismuthate, zinc
Pregnancy category: D
Important contra-indications noted in the prescribing guidelines for: nursing mothers; pediatric patients

---

Skin
AGEP [2]
Angioedema [2]
Candidiasis [3]
Erythema multiforme [4]
Exanthems [2]
Fixed eruption [9]
Hypersensitivity [2]
Photosensitivity [20]
Phototoxicity [8]
Pigmentation [5]
Pruritus [3]
Rash [5]
Stevens–Johnson syndrome [6]
Sweet's syndrome [2]
Toxic epidermal necrolysis [2]
Urticaria [6]

Nails
Photo-onycholysis [12]

Mucosal
Black tongue [2]
Mucosal candidiasis [2]

Central Nervous System
Anosmia [2]
Fever [2]
Headache [4]
Intracranial pressure increased [2]
Paresthesias [4]
Vertigo (dizziness) [3]

Neuromuscular/Skeletal
Myalgia/Myopathy [2]

Gastrointestinal/Hepatic
Abdominal pain [3]
Diarrhea [3]
Esophagitis [2]
Hepatotoxicity [2]
Nausea [5]
Pancreatitis [3]
Ulcerative esophagitis [2]
Vomiting [3]

Endocrine/Metabolic
Hypoglycemia [2]

Genitourinary
Vaginitis [2]

Other
Adverse effects [5]
Allergic reactions [3]
Tooth pigmentation (>10%) [5]

DRONABINOL

Synonyms: tetrahydrocannabinol; THC
Trade names: Marinol (AbbVie), Syndros (Insys)
Indications: Chemotherapy-induced nausea, anorexia associated with weight loss in patients with AIDS
Class: Antiemetic, Cannabinoid
Half-life: 19–24 hours
Clinically important, potentially hazardous interactions with: disulfiram, metronidazole
Pregnancy category: C
Important contra-indications noted in the prescribing guidelines for: the elderly; nursing mothers; pediatric patients

Mucosal
Xerostomia (<10%)

Central Nervous System
Euphoria (<10%)
Paranoia (<10%)
Somnolence (drowsiness) (<10%)
Vertigo (dizziness) (<10%) [4]

Gastrointestinal/Hepatic
Abdominal pain (<10%)
Nausea (<10%) [2]
Vomiting (<10%)

Other
Adverse effects [4]

DRONEDARONE

Trade name: Multaq (Sanofi-Aventis)
Indications: Atrial fibrillation and atrial flutter
Class: Antiarrhythmic, Antiarrhythmic class III
Half-life: 13–19 hours
Clinically important, potentially hazardous interactions with: amiodarone, amitriptyline, amoxapine, antiarrhythmics, antipsychotics prolonging QT interval, arsenic, atorvastatin, beta blockers, bupivacaine, calcium channel blockers, carbamazepine, citalopram, clarithromycin, conivaptan, coumarins, cyclosporine, CYP3A inducers, dabigatran, darunavir, dasatinib, degarelix, delavirdine, digoxin, diltiazem, disopyramide, dolasetron, efavirenz, erythromycin, fingolimod, grapefruit juice, indinavir, itraconazole, ketoconazole, lapatinib, levobupivacaine, levofloxacin, levomepromazine, metoprolol, moxifloxacin, nefazodone, nifedipine, ombitasvir/paritaprevir/ritonavir, oxcarbazepine, pazopanib, phenindione, phenobarbital, phenothiazines, phenytoin, posaconazole, prilocaine, propranolol, rifampin, rifapentine, ritonavir, ropivacaine, rosuvastatin, saquinavir, simvastatin, sirolimus, sotalol, St John's wort, statins, tacrolimus, telavancin, telithromycin, tricyclic antidepressants, venetoclax, verapamil, voriconazole, vorinostat, warfarin, ziprasidone
Pregnancy category: X
Important contra-indications noted in the prescribing guidelines for: nursing mothers; pediatric patients
Black Box Warning: INCREASED RISK OF DEATH, STROKE AND HEART FAILURE IN PATIENTS WITH DECOMPENSATED HEART FAILURE OR PERMANENT ATRIAL FIBRILLATION

Skin
Dermatitis (5%)
Eczema (5%)
Erythema (5%)
Pruritus (5%)
Rash (5%) [7]

Cardiovascular
Arrhythmias [3]
Bradycardia (3%) [7]
Cardiac failure (new or worsening) [9]
Cardiotoxicity [3]
QT prolongation (28%) [9]
Torsades de pointes [3]

Central Nervous System
Vertigo (dizziness) [2]

Neuromuscular/Skeletal
Asthenia (fatigue) (7%) [2]

Gastrointestinal/Hepatic
Abdominal pain (4%)
Diarrhea (9%) [13]
Dyspepsia (2%)
Gastrointestinal disorder [4]
Hepatic failure [4]
Hepatotoxicity [8]
Nausea (5%) [11]
Vomiting (2%) [5]

Respiratory
Pulmonary toxicity [9]

Endocrine/Metabolic
Creatine phosphokinase increased (51%) [6]

Renal
Nephrotoxicity [2]
Renal failure [2]

Other
Adverse effects [2]
Death [2]
Side effects [2]

DROPERIDOL

Trade names: Inapsine (Akorn), Xomolix (ProStrakan)
Indications: Tranquilizer and antiemetic in surgical procedures
Class: Antiemetic, Antipsychotic, Butyrophenone
Half-life: 2.3 hours
Clinically important, potentially hazardous interactions with: amiodarone, amisulpride, amitriptyline, arsenic, atomoxetine, azithromycin, chloroquine, CNS depressants, cyclobenzaprine, disopyramide, duloxetine, eszopiclone, fluoxetine, fluvoxamine, hydromorphone, hydroxychloroquine, levomepromazine, lurasidone, macrolides, metaxalone, milnacipran, moxifloxacin, paliperidone, pentamidine, pimozide, QT prolonging agents, quinine, ramelteon, sertraline, sotalol, sulpiride, tamoxifen, tapentadol, thiopental, tiagabine, tricyclic antidepressants
Pregnancy category: C
Important contra-indications noted in the prescribing guidelines for: nursing mothers; pediatric patients
Note: Contraindicated in patients with known or suspected QT prolongation.
This product is not available in the European market.
Black Box Warning: QT PROLONGATION AND TORSADE DE POINTES

Skin
Anaphylactoid reactions/Anaphylaxis [3]
Angioedema [2]

Cardiovascular
Arrhythmias [2]
QT prolongation [13]
Torsades de pointes [6]

Central Nervous System
Akathisia [5]
Extrapyramidal symptoms [2]
Neuroleptic malignant syndrome [2]
Restlessness [2]
Sedation [2]

Neuromuscular/Skeletal
Dystonia [6]

Other
Death [3]

DROXIDOPA

Synonym: L-DOPS
Trade name: Northera (Chelsea Therapeutics)
Indications: Neurogenic orthostatic hypotension
Class: Amino acid analog (synthetic)
Half-life: 2.5 hours
Clinically important, potentially hazardous interactions with: none known
Pregnancy category: C
Important contra-indications noted in the prescribing guidelines for: nursing mothers; pediatric patients
Black Box Warning: SUPINE HYPERTENSION

Cardiovascular
Hypertension (2–7%)

Central Nervous System
Gait instability (15%) [2]
Headache (6–15%) [3]
Syncope (13%)
Vertigo (dizziness) (4–10%) [2]

Gastrointestinal/Hepatic
Nausea (2–9%)

Genitourinary
Urinary tract infection (15%) [2]

DULAGLUTIDE

Trade name: Trulicity (Lilly)
Indications: To improve glycemic control in adults with Type II diabetes mellitus
Class: Glucagon-like peptide-1 (GLP-1) receptor agonist
Half-life: 5 days
Clinically important, potentially hazardous interactions with: none known
Pregnancy category: C
Important contra-indications noted in the prescribing guidelines for: nursing mothers; pediatric patients
Note: Contraindicated in patients with a personal or family history of medullary thyroid carcinoma or in patients with multiple endocrine neoplasia syndrome Type 2.
Black Box Warning: RISK OF THYROID C-CELL TUMORS

Cardiovascular
- Atrioventricular block (2%)
- Tachycardia (3–6%)

Central Nervous System
- Headache [3]

Neuromuscular/Skeletal
- Asthenia (fatigue) (4–6%)

Gastrointestinal/Hepatic
- Abdominal pain (7–9%)
- Constipation [4]
- Diarrhea [20]
- Dyspepsia (4–6%) [2]
- Nausea (12–21%) [21]
- Pancreatitis [2]
- Vomiting (6–13%) [14]

Respiratory
- Nasopharyngitis [6]

Endocrine/Metabolic
- Appetite decreased (5–9%) [2]

Local
- Injection-site reactions [5]

Other
- Adverse effects (gastrointestinal) [4]

DULOXETINE

Trade names: Cymbalta (Lilly), Yentreve (Lilly)
Indications: Depression
Class: Antidepressant, Noradrenaline reuptake inhibitor, Serotonin reuptake inhibitor
Half-life: 8–17 hours
Clinically important, potentially hazardous interactions with: 5HT1 agonists, alcohol, amitriptyline, artemether/lumefantrine, aspirin, atomoxetine, cimetidine, ciprofloxacin, citalopram, clomipramine, CYP1A2 inducers, CYP2D6 inhibitors and substrates, darunavir, droperidol, enoxacin, fesoterodine, fluoxetine, fluvoxamine, iobenguane, levomepromazine, MAO inhibitors, meperidine, moclobemide, naratriptan, nebivolol, NSAIDs, paroxetine hydrochloride, PEG-interferon, quinidine, sibutramine, SSRIs, St John's wort, tamoxifen, teriflunomide, thioridazine, tramadol, tricyclic antidepressants, tryptophan, venlafaxine, warfarin
Pregnancy category: C
Important contra-indications noted in the prescribing guidelines for: nursing mothers; pediatric patients
Black Box Warning: SUICIDAL THOUGHTS AND BEHAVIORS

Skin
- Diaphoresis (6%) [2]
- Hot flashes (>2%)
- Hyperhidrosis (7%) [7]

Mucosal
- Oropharyngeal pain (>2%)
- Xerostomia (13%) [22]

Cardiovascular
- Flushing (3%)
- Palpitation (>2%)

Central Nervous System
- Agitation (5%)
- Anxiety (3%)
- Headache (14%) [11]
- Insomnia (10%) [13]
- Paresthesias (>2%)
- Restless legs syndrome [2]
- Serotonin syndrome [4]
- Somnolence (drowsiness) (10%) [15]
- Suicidal ideation [4]
- Tardive dyskinesia [2]
- Tremor (3%)
- Vertigo (dizziness) (10%) [15]
- Yawning (>2%) [2]

Neuromuscular/Skeletal
- Arthralgia (>2%)
- Asthenia (fatigue) (10%) [14]
- Back pain (>2%)
- Bone or joint pain (4%)
- Muscle spasm (3%)

Gastrointestinal/Hepatic
- Abdominal pain (>2%)
- Colitis [2]
- Constipation (10%) [7]
- Diarrhea (9%) [6]
- Hepatotoxicity (rare) [4]
- Nausea (24%) [23]
- Vomiting (>2%) [3]

Respiratory
- Cough (>2%)
- Influenza (3%)
- Nasopharyngitis (5%)
- Upper respiratory tract infection (4%)

Endocrine/Metabolic
- ALT increased [2]
- Appetite decreased (8–9%) [2]
- Hyponatremia [2]
- Libido decreased (4%)
- SIADH [6]
- Weight loss (>2%)

Genitourinary
- Ejaculatory dysfunction (2–5%)
- Sexual dysfunction [6]

Ocular
- Vision blurred (>2%)

Other
- Adverse effects [11]
- Bruxism [3]
- Death [2]

DUTASTERIDE

Trade names: Avodart (GSK), Jalyn (GSK)
Indications: Benign prostatic hyperplasia, male pattern baldness (anecdotal)
Class: 5-alpha reductase inhibitor, Androgen antagonist
Half-life: 3–5 weeks
Clinically important, potentially hazardous interactions with: cimetidine, ciprofloxacin, conivaptan, darunavir, delavirdine, diltiazem, indinavir, ketoconazole, ritonavir, telithromycin, troleandomycin, verapamil, voriconazole
Pregnancy category: X
Important contra-indications noted in the prescribing guidelines for: nursing mothers; pediatric patients
Note: Jalyn is dutasteride and tamsulosin.

Endocrine/Metabolic
- Gynecomastia [2]
- Libido decreased (<3%) [3]

Genitourinary
- Ejaculatory dysfunction [3]
- Erectile dysfunction [7]
- Impotence (<5%)
- Sexual dysfunction [6]

Other
- Adverse effects [2]

ECULIZUMAB

Trade name: Soliris (Alexion)
Indications: Paroxysmal nocturnal hemoglobinuria, atypical hemolytic uremic syndrome
Class: Complement inhibitor, Monoclonal antibody
Half-life: ~12 days
Clinically important, potentially hazardous interactions with: none known
Pregnancy category: C
Important contra-indications noted in the prescribing guidelines for: nursing mothers; pediatric patients
Black Box Warning: SERIOUS MENINGOCOCCAL INFECTIONS

Skin
Peripheral edema [2]
Pruritus [2]

Mucosal
Nasal congestion [2]

Cardiovascular
Hypertension [2]

Central Nervous System
Fever [3]
Headache (44%) [5]
Insomnia [2]
Meningococcal infection [4]
Vertigo (dizziness) [3]

Neuromuscular/Skeletal
Asthenia (fatigue) (12%) [4]
Back pain (19%) [3]
Pain in extremities [2]

Gastrointestinal/Hepatic
Abdominal pain [2]
Diarrhea [3]
Nausea [4]
Vomiting [3]

Respiratory
Cough (12%) [4]
Nasopharyngitis (23%) [5]
Pharyngolaryngeal pain [2]
Upper respiratory tract infection [2]

Genitourinary
Urinary tract infection [3]

Hematologic
Anemia [2]
Leukopenia [2]

EDOXABAN

Trade name: Savaysa (Daiichi Sankyo)
Indications: Reduce the risk of stroke and systemic embolism in patients with nonvalvular atrial fibrillation, treatment of deep vein thrombosis and pulmonary embolism
Class: Direct factor Xa inhibitor
Half-life: 10–14 hours
Clinically important, potentially hazardous interactions with: anticoagulants, rifampin
Pregnancy category: C
Important contra-indications noted in the prescribing guidelines for: nursing mothers; pediatric patients
Note: Contraindicated in patients with active pathological bleeding.
Black Box Warning: REDUCED EFFICACY IN NONVALVULAR ATRIAL FIBRILLATION PATIENTS WITH CrCL>95ml/min
ISCHEMIC EVENTS ON PREMATURE DISCONTINUATION
SPINAL / EDPIDURAL HEMATOMA

Skin
Rash (4%)

Mucosal
Epistaxis (nosebleed) (5%)
Gingival bleeding [2]
Oral bleeding (3%)

Gastrointestinal/Hepatic
Diarrhea [2]
Gastrointestinal bleeding (4%)
Hepatotoxicity (5–8%) [2]

Genitourinary
Hematuria (2%) [2]

Hematologic
Anemia (2–10%)
Bleeding (>5%) [13]

Other
Adverse effects [4]

EFAVIRENZ

Trade names: Atripla (Gilead), Sustiva (Bristol-Myers Squibb)
Indications: HIV infection
Class: Antiretroviral, CYP1A2 inhibitor, CYP3A4 inducer, Non-nucleoside reverse transcriptase inhibitor
Half-life: 52–76 hours
Clinically important, potentially hazardous interactions with: alcohol, alprazolam, amprenavir, aripiprazole, artesunate, atazanavir, atorvastatin, atovaquone, benzodiazepines, bepridil, boceprevir, bortezomib, brentuximab vedotin, budesonide, buprenorphine, bupropion, carbamazepine, carvedilol, caspofungin, chlordiazepoxide, cisapride, citalopram, clarithromycin, clonazepam, clopidogrel, clorazepate, CNS depressants, cobimetinib, colchicine, conivaptan, crizotinib, cyclosporine, CYP2B6 inhibitors and inducers, CYP2C19 substrates, CYP2C9 substrates, CYP3A4 substrates and inducers, darunavir, dasatinib, deferasirox, diazepam, dihydroergotamine, diltiazem, dronedarone, enzalutamide, eplerenone, ergot, etravirine, everolimus, exemestane, fentanyl, flurazepam, fosamprenavir, fosphenytoin, gefitinib, grapefruit juice, guanfacine, halofantrine, hydroxyzine, imatinib, indinavir, itraconazole, ixabepilone, lapatinib, levomepromazine, levonorgestrel, linagliptin, lopinavir, lorazepam, lovastatin, lurasidone, maraviroc, methadone, methysergide, midazolam, mifepristone, nevirapine, nifedipine, nilotinib, nisoldipine, ombitasvir/paritaprevir/ritonavir, oral contraceptives, oxazepam, paclitaxel, pazopanib, phenytoin, pimecrolimus, pimozide, posaconazole, pravastatin, praziquantel, progestogens, propafenone, protease inhibitors, quazepam, raltegravir, ranolazine, rifabutin, rifampin, rilpivirine, ritonavir, rivaroxaban, roflumilast, romidepsin, salmeterol, saquinavir, saxagliptin, sertraline, simeprevir, simvastatin, sirolimus, sorafenib, SSRIs, St John's wort, sunitinib, tacrolimus, tadalafil, telaprevir, temazepam, ticagrelor, tipranavir, tocilizumab, tolvaptan, toremifene, triazolam, ulipristal, vandetanib, vemurafenib, vilazodone, vitamin K antagonists, voriconazole, warfarin, zuclopenthixol
Pregnancy category: D
Important contra-indications noted in the prescribing guidelines for: the elderly; nursing mothers; pediatric patients
Note: Atripla is efavirenz, emtricitabine and tenofovir disoproxil.

Skin
DRESS syndrome [2]
Eczema (<2%)
Erythema (11%)
Exanthems (27%) [3]
Exfoliative dermatitis (<2%)
Folliculitis (<2%)
Hot flashes (<2%)
Hypersensitivity [5]
Lipodystrophy [2]
Peripheral edema (<2%)
Photosensitivity [3]
Pruritus (11%)
Rash (26%) [15]
Stevens–Johnson syndrome [3]
Toxicity [2]
Urticaria (<2%)

Hair
Alopecia (<2%)

Mucosal
Xerostomia (<2%)

Cardiovascular
Flushing (<2%)
Thrombophlebitis (<2%)

Central Nervous System
Abnormal dreams (<3%) [9]
Aggression [2]
Anorexia (<2%)
Anxiety (13%) [4]
Depression (19%) [9]
Dysgeusia (taste perversion) (<2%)
Hallucinations [2]
Headache (2–8%) [2]
Impaired concentration (3–5%) [4]
Insomnia (7%) [4]
Nervousness (7%)
Neuropsychiatric disturbances [2]
Neurotoxicity [14]
Nightmares [3]
Pain (<13%)
Paresthesias (<2%)
Parosmia (<2%)
Psychosis [6]
Sleep related disorder [2]
Somnolence (drowsiness) (2%) [3]
Suicidal ideation [5]
Tremor (<2%)
Vertigo (dizziness) (2–9%) [14]

Neuromuscular/Skeletal
- Asthenia (fatigue) (2–8%) [3]
- Myalgia/Myopathy (<2%)

Gastrointestinal/Hepatic
- Abdominal pain (2–3%)
- Diarrhea (3–14%) [2]
- Dyspepsia (4%)
- Hepatic failure [2]
- Hepatotoxicity [12]
- Nausea (2–10%) [2]
- Vomiting (3–6%)

Endocrine/Metabolic
- ALT increased [2]
- Gynecomastia [13]

Genitourinary
- Urolithiasis [3]

Hematologic
- Dyslipidemia [2]

Other
- Adverse effects [10]
- Teratogenicity [4]

EFINACONAZOLE

Trade name: Jublia (Valeant)
Indications: Onychomycosis
Class: Antifungal
Half-life: 30 hours
Clinically important, potentially hazardous interactions with: none known
Pregnancy category: C
Important contra-indications noted in the prescribing guidelines for: nursing mothers; pediatric patients

---

Nails
- Onychocryptosis (2%)

Local
- Application-site dermatitis (2%)
- Application-site reactions [4]
- Application-site vesicles (2%)

EFLORNITHINE

Trade name: Vaniqa (Women First)
Indications: Sleeping sickness, hypertrichosis
Class: Ornithine decarboxylase inhibitor
Half-life: 3–3.5 hours (intravenous); 8 hours (topical)
Clinically important, potentially hazardous interactions with: none known
Pregnancy category: C
Important contra-indications noted in the prescribing guidelines for: nursing mothers; pediatric patients

---

Skin
- Acneform eruption (24%)
- Burning (4%)
- Facial edema (3%)
- Pruritus (4%) [2]
- Rash (3%)
- Stinging (8%)
- Xerosis (2%)

Hair
- Alopecia (5–10%)
- Ingrown (2%)
- Pseudofolliculitis barbae (5–15%)

Central Nervous System
- Headache (5%)
- Paresthesias (4%)
- Seizures (7%) [2]
- Vertigo (dizziness) (<10%)

Gastrointestinal/Hepatic
- Diarrhea (<10%)
- Vomiting (<10%)

Hematologic
- Eosinophilia (<10%)

Otic
- Hearing impairment (<10%)

ELBASVIR & GRAZOPREVIR *

Trade name: Zepatier (Merck)
Indications: Chronic hepatitis C virus genotypes 1 or 4 (with or without ribavirin)
Class: Hepatitis C virus NS3/4A protease inhibitor (grazoprevir), Hepatitis C virus NS5A inhibitor (elbasvir)
Half-life: 24 hours (elbasvir); 31 hours (grazoprevir)
Clinically important, potentially hazardous interactions with: atazanavir, atorvastatin, bosentan, carbamazepine, cobicistat/elvitegravir/emtricitabine/tenofovir disoproxil, cyclosporine, darunavir, efavirenz, fluvastatin, ketoconazole, lopinavir, lovastatin, modafinil, moderate CYP3A inducers, nafcillin, OATP1B1/3 inhibitors, phenytoin, rifampin, rosuvastatin, saquinavir, simvastatin, strong CYP3A inducers, tacrolimus, tipranavir
Pregnancy category: N/A (No available data; contraindicated in pregnant women and in men with pregnant partners when administered with ribavirin)
Important contra-indications noted in the prescribing guidelines for: pediatric patients
Note: Contraindicated in patients with moderate or severe hepatic impairment (Child-Pugh B or C).

Central Nervous System
- Headache (10–11%) [7]

Neuromuscular/Skeletal
- Asthenia (fatigue) (5–11%) [7]

Gastrointestinal/Hepatic
- Abdominal pain (2%)
- Diarrhea (2%) [2]
- Nausea (11%) [6]

ELETRIPTAN

Trade name: Relpax (Pfizer)
Indications: Migraine headaches
Class: 5-HT1 agonist, Serotonin receptor agonist, Triptan
Half-life: 4–5 hours
Clinically important, potentially hazardous interactions with: clarithromycin, dihydroergotamine, itraconazole, ketoconazole, methysergide, nefazodone, nelfinavir, paclitaxel, ritonavir, SNRIs, SSRIs, telithromycin, triptans, troleandomycin, voriconazole
Pregnancy category: C
Important contra-indications noted in the prescribing guidelines for: nursing mothers; pediatric patients
Note: Contraindicated in patients with history, symptoms, or signs of ischemic cardiac, cerebrovascular, or peripheral vascular syndromes, or in patients with uncontrolled hypertension.

Mucosal
- Xerostomia (2–4%)

Cardiovascular
- Chest pain (<4%) [3]
- Flushing (2%)

Central Nervous System
- Headache (3–4%)
- Neurotoxicity [2]
- Paresthesias (3–4%)
- Somnolence (drowsiness) (3–7%) [2]
- Vertigo (dizziness) (3–7%)
- Warm feeling (2%)

Neuromuscular/Skeletal
- Asthenia (fatigue) (4–10%) [4]

Gastrointestinal/Hepatic
- Abdominal pain (<2%)
- Dyspepsia (<2%)
- Dysphagia (<2%)
- Nausea (3–7%) [5]
- Vomiting [2]

Other
- Adverse effects [2]

ELIGLUSTAT

Trade name: Cerdelga (Genzyme)
Indications: Gaucher disease
Class: Glucosylceramide synthase inhibitor
Half-life: 7–9 hours
Clinically important, potentially hazardous interactions with: carbamazepine, grapefruit juice, phenobarbital, phenytoin, rifampin, St John's wort, strong or moderate CYP2D6 inhibitors
Pregnancy category: C
Important contra-indications noted in the prescribing guidelines for: nursing mothers; pediatric patients

---

Skin
- Rash (5%)

Mucosal
- Oropharyngeal pain (10%)

Cardiovascular
Palpitation (5%) [3]

Central Nervous System
Headache (13–40%) [2]
Migraine (10%)
Vertigo (dizziness) (8%)

Neuromuscular/Skeletal
Asthenia (fatigue) (8–14%)
Back pain (12%)
Pain in extremities (11%)

Gastrointestinal/Hepatic
Abdominal pain (10%) [2]
Constipation (5%)
Diarrhea (12%) [2]
Dyspepsia (7%)
Flatulence (10%)
Gastroesophageal reflux (7%)
Nausea (10–12%)

Respiratory
Cough (7%)

Other
Adverse effects [2]

ELOSULFASE ALFA

Trade name: Vimizim (BioMarin)
Indications: Mucopolysaccharidosis IVA (Morquio A syndrome)
Class: Enzyme
Half-life: 8–36 minutes
Clinically important, potentially hazardous interactions with: none known
Pregnancy category: C
Important contra-indications noted in the prescribing guidelines for: nursing mothers; pediatric patients
Black Box Warning: RISK OF ANAPHYLAXIS

Skin
Anaphylactoid reactions/Anaphylaxis (8%)
Hypersensitivity (19%)

Central Nervous System
Chills (10%)
Fever (33%)
Headache (26%)

Neuromuscular/Skeletal
Asthenia (fatigue) (10%)

Gastrointestinal/Hepatic
Abdominal pain (21%)
Nausea (24%)
Vomiting (31%) [2]

Local
Infusion-related reactions [2]

ELOTUZUMAB *

Trade name: Empliciti (Bristol-Myers Squibb)
Indications: Multiple myeloma (in combination with lenalidomide and dexamethasone) in patients who have received one to three prior therapies
Class: Monoclonal antibody
Half-life: N/A
Clinically important, potentially hazardous interactions with: none known
Pregnancy category: N/A (Embryo-fetal toxicity with combination dosage)
Important contra-indications noted in the prescribing guidelines for: nursing mothers; pediatric patients
Note: See separate entries for dexamethasone and lenalidomide.

Skin
Herpes zoster (14%)
Hyperhidrosis (>5%)
Hypersensitivity (>5%) [2]
Peripheral edema [5]
Rash [2]

Mucosal
Oropharyngeal pain (10%)

Cardiovascular
Chest pain (>5%) [2]

Central Nervous System
Anorexia [2]
Chills [3]
Fever (37%) [4]
Headache (15%) [4]
Hypoesthesia (>5%)
Insomnia [4]
Mood changes (>5%)
Neurotoxicity [2]
Peripheral neuropathy (27%) [3]

Neuromuscular/Skeletal
Arthralgia [2]
Asthenia (fatigue) (62%) [8]
Back pain [3]
Muscle spasm [3]
Pain in extremities (16%)

Gastrointestinal/Hepatic
Constipation (36%) [4]
Diarrhea (47%) [5]
Nausea [4]
Vomiting (15%) [4]

Respiratory
Cough [3]
Dyspnea [4]
Nasopharyngitis (25%)
Pneumonia (20%) [4]
Upper respiratory tract infection (23%) [2]

Endocrine/Metabolic
ALP increased (39%)
Appetite decreased (21%)
Hyperglycemia (89%) [2]
Hyperkalemia (32%)
Hypocalcemia (78%)
Hypokalemia [4]
Serum creatinine increased [3]
Weight loss (14%) [2]

Hematologic
Anemia [3]
Leukopenia (91%) [2]
Lymphocytopenia [2]
Lymphopenia (13–99%) [3]
Neutropenia [6]
Thrombocytopenia (84%) [4]

Ocular
Cataract (12%)

Local
Infusion-related reactions (10%) [7]

ELTROMBOPAG

Trade names: Promacta (Novartis), Revolade (Novartis)
Indications: Thrombocytopenic purpura, severe aplastic anemia in patients with insufficient response to immunosuppressive therapy
Class: Thrombopoietin receptor (TPO) agonist
Half-life: 21–32 hours
Clinically important, potentially hazardous interactions with: antacids, atorvastatin, dairy products, lopinavir, mineral supplements, olmesartan, rosuvastatin, selenium, zinc
Pregnancy category: C
Important contra-indications noted in the prescribing guidelines for: nursing mothers; pediatric patients
Black Box Warning: RISK FOR HEPATIC DECOMPENSATION IN PATIENTS WITH CHRONIC HEPATITIS C

Skin
Peripheral edema (3–4%)
Pigmentation [2]
Rash (3–7%)

Hair
Alopecia (2%)

Mucosal
Oropharyngeal pain (4%)
Xerostomia (2%)

Cardiovascular
Thromboembolism [5]
Venous thromboembolism [2]

Central Nervous System
Dysgeusia (taste perversion) (4%)
Headache (10–21%) [9]
Paresthesias (3%)

Neuromuscular/Skeletal
Arthralgia (3%) [2]
Asthenia (fatigue) (3–4%) [4]
Back pain (3%)
Myalgia/Myopathy (5%)
Pain in extremities (7%)

Gastrointestinal/Hepatic
Abdominal pain [2]
Constipation [2]
Diarrhea (9%)
Hepatotoxicity [3]
Nausea (4–9%) [5]
Vomiting (6%)

Respiratory
Cough (5%)
Nasopharyngitis [2]
Pharyngitis (4%)
Upper respiratory tract infection (7%)

Endocrine/Metabolic
ALP increased (2%)
ALT increased (5–6%) [4]
AST increased (4%)

Genitourinary
Urinary tract infection (5%)

Renal
Renal failure [3]

Hematologic
Bleeding [3]
Neutropenia [2]

Thrombocytopenia [2]
Thrombosis [5]

Ocular
Cataract (5%) [2]

Other
Adverse effects [7]

ELUXADOLINE

Trade name: Viberzi (Forest)
Indications: Irritable bowel syndrome with diarrhea
Class: Opioid mu receptor agonist
Half-life: 4–6 hours
Clinically important, potentially hazardous interactions with: alfentanil, alosetron, anticholinergics, atazanavir, bupropion, ciprofloxacin, clarithromycin, cyclosporine, dihydroergotamine, eltrombopag, ergotamine, fentanyl, fluconazole, gemfibrozil, lopinavir, opioids, paroxetine hydrochloride, paroxetine mesylate, pimozide, quinidine, rifampin, ritonavir, rosuvastatin, saquinavir, sirolimus, tacrolimus, tipranavir
Pregnancy category: N/A (Insufficient evidence to inform drug-associated risk)
Important contra-indications noted in the prescribing guidelines for: pediatric patients
Note: Contraindicated in patients with known or suspected biliary duct obstruction, or sphincter of Oddi disease or dysfunction; alcoholism, alcohol abuse, alcohol addiction, or drink more than 3 alcoholic beverages/day; a history of pancreatitis; structural diseases of the pancreas, including known or suspected pancreatic duct obstruction; severe hepatic impairment (Child-Pugh Class C); severe constipation or sequelae from constipation, or known or suspected mechanical gastrointestinal obstruction.

Skin
Rash (3%)

Central Nervous System
Euphoria (<2%)
Sedation (<2%)
Somnolence (drowsiness) (<2%)
Vertigo (dizziness) (3%) [2]

Gastrointestinal/Hepatic
Abdominal distension (3%) [2]
Abdominal pain (6–7%) [3]
Constipation (7–8%) [4]
Flatulence (3%)
Gastroenteritis (<3%) [2]
Gastroesophageal reflux (<2%)
Nausea (7–8%) [3]
Pancreatitis [4]
Vomiting (4%) [3]

Respiratory
Asthma (<2%)
Bronchitis (3%)
Bronchospasm (<2%)
Nasopharyngitis (3–4%) [2]
Respiratory failure (<2%)
Wheezing (<2%)

Endocrine/Metabolic
ALT increased (2–3%)
AST increased (<2%)

EMPAGLIFLOZIN

Trade names: Glyxambi (Boehringer Ingelheim), Jardiance (Boehringer Ingelheim), Synjardy (Boehringer Ingelheim)
Indications: Type II diabetes mellitus
Class: Sodium-glucose co-transporter 2 (SGLT2) inhibitor
Half-life: 12 hours
Clinically important, potentially hazardous interactions with: none known
Pregnancy category: C
Important contra-indications noted in the prescribing guidelines for: nursing mothers; pediatric patients
Note: Contraindicated in patients with severe renal impairment, end stage renal disease, or on dialysis. Glyxambi is empagliflozin and linagliptin; Synjardy is empagliflozin and metformin.

Central Nervous System
Headache [2]

Gastrointestinal/Hepatic
Constipation [2]

Respiratory
Nasopharyngitis [4]

Endocrine/Metabolic
Hypoglycemia [3]

Genitourinary
Genital mycotic infections (2–6%) [5]
Pollakiuria [3]
Urinary frequency (3%)
Urinary tract infection (8–9%) [5]

Other
Adverse effects [7]
Dipsia (thirst) (2%)

EMTRICITABINE

Trade names: Atripla (Gilead), Complera (Gilead), Descovy (Gilead), Emtriva (Gilead), Truvada (Gilead)
Indications: HIV-1 infection
Class: Antiretroviral, Nucleoside analog reverse transcriptase inhibitor
Half-life: ~10 hours
Clinically important, potentially hazardous interactions with: cobicistat/elvitegravir/emtricitabine/tenofovir disoproxil, ganciclovir, lamivudine, ribavirin, valganciclovir
Pregnancy category: B
Important contra-indications noted in the prescribing guidelines for: nursing mothers
Note: Emtricitabine is a fluorinated derivative of lamivudine. Atripla is emtricitabine, efavirenz and tenofovir disoproxil; Complera is emtricitabine, rilpivirine and tenofovir disoproxil; Descovy is emtricitabine and tenofovir alafenamide; Truvada is emtricitabine and tenofovir disoproxil. See also separate profiles for emtricitabine in combination with cobicistat, elvitegravir and tenofovir disoproxil or tenofovir alafenamide.
Black Box Warning: LACTIC ACIDOSIS / SEVERE HEPATOMEGALY WITH STEATOSIS and POST TREATMENT EXACERBATION OF HEPATITIS B

Skin
Exanthems (17%)
Pigmentation (palms and soles) (32%)
Pruritus (17–30%)
Pustules (17–30%)
Rash (17–30%) [5]
Urticaria (17–30%)
Vesiculobullous eruption (17–30%)

Central Nervous System
Abnormal dreams (2–11%) [3]
Anxiety [2]
Depression (6–9%)
Fever (18%)
Headache (13–22%) [3]
Insomnia (7–16%)
Neurotoxicity [5]
Paresthesias (6%)
Peripheral neuropathy (4%)
Somnolence (drowsiness) [2]
Vertigo (dizziness) (4–25%) [4]

Neuromuscular/Skeletal
Arthralgia (3–5%)
Asthenia (fatigue) (12–16%) [3]
Myalgia/Myopathy (4–6%) [2]

Gastrointestinal/Hepatic
Abdominal pain (8–14%) [2]
Diarrhea (20–23%) [4]
Dyspepsia (4–8%)
Gastroenteritis (11%)
Hepatic failure [2]
Hepatotoxicity [2]
Nausea (13–18%) [4]
Vomiting (9–23%) [3]

Respiratory
Cough (14–28%)
Pneumonia (15%)
Rhinitis (12–20%)

Hematologic
Anemia (7%)

Otic
Otitis media (23%)

Other
Adverse effects [5]
Allergic reactions (17–30%)
Infection (44%)

EMTRICITABINE/ RILPIVIRINE/ TENOFOVIR ALAFENAMIDE *

Trade name: Odefsey (Gilead)
Indications: HIV-1 infection
Class: Hepatitis B virus necleoside analog reverse transcriptase inhibitor (tenofovir alafenamide), Non-nucleoside reverse transcriptase inhibitor (rilpivirine), Nucleoside analog reverse transcriptase inhibitor (emtricitabine)
Half-life: 10 hours (emtricitabine); 50 hours (rilpivirine); <1 hour (tenofovir alafenamide)
Clinically important, potentially hazardous interactions with: carbamazepine, dexamethasone, dexlansoprazole, esomeprazole, lansoprazole, omeprazole, oxcarbazepine, pantoprazole, phenobarbital, phenytoin,

rabeprazole, rifampin, rifapentine, St John's wort
Pregnancy category: N/A (Insufficient evidence to inform drug-associated risk)
Important contra-indications noted in the prescribing guidelines for: nursing mothers; pediatric patients
Black Box Warning: LACTIC ACIDOSIS/ SEVERE HEPATOMEGALY WITH STEATOSIS and POST TREATMENT ACUTE EXACERBATION OF HEPATITIS B

Central Nervous System
Depression (<2%)
Headache (<2%)
Insomnia (<2%)

ENALAPRIL

Trade names: Innovace (Merck Sharpe & Dohme), Lexxel (AstraZeneca), Teczem (Sanofi-Aventis), Vaseretic (Valeant), Vasotec (Valeant)
Indications: Hypertension, symptomatic congestive heart failure, asymptomatic left ventricular dysfunction
Class: Angiotensin-converting enzyme (ACE) inhibitor, Antihypertensive, Vasodilator
Half-life: 11 hours
Clinically important, potentially hazardous interactions with: alcohol, aldesleukin, allopurinol, alpha blockers, alprostadil, amifostine, amiloride, angiotensin II receptor antagonists, antacids, antidiabetics, antihypertensives, antipsychotics, anxiolytics and hypnotics, aprotinin, azathioprine, baclofen, beta blockers, calcium channel blockers, clonidine, conivaptan, corticosteroids, cyclosporine, CYP3A4 inducers, deferasirox, diazoxide, diuretics, eplerenone, estrogens, everolimus, general anesthetics, gold & gold compounds, grapefruit juice, heparins, hydralazine, hypotensives, insulin, levodopa, lithium, MAO inhibitors, metformin, methyldopa, methylphenidate, minoxidil, moxisylyte, moxonidine, nitrates, nitroprusside, NSAIDs, pentoxifylline, phosphodiesterase 5 inhibitors, potassium salts, prostacyclin analogues, quinine, rituximab, salicylates, sirolimus, spironolactone, sulfonylureas, tadalafil, temsirolimus, tizanidine, tolvaptan, triamterene, trimethoprim
Pregnancy category: D (category C in first trimester; category D in second and third trimesters)
Important contra-indications noted in the prescribing guidelines for: nursing mothers
Note: Lexxel is enalapril and felodipine; Teczem is enalapril and diltiazem; Vaseretic is enalapril and hydrochlorothiazide. Hydrochlorothiazide is a sulfonamide and can be absorbed systemically. Sulfonamides can produce severe, possibly fatal, reactions such as toxic epidermal necrolysis and Stevens-Johnson syndrome.
Contraindicated in patients with a history of angioedema with or without previous ACE inhibitor treatment.
Black Box Warning: FETAL TOXICITY

Skin
Angioedema [73]
Bullous pemphigoid [2]
Exanthems [9]
Lichenoid eruption [2]
Lupus erythematosus [2]
Pemphigus [10]
Pemphigus foliaceus [2]
Peripheral edema [2]
Photosensitivity [2]
Pruritus [3]
Psoriasis [3]
Rash [5]
Urticaria [5]
Vasculitis [2]

Mucosal
Oral lesions [4]
Oral ulceration [2]
Tongue edema [2]

Cardiovascular
Flushing [4]

Central Nervous System
Ageusia (taste loss) [4]
Dysgeusia (taste perversion) (<10%) [7]
Headache (5%)
Vertigo (dizziness) (4–8%) [2]

Neuromuscular/Skeletal
Asthenia (fatigue) (<3%)
Pseudopolymyalgia [2]

Gastrointestinal/Hepatic
Hepatotoxicity [3]
Pancreatitis [2]

Respiratory
Cough (8–23%) [40]

Endocrine/Metabolic
Hyperkalemia [4]
SIADH [3]

Renal
Nephrotoxicity [2]

Other
Adverse effects [9]
Death [4]

ENFUVIRTIDE

Trade name: Fuzeon (Roche)
Indications: HIV-1 infection (in combination with other antiretroviral agents)
Class: Antiretroviral, HIV cell fusion inhibitor
Half-life: 3.8 hours
Clinically important, potentially hazardous interactions with: darunavir, indinavir, tipranavir
Pregnancy category: B
Important contra-indications noted in the prescribing guidelines for: the elderly; nursing mothers

---

Skin
Folliculitis (2%)
Herpes simplex (4%)
Hypersensitivity [3]
Papillomas (4%)
Pruritus (62%)

Mucosal
Xerostomia (2%)

Central Nervous System
Anorexia (2%)
Depression (9%)

Neuromuscular/Skeletal
Asthenia (fatigue) (16%) [2]
Myalgia/Myopathy (3%)
Pain in extremities (3%)

Gastrointestinal/Hepatic
Abdominal pain (4%)
Pancreatitis (3%)

Respiratory
Cough (4%)
Flu-like syndrome (2%)
Pneumonia (3%)
Sinusitis (6%)

Endocrine/Metabolic
ALT increased (<4%)
Appetite decreased (3%)
Creatine phosphokinase increased (3–7%)
Weight loss (7%)

Hematologic
Eosinophilia (2–9%)

Ocular
Conjunctivitis (2%)

Local
Injection-site bruising (52%)
Injection-site erythema (91%)
Injection-site induration (90%)
Injection-site nodules (80%) [4]
Injection-site pain (96%)
Injection-site pruritus (65%)
Injection-site reactions (98%) [27]
Injection-site scleroderma [2]

Other
Infection [3]

ENOXAPARIN

Trade names: Clexane (Sanofi-Aventis), Lovenox (Sanofi-Aventis)
Indications: Prevention of deep vein thrombosis, ischemic complications of unstable angina and non-Q wave myocardial infarction, treatment of acute ST-segment elevation myocardial infarction
Class: Heparin, low molecular weight
Half-life: 4.5 hours
Clinically important, potentially hazardous interactions with: ACE inhibitors, angiotensin II receptor antagonists, anticoagulants, aspirin, butabarbital, clopidogrel, danaparoid, diclofenac, dipyridamole, drotrecogin alfa, iloprost, infused nitrates, ketorolac, NSAIDs, platelet inhibitors, rivaroxaban, salicylates, sulfinpyrazone
Pregnancy category: B
Important contra-indications noted in the prescribing guidelines for: nursing mothers; pediatric patients
Note: Epidural or spinal hematomas may occur in patients who are anticoagulated with low molecular weight heparins or heparinoids and are receiving neuraxial anesthesia or undergoing spinal puncture. Contraindicated in patients with active major bleeding; thrombocytopenia with a positive *in vitro* test for anti-platelet antibody in the presence of enoxaparin; hypersensitivity to heparin or pork products; hypersensitivity to benzyl alcohol (multi-dose formulation only).
Black Box Warning: SPINAL/EPIDURAL HEMATOMA

Skin
Anaphylactoid reactions/Anaphylaxis [3]
Angioedema [2]
Bullous dermatitis [5]
Ecchymoses (2%)
Edema (3%)
Erythema (<10%)
Exanthems [2]
Hematoma [11]
Hypersensitivity [7]
Necrosis [4]
Peripheral edema (3%)
Purpura (<10%)

Cardiovascular
Venous thromboembolism [2]

Gastrointestinal/Hepatic
Hepatotoxicity [5]

Endocrine/Metabolic
ALT increased [4]
AST increased [3]

Genitourinary
Hematuria [2]

Hematologic
Bleeding [8]
Hemorrhage [4]
Thrombocytopenia [5]

Local
Injection-site necrosis [4]
Injection-site plaques [2]

Other
Adverse effects [3]
Death [2]

ENTACAPONE

Trade names: Comtan (Orion), Comtess (Orion), Stalevo (Orion)
Indications: Parkinsonism
Class: Catechol-O-methyl transferase inhibitor
Half-life: 2.4 hours
Clinically important, potentially hazardous interactions with: amitriptyline, MAO inhibitors, paroxetine hydrochloride, phenelzine, rasagiline, tranylcypromine, venlafaxine
Pregnancy category: C
Important contra-indications noted in the prescribing guidelines for: nursing mothers; pediatric patients

---

Skin
Diaphoresis (2%)
Purpura (2%)

Mucosal
Xerostomia (3%)

Central Nervous System
Anxiety (2%)
Dyskinesia (25%) [2]
Hyperactivity (10%)
Hypokinesia (9%)
Parkinsonism (17%)
Somnolence (drowsiness) (2%)
Vertigo (dizziness) (8%) [2]

Neuromuscular/Skeletal
Asthenia (fatigue) (8%)
Back pain (4%)

Gastrointestinal/Hepatic
Abdominal pain (8%)
Constipation (6%)
Diarrhea (10%) [3]
Dyspepsia (2%)
Flatulence (2%)
Nausea (14%)
Vomiting (4%)

Respiratory
Dyspnea (3%)

Genitourinary
Melanuria (10%)

ENTECAVIR

Trade name: Baraclude (Bristol-Myers Squibb)
Indications: Chronic hepatitis B virus infection
Class: Antiviral, Guanosine nucleoside analog
Half-life: ~24 hours
Clinically important, potentially hazardous interactions with: none known
Pregnancy category: C
Important contra-indications noted in the prescribing guidelines for: nursing mothers; pediatric patients
Black Box Warning: SEVERE ACUTE EXACERBATIONS OF HEPATITIS B, PATIENTS CO-INFECTED WITH HIV AND HBV, and LACTIC ACIDOSIS AND HEPATOMEGALY

Skin
Rash [2]

Hair
Alopecia [2]

Central Nervous System
Headache (2–4%) [3]
Neurotoxicity [3]
Peripheral neuropathy [2]

Neuromuscular/Skeletal
Asthenia (fatigue) (<3%) [6]
Myalgia/Myopathy [3]

Gastrointestinal/Hepatic
Abdominal pain [2]
Diarrhea [2]
Pancreatitis [3]

Respiratory
Cough [2]
Upper respiratory tract infection [2]

Endocrine/Metabolic
Acidosis [6]
ALT increased (2–12%) [2]
Creatine phosphokinase increased (<2%)
Hypophosphatemia [2]

Genitourinary
Hematuria (9%)

Other
Adverse effects [4]

ENZALUTAMIDE

Trade name: Xtandi (Medivation)
Indications: Metastatic castration-resistant prostate cancer in patients who have previously received docetaxel
Class: Androgen antagonist
Half-life: 8–9 days
Clinically important, potentially hazardous interactions with: alfentanil, bosentan, carbamazepine, cyclosporine, dihydroergotamine, efavirenz, ergotamine, fentanyl, gemfibrozil, itraconazole, midazolam, modafinil, nafcillin, omeprazole, phenobarbital, phenytoin, pimozide, quinidine, rifabutin, rifampin, rifapentine, sirolimus, St John's wort, tacrolimus, warfarin
Pregnancy category: X (not indicated for use in women)
Important contra-indications noted in the prescribing guidelines for: nursing mothers; pediatric patients

---

Skin
Hot flashes (20%) [10]
Peripheral edema (15%) [3]
Pruritus (4%)
Xerosis (4%)

Mucosal
Epistaxis (nosebleed) (3%)

Cardiovascular
Hypertension (6%) [5]

Central Nervous System
Amnesia (>2%)
Anxiety (7%)
Cognitive impairment (4%)
Gait instability [2]
Hallucinations (2%)
Headache (12%) [4]
Hypoesthesia (4%)
Insomnia (9%)
Paresthesias (7%) [2]
Seizures [12]
Spinal cord compression (7%)
Vertigo (dizziness) (10%) [2]

Neuromuscular/Skeletal
Arthralgia (21%) [3]
Asthenia (fatigue) (51%) [18]
Back pain (26%) [4]
Bone or joint pain (15%) [7]
Fractures (4%) [2]

Gastrointestinal/Hepatic
Constipation [3]
Diarrhea (22%) [9]
Nausea [3]

Respiratory
Bronchitis (>2%)
Laryngitis (>2%)
Nasopharyngitis (>2%)
Pharyngitis (>2%)
Pneumonia (>2%)
Sinusitis (>2%)
Upper respiratory tract infection (11%) [3]

Endocrine/Metabolic
ALT increased (10%)
Appetite decreased [3]
Weight loss [3]

Genitourinary
- Hematuria (7%)
- Pollakiuria (5%)

Hematologic
- Anemia [2]
- Neutropenia (15%)

Other
- Adverse effects [4]

EPHEDRINE

Trade names: Rynatuss (MedPointe), Vicks Vatronol (Procter & Gamble)
Indications: Nasal congestion, acute hypotensive states, asthma
Class: Adrenergic alpha-receptor agonist, Sympathomimetic
Half-life: 3–6 hours
Clinically important, potentially hazardous interactions with: antihypertensives, dexamethasone, furazolidone, guanethidine, iobenguane, levomepromazine, MAO inhibitors, methyldopa, oxprenolol, phenelzine, phenylpropanolamine, selegiline, tranylcypromine, tricyclic antidepressants
Pregnancy category: C
Important contra-indications noted in the prescribing guidelines for: nursing mothers

---

Skin
- Dermatitis [5]
- Diaphoresis (<10%)
- Fixed eruption [6]
- Pallor (<10%)
- Urticaria [2]

Mucosal
- Xerostomia (<10%)

Central Nervous System
- Trembling (<10%)
- Tremor (<10%)

EPINEPHRINE

Synonym: adrenaline
Trade names: Adrenaclick (Amedra), Adrenalin (JHP Pharmaceuticals), Auvi-Q (Sanofi-Aventis), Epipen (Mylan)
Indications: Cardiac arrest, hay fever, asthma, anaphylaxis
Class: Catecholamine, Sympathomimetic
Half-life: N/A
Clinically important, potentially hazardous interactions with: albuterol, alpha blockers, amitriptyline, amoxapine, atenolol, beta blockers, carteolol, chlorpromazine, clomipramine, clozapine, cocaine, desipramine, doxepin, ergotamine, furazolidone, halothane, imipramine, insulin aspart, insulin degludec, insulin detemir, insulin glargine, insulin glulisine, levalbuterol, lisdexamfetamine, lurasidone, MAO inhibitors, metoprolol, milnacipran, nadolol, nortriptyline, oxprenolol, penbutolol, phenelzine, phenoxybenzamine, phenylephrine, pindolol, prazosin, propranolol, protriptyline, sympathomimetics, terbutaline, thioridazine, timolol, tranylcypromine, tricyclic antidepressants, trimipramine, vasopressors
Pregnancy category: C
Important contra-indications noted in the prescribing guidelines for: the elderly; nursing mothers

---

Skin
- Dermatitis [4]
- Diaphoresis (<10%)
- Necrosis [3]
- Pemphigus (cicatricial) [2]

Cardiovascular
- Arrhythmias [3]
- Flushing (<10%)
- Hypertension [2]
- Hypotension [3]
- Myocardial infarction [5]
- QT prolongation [2]
- Ventricular tachycardia [2]

Central Nervous System
- Trembling (<10%)
- Tremor [2]

EPIRUBICIN

Trade name: Ellence (Pfizer)
Indications: Adjuvant therapy in primary breast cancer
Class: Antibiotic, anthracycline
Half-life: 33 hours
Clinically important, potentially hazardous interactions with: amlodipine, bepridil, cimetidine, diltiazem, felodipine, isradipine, nicardipine, nifedipine, nimodipine, nisoldipine, verapamil
Pregnancy category: D
Important contra-indications noted in the prescribing guidelines for: nursing mothers
Black Box Warning: SEVERE OR LIFE-THREATENING HEMATOLOGICAL AND OTHER ADVERSE REACTIONS

Skin
- Erythroderma (5%)
- Hand–foot syndrome [5]
- Hot flashes (5–39%)
- Pruritus (9%)
- Rash (<9%) [2]
- Vasculitis [2]

Hair
- Alopecia (69–95%) [17]

Mucosal
- Mucositis [5]
- Stomatitis [9]

Cardiovascular
- Cardiotoxicity [3]
- QT prolongation [3]

Central Nervous System
- Anorexia [5]
- Dysgeusia (taste perversion) [2]
- Fever [2]
- Headache [2]
- Neurotoxicity [2]
- Peripheral neuropathy [3]

Neuromuscular/Skeletal
- Arthralgia [2]
- Asthenia (fatigue) (6%) [9]
- Myalgia/Myopathy (55%) [5]

Gastrointestinal/Hepatic
- Abdominal pain [2]
- Constipation [2]
- Diarrhea [7]
- Hepatotoxicity [2]
- Nausea [12]
- Vomiting [11]

Endocrine/Metabolic
- ALT increased [2]
- Amenorrhea [2]
- AST increased [2]

Hematologic
- Anemia [9]
- Febrile neutropenia [4]
- Leukopenia [4]
- Neutropenia [11]
- Thrombocytopenia [5]

Local
- Injection-site reactions (3–20%)

Other
- Allergic reactions [2]

EPOETIN ALFA

Synonyms: erythropoietin; EPO
Trade names: Epogen (Amgen), Eprex (Janssen-Cilag), Procrit (Ortho)
Indications: Anemia
Class: Erythropoiesis-stimulating agent (ESA), Erythropoietin
Half-life: 4–13 hours (in patients with chronic renal failure)
Clinically important, potentially hazardous interactions with: none known
Pregnancy category: C
Important contra-indications noted in the prescribing guidelines for: nursing mothers
Black Box Warning: ERYTHROPOIESIS-STIMULATING AGENTS (ESAs) INCREASE THE RISK OF DEATH, MYOCARDIAL INFARCTION, STROKE, VENOUS THROMBOEMBOLISM, THROMBOSIS OF VASCULAR ACCESS AND TUMOR PROGRESSION OR RECURRENCE

Skin
- Angioedema (<5%)
- Edema (17%)
- Pruritus (12–21%) [2]
- Rash (2–19%)

Cardiovascular
- Hypertension (3–28%)

Central Nervous System
- Fever (10–42%) [2]
- Headache (5–18%)
- Paresthesias (11%)

Neuromuscular/Skeletal
- Arthralgia (10–16%)

Gastrointestinal/Hepatic
- Constipation [2]
- Nausea (35–56%)

Respiratory
- Cough (4–26%)
- Dyspnea [2]

Hematologic
Thrombocytopenia [2]

Ocular
Hallucinations, visual [2]

Local
Injection-site reactions (7%)

EPOPROSTENOL

Trade names: Flolan (GSK), Veletri (Actelion)
Indications: Pulmonary arterial hypertension
Class: Peripheral vasodilator
Half-life: 6 minutes
Clinically important, potentially hazardous interactions with: anticoagulants, antihypertensives, diuretics, vasodilators
Pregnancy category: B
Important contra-indications noted in the prescribing guidelines for: the elderly; nursing mothers; pediatric patients
Note: Contraindicated in patients with heart failure induced by reduced left ventricular ejection fraction.

Skin
Diaphoresis (41%)
Pruritus (4%)
Rash (10%) [2]

Cardiovascular
Bradycardia (5%) [2]
Cardiac failure (31%)
Chest pain (11%) [2]
Flushing [6]
Hypotension (16%) [5]
Tachycardia (35%) [2]

Central Nervous System
Agitation (11%)
Anxiety (21%) [2]
Chills (25%)
Fever (25%)
Headache (83%) [13]
Insomnia (9%)
Paresthesias (12%)
Seizures (4%)
Somnolence (drowsiness) (4%)
Syncope (13%)
Tremor (21%)

Neuromuscular/Skeletal
Back pain (13%)
Jaw pain (54%) [6]
Myalgia/Myopathy (44%)

Gastrointestinal/Hepatic
Abdominal pain (14%)
Diarrhea [2]
Nausea [4]

Respiratory
Alveolar hemorrhage (pulmonary) [2]
Dyspnea (2%)
Flu-like syndrome (25%)
Pneumonia [2]

Endocrine/Metabolic
Weight loss (27%)

Hematologic
Sepsis (25%)

Local
Injection-site infection (21%)
Injection-site pain (13%)

Other
Adverse effects [3]

EPROSARTAN

Trade name: Teveten (AbbVie)
Indications: Hypertension
Class: Angiotensin II receptor antagonist (blocker), Antihypertensive
Half-life: 5–9 hours
Clinically important, potentially hazardous interactions with: none known
Pregnancy category: D (category C in first trimester; category D in second and third trimesters)
Important contra-indications noted in the prescribing guidelines for: nursing mothers; pediatric patients
Black Box Warning: FETAL TOXICITY

Central Nervous System
Dysgeusia (taste perversion) [2]
Vertigo (dizziness) [2]

Neuromuscular/Skeletal
Arthralgia (2%)
Asthenia (fatigue) (2%)

Gastrointestinal/Hepatic
Abdominal pain (2%)

Respiratory
Cough (4%) [3]
Pharyngitis (4%)
Rhinitis (4%)
Upper respiratory tract infection (8%) [2]

Other
Adverse effects [3]

EPTIFIBATIDE

Trade name: Integrilin (Merck)
Indications: Acute coronary syndrome, unstable angina
Class: Antiplatelet, Glycoprotein IIb/IIIa inhibitor
Half-life: 2.5 hours
Clinically important, potentially hazardous interactions with: anticoagulants, antiplatelet agents, collagenase, dasatinib, drotrecogin alfa, fondaparinux, glucosamine, ibritumomab, iloprost, lepirudin, NSAIDs, pentoxifylline, salicylates, thrombolytic agents, tositumomab & iodine^{131}
Pregnancy category: B
Important contra-indications noted in the prescribing guidelines for: nursing mothers; pediatric patients
Note: Contraindicated in patients with a history of bleeding diathesis, or evidence of active abnormal bleeding within the previous 30 days; severe hypertension not adequately controlled on antihypertensive therapy; major surgery within the preceding 6 weeks; history of stroke within 30 days or any history of hemorrhagic stroke; current or planned administration of another parenteral GP IIb/IIIa inhibitor; or dependency on renal dialysis.

Cardiovascular
Hypotension (7%)

Hematologic
Bleeding [3]
Hemorrhage (<10%)
Thrombocytopenia [16]
Thrombosis [3]

Other
Death [2]

ERGOMETRINE

Trade name: Ergometrine (Hameln)
Indications: Management of the third stage of labor and in the treatment of postpartum hemorrhage
Class: Amine alkaloid
Half-life: N/A
Clinically important, potentially hazardous interactions with: halothane, sympathomimetic agents
Important contra-indications noted in the prescribing guidelines for: nursing mothers

---

Cardiovascular
Myocardial infarction [4]
Myocardial ischemia [3]

ERGOTAMINE

Trade name: Wigrettes (Organon)
Indications: Migraine, migraine variants
Class: Ergot alkaloid
Half-life: 2 hours
Clinically important, potentially hazardous interactions with: acebutolol, almotriptan, amprenavir, azithromycin, boceprevir, chlortetracycline, crizotinib, darunavir, dasatinib, delavirdine, demeclocycline, doxycycline, enzalutamide, epinephrine, erythromycin, indinavir, itraconazole, lopinavir, lymecycline, methylergonovine, mifepristone, minocycline, naratriptan, nelfinavir, nilotinib, ombitasvir/paritaprevir/ritonavir, oxytetracycline, posaconazole, propyphenazone, ritonavir, telaprevir, telithromycin, tetracycline, tigecycline, tipranavir, troleandomycin, voriconazole, warfarin
Pregnancy category: X
Important contra-indications noted in the prescribing guidelines for: nursing mothers
Note: Ergotamine is excreted in breast milk and may cause symptoms of vomiting, diarrhea, weak pulse and unstable blood pressure in nursing infants.

Skin
Toxicity [4]

Cardiovascular
Valvulopathy [3]

Respiratory
Pleural effusion [2]

ERIBULIN

Trade name: Halaven (Eisai)
Indications: Metastatic breast cancer in patients who have previously received at least two chemotherapeutic regimens (prior therapy should have included an anthracycline and a taxane in either the adjuvant or metastatic setting), unresectable or metastatic liposarcoma in patients who have received a prior anthracycline-containing regimen
Class: Antineoplastic, Microtubule inhibitor
Half-life: 40 hours
Clinically important, potentially hazardous interactions with: none known
Pregnancy category: N/A (No available data but caused embryo-fetal toxicity in animal studies)
Important contra-indications noted in the prescribing guidelines for: nursing mothers; pediatric patients

---

Skin
- Peripheral edema (5–10%)
- Rash (5–10%)

Hair
- Alopecia (45%) [10]

Mucosal
- Mucosal inflammation (9%)
- Stomatitis (5–10%)
- Xerostomia (5–10%)

Central Nervous System
- Anorexia (20%) [3]
- Depression (5–10%)
- Dysgeusia (taste perversion) (5–10%)
- Fever (21%)
- Headache (19%)
- Insomnia (5–10%)
- Neurotoxicity [6]
- Peripheral neuropathy (35%) [22]
- Vertigo (dizziness) (5–10%)

Neuromuscular/Skeletal
- Arthralgia (22%)
- Asthenia (fatigue) (54%) [29]
- Back pain (16%)
- Muscle spasm (5–10%)
- Myalgia/Myopathy (22%)
- Pain in extremities (11%)

Gastrointestinal/Hepatic
- Abdominal pain (5–10%)
- Constipation (25%) [2]
- Diarrhea (18%) [3]
- Dyspepsia (5–10%)
- Nausea (35%) [9]
- Vomiting (18%)

Respiratory
- Cough (14%)
- Dyspnea (16%) [2]
- Upper respiratory tract infection (5–10%)

Endocrine/Metabolic
- Appetite decreased [2]
- Hypokalemia (5–10%)
- Weight loss (21%)

Genitourinary
- Urinary tract infection (10%)

Hematologic
- Anemia (58%) [10]
- Febrile neutropenia (5%) [10]
- Leukopenia [13]
- Neutropenia (82%) [41]

Ocular
- Lacrimation (increased) (5–10%)

Other
- Adverse effects [3]
- Death [2]

ERLOTINIB

Trade name: Tarceva (OSI)
Indications: Non-small cell lung cancer, pancreatic cancer (with gemcitabine)
Class: Antineoplastic, Biologic, Epidermal growth factor receptor (EGFR) inhibitor, Tyrosine kinase inhibitor
Half-life: ~36 hours
Clinically important, potentially hazardous interactions with: atazanavir, capecitabine, carbamazepine, ciprofloxacin, clarithromycin, diclofenac, itraconazole, ketoconazole, meloxicam, nefazodone, nelfinavir, omeprazole, pantoprazole, phenobarbital, phenytoin, rifabutin, rifampin, rifapentine, ritonavir, saquinavir, St John's wort, troleandomycin, voriconazole, warfarin
Pregnancy category: D
Important contra-indications noted in the prescribing guidelines for: nursing mothers; pediatric patients

---

Skin
- Acne keloid [2]
- Acneform eruption [26]
- Dermatitis [2]
- DRESS syndrome [2]
- Erythema (18%)
- Exanthems [3]
- Folliculitis [9]
- Hand–foot syndrome [3]
- Papulopustular eruption [7]
- Pruritus (13%) [8]
- Purpura [3]
- Rash (75%) [105]
- Rosacea [2]
- Toxicity [7]
- Xerosis (12%) [11]

Hair
- Alopecia [10]
- Hair changes [3]
- Hypertrichosis [4]

Nails
- Nail changes [2]
- Paronychia [11]

Mucosal
- Mucositis [9]
- Stomatitis (17%) [9]

Cardiovascular
- Hypertension [2]

Central Nervous System
- Anorexia [8]
- Fever [2]

Neuromuscular/Skeletal
- Asthenia (fatigue) (52%) [28]
- Rhabdomyolysis [2]

Gastrointestinal/Hepatic
- Abdominal pain (11%)
- Cholangitis [2]
- Diarrhea [60]
- Gastrointestinal bleeding [2]
- Hepatotoxicity [9]
- Nausea [14]
- Vomiting [7]

Respiratory
- Cough (33%)
- Dyspnea [4]
- Pneumonia [2]
- Pneumonitis [4]
- Pneumothorax [2]
- Pulmonary toxicity [14]

Endocrine/Metabolic
- ALT increased [2]
- Appetite decreased [3]
- AST increased [3]
- Dehydration [3]
- Hyperglycemia [3]

Hematologic
- Anemia [12]
- Febrile neutropenia [2]
- Hemotoxicity [2]
- Leukopenia [4]
- Neutropenia [13]
- Thrombocytopenia [10]

Ocular
- Conjunctivitis (12%) [3]
- Corneal perforation [2]
- Ectropion [4]
- Ocular adverse effects [3]
- Periorbital rash [2]
- Trichomegaly [13]

Other
- Adverse effects [11]
- Death [9]
- Infection (24%) [7]

ERTAPENEM

Trade name: Invanz (Merck)
Indications: Severe resistant bacterial infections caused by susceptible organisms
Class: Antibiotic, carbapenem
Half-life: 4 hours
Clinically important, potentially hazardous interactions with: probenecid
Pregnancy category: B
Important contra-indications noted in the prescribing guidelines for: the elderly; nursing mothers

---

Skin
- Edema (3%)
- Erythema (<2%)
- Pruritus (<2%)
- Rash (2–3%)
- Wound complications [2]

Cardiovascular
- Phlebitis (2%)
- Thrombophlebitis (2%)

Central Nervous System
- Seizures [6]

Gastrointestinal/Hepatic
Nausea [2]

Respiratory
Cough (<2%)

Genitourinary
Vaginitis (<3%)

Local
Injection-site extravasation (2%)

Other
Death (2%)

ERYTHROMYCIN

Trade names: Eryc (Warner Chilcott), PCE (AbbVie)
Indications: Various infections caused by susceptible organisms
Class: Antibiotic, macrolide, CYP3A4 inhibitor
Half-life: 1.4–2 hours
Clinically important, potentially hazardous interactions with: afatinib, alfentanil, aminophylline, amisulpride, amoxicillin, ampicillin, anticonvulsants, arsenic, astemizole, atorvastatin, avanafil, benzodiazepines, bosentan, bromocriptine, buprenorphine, bupropion, carbamazepine, cilostazol, ciprofloxacin, cisapride, clindamycin, clindamycin/tretinoin, clopidogrel, clozapine, colchicine, cyclosporine, CYP3A inhibitors, darifenacin, dasatinib, digoxin, dihydroergotamine, diltiazem, disopyramide, docetaxel, doxercalciferol, dronedarone, enoxacin, eplerenone, ergotamine, estradiol, eszopiclone, everolimus, flibanserin, fluconazole, fluoxetine, fluvastatin, gatifloxacin, HMG-CoA reductase inhibitors, imatinib, indacaterol, itraconazole, ketoconazole, levodopa, lomefloxacin, lorazepam, lovastatin, methadone, methylergonovine, methylprednisolone, methysergide, midazolam, mifepristone, mizolastine, moxifloxacin, nitrazepam, norfloxacin, ofloxacin, oxtriphylline, paroxetine hydrochloride, pentamidine, pimecrolimus, pimozide, pitavastatin, pravastatin, quetiapine, quinolones, ranolazine, repaglinide, rilpivirine, rivaroxaban, roflumilast, rosuvastatin, rupatadine, sertraline, sildenafil, silodosin, simeprevir, simvastatin, sparfloxacin, sulpiride, tacrolimus, tadalafil, tamsulosin, terfenadine, tramadol, triamcinolone, triazolam, troleandomycin, vardenafil, venetoclax, verapamil, vilazodone, vinblastine, warfarin, zafirlukast, zaleplon, zolpidem, zuclopenthixol
Pregnancy category: B
Important contra-indications noted in the prescribing guidelines for: the elderly; nursing mothers

---

Skin
AGEP [2]
Anaphylactoid reactions/Anaphylaxis [2]
Baboon syndrome (SDRIFE) [2]
Dermatitis (systemic) [4]
Exanthems (<5%) [4]
Fixed eruption [6]
Hypersensitivity (<10%) [3]
Rash [3]
Stevens–Johnson syndrome [7]
Toxic epidermal necrolysis [7]
Urticaria [4]

Mucosal
Oral candidiasis (<10%)

Cardiovascular
QT prolongation [5]
Torsades de pointes [8]

Neuromuscular/Skeletal
Rhabdomyolysis [4]

Gastrointestinal/Hepatic
Abdominal pain [3]
Diarrhea [4]
Nausea [4]

Otic
Tinnitus [3]

Local
Injection-site phlebitis (<10%) [2]

Other
Allergic reactions (<2%) [3]

ESCITALOPRAM

Trade name: Lexapro (Forest)
Indications: Major depressive disorders, anxiety
Class: Antidepressant, Selective serotonin reuptake inhibitor (SSRI)
Half-life: 27–32 hours
Clinically important, potentially hazardous interactions with: alcohol, bupropion, MAO inhibitors, methylphenidate, omeprazole, selegiline, St John's wort, sumatriptan, telaprevir, valerian
Pregnancy category: C
Important contra-indications noted in the prescribing guidelines for: the elderly; nursing mothers; pediatric patients
Black Box Warning: SUICIDALITY AND ANTIDEPRESSANT DRUGS

Skin
Diaphoresis (5%)
Hot flashes (<10%)
Rash (<10%)

Mucosal
Oral vesiculation (<19%)
Xerostomia (6%) [3]

Cardiovascular
QT prolongation [9]
Torsades de pointes [2]

Central Nervous System
Headache (24%) [4]
Insomnia (9–12%) [3]
Paresthesias (<10%)
Restless legs syndrome [5]
Serotonin syndrome [5]
Somnolence (drowsiness) (6–13%) [4]
Tremor (<10%)
Vertigo (dizziness) (5%) [3]

Neuromuscular/Skeletal
Asthenia (fatigue) [3]
Myalgia/Myopathy (<10%)

Gastrointestinal/Hepatic
Abdominal pain [3]
Nausea [6]
Vomiting [2]

Respiratory
Cough (<10%)
Flu-like syndrome (5%)

Endocrine/Metabolic
Galactorrhea [2]
Hyponatremia [2]
SIADH [5]
Weight gain [2]

Genitourinary
Ejaculatory dysfunction (9–14%)
Sexual dysfunction [4]

Otic
Tinnitus (<10%)

Ocular
Glaucoma [3]

Other
Adverse effects [2]
Allergic reactions (<10%)
Toothache (<10%)

ESLICARBAZEPINE

Trade names: Aptiom (Sunovion), Zebinix (Eisai)
Indications: Partial-onset seizures
Class: Antiepileptic
Half-life: 13–20 hours
Clinically important, potentially hazardous interactions with: carbamazepine, digoxin, lamotrigine, levetiracetam, MAO inhibitors, oral contraceptives, oxcarbazepine, phenytoin, topiramate, valproic acid, warfarin
Pregnancy category: C
Important contra-indications noted in the prescribing guidelines for: nursing mothers; pediatric patients

---

Skin
Peripheral edema (<2%)
Rash (<3%)

Cardiovascular
Hypertension (<2%)

Central Nervous System
Balance disorder (3%)
Depression (<3%)
Dysarthria (<2%)
Gait instability (2%)
Headache (13–15%) [10]
Incoordination [3]
Insomnia (2%)
Somnolence (drowsiness) (11–18%) [12]
Tremor (2–4%)
Vertigo (dizziness) (20–28%) [16]

Neuromuscular/Skeletal
Asthenia (fatigue) (4–7%) [5]
Ataxia (4–6%)

Gastrointestinal/Hepatic
Constipation (2%)
Diarrhea (2–4%)
Nausea (10–16%) [8]
Vomiting (6–10%) [4]

Respiratory
Cough (<2%)
Nasopharyngitis [2]

Endocrine/Metabolic
Hyponatremia (2%)

Genitourinary
Urinary tract infection (2%)

Ocular
Diplopia (9–11%) [7]
Nystagmus (<2%)
Vision blurred (5–6%) [3]
Vision impaired (<2%)

ESMOLOL

Trade name: Brevibloc (Baxter)
Indications: Tachyarrhythmias, tachycardia
Class: Adrenergic beta-receptor antagonist, Antiarrhythmic class II
Half-life: 9 minutes
Clinically important, potentially hazardous interactions with: clonidine, verapamil
Pregnancy category: C
Important contra-indications noted in the prescribing guidelines for: nursing mothers; pediatric patients

Skin
Diaphoresis (>10%)

Cardiovascular
Bradycardia [5]
Hypotension [12]

Local
Injection-site pain (8%)
Injection-site reactions (<10%)

Other
Death [2]

ESOMEPRAZOLE

Trade name: Nexium (AstraZeneca)
Indications: Gastroesophageal reflux disease
Class: Proton pump inhibitor (PPI)
Half-life: 1.5 hours
Clinically important, potentially hazardous interactions with: benzodiazepines, chlordiazepoxide, cilostazol, clonazepam, clopidogrel, clorazepate, diazepam, digoxin, flurazepam, lorazepam, midazolam, oxazepam, posaconazole, quazepam, rifampin, rilpivirine, St John's wort, temazepam, tipranavir, voriconazole
Pregnancy category: C
Important contra-indications noted in the prescribing guidelines for: nursing mothers; pediatric patients

Skin
DRESS syndrome [2]
Fixed eruption [2]
Lupus erythematosus [2]

Central Nervous System
Dysgeusia (taste perversion) [3]
Fever [2]
Headache (8–11%) [5]
Vertigo (dizziness) [3]

Neuromuscular/Skeletal
Rhabdomyolysis [2]

Gastrointestinal/Hepatic
Abdominal pain [3]
Constipation [2]
Diarrhea [6]
Nausea [4]
Vomiting [3]

Respiratory
Bronchitis (4%)

Endocrine/Metabolic
Hypomagnesemia [2]

Other
Adverse effects [5]

ESTRADIOL

Trade names: Alora (Watson), Climara (Bayer), Divigel (Upsher-Smith), Elestrin (Azur Pharma), Esclim (Women First), Estrace (Bristol-Myers Squibb) (Warner Chilcott), Estraderm (Novartis), Estring (Pharmacia & Upjohn), Estrogel (Ascend), Evamist (KV Pharm), Fempatch (Pfizer), Gynodiol (Barr), Innofem (Novo Nordisk), Menostar (Bayer), Vagifem (Novo Nordisk), Vivelle (Novartis), Vivelle-Dot (Novartis)
Indications: Menopausal symptoms, hypoestrogenism due to hypogonadism, castration or primary ovarian failure, postmenopausal osteoporosis
Class: Estrogen, Hormone
Half-life: 1.75±2.87 hours
Clinically important, potentially hazardous interactions with: alcohol, amprenavir, anastrozole, ascorbic acid, atorvastatin, boceprevir, carbamazepine, chenodiol, clarithromycin, colesevelam, conivaptan, corticosteroids, CYP1A2 inducers, CYP3A4 inducers, deferasirox, delavirdine, erythromycin, folic acid, grapefruit juice, itraconazole, ketoconazole, lopinavir, minocycline, oxtriphylline, P-glycoprotein inhibitors or inducers, PEG-interferon, phenobarbital, rifampin, ritonavir, ropinirole, saxagliptin, somatropin, St John's wort, telaprevir, thyroid products, tipranavir, ursodiol
Pregnancy category: X
Important contra-indications noted in the prescribing guidelines for: the elderly; nursing mothers; pediatric patients
Black Box Warning: ENDOMETRIAL CANCER, CARDIOVASCULAR DISORDERS, BREAST CANCER and PROBABLE DEMENTIA

Central Nervous System
Headache [2]

Gastrointestinal/Hepatic
Nausea [3]

Respiratory
Nasopharyngitis (10%)
Upper respiratory tract infection (6%)

Endocrine/Metabolic
Mastodynia (7%)

Genitourinary
Metrorrhagia (4%)

Other
Adverse effects [3]

ESTRAMUSTINE

Trade name: Emcyt (Pfizer)
Indications: Prostate carcinoma
Class: Alkylating agent, Nitrosourea
Half-life: 20 hours
Clinically important, potentially hazardous interactions with: aldesleukin
Pregnancy category: X (not indicated for use in women)

Skin
Angioedema [2]
Edema (>10%) [4]
Peripheral edema [2]
Pruritus (2%) [2]
Purpura (3%)
Xerosis (2%)

Cardiovascular
Thrombophlebitis (3%)

Neuromuscular/Skeletal
Asthenia (fatigue) [3]

Gastrointestinal/Hepatic
Diarrhea [3]
Nausea [3]

Endocrine/Metabolic
Gynecomastia (>10%) [5]
Mastodynia (66%)

Hematologic
Anemia [3]
Febrile neutropenia [2]
Leukopenia [2]
Neutropenia [5]

Local
Injection-site thrombophlebitis (<10%) [3]

Other
Allergic reactions [2]
Death [2]

ESZOPICLONE

Trade names: Imovane (Sanofi-Aventis), Lunesta (Sunovion), Zimovane (Sanofi-Aventis)
Indications: Insomnia
Class: Hypnotic, non-benzodiazepine
Half-life: 6 hours
Clinically important, potentially hazardous interactions with: alcohol, antifungals, cimetidine, CNS depressants, conivaptan, CYP3A4 inhibitors and inducers, dasatinib, deferasirox, droperidol, erythromycin, ethanol, flumazenil, ketoconazole, levomepromazine, lorazepam, nefazodone, nelfinavir, olanzapine, rifampin, ritonavir, St John's wort, telithromycin, tricyclic antidepressants, valerian, voriconazole
Pregnancy category: C
Important contra-indications noted in the prescribing guidelines for: the elderly; nursing mothers; pediatric patients

Skin
Pruritus (<4%)
Rash (<5%)

Mucosal
Xerostomia (3–7%) [5]

Central Nervous System
Abnormal dreams (<3%)
Amnesia [3]
Anxiety (<3%)
Confusion (<3%)
Depression (<4%)
Dysgeusia (taste perversion) (8–34%) [21]
Hallucinations (<3%)
Headache (13–21%) [8]
Nervousness (<5%)
Neurotoxicity (<3%)
Pain (4–5%)
Somnolence (drowsiness) (8–10%) [2]
Vertigo (dizziness) [3]

Gastrointestinal/Hepatic
Diarrhea (2–4%)
Dyspepsia (2–6%)
Nausea (4–5%) [2]
Vomiting (<3%)

Endocrine/Metabolic
Gynecomastia (<3%)
Libido decreased (<3%)

Genitourinary
Dysmenorrhea (<3%)
Urinary tract infection (<3%)

Other
Adverse effects [4]
Infection (3–10%)

ETANERCEPT

Trade names: Enbrel (Amgen), Erelzi (Sandoz)
Indications: Rheumatoid arthritis, polyarticular juvenile idiopathic arthritis in patients aged 2 years or older, psoriatic arthritis, ankylosing spondylitis, plaque psoriasis
Class: Cytokine inhibitor, Disease-modifying antirheumatic drug (DMARD), TNF inhibitor
Half-life: 4–13 days
Clinically important, potentially hazardous interactions with: abatacept, anakinra, cyclophosphamide, live vaccines
Pregnancy category: B
Important contra-indications noted in the prescribing guidelines for: the elderly; nursing mothers; pediatric patients
Note: TNF inhibitors should be used in patients with heart failure only after consideration of other treatment options. Contraindicated in patients with sepsis. TNF inhibitors are contraindicated in patients with a personal or family history of multiple sclerosis or demyelinating disease. TNF inhibitors should not be administered to patients with moderate to severe heart failure (New York Heart Association Functional Class III/IV).
Black Box Warning: SERIOUS INFECTIONS AND MALIGNANCIES

Skin
Abscess [2]
Anaphylactoid reactions/Anaphylaxis [2]
Carcinoma [2]
Cellulitis [2]
Dermatitis [3]
Dermatomyositis [4]
Exanthems [2]
Granulomas [2]
Granulomatous reaction [5]
Henoch-Schönlein purpura [3]
Herpes zoster [5]
Hidradenitis [2]
Leprosy [2]
Lichen planus [2]
Lichenoid eruption [3]
Lupus erythematosus [25]
Lupus syndrome [2]
Lymphoma [3]
Malignancies (<3%) [3]
Melanoma [2]
Neoplasms [2]
Nodular eruption [3]
Pruritus (2–5%) [2]
Psoriasis [19]
Pustules [2]
Rash (3–13%) [7]
Sarcoidosis [8]
Squamous cell carcinoma [4]
Urticaria (2%) [2]
Vasculitis [21]

Hair
Alopecia [4]

Cardiovascular
Atrial fibrillation [2]
Cardiotoxicity [2]
Hypertension [2]

Central Nervous System
Fever (2–3%)
Headache [15]
Leukoencephalopathy [3]
Multiple sclerosis [2]
Neurotoxicity [3]
Paresthesias [2]
Vertigo (dizziness) [2]

Neuromuscular/Skeletal
Asthenia (fatigue) [6]
Back pain [2]
Myalgia/Myopathy [2]
Myasthenia gravis [3]

Gastrointestinal/Hepatic
Abdominal pain [3]
Crohn's disease [4]
Diarrhea (8–16%) [4]
Gastroenteritis [3]
Hepatotoxicity [4]
Nausea [5]

Respiratory
Asthma [2]
Bronchitis [4]
Cough [3]
Flu-like syndrome [3]
Laryngitis [2]
Nasopharyngitis [2]
Pharyngitis [4]
Pneumonia [5]
Pneumonitis [2]
Pulmonary toxicity [3]
Rhinitis [4]
Sinusitis [5]
Tuberculosis [2]
Upper respiratory tract infection (38–65%) [9]

Endocrine/Metabolic
ALT increased [3]
Hypertriglyceridemia [2]
Thyroiditis [2]

Genitourinary
Cystitis [2]
Urinary tract infection [2]

Renal
Nephrotoxicity [2]

Hematologic
Leukopenia [2]
Macrophage activation syndrome [2]
Neutropenia [2]
Pancytopenia [2]
Thrombocytopenia [2]

Otic
Otitis media [2]

Ocular
Uveitis [12]

Local
Injection-site reactions (37–43%) [56]

Other
Adverse effects [34]
Allergic reactions (<3%)
Death [6]
Infection (50–81%) [43]

ETHAMBUTOL

Trade name: Myambutol (Stat Trade)
Indications: Tuberculosis
Class: Antimycobacterial
Half-life: 3–4 hours
Clinically important, potentially hazardous interactions with: cortisone, zinc
Pregnancy category: C
Important contra-indications noted in the prescribing guidelines for: nursing mothers; pediatric patients

---

Skin
Bullous dermatitis [2]
Dermatitis [2]
DRESS syndrome [4]
Erythema multiforme [2]
Exanthems (<5%) [4]
Hypersensitivity [3]
Lichenoid eruption [2]
Lupus erythematosus [2]
Pruritus [3]
Rash [2]
Toxic epidermal necrolysis [2]
Urticaria [2]

Renal
Nephrotoxicity [2]

Ocular
Amblyopia [2]
Ocular toxicity [9]
Optic neuritis [4]
Optic neuropathy [8]
Vision impaired [2]

Other
Adverse effects [3]

ETHOSUXIMIDE

Trade name: Zarontin (Pfizer)
Indications: Absence (petit mal) seizures
Class: Antiepileptic, succinimide
Half-life: 50–60 hours
Clinically important, potentially hazardous interactions with: antipsychotics, carbamazepine, chloroquine, cobicistat/elvitegravir/emtricitabine/tenofovir disoproxil, hydroxychloroquine, isoniazid, levomepromazine, lisdexamfetamine, MAO inhibitors, mefloquine, nevirapine, orlistat, phenobarbital, phenytoin, primidone, risperidone, SSRIs, St John's wort, tricyclic antidepressants, valproic acid, zuclopenthixol
Pregnancy category: C
Important contra-indications noted in the prescribing guidelines for: nursing mothers
Note: Cases of birth defects have been reported with ethosuximide.

Skin
Exanthems (<5%) [2]
Lupus erythematosus (>10%) [22]
Raynaud's phenomenon [3]
Stevens–Johnson syndrome (>10%)
Urticaria (<5%)

Hematologic
Agranulocytosis [2]

Other
Side effects (3%)

ETIDRONATE

Trade name: Didronel (Procter & Gamble)
Indications: Paget's disease, osteoporosis
Class: Bisphosphonate
Half-life: 6 hours
Clinically important, potentially hazardous interactions with: ferrous sulfate
Pregnancy category: C
Important contra-indications noted in the prescribing guidelines for: nursing mothers; pediatric patients

Neuromuscular/Skeletal
Fractures [6]
Osteomalacia [3]
Pseudogout [2]
Skeletal toxicity [2]

Gastrointestinal/Hepatic
Esophagitis [2]

ETODOLAC

Trade name: Lodine (Wyeth)
Indications: Pain
Class: COX-2 inhibitor, Non-steroidal anti-inflammatory (NSAID)
Half-life: 7 hours
Clinically important, potentially hazardous interactions with: aspirin, methotrexate
Pregnancy category: C
Important contra-indications noted in the prescribing guidelines for: the elderly; nursing mothers; pediatric patients
Note: NSAIDs may cause an increased risk of serious cardiovascular and gastrointestinal adverse events, which can be fatal. This risk may increase with duration of use.

Skin
Exanthems [2]
Facial edema [2]
Fixed eruption [2]
Pruritus (<10%) [7]
Rash (>10%) [5]
Vasculitis [2]

Gastrointestinal/Hepatic
Abdominal pain [2]
Constipation [2]
Dyspepsia [3]
Nausea [2]

Other
Adverse effects [2]

ETOPOSIDE

Trade name: VePesid (Bristol-Myers Squibb)
Indications: Lymphomas, carcinomas
Class: Topoisomerase 2 inhibitor
Half-life: 4–11 hours
Clinically important, potentially hazardous interactions with: aldesleukin, atovaquone, atovaquone/proguanil, cyclosporine, gadobenate, prednisolone, St John's wort
Pregnancy category: D
Important contra-indications noted in the prescribing guidelines for: the elderly; nursing mothers; pediatric patients

Skin
Anaphylactoid reactions/Anaphylaxis (<2%) [3]
Erythema [3]
Exanthems [4]
Hand–foot syndrome [3]
Hypersensitivity [8]
Pigmentation [2]
Radiation recall dermatitis [3]
Rash [2]
Stevens–Johnson syndrome [3]

Hair
Alopecia (8–66%) [8]

Mucosal
Mucositis (>10%)
Oral lesions (<5%) [2]
Stomatitis (<10%) [2]

Cardiovascular
Flushing [3]

Central Nervous System
Anorexia [2]
Leukoencephalopathy [2]
Neurotoxicity [3]

Neuromuscular/Skeletal
Asthenia (fatigue) [2]

Gastrointestinal/Hepatic
Diarrhea [2]
Hepatotoxicity [2]
Nausea [5]
Vomiting [7]

Respiratory
Pulmonary toxicity [2]

Endocrine/Metabolic
Hyponatremia [2]

Renal
Nephrotoxicity [3]

Hematologic
Anemia [5]
Febrile neutropenia [5]
Leukopenia [3]
Neutropenia [11]
Thrombocytopenia [9]

Other
Adverse effects [3]
Allergic reactions (<2%)
Death [2]
Infection [4]

ETRAVIRINE

Trade name: Intelence (Tibotec)
Indications: HIV infection
Class: Non-nucleoside reverse transcriptase inhibitor
Half-life: 41 hours
Clinically important, potentially hazardous interactions with: atazanavir, atorvastatin, carbamazepine, clarithromycin, clopidogrel, darunavir, delavirdine, digoxin, efavirenz, fosamprenavir, indinavir, maraviroc, nelfinavir, nevirapine, non-nucleoside reverse transcriptase inhibitors, phenobarbital, phenytoin, rifabutin, rifampin, rifapentine, rilpivirine, ritonavir, sildenafil, simeprevir, St John's wort, tadalafil, telithromycin, tipranavir, vardenafil, voriconazole
Pregnancy category: B
Important contra-indications noted in the prescribing guidelines for: nursing mothers; pediatric patients

Skin
Facial edema (<2%)
Hyperhidrosis (<2%)
Lipohypertrophy (<2%)
Prurigo (<2%)
Rash (9%) [17]
Xerosis (<2%)

Mucosal
Stomatitis (<2%)
Xerostomia (<2%)

Cardiovascular
Angina (<2%)
Atrial fibrillation (<2%)
Hypertension (3%)
Myocardial infarction (<2%)

Central Nervous System
Abnormal dreams (<2%)
Amnesia (<2%)
Anorexia (<2%)
Anxiety (<2%)
Confusion (<2%)
Disorientation (<2%)
Headache (3%) [3]

Hypersomnia (<2%)
Hypoesthesia (<2%)
Insomnia (<2%)
Nervousness (<2%)
Neurotoxicity [3]
Nightmares (<2%)
Paresthesias (<2%)
Peripheral neuropathy (3%)
Seizures (<2%)
Sleep related disorder (<2%)
Somnolence (drowsiness) (<2%)
Syncope (<2%)
Tremor (<2%)
Vertigo (dizziness) (<2%)

Neuromuscular/Skeletal
Asthenia (fatigue) (3%)

Gastrointestinal/Hepatic
Abdominal distension (<2%)
Abdominal pain (3%)
Constipation (<2%)
Diarrhea [3]
Flatulence (<2%)
Gastritis (<2%)
Gastroesophageal reflux (<2%)
Hematemesis (<2%)
Hepatic failure (<2%)
Hepatomegaly (<2%)
Hepatotoxicity [2]
Nausea [4]
Pancreatitis (<2%)
Retching (<2%)

Respiratory
Bronchospasm (<2%)
Dyspnea (<2%)

Endocrine/Metabolic
Diabetes mellitus (<2%)
Gynecomastia (<2%)

Renal
Renal failure (<2%)

Hematologic
Dyslipidemia (<2%)
Hemolytic anemia (<2%)

Ocular
Vision blurred (<2%)

Other
Adverse effects [6]

EVEROLIMUS

Trade names: Afinitor (Novartis), Certican (Novartis), Zortress (Novartis)
Indications: Prophylaxis of organ rejection in adults following kidney or liver transplant, advanced renal cell carcinoma, neuroendocrine tumors of pancreatic, gastrointestinal or lung origin, breast cancer in post-menopausal women with advanced hormone-receptor positive, HER2-negative type cancer, renal angiomyolipoma and tuberous sclerosis complex, subependymal giant cell astrocytoma associated with tuberous sclerosis
Class: Antineoplastic, Immunosuppressant, mTOR inhibitor
Half-life: ~30 hours
Clinically important, potentially hazardous interactions with: aprepitant, atazanavir, atorvastatin, benazepril, captopril, clarithromycin, clozapine, conivaptan, cyclosporine, darunavir, delavirdine, digoxin, efavirenz, enalapril, erythromycin, grapefruit juice, indinavir, itraconazole, ketoconazole, lapatinib, lisinopril, live vaccines, nelfinavir, oxcarbazepine, phenytoin, posaconazole, quinapril, ramipril, rifampin, rifapentine, ritonavir, saquinavir, St John's wort, telithromycin, verapamil, voriconazole
Pregnancy category: D
Important contra-indications noted in the prescribing guidelines for: nursing mothers; pediatric patients
Black Box Warning: In immunosuppression therapy: MALIGNANCIES AND SERIOUS INFECTIONS, KIDNEY GRAFT THROMBOSIS; NEPHROTOXICITY; AND MORTALITY IN HEART TRANSPLANTATION

Skin
Acneform eruption (3–25%) [3]
Angioedema [3]
Cellulitis (21%)
Contact dermatitis (14%)
Edema (39%) [4]
Erythema (4%)
Excoriations (14%)
Hand–foot syndrome (5%) [9]
Lymphedema [2]
Peripheral edema (4–39%) [6]
Pityriasis rosea (4%)
Pruritus (14–21%) [5]
Rash (18–59%) [39]
Tinea (18%)
Toxicity [9]
Xerosis (13–18%)

Nails
Nail disorder (4–22%) [2]

Mucosal
Aphthous stomatitis [3]
Epistaxis (nosebleed) (18–22%) [3]
Mucosal inflammation (19%) [3]
Mucositis [14]
Nasal congestion (14%)
Oral ulceration [3]
Oropharyngeal pain (11%)
Rhinorrhea (3%)
Stomatitis (44–86%) [58]
Xerostomia (8–11%)

Cardiovascular
Chest pain (5%)
Hypertension (4–13%) [11]
Tachycardia (3%)

Central Nervous System
Anorexia (25%) [10]
Anxiety (7%)
Chills (4%)
Dysgeusia (taste perversion) (10–19%) [2]
Fever (20–32%) [5]
Headache (18–30%) [4]
Insomnia (9%)
Migraine (30%)
Seizures (29%)
Somnolence (drowsiness) (7%)
Vertigo (dizziness) (7–14%)

Neuromuscular/Skeletal
Arthralgia (15%)
Asthenia (fatigue) (7–45%) [50]
Back pain (15%)
Jaw pain (3%)
Muscle spasm (10%)
Pain in extremities (10–14%)

Gastrointestinal/Hepatic
Abdominal pain (9–36%) [3]
Constipation (11–14%)
Diarrhea (25–50%) [27]
Dysphagia (4%)
Gastritis (7%)
Gastroenteritis (18%)
Hemorrhoids (5%)
Hepatotoxicity [5]
Nausea (26–32%) [8]
Vomiting (20–29%) [3]

Respiratory
Cough (21–30%) [4]
Dyspnea (20–24%) [5]
Nasopharyngitis (25%)
Pharyngitis (11%)
Pharyngolaryngeal pain (4%)
Pleural effusion (7%)
Pneumonia [7]
Pneumonitis (14–17%) [35]
Pulmonary toxicity [8]
Rhinitis (25%)
Sinusitis (39%)
Upper respiratory tract infection (25–82%) [2]

Endocrine/Metabolic
ALT increased (21–48%) [3]
Appetite decreased (30%) [3]
AST increased (25–56%) [2]
Diabetes mellitus (2–10%) [2]
Hypercholesterolemia [5]
Hyperglycemia [27]
Hyperlipidemia [6]
Hypertriglyceridemia [2]
Hypokalemia [3]
Hypomagnesemia [2]
Hyponatremia [3]
Hypophosphatemia [4]
Hypothyroidism [2]
Serum creatinine increased (19–50%) [3]
Weight loss (9–28%) [2]

Genitourinary
Urinary tract infection (15%)

Renal
Nephrotoxicity [2]
Proteinuria (7%) [12]
Renal failure (3%) [2]

Hematologic
Anemia [30]
Febrile neutropenia [3]
Hemoglobin decreased (86–92%)
Hemolytic uremic syndrome [2]
Hemorrhage (3%) [2]
Hemotoxicity [5]
Immunosupression [2]
Leukopenia [3]
Lymphopenia [6]
Neutropenia [12]
Platelets decreased (23–45%)
Thrombocytopenia [18]

Otic
Otitis media (36%)

Ocular
Conjunctivitis (2%)
Eyelid edema (4%)
Ocular hyperemia (4%)

Other
Adverse effects [28]
Death [8]
Infection (18%) [26]
Side effects [2]

EVOLOCUMAB

Trade name: Repatha (Amgen)
Indications: Heterozygous or homozygous familial hypercholesterolemia where additional lowering of low density lipoprotein cholesterol is required
Class: Monoclonal antibody, Proprotein convertase subtilisin kexin type 9 (PCSK9) inhibitor
Half-life: 11–17 days
Clinically important, potentially hazardous interactions with: none known
Pregnancy category: N/A (No data available but likely to cross the placenta in second and third trimester)
Important contra-indications noted in the prescribing guidelines for: pediatric patients

---

Mucosal
Nasal congestion [2]
Oropharyngeal pain [2]

Cardiovascular
Hypertension (2%)

Central Nervous System
Headache (4%) [9]
Neurotoxicity [2]
Vertigo (dizziness) (3%)

Neuromuscular/Skeletal
Arthralgia (2%) [8]
Asthenia (fatigue) [3]
Back pain (2–6%) [10]
Bone or joint pain (3%) [3]
Muscle spasm [6]
Myalgia/Myopathy (3%) [9]
Pain in extremities [5]

Gastrointestinal/Hepatic
Diarrhea (3%) [5]
Gastroenteritis (2%) [2]
Hepatotoxicity [5]
Nausea [4]

Respiratory
Cough (<4%) [3]
Influenza (<6%) [9]
Nasopharyngitis (4–10%) [13]
Pharyngitis [2]
Sinusitis (3%) [2]
Upper respiratory tract infection (2–6%) [9]

Endocrine/Metabolic
Creatine phosphokinase increased [9]

Genitourinary
Urinary tract infection (<4%)

Local
Injection-site bruising [4]
Injection-site edema [2]
Injection-site erythema [3]
Injection-site pain [7]
Injection-site reactions (3–5%) [6]

Other
Adverse effects [6]
Allergic reactions (5%)

EXEMESTANE

Trade name: Aromasin (Pfizer)
Indications: Advanced breast cancer
Class: Aromatase inhibitor
Half-life: 24 hours
Clinically important, potentially hazardous interactions with: efavirenz, oxcarbazepine, rifapentine
Pregnancy category: X
Important contra-indications noted in the prescribing guidelines for: nursing mothers; pediatric patients

---

Skin
Diaphoresis (6–12%) [2]
Edema (7%)
Hot flashes (30%) [7]
Lymphedema (2–5%)
Peripheral edema (9%) [2]
Pruritus (2–5%)
Radiation recall dermatitis [2]
Rash (2–5%) [5]

Hair
Alopecia (2–5%)

Mucosal
Stomatitis [5]

Central Nervous System
Dysgeusia (taste perversion) [2]
Headache [3]
Insomnia [2]
Paresthesias (2–5%)
Tumor pain (30%)

Neuromuscular/Skeletal
Arthralgia [4]
Asthenia (fatigue) [5]
Back pain [2]
Bone or joint pain [2]
Myalgia/Myopathy [2]

Gastrointestinal/Hepatic
Diarrhea [4]

Respiratory
Pneumonitis [3]

Endocrine/Metabolic
Hyperglycemia [3]

Other
Adverse effects [2]

EXENATIDE

Trade names: Bydureon (Amylin), Byetta (Amylin)
Indications: Type II diabetes mellitus
Class: Glucagon-like peptide-1 (GLP-1) receptor agonist, Incretin mimetic, Insulin secretagogue
Half-life: 2.4 hours
Clinically important, potentially hazardous interactions with: acetaminophen, alcohol, antibiotics, corticosteroids, lovastatin, oral contraceptives, pegvisomant, prandial insulin, somatropin, sulfonylureas, thiazide diuretics, vitamin K antagonists, warfarin
Pregnancy category: C
Important contra-indications noted in the prescribing guidelines for: nursing mothers; pediatric patients
Note: Risk of thyroid C-cell tumors with exenatide extended release formulations. Bydureon is contraindicated in patients with a personal or family history of medullary thyroid carcinoma or in patients with multiple endocrine neoplasia syndrome Type 2.

Skin
Hyperhidrosis (<10%)
Urticaria [2]

Cardiovascular
Cardiotoxicity [2]

Central Nervous System
Chills (<2%)
Headache (<10%) [8]
Vertigo (dizziness) (<10%) [3]

Neuromuscular/Skeletal
Asthenia (fatigue) (<10%)

Gastrointestinal/Hepatic
Abdominal distension (<10%)
Abdominal pain (<10%) [2]
Constipation (>5%)
Diarrhea (<11%) [18]
Dyspepsia (<10%)
Flatulence (2%)
Gastroenteritis (<10%)
Gastroesophageal reflux (3%)
Nausea (<11%) [39]
Pancreatitis [10]
Vomiting (~10%) [24]

Respiratory
Nasopharyngitis [2]

Endocrine/Metabolic
Appetite decreased (<10%) [3]
Hypoglycemia (>5%) [4]

Genitourinary
Urinary tract infection [2]

Renal
Nephrotoxicity [2]
Renal failure [3]

Local
Injection-site erythema (5–7%)
Injection-site nodules (~10%) [4]
Injection-site pruritus (5–6%)
Injection-site reactions [6]

Other
Adverse effects [9]
Cancer [2]

EZETIMIBE

Trade names: Ezetrol (Merck), Liptruzet (Merck Sharpe & Dohme), Vytorin (MSD), Zetia (Merck)
Indications: Hypercholesterolemia
Class: Cholesterol inhibitor
Half-life: 22 hours
Clinically important, potentially hazardous interactions with: cholestyramine, cyclosporine, fenofibrate, gemfibrozil, HMG-CoA reductase inhibitors, ritonavir

Pregnancy category: C (Pregnancy category is X when combined with a statin.)
Important contra-indications noted in the prescribing guidelines for: nursing mothers
Note: Liptruzet is ezetimibe and atorvastatin; vytorin is ezetimibe and simvastatin.

Skin
Rash [3]

Central Nervous System
Headache [5]
Vertigo (dizziness) [4]

Neuromuscular/Skeletal
Arthralgia (4%) [3]
Asthenia (fatigue) [2]
Back pain (4%) [4]
Bone or joint pain [3]
Muscle spasm [3]
Myalgia/Myopathy (5%) [15]
Pain in extremities [2]

Gastrointestinal/Hepatic
Abdominal pain (2%)
Diarrhea [4]
Hepatotoxicity [5]
Nausea [4]
Pancreatitis [3]

Respiratory
Cough (2%)
Influenza [3]
Nasopharyngitis [5]
Upper respiratory tract infection [2]

Endocrine/Metabolic
Creatine phosphokinase increased [7]

Genitourinary
Urinary tract infection [2]

Hematologic
Thrombocytopenia [2]

Local
Injection-site erythema [2]
Injection-site reactions [4]

Other
Adverse effects [4]

EZOGABINE

Synonym: retigabine
Trade names: Potiga (GSK), Trobalt (GSK)
Indications: Epilepsy
Class: Anticonvulsant, Potassium channel opener
Half-life: 7–11 hours
Clinically important, potentially hazardous interactions with: alcohol, carbamazepine, digoxin, phenytoin
Pregnancy category: C
Important contra-indications noted in the prescribing guidelines for: the elderly; nursing mothers; pediatric patients
Black Box Warning: RETINAL ABNORMALITIES AND POTENTIAL VISION LOSS

Skin
Hyperhidrosis (<2%)
Peripheral edema (<2%)
Pigmentation [2]

Mucosal
Mucosal membrane pigmentation [4]
Xerostomia (<2%)

Central Nervous System
Amnesia (2%)
Anxiety (3%)
Aphasia (4%)
Balance disorder (4%)
Confusion (9%) [6]
Disorientation (2%)
Dysarthria (4%) [3]
Dysphasia (2%)
Gait instability (4%)
Hallucinations (<2%)
Headache [6]
Hypokinesia (<2%)
Impaired concentration (6%)
Incoordination (7%)
Memory loss (6%)
Neurotoxicity [3]
Paresthesias (3%)
Somnolence (drowsiness) (22%) [14]
Speech disorder [3]
Tremor (8%) [3]
Vertigo (dizziness) (31%) [14]

Neuromuscular/Skeletal
Asthenia (fatigue) (20%) [11]
Ataxia [3]
Myoclonus (<2%)

Gastrointestinal/Hepatic
Constipation (3%)
Dyspepsia (2%)
Dysphagia (<2%)
Nausea (7%) [5]

Respiratory
Influenza (3%)

Endocrine/Metabolic
Appetite increased (<2%)
Weight gain (dose related) (3%)

Genitourinary
Dysuria (2%)
Hematuria (2%)
Urinary hesitancy (2%)
Urinary retention (<2%) [6]
Urinary tract infection [3]

Renal
Chromaturia (2%)

Ocular
Diplopia (7%) [2]
Ocular pigmentation [4]
Vision blurred (5%) [2]

Other
Adverse effects [2]

FAMCICLOVIR

Trade name: Famvir (Novartis)
Indications: Acute herpes zoster, recurrent genital herpes
Class: Antiviral, Guanine nucleoside analog
Half-life: 2–3 hours
Clinically important, potentially hazardous interactions with: none known
Pregnancy category: B
Important contra-indications noted in the prescribing guidelines for: nursing mothers; pediatric patients

---

Skin
Pruritus (4%)
Rash (<4%)
Vasculitis [3]

Central Nervous System
Headache (9–39%) [5]
Paresthesias (<3%)

Neuromuscular/Skeletal
Asthenia (fatigue) (<5%)

Gastrointestinal/Hepatic
Abdominal pain (<8%) [2]
Diarrhea (2–9%)
Flatulence (<5%)
Nausea (2–13%) [3]
Vomiting (<5%) [2]

Genitourinary
Dysmenorrhea (<8%)

Other
Adverse effects [4]

FAMOTIDINE

Trade names: Duexis (Horizon), Pepcid (Valeant)
Indications: Duodenal ulcer, gastric ulcer, gastroesophageal reflux disease
Class: Histamine H2 receptor antagonist
Half-life: 2.5–3.5 hours
Clinically important, potentially hazardous interactions with: atazanavir, cefditoren, dasatinib, delavirdine, rilpivirine, thalidomide
Pregnancy category: B
Important contra-indications noted in the prescribing guidelines for: nursing mothers
Note: Duexis is famotidine and ibuprofen.

Skin
Dermatitis [3]
Peripheral edema [2]
Pruritus [2]
Rash [3]
Urticaria [3]
Vasculitis [2]

Cardiovascular
Hypertension [3]

Central Nervous System
Delirium [2]
Fever [2]
Headache (5%) [4]
Neurotoxicity [2]
Somnolence (drowsiness) [2]

Neuromuscular/Skeletal
Arthralgia [2]
Back pain [2]

Gastrointestinal/Hepatic
Abdominal pain [2]
Diarrhea (2%) [3]
Dyspepsia [3]
Gastroesophageal reflux [2]
Nausea [4]
Vomiting [4]

Respiratory
Influenza [2]
Sinusitis [2]
Upper respiratory tract infection [2]

Endocrine/Metabolic
Hypomagnesemia [2]
Hypophosphatemia [2]

Genitourinary
Urinary tract infection [2]

Hematologic
Eosinophilia [2]
Thrombocytopenia [2]

FEBUXOSTAT

Trade name: Uloric (Takeda)
Indications: Hyperuricemia in gout
Class: Xanthine oxidase inhibitor
Half-life: 5–8 hours
Clinically important, potentially hazardous interactions with: aminophylline, azathioprine, didanosine, mercaptopurine, oxtriphylline, theophylline
Pregnancy category: C

Skin
Rash (2%) [6]

Cardiovascular
Cardiotoxicity [2]

Central Nervous System
Headache [5]
Vertigo (dizziness) [5]

Neuromuscular/Skeletal
Arthralgia [5]
Bone or joint pain [2]
Gouty tophi (flare) [3]
Joint disorder [2]

Gastrointestinal/Hepatic
Diarrhea [8]
Hepatotoxicity (5%) [11]
Nausea [7]
Vomiting [2]

Respiratory
Upper respiratory tract infection [2]

Other
Adverse effects [7]

FENOFIBRATE

Trade name: Tricor (AbbVie)
Indications: Hyperlipidemia
Class: Fibrate, Lipid regulator
Half-life: 20 hours
Clinically important, potentially hazardous interactions with: atorvastatin, colchicine, dicumarol, ezetimibe, lovastatin, nicotinic acid, rosuvastatin, statins, warfarin
Pregnancy category: C
Important contra-indications noted in the prescribing guidelines for: the elderly; nursing mothers; pediatric patients

---

Skin
Photosensitivity [11]
Phototoxicity [2]
Pruritus (4%)
Rash (2–8%) [3]

Neuromuscular/Skeletal
Myalgia/Myopathy [11]
Rhabdomyolysis [18]

Gastrointestinal/Hepatic
Hepatotoxicity [15]
Pancreatitis [3]

Endocrine/Metabolic
Gynecomastia [2]

Renal
Nephrotoxicity [3]
Renal failure [2]

Other
Adverse effects (<10%)

FENTANYL

Trade names: Actiq (Cephalon), Duragesic (Janssen)
Indications: Chronic pain
Class: Analgesic, opioid, Anesthetic
Half-life: ~7 hours
Clinically important, potentially hazardous interactions with: amiodarone, amprenavir, aprepitant, atazanavir, cimetidine, conivaptan, crizotinib, darunavir, dasatinib, delavirdine, efavirenz, enzalutamide, indinavir, itraconazole, ketoconazole, lapatinib, lopinavir, mifepristone, nelfinavir, nevirapine, nifedipine, osimertinib, ranitidine, rifapentine, ritonavir, saquinavir, telithromycin, voriconazole
Pregnancy category: C
Important contra-indications noted in the prescribing guidelines for: nursing mothers; pediatric patients
Note: Contraindicated in opioid non-tolerant patients, and for the management of acute or postoperative pain including headache/migraines and dental pain.
Black Box Warning: ADDICTION, ABUSE, and MISUSE; LIFE-THREATENING RESPIRATORY DEPRESSION; ACCIDENTAL EXPOSURE; NEONATAL OPIOID WITHDRAWAL SYNDROME; CYTOCHROME P450 3A4 INTERACTION
EXPOSURE TO HEAT (for topical patches)

Skin
Anaphylactoid reactions/Anaphylaxis [6]
Diaphoresis (>10%) [2]
Edema (>10%)
Erythema (at application site) [3]
Pruritus (3–44%) [30]
Rash [3]

Mucosal
Xerostomia (>10%) [3]

Cardiovascular
Bradycardia (>10%) [3]
Flushing (3–10%)
Hypotension [7]
Tachycardia [2]

Central Nervous System
Agitation [2]
Anorexia [2]
Confusion (>10%)
Delirium [2]
Depression (>10%)
Hallucinations [2]
Headache (>10%)
Neuroleptic malignant syndrome [2]
Serotonin syndrome [4]
Somnolence (drowsiness) [12]
Vertigo (dizziness) [12]

Neuromuscular/Skeletal
Asthenia (fatigue) (>10%) [2]
Myoclonus [3]

Gastrointestinal/Hepatic
Constipation (>10%) [11]
Nausea (>10%) [30]
Vomiting (>10%) [20]

Respiratory
Cough [15]
Respiratory depression [7]

Ocular
Miosis (>10%)

Local
Application-site erythema [2]

Other
Adverse effects [5]
Death [7]

FERUMOXYTOL

Trade name: Feraheme (AMG Pharma)
Indications: Iron deficiency anemia in adults with chronic kidney disease
Class: Iron supplement
Half-life: 15 hours
Clinically important, potentially hazardous interactions with: none known
Pregnancy category: C
Important contra-indications noted in the prescribing guidelines for: the elderly; nursing mothers; pediatric patients
Note: May cause hypersensitivity reactions, hypotension and iron overload. Feraheme may transiently affect magnetic resonance (MRI) imaging for up to 3 months following dosage. Contraindicated in patients with evidence of iron overload or anemia not caused by iron deficiency.

Skin
Anaphylactoid reactions/Anaphylaxis [3]
Hypersensitivity [3]
Pruritus [4]
Rash [2]

Cardiovascular
Hypotension (3%) [3]

Central Nervous System
Headache [5]
Vertigo (dizziness) (3%) [3]

Neuromuscular/Skeletal
Asthenia (fatigue) [2]

Gastrointestinal/Hepatic
Nausea (3%) [5]
Vomiting [2]

Respiratory
Dyspnea [2]

Local
Injection-site pain [3]

Other
Adverse effects [2]

FESOTERODINE

Trade name: Toviaz (Pfizer)
Indications: Overactive bladder syndrome, urinary incontinence, urgency and frequency
Class: Antimuscarinic, Muscarinic antagonist
Half-life: 7 hours; 4 hours (oral)
Clinically important, potentially hazardous interactions with: alcohol, amantadine, anticholinergics, antidepressants, antimuscarinics, atazanavir, botulinum toxin (A & B), carbamazepine, cinacalcet, clarithromycin, conivaptan, CYP2D6 inhibitors, CYP3A4 inhibitors, CYP3AF inhibitors, darunavir, dasatinib, deferasirox, delavirdine, duloxetine, indinavir, itraconazole, ketoconazole, nefazodone, nelfinavir, PEG-interferon, phenobarbital, phenytoin, pramlintide, rifampin, ritonavir, saquinavir, secretin, St John's wort, telithromycin, terbinafine, tipranavir, tocilizumab, voriconazole
Pregnancy category: C
Important contra-indications noted in the prescribing guidelines for: nursing mothers; pediatric patients
Note: Contraindicated in patients with urinary retention, gastric retention, or uncontrolled narrow-angle glaucoma.

Mucosal
Xerostomia (19–35%) [28]

Central Nervous System
Headache [3]

Neuromuscular/Skeletal
Back pain (2%)

Gastrointestinal/Hepatic
Constipation (4–6%) [16]
Diarrhea (<10%)
Dyspepsia (<2%)
Nausea (<2%) [2]

Respiratory
Upper respiratory tract infection (2–3%)

Genitourinary
Dysuria (<2%)
Urinary tract infection (3–4%) [3]

Ocular
Vision blurred [2]
Xerophthalmia (<4%) [2]

Other
Adverse effects [3]

FEXOFENADINE

Trade name: Allegra (Sanofi-Aventis)
Indications: Allergic rhinitis, pruritus, urticaria
Class: Histamine H1 receptor antagonist
Half-life: 14.4 hours
Clinically important, potentially hazardous interactions with: St John's wort
Pregnancy category: C
Important contra-indications noted in the prescribing guidelines for: the elderly; nursing mothers; pediatric patients

---

Skin
Urticaria [3]

Central Nervous System
Headache (5–11%) [2]

FINAFLOXACIN

Trade name: Xtoro (Alcon)
Indications: Acute otitis externa caused by susceptible strains of *Pseudomonas aeruginosa* and *Staphylococcus aureus*
Class: Antibiotic, fluoroquinolone
Half-life: N/A
Clinically important, potentially hazardous interactions with: none known
Pregnancy category: C
Important contra-indications noted in the prescribing guidelines for: nursing mothers; pediatric patients

---

Central Nervous System
Headache [2]

Gastrointestinal/Hepatic
Diarrhea [2]
Flatulence [2]
Loose stools [2]
Nausea [2]

Respiratory
Nasopharyngitis [2]
Rhinitis [2]

FINASTERIDE

Trade names: Propecia (Merck), Proscar (Merck)
Indications: Benign prostatic hypertrophy, male-pattern baldness
Class: 5-alpha reductase inhibitor, Androgen antagonist, Enzyme inhibitor
Half-life: 5–8 hours
Clinically important, potentially hazardous interactions with: none known

Pregnancy category: X
Important contra-indications noted in the prescribing guidelines for: nursing mothers; pediatric patients
Note: Contraindicated for use in women and pediatric patients.

Skin
- Folliculitis [2]
- Rash [3]
- Urticaria [2]
- Xerosis [2]

Hair
- Hirsutism [3]

Cardiovascular
- Postural hypotension [2]

Central Nervous System
- Depression [5]
- Headache [2]
- Vertigo (dizziness) (7%) [3]

Neuromuscular/Skeletal
- Asthenia (fatigue) (5%) [2]
- Myalgia/Myopathy (severe) [2]

Endocrine/Metabolic
- Gynecomastia (<2%) [14]
- Libido decreased (2–10%) [7]
- Mastodynia (<2%)
- Menstrual irregularities [2]

Genitourinary
- Ejaculatory dysfunction [8]
- Erectile dysfunction [7]
- Impotence (5–19%)
- Sexual dysfunction [5]

Other
- Adverse effects [5]

FINGOLIMOD

Trade name: Gilenya (Novartis)
Indications: Multiple sclerosis
Class: Immunosuppressant
Half-life: 6–9 days
Clinically important, potentially hazardous interactions with: BCG vaccine, beta blockers, class Ia antiarrhythmics, class III antiarrhythmics, conivaptan, cyproterone, denosumab, digoxin, diltiazem, dronedarone, ketoconazole, leflunomide, live vaccines, natalizumab, PEG-interferon, pimecrolimus, QT prolonging drugs, roflumilast, sipuleucel-T, tacrolimus, tocilizumab, trastuzumab, typhoid vaccine, verapamil, yellow fever vaccine
Pregnancy category: C
Important contra-indications noted in the prescribing guidelines for: nursing mothers; pediatric patients
Note: Contraindicated in patients with recent (within the last 6 months) occurrence of: myocardial infarction, unstable angina, stroke, transient ischemic attack, decompensated heart failure requiring hospitalization, or Class III/IV heart failure; history or presence of Mobitz Type II 2nd degree or 3rd degree AV block or sick sinus syndrome, unless patient has a pacemaker; baseline QT interval ≥500 ms; or is receiving treatment with Class Ia or Class III anti-arrhythmic drugs.

Skin
- Basal cell carcinoma [3]
- Eczema (3%)
- Herpes (9%) [6]
- Herpes simplex [2]
- Herpes zoster [2]
- Kaposi's sarcoma [2]
- Lymphoma [2]
- Melanoma [2]
- Neoplasms [2]
- Pruritus (3%)
- Skin cancer [3]
- Tinea (4%)
- Varicella zoster [5]

Hair
- Alopecia (4%)

Cardiovascular
- Asystole [2]
- Atrial fibrillation [2]
- Atrioventricular block [17]
- Bradycardia (4%) [20]
- Cardiac failure [2]
- Cardiotoxicity [2]
- Hypertension (6%) [9]

Central Nervous System
- Depression (8%)
- Headache (25%) [7]
- Leukoencephalopathy [3]
- Migraine (5%)
- Paresthesias (5%)
- Vertigo (dizziness) (7%)

Neuromuscular/Skeletal
- Asthenia (fatigue) (3%) [4]
- Back pain (12%) [4]

Gastrointestinal/Hepatic
- Diarrhea (12%) [3]
- Gastroenteritis (5%)
- Hepatotoxicity [7]

Respiratory
- Bronchitis (8%)
- Cough (10%) [3]
- Dyspnea (8%)
- Influenza (13%) [3]
- Nasopharyngitis [3]
- Pulmonary toxicity [2]
- Respiratory tract infection [2]
- Sinusitis (7%)

Endocrine/Metabolic
- ALT increased (14%) [2]
- AST increased (14%)
- GGT increased (5%)
- Weight loss (5%)

Hematologic
- Leukopenia (3%)
- Lymphocytopenia [2]
- Lymphopenia (4%) [6]

Ocular
- Macular edema [18]
- Ocular pain (3%)
- Vision blurred (4%)

Other
- Adverse effects [9]
- Death [7]
- Infection [13]

FLECAINIDE

Trade name: Tambocor (3M)
Indications: Atrial fibrillation
Class: Antiarrhythmic, Antiarrhythmic class Ic
Half-life: 12–16 hours
Clinically important, potentially hazardous interactions with: acebutolol, amiodarone, amisulpride, amitriptyline, artemether/lumefantrine, boceprevir, cinacalcet, clozapine, cobicistat/elvitegravir/emtricitabine/tenofovir alafenamide, cobicistat/elvitegravir/emtricitabine/tenofovir disoproxil, darifenacin, delavirdine, fosamprenavir, lopinavir, mirabegron, quinine, ritonavir, telaprevir, tipranavir
Pregnancy category: C
Important contra-indications noted in the prescribing guidelines for: nursing mothers; pediatric patients

Skin
- Diaphoresis (<3%)
- Edema (4%)
- Psoriasis [2]
- Rash (<3%)

Cardiovascular
- Arrhythmias [7]
- Atrial fibrillation [3]
- Atrial flutter [2]
- Atrioventricular block [2]
- Bradycardia [4]
- Brugada syndrome [4]
- Bundle branch block [2]
- Cardiotoxicity [2]
- Chest pain (5%)
- Congestive heart failure [2]
- Extrasystoles [2]
- Flushing (<3%)
- Hypotension [2]
- Palpitation (6%)
- QT prolongation [7]
- Supraventricular tachycardia [2]
- Torsades de pointes [4]

Central Nervous System
- Headache (10%) [4]
- Hyperesthesia (<10%)
- Neurotoxicity [3]
- Syncope [2]
- Tremor (5%)
- Vertigo (dizziness) (19%) [5]

Neuromuscular/Skeletal
- Asthenia (fatigue) (5–8%)

Gastrointestinal/Hepatic
- Abdominal pain (3%)
- Constipation (4%)
- Diarrhea (<3%) [2]
- Nausea (9%) [3]

Respiratory
- Dyspnea (10%)

Ocular
- Vision blurred [2]
- Visual disturbances (16%) [3]

Other
- Adverse effects [2]

FLIBANSERIN

Trade name: Addyi (Sprout)
Indications: Hypoactive sexual desire disorder in premenopausal women
Class: Serotonin type 1A receptor agonist, Serotonin type 2A receptor antagonist
Half-life: 11 hours
Clinically important, potentially hazardous interactions with: alcohol, amprenavir, atazanavir, boceprevir, carbamazepine, ciprofloxacin, clarithromycin, conivaptan, digoxin, diltiazem, erythromycin, fluconazole, fosamprenavir, grapefruit juice, indinavir, itraconazole, ketoconazole, nefazodone, nelfinavir, phenobarbital, phenytoin, posaconazole, rifabutin, rifampin, rifapentine, ritonavir, saquinavir, St John's wort, telaprevir, telithromycin, verapamil
Pregnancy category: N/A (No data available)
Important contra-indications noted in the prescribing guidelines for: the elderly; nursing mothers; pediatric patients
Black Box Warning: HYPOTENSION AND SYNCOPE IN CERTAIN SETTINGS

Mucosal
Xerostomia (2%)

Central Nervous System
Anxiety (2%)
Insomnia (5%)
Sedation [2]
Somnolence (drowsiness) (11%) [8]
Vertigo (dizziness) (2%) [8]

Neuromuscular/Skeletal
Asthenia (fatigue) (9%) [5]

Gastrointestinal/Hepatic
Abdominal pain (2%)
Constipation (2%)
Nausea (10%) [6]

FLUCONAZOLE

Trade name: Diflucan (Pfizer)
Indications: Candidiasis
Class: Antibiotic, triazole, Antifungal, azole, CYP3A4 inhibitor
Half-life: 25–30 hours
Clinically important, potentially hazardous interactions with: alprazolam, amphotericin B, anisindione, anticoagulants, atorvastatin, avanafil, betamethasone, bosentan, celecoxib, citalopram, clobazam, clopidogrel, dicumarol, eplerenone, erythromycin, flibanserin, irbesartan, ivacaftor, lesinurad, methadone, midazolam, mifepristone, nevirapine, ospemifene, pantoprazole, phenobarbital, phenytoin, pimecrolimus, propranolol, quetiapine, ramelteon, rifapentine, rilpivirine, ruxolitinib, simeprevir, sulfonylureas, temsirolimus, terbinafine, tipranavir, tofacitinib, trabectedin, triamcinolone, venetoclax, vinblastine, vincristine, warfarin, zidovudine
Pregnancy category: D (fluconazole is pregnancy category C for vaginal candidiasis)
Important contra-indications noted in the prescribing guidelines for: the elderly; nursing mothers

---

Skin
AGEP [3]
Erythema multiforme [3]
Exfoliative dermatitis [2]
Fixed eruption [10]
Hypersensitivity (<4%)
Rash (2%) [4]
Stevens–Johnson syndrome [6]
Toxic epidermal necrolysis [4]

Hair
Alopecia [4]

Nails
Nail changes [2]

Mucosal
Oral ulceration [2]

Cardiovascular
Hypotension [2]
QT prolongation [7]
Torsades de pointes [11]

Central Nervous System
Dysgeusia (taste perversion) [2]
Headache (2–13%) [3]
Neurotoxicity [2]

Neuromuscular/Skeletal
Rhabdomyolysis [4]

Gastrointestinal/Hepatic
Abdominal pain [2]
Diarrhea [2]
Hepatotoxicity [2]
Nausea (2–7%)

Renal
Renal failure [2]

Other
Adverse effects [5]

FLUDARABINE

Trade names: Fludara (Genzyme), Oforta (Sanofi-Aventis)
Indications: Chronic lymphocytic leukemia (B-cell)
Class: Antimetabolite, Antineoplastic
Half-life: 9 hours
Clinically important, potentially hazardous interactions with: aldesleukin, clofazimine, live vaccines, pentostatin
Pregnancy category: D
Important contra-indications noted in the prescribing guidelines for: nursing mothers; pediatric patients
Note: Severe neurologic effects, including blindness, coma, and death were observed in dose-ranging studies in patients with acute leukemia when fludarabine phosphate was administered at high doses. Instances of life-threatening and sometimes fatal autoimmune hemolytic anemia have been reported after one or more cycles of treatment with fludarabine phosphate.
Black Box Warning: CNS TOXICITY, HEMOLYTIC ANEMIA, AND PULMONARY TOXICITY

Skin
Anaphylactoid reactions/Anaphylaxis (<3%)
Diaphoresis (14%)
Edema (8–19%)
Herpes simplex (7–8%)
Herpes zoster [2]
Paraneoplastic pemphigus [4]
Peripheral edema (7%)
Pruritus (<3%)
Rash (4–15%)

Hair
Alopecia (<10%)

Mucosal
Mucositis (2%)
Stomatitis (9%)

Cardiovascular
Angina (6%)
Arrhythmias (<4%)
Chest pain (5%)
Congestive heart failure (<4%)
Myocardial infarction (<4%)
Phlebitis (<3%)
Supraventricular tachycardia (<4%)

Central Nervous System
Aneurysm (<2%)
Anorexia (7–34%)
Cerebrovascular accident (<4%)
Chills (11–19%)
Fever (11–69%) [2]
Headache (3–9%)
Leukoencephalopathy [9]
Neurotoxicity [3]
Pain (5–22%)
Paresthesias (4–12%)
Sleep related disorder (<3%)

Neuromuscular/Skeletal
Asthenia (fatigue) (6–65%)
Back pain (4–9%)
Myalgia/Myopathy (>10%)

Gastrointestinal/Hepatic
Abdominal pain (8–10%)
Cholelithiasis (gallstones) (3%)
Constipation (<3%)
Diarrhea (5–15%)
Esophagitis (3%)
Gastrointestinal bleeding (3–13%) [2]
Hepatotoxicity [2]
Nausea (<36%)

Respiratory
Bronchitis (<9%)
Cough (6–44%)
Dyspnea (<22%)
Flu-like syndrome (5–8%)
Hemoptysis (<6%)
Pharyngitis (9%)
Pneumonia (3–22%) [3]
Pneumonitis (6%)
Pulmonary toxicity [4]
Rhinitis (3–11%)
Sinusitis (<5%)
Upper respiratory tract infection (2–14%)

Endocrine/Metabolic
Hyperglycemia (<6%)
Weight loss (<6%)

Genitourinary
- Dysuria (3–4%)
- Hematuria (<3%)
- Urinary hesitancy (3%)
- Urinary tract infection (4–15%)

Hematologic
- Anemia [3]
- Cytopenia [2]
- Febrile neutropenia [2]
- Hemolytic anemia [2]
- Hemotoxicity [3]
- Leukopenia [2]
- Myelosuppression [3]
- Myelotoxicity [2]
- Neutropenia [6]
- Sepsis [2]
- Thrombocytopenia [4]
- Thrombosis (<3%)

Otic
- Hearing loss (2–6%)

Ocular
- Visual disturbances (3–15%)

Other
- Adverse effects [2]
- Death [4]
- Infection (12–44%) [6]

FLUORIDES

Indications: Caries prevention (topical), osteoporosis prevention (oral)
Class: Chemical
Half-life: N/A
Clinically important, potentially hazardous interactions with: caffeine
Pregnancy category: C

Skin
- Acneform eruption [2]
- Burning [12]
- Dermatitis [4]
- Edema [2]
- Erythema [2]
- Hypersensitivity [6]
- Necrosis [2]
- Pruritus [5]
- Toxicity [27]
- Urticaria [7]

Mucosal
- Oral ulceration [2]
- Stomatitis [3]

Central Nervous System
- Headache [2]

Neuromuscular/Skeletal
- Arthralgia [5]
- Bone or joint pain [12]
- Skeletal fluorosis [35]

Gastrointestinal/Hepatic
- Abdominal pain [2]

Ocular
- Cataract [2]

Other
- Adverse effects [9]
- Death [7]
- Tooth fluorosis [39]

FLUOROURACIL

Trade names: 5-fluorouracil (Taj), Carac (Valeant), Efudex (Valeant), Fluoroplex (Allergan), Fluorouracil Injection, USP (Bioniche), Tolak (Hill Dermac)
Indications: Palliative management of malignant neoplasms especially of the gastrointestinal tract, breast, liver and pancreas, topical therapy for actinic keratoses
Class: Antimetabolite, Antineoplastic
Half-life: 8–20 minutes
Clinically important, potentially hazardous interactions with: aldesleukin, bromelain, cimetidine, granulocyte colony-stimulating factor (G-CSF), metronidazole, tinidazole
Pregnancy category: X
Important contra-indications noted in the prescribing guidelines for: nursing mothers; pediatric patients
Note: Contraindicated in patients with dihydropyrimidine dehydrogenase deficiency. Tolak cream contains peanut oil and should be used with caution in peanut-sensitive individuals.

Skin
- Acneform eruption [3]
- Acral erythema [4]
- Actinic keratoses [4]
- Anaphylactoid reactions/Anaphylaxis [2]
- Dermatitis (>10%) [4]
- Eczema [2]
- Edema [2]
- Erythema [4]
- Erythema multiforme [3]
- Exanthems (<10%) [3]
- Hand–foot syndrome (<38%) [49]
- Lupus erythematosus (systemic) [5]
- Palmar–plantar pigmentation [2]
- Peripheral edema [2]
- Photosensitivity [3]
- Pigmentation [10]
- Pruritus [4]
- Radiation recall dermatitis [3]
- Rash [8]
- Recall reaction [3]
- Seborrheic dermatitis [3]
- Toxicity [3]
- Ulcerations [2]
- Xerosis (<10%) [2]

Hair
- Alopecia (>10%) [15]

Nails
- Nail pigmentation [3]
- Paronychia [2]

Mucosal
- Epistaxis (nosebleed) [2]
- Mucosal inflammation [2]
- Mucositis (<79%) [14]
- Oral mucositis [5]
- Oral ulceration [2]
- Stomatitis (>10%) [19]

Cardiovascular
- Angina [9]
- Bradycardia [2]
- Cardiac failure [5]
- Cardiomyopathy [3]
- Cardiotoxicity [12]
- Hypertension [9]
- Myocardial infarction [4]
- QT prolongation [3]
- Thromboembolism [2]
- Venous thromboembolism [2]
- Ventricular tachycardia [2]

Central Nervous System
- Anorexia [8]
- Dysgeusia (taste perversion) [2]
- Encephalopathy [3]
- Fever [5]
- Headache [2]
- Insomnia [2]
- Leukoencephalopathy [26]
- Neurotoxicity [11]
- Peripheral neuropathy [3]
- Vertigo (dizziness) [2]

Neuromuscular/Skeletal
- Asthenia (fatigue) [15]

Gastrointestinal/Hepatic
- Abdominal pain [4]
- Constipation [3]
- Diarrhea [25]
- Hepatotoxicity [7]
- Nausea [20]
- Vomiting [16]

Respiratory
- Dysphonia [2]
- Pulmonary embolism [2]

Endocrine/Metabolic
- Acidosis [2]
- Hyperammonemia [2]
- Hypocalcemia [2]
- Hypokalemia [3]
- Hypomagnesemia [3]
- Hyponatremia [3]
- SIADH [4]
- Weight loss [2]

Renal
- Proteinuria [3]

Hematologic
- Anemia [17]
- Febrile neutropenia [13]
- Hemolytic uremic syndrome [3]
- Leukopenia [13]
- Lymphopenia [2]
- Myelosuppression [4]
- Neutropenia [37]
- Thrombocytopenia [18]

Ocular
- Ectropion [2]
- Epiphora [2]
- Ocular inflammation [2]

Local
- Application-site edema [2]
- Application-site pruritus [3]
- Injection-site burning [2]
- Injection-site desquamation [4]
- Injection-site edema [3]
- Injection-site erythema [4]
- Injection-site necrosis [2]
- Injection-site pain [2]
- Injection-site ulceration [2]

Other
- Adverse effects [8]
- Death [4]

Infection [6]
Side effects [2]

FLUOXETINE

Trade names: Prozac (Lilly), Sarafem (Warner Chilcott), Symbyax (Lilly)
Indications: Depression, obsessive-compulsive disorder
Class: Antidepressant, Selective serotonin reuptake inhibitor (SSRI)
Half-life: 2–3 days
Clinically important, potentially hazardous interactions with: alprazolam, amoxapine, amphetamines, astemizole, clarithromycin, clopidogrel, clozapine, desipramine, dexibuprofen, dextroamphetamine, diethylpropion, droperidol, duloxetine, erythromycin, haloperidol, iloperidone, imipramine, insulin aspart, insulin degludec, insulin glargine, insulin glulisine, isocarboxazid, linezolid, lithium, MAO inhibitors, mazindol, meperidine, methamphetamine, midazolam, moclobemide, nifedipine, nortriptyline, olanzapine, PEG-interferon, phendimetrazine, phenelzine, phentermine, phenylpropanolamine, phenytoin, pimozide, propranolol, pseudoephedrine, rasagiline, risperidone, selegiline, serotonin agonists, sibutramine, St John's wort, sumatriptan, sympathomimetics, tramadol, tranylcypromine, trazodone, tricyclic antidepressants, troleandomycin, tryptophan, vortioxetine, zolmitriptan
Pregnancy category: C
Important contra-indications noted in the prescribing guidelines for: the elderly; nursing mothers; pediatric patients
Note: Increased risk of suicidal thinking and behavior in children, adolescents, and young adults taking antidepressants for Major Depressive Disorder (MDD) and other psychiatric disorders. Sarafem is not approved for use in pediatric patients with MDD and obsessive compulsive disorder. Symbyax is not approved for use in children and adolescents.
Symbyax is fluoxetine and olanzapine.
Black Box Warning: SUICIDAL THOUGHTS AND BEHAVIORS

Skin
Diaphoresis (8%) [2]
Exanthems (4%) [7]
Mycosis fungoides [2]
Phototoxicity [2]
Pruritus (2%) [4]
Pseudolymphoma [4]
Rash (6%) [3]
Raynaud's phenomenon [2]
Serum sickness [3]
Toxic epidermal necrolysis [2]
Toxicity [2]
Urticaria (4%) [5]
Vasculitis [2]

Hair
Alopecia [7]

Mucosal
Black tongue [2]
Xerostomia (12%) [7]

Cardiovascular
Flushing (<2%)
Orthostatic hypotension [2]
QT prolongation [6]

Central Nervous System
Akathisia [6]
Amnesia [2]
Delirium [3]
Depression [2]
Dysgeusia (taste perversion) (2%)
Extrapyramidal symptoms [3]
Hallucinations [3]
Headache (<27%) [3]
Neuroleptic malignant syndrome [2]
Paresthesias [2]
Restless legs syndrome [4]
Serotonin syndrome [13]
Somnolence (drowsiness) [4]
Suicidal ideation [11]
Tremor (2–10%)
Vertigo (dizziness) [3]

Neuromuscular/Skeletal
Asthenia (fatigue) [2]
Rhabdomyolysis [2]

Gastrointestinal/Hepatic
Nausea [3]

Endocrine/Metabolic
Gynecomastia [2]
SIADH [20]
Weight gain [4]

Genitourinary
Priapism [2]
Sexual dysfunction [5]

Ocular
Hallucinations, visual [4]

Other
Adverse effects [3]
Bruxism [4]
Death [3]

FLUPHENAZINE

Trade name: Prolixin (Bristol-Myers Squibb)
Indications: Psychoses
Class: Antipsychotic, Phenothiazine
Half-life: 84–96 hours
Clinically important, potentially hazardous interactions with: antihistamines, arsenic, chlorpheniramine, clozapine, dofetilide, evening primrose, quinolones, sparfloxacin
Pregnancy category: C
Important contra-indications noted in the prescribing guidelines for: nursing mothers

---

Skin
Rash (<10%)
Vitiligo [2]

Central Nervous System
Neuroleptic malignant syndrome [14]
Parkinsonism [2]
Somnolence (drowsiness) [3]

Neuromuscular/Skeletal
Dystonia [3]

Endocrine/Metabolic
Galactorrhea (<10%)
Gynecomastia (<10%)
Mastodynia (<10%)

Genitourinary
Priapism [2]

Ocular
Maculopathy [3]

FLURBIPROFEN

Trade name: Ansaid (Pfizer)
Indications: Rheumatoid arthritis, osteoarthritis
Class: Non-steroidal anti-inflammatory (NSAID)
Half-life: 3–4 hours
Clinically important, potentially hazardous interactions with: ACE inhibitors, aspirin, furosemide, lithium, methotrexate
Pregnancy category: C
Important contra-indications noted in the prescribing guidelines for: the elderly; nursing mothers
Note: NSAIDs may cause an increased risk of serious cardiovascular and gastrointestinal adverse events, which can be fatal. This risk may increase with duration of use.
Elderly patients are at greater risk for serious gastrointestinal events.
Black Box Warning: CARDIOVASCULAR AND GASTROINTESTINAL RISKS

Skin
Eczema (3–9%)
Edema (3–9%)
Exanthems [3]
Fixed eruption [2]
Hypersensitivity [4]
Pruritus (<5%)
Rash (<3%)

Mucosal
Oral lichenoid eruption [2]

Central Nervous System
Headache [4]

Renal
Nephrotoxicity [2]

Other
Side effects (6%) [2]

FLUTAMIDE

Indications: Metastatic prostate carcinoma
Class: Androgen antagonist
Half-life: 8–10 hours
Clinically important, potentially hazardous interactions with: none known
Pregnancy category: D (not indicated for use in women)
Important contra-indications noted in the prescribing guidelines for: nursing mothers; pediatric patients
Black Box Warning: HEPATIC INJURY

Skin
Edema (4%)
Hot flashes (61%)
Photosensitivity [9]
Rash (3%)
Xerosis [2]

Central Nervous System
Paresthesias (<10%)

Gastrointestinal/Hepatic
Hepatotoxicity [11]

Endocrine/Metabolic
Gynecomastia (9%) [4]
Pseudoporphyria [3]

Local
Injection-site irritation (3%)

FLUVASTATIN

Trade name: Lescol (Novartis)
Indications: Hypercholesterolemia
Class: HMG-CoA reductase inhibitor, Statin
Half-life: 1.2 hours
Clinically important, potentially hazardous interactions with: azithromycin, bosentan, ciprofibrate, clarithromycin, colchicine, cyclosporine, delavirdine, erythromycin, gemfibrozil, imatinib, mifepristone, red rice yeast
Pregnancy category: X
Important contra-indications noted in the prescribing guidelines for: nursing mothers

---

Skin
Lupus erythematosus [2]
Rash (3%)

Central Nervous System
Headache (9%)

Neuromuscular/Skeletal
Asthenia (fatigue) (3%)
Myalgia/Myopathy (5%) [4]
Rhabdomyolysis [13]

Gastrointestinal/Hepatic
Diarrhea (5%)
Dyspepsia (8%)
Hepatotoxicity [5]

Respiratory
Sinusitis (3%)
Upper respiratory tract infection (16%)

Endocrine/Metabolic
Creatine phosphokinase increased [2]

Other
Allergic reactions (3%)

FLUVOXAMINE

Trade name: Luvox (Solvay)
Indications: Obsessive-compulsive disorder, depression
Class: Antidepressant, CYP1A2 inhibitor, CYP3A4 inhibitor, Selective serotonin reuptake inhibitor (SSRI)
Half-life: 15 hours
Clinically important, potentially hazardous interactions with: alosetron, alprazolam, aminophylline, amphetamines, anagrelide, asenapine, astemizole, bendamustine, clobazam, clopidogrel, clozapine, dextroamphetamine, diethylpropion, droperidol, duloxetine, isocarboxazid, linezolid, MAO inhibitors, mazindol, methadone, methamphetamine, olanzapine, oxtriphylline, phendimetrazine, phenelzine, phentermine, phenylpropanolamine, pirfenidone, propranolol, pseudoephedrine, ramelteon, rasagiline, roflumilast, ropivacaine, selegiline, sibutramine, St John's wort, sumatriptan, sympathomimetics, tacrine, tasimelteon, tizanidine, tramadol, tranylcypromine, trazodone, troleandomycin, tryptophan, zolmitriptan
Pregnancy category: C
Important contra-indications noted in the prescribing guidelines for: the elderly; nursing mothers; pediatric patients
Black Box Warning: SUICIDALITY AND ANTIDEPRESSANT DRUGS

Skin
Diaphoresis (<7%)
Photosensitivity [3]

Mucosal
Oral lesions (10%)
Xerostomia (<14%) [2]

Cardiovascular
Chest pain (3%)
Palpitation (3%)
QT prolongation [2]

Central Nervous System
Anorexia (6–14%)
Anxiety (5–8%)
Dysgeusia (taste perversion) (3%)
Headache (22–35%)
Insomnia (21–35%)
Neuroleptic malignant syndrome [2]
Pain (10%)
Seizures [2]
Serotonin syndrome [6]
Somnolence (drowsiness) (22–27%)
Tremor (5–8%)
Vertigo (dizziness) (11–15%)
Yawning (2–5%)

Neuromuscular/Skeletal
Asthenia (fatigue) (14–26%) [3]
Myalgia/Myopathy (5%)

Gastrointestinal/Hepatic
Diarrhea (16–18%)
Dyspepsia (8–10%)
Nausea (34–40%)

Respiratory
Pharyngitis (6%)
Upper respiratory tract infection (9%)

Endocrine/Metabolic
Galactorrhea [2]
Libido decreased (2–10%)
SIADH [2]

Genitourinary
Ejaculatory dysfunction (8–11%)

FOLIC ACID

Synonyms: folacin; folate; vitamin B_9
Indications: Anemias
Class: Vitamin
Half-life: N/A
Clinically important, potentially hazardous interactions with: balsalazide, estradiol, raltitrexed
Pregnancy category: A

Skin
Anaphylactoid reactions/Anaphylaxis [3]
Exanthems [2]
Pruritus [2]
Urticaria [2]

FONDAPARINUX

Trade name: Arixtra (Mylan)
Indications: Prophylaxis of deep vein thrombosis
Class: Anticoagulant, Heparinoid
Half-life: 17–21 hours
Clinically important, potentially hazardous interactions with: abciximab, anagrelide, anticoagulants, cilostazol, clopidogrel, dabigatran, dipyridamole, eptifibatide, nandrolone, salicylates, ticlopidine, tirofiban
Pregnancy category: B
Important contra-indications noted in the prescribing guidelines for: the elderly; nursing mothers; pediatric patients
Black Box Warning: SPINAL/EPIDURAL HEMATOMAS

Skin
Bullous dermatitis (3%)
Edema (9%)
Hematoma [2]
Hypersensitivity [4]
Purpura (4%)
Rash (8%)

Central Nervous System
Pain (2%)

Gastrointestinal/Hepatic
Hepatotoxicity [2]

Local
Injection-site bleeding (<10%)
Injection-site pruritus (<10%)

FORMOTEROL

Trade names: Dulera (Merck Sharpe & Dohme), Foradil (Novartis), Perforomist (Mylan), Symbicort (AstraZeneca)
Indications: Asthma, bronchospasm
Class: Beta-2 adrenergic agonist, Bronchodilator
Half-life: 10–14 hours
Clinically important, potentially hazardous interactions with: beta blockers, clomipramine, desipramine, doxepin, imipramine, iobenguane, nortriptyline, protriptyline, trimipramine
Pregnancy category: C
Important contra-indications noted in the prescribing guidelines for: nursing mothers; pediatric patients
Note: Dulera is formoterol and mometasone; Symbicort is formoterol and budesonide.
Black Box Warning: ASTHMA-RELATED DEATH

Skin
Pruritus (2%)

Mucosal
Xerostomia (<3%) [3]

Cardiovascular
Chest pain (2%)

Central Nervous System
Anxiety (2%)
Fever (2%)
Headache [8]
Insomnia (2%)
Tremor (2%) [6]
Vertigo (dizziness) (2–3%) [2]

Neuromuscular/Skeletal
Back pain (4%)
Cramps (2%)
Leg cramps (2%)

Gastrointestinal/Hepatic
Diarrhea (5%) [2]
Nausea (5%)
Vomiting (2%)

Respiratory
Asthma (exacerbation) [3]
Bronchitis (5%)
Cough [5]
Dysphonia [2]
Dyspnea (2%) [2]
Nasopharyngitis [6]
Pharyngitis (4%) [2]
Pneumonia [2]
Rhinitis [2]
Upper respiratory tract infection (7%) [3]

Other
Adverse effects [2]
Death [2]
Infection (17%)

FOSAMPRENAVIR

Trade name: Lexiva (ViiV)
Indications: HIV infections (in combination with other antiretrovirals)
Class: Antiretroviral, HIV-1 protease inhibitor
Half-life: 7.7 hours
Clinically important, potentially hazardous interactions with: amiodarone, atorvastatin, avanafil, bepridil, carbamazepine, darifenacin, delavirdine, dihydroergotamine, efavirenz, etravirine, flecainide, flibanserin, itraconazole, ketoconazole, lidocaine, lopinavir, lovastatin, midazolam, mifepristone, nevirapine, phenobarbital, phenytoin, pimozide, posaconazole, propafenone, quinidine, quinine, rifabutin, rifampin, rilpivirine, ritonavir, rivaroxaban, rosuvastatin, sildenafil, simeprevir, simvastatin, St John's wort, tadalafil, telaprevir, telithromycin, tipranavir, triazolam, vardenafil, warfarin
Pregnancy category: C
Important contra-indications noted in the prescribing guidelines for: the elderly; nursing mothers; pediatric patients
Note: Fosamprenavir is a sulfonamide and can be absorbed systemically. Sulfonamides can produce severe, possibly fatal, reactions such as toxic epidermal necrolysis and Stevens-Johnson syndrome.
Fosamprenavir is a prodrug of amprenavir.

Skin
Hypersensitivity [2]
Pruritus (7%)
Rash (~19%) [5]

Central Nervous System
Depression (8%)
Headache (19%)
Paresthesias (oral) (2%)

Neuromuscular/Skeletal
Asthenia (fatigue) (10%)

Gastrointestinal/Hepatic
Abdominal pain (5%)
Diarrhea [2]
Hepatotoxicity [2]
Vomiting [2]

Respiratory
Bronchitis [2]
Cough [2]
Nasopharyngitis [3]
Rhinitis [2]
Upper respiratory tract infection [2]

Other
Adverse effects [3]

FOSINOPRIL

Trade name: Monopril (Bristol-Myers Squibb)
Indications: Hypertension, heart failure
Class: Angiotensin-converting enzyme (ACE) inhibitor, Antihypertensive, Vasodilator
Half-life: 12 hours
Clinically important, potentially hazardous interactions with: alcohol, aldesleukin, allopurinol, alpha blockers, alprostadil, amifostine, amiloride, angiotensin II receptor blocking agents, antacids, antidiabetics, antihypertensives, antipsychotics, anxiolytics and hypnotics, azathioprine, baclofen, beta blockers, calcium channel blockers, clonidine, corticosteroids, cyclosporine, diazoxide, diuretics, estrogens, general anesthetics, gold & gold compounds, heparins, hydralazine, hypotensives, insulin, levodopa, lithium, MAO inhibitors, metformin, methyldopa, minoxidil, moxisylyte, moxonidine, nitrates, nitroprusside, NSAIDs, pentoxifylline, phosphodiesterase 5 inhibitors, potassium salts, prostacyclin analogues, rituximab, sirolimus, spironolactone, sulfonylureas, temsirolimus, tizanidine, tolvaptan, triamterene, trimethoprim
Pregnancy category: D (category C in first trimester; category D in second and third trimesters)
Important contra-indications noted in the prescribing guidelines for: nursing mothers
Black Box Warning: USE IN PREGNANCY

Skin
Angioedema [3]

Respiratory
Cough [3]

FUROSEMIDE

Trade name: Lasix (Sanofi-Aventis)
Indications: Edema
Class: Diuretic, loop
Half-life: ~2 hours
Clinically important, potentially hazardous interactions with: acemetacin, aliskiren, amikacin, amyl nitrite, celecoxib, diclofenac, digoxin, flurbiprofen, gentamicin, hyaluronic acid, hydrocortisone, kanamycin, mivacurium, neomycin, piroxicam, probenecid, streptomycin, tobramycin, tolmetin
Pregnancy category: C
Important contra-indications noted in the prescribing guidelines for: the elderly; nursing mothers; pediatric patients
Note: Furosemide is a sulfonamide and can be absorbed systemically. Sulfonamides can produce severe, possibly fatal, reactions such as toxic epidermal necrolysis and Stevens-Johnson syndrome.

Skin
AGEP [2]
Anaphylactoid reactions/Anaphylaxis [2]
Bullous dermatitis [16]
Bullous pemphigoid [11]
Erythema multiforme [3]
Exanthems (12%) [7]
Exfoliative dermatitis [3]
Lichenoid eruption [2]
Linear IgA bullous dermatosis [2]
Photosensitivity (<10%) [2]
Phototoxicity [4]
Pruritus [2]
Purpura [3]
Pustules [3]
Stevens–Johnson syndrome [3]
Sweet's syndrome [2]
Urticaria [3]
Vasculitis [7]

Mucosal
Xerostomia [3]

Cardiovascular
Hypotension [2]

Gastrointestinal/Hepatic
Pancreatitis [3]

Endocrine/Metabolic
Porphyria cutanea tarda [3]

Otic
Hearing loss [2]
Ototoxicity [3]

Other
Adverse effects [3]
Side effects [2]

GABAPENTIN

Trade names: Horizant (GSK), Neurontin (Pfizer)
Indications: Postherpetic neuralgia in adults, seizures
Class: Anticonvulsant
Half-life: 5–7 hours
Clinically important, potentially hazardous interactions with: none known
Pregnancy category: C
Important contra-indications noted in the prescribing guidelines for: the elderly; nursing mothers; pediatric patients

---

Skin
Anticonvulsant hypersensitivity syndrome [2]
Edema [5]
Exanthems [2]
Peripheral edema (8%) [11]
Rash [2]
Stevens–Johnson syndrome [2]

Hair
Alopecia [2]

Mucosal
Xerostomia (5%)

Central Nervous System
Aggression [2]
Coma [3]
Confusion [3]
Delirium [2]
Fever (10%)
Gait instability (2%) [3]
Headache (3%) [9]
Incoordination (2%)
Neurotoxicity [4]
Psychosis [2]
Sedation [5]
Seizures [4]
Somnolence (drowsiness) (21%) [36]
Tremor [3]
Vertigo (dizziness) (17–28%) [47]

Neuromuscular/Skeletal
Asthenia (fatigue) (6%) [12]
Ataxia (3%) [10]
Dystonia [2]
Myalgia/Myopathy [3]
Myasthenia gravis [3]
Myoclonus [5]
Rhabdomyolysis [4]

Gastrointestinal/Hepatic
Abdominal pain (3%)
Constipation (4%) [2]
Diarrhea (6%)
Flatulence (2%) [2]
Nausea (4%) [5]
Vomiting (3%) [3]

Respiratory
Respiratory depression [2]

Endocrine/Metabolic
Weight gain (2%) [8]

Genitourinary
Sexual dysfunction [5]

Ocular
Diplopia [2]
Hallucinations, visual [2]
Vision blurred (3%)

Other
Adverse effects [7]
Infection (5%)

GALANTAMINE

Trade names: Razadyne (Janssen), Reminyl (Janssen)
Indications: Alzheimer's disease
Class: Acetylcholinesterase inhibitor, Cholinesterase inhibitor
Half-life: ~7 hours
Clinically important, potentially hazardous interactions with: bethanechol, cimetidine, donepezil, edrophonium, paroxetine hydrochloride, physostigmine, pilocarpine, rivastigmine, succinylcholine, tacrine
Pregnancy category: C
Important contra-indications noted in the prescribing guidelines for: nursing mothers; pediatric patients
Note: Originally derived from snowdrop (*Galanthus* sp) bulbs.

Skin
Peripheral edema (>2%)
Purpura (>2%)

Cardiovascular
Bradycardia (2%) [5]
QT prolongation [5]

Central Nervous System
Anorexia (7–9%) [2]
Depression (7%)
Headache (8%) [2]
Insomnia (5%)
Somnolence (drowsiness) (4%)
Syncope (2%) [3]
Tremor (3%)
Vertigo (dizziness) (9%) [4]

Neuromuscular/Skeletal
Asthenia (fatigue) (5%)

Gastrointestinal/Hepatic
Abdominal pain (5%)
Diarrhea (6–12%) [4]
Dyspepsia (5%)
Nausea (6–24%) [5]
Vomiting (4–13%) [5]

Respiratory
Rhinitis (4%)
Upper respiratory tract infection (>2%)

Endocrine/Metabolic
Weight loss (5–7%)

Genitourinary
Hematuria (3%)
Urinary tract infection (8%)

Hematologic
Anemia (3%)

Other
Adverse effects [3]

GEFITINIB

Trade name: Iressa (AstraZeneca)
Indications: Advanced non-small cell lung cancer
Class: Antineoplastic, Biologic, Epidermal growth factor receptor (EGFR) inhibitor, Tyrosine kinase inhibitor
Half-life: 48 hours
Clinically important, potentially hazardous interactions with: antifungals, BCG vaccine, boceprevir, carbamazepine, cardiac glycosides, clozapine, conivaptan, CYP3A4 inhibitors and inducers, dasatinib, deferasirox, denosumab, echinacea, efavirenz, grapefruit juice, itraconazole, leflunomide, natalizumab, phenobarbital, phenytoin, pimecrolimus, ranitidine, rifampin, rifapentine, sipuleucel-T, St John's wort, tacrolimus, topotecan, trastuzumab, vaccines, vitamin K antagonists, voriconazole, warfarin
Pregnancy category: D
Important contra-indications noted in the prescribing guidelines for: nursing mothers; pediatric patients

---

Skin
Acneform eruption (25–33%) [32]
Desquamation (39%) [2]
Exanthems [3]
Folliculitis [4]
Hand–foot syndrome [2]
Papulopustular eruption [3]
Peripheral edema (2%)
Pruritus (8–9%) [4]
Rash (43–54%) [59]
Seborrhea [2]
Toxicity [9]
Ulcerations [2]
Xerosis (13–26%) [11]

Hair
Alopecia [6]
Hypertrichosis [2]

Nails
Nail changes (17%)
Paronychia (6%) [13]
Pyogenic granuloma [2]

Mucosal
Mucositis [4]
Stomatitis [7]

Cardiovascular
Hypertension [2]

Central Nervous System
Anorexia (7–10%) [2]

Neuromuscular/Skeletal
Asthenia (fatigue) [11]

Gastrointestinal/Hepatic
Abdominal pain [3]
Diarrhea (48–67%) [33]
Gastrointestinal perforation [2]
Hepatotoxicity [21]
Nausea (13–18%) [8]
Vomiting (9–12%) [5]

Respiratory
Dyspnea (2%)
Pneumonia [2]
Pneumonitis [3]
Pulmonary toxicity [15]

Endocrine/Metabolic
- ALT increased [6]
- Appetite decreased [2]
- AST increased [5]
- Dehydration [2]
- Weight loss (3–5%)

Genitourinary
- Cystitis [2]

Renal
- Nephrotoxicity [2]

Hematologic
- Anemia [4]
- Neutropenia [6]
- Thrombocytopenia [3]

Ocular
- Amblyopia (2%)
- Blepharitis [2]
- Conjunctivitis [2]

Other
- Adverse effects [11]
- Death [7]

GEMCITABINE

Trade name: Gemzar (Lilly)
Indications: Pancreatic carcinoma as a single agent, ovarian cancer (with carboplatin), breast cancer (with paclitaxel), non-small cell lung cancer (with cisplatin)
Class: Antimetabolite, Antineoplastic
Half-life: 42–94 minutes for short infusions; 4–11 hours for longer infusions
Clinically important, potentially hazardous interactions with: aldesleukin
Pregnancy category: D
Important contra-indications noted in the prescribing guidelines for: nursing mothers; pediatric patients

---

Skin
- Acneform eruption [3]
- Bullous dermatitis [2]
- Cellulitis [5]
- Dermatitis [5]
- Eczema (13%)
- Edema (13%) [4]
- Exanthems [2]
- Hand–foot syndrome [19]
- Hypersensitivity [3]
- Livedo reticularis [2]
- Necrosis [2]
- Peripheral edema (20%) [4]
- Petechiae (16%)
- Pruritus (13%) [2]
- Radiation recall dermatitis (<74%) [17]
- Rash (30%) [33]
- Raynaud's phenomenon [2]
- Thrombocytopenic purpura [5]
- Toxic epidermal necrolysis [3]
- Toxicity [5]
- Vasculitis [3]

Hair
- Alopecia (15%) [15]

Mucosal
- Mucositis [5]
- Stomatitis (11%) [13]

Cardiovascular
- Arrhythmias [3]
- Atrial fibrillation [4]
- Capillary leak syndrome [8]
- Cardiotoxicity [3]
- Hypertension [3]
- Hypotension [2]
- Myocardial infarction [3]
- Venous thromboembolism [3]

Central Nervous System
- Anorexia [11]
- Fever (41%) [12]
- Leukoencephalopathy [4]
- Neurotoxicity [9]
- Paresthesias (10%)
- Peripheral neuropathy [5]
- Somnolence (drowsiness) (11%)

Neuromuscular/Skeletal
- Asthenia (fatigue) (18%) [39]
- Myalgia/Myopathy (>10%) [6]

Gastrointestinal/Hepatic
- Abdominal pain [2]
- Cholangitis [2]
- Constipation [3]
- Diarrhea (19%) [23]
- Gastrointestinal bleeding [2]
- Hepatic disorder [2]
- Hepatotoxicity [11]
- Nausea (69%) [24]
- Vomiting (69%) [18]

Respiratory
- Dyspnea (10–23%) [2]
- Flu-like syndrome (19%) [2]
- Pneumonitis [4]
- Pulmonary toxicity [10]

Endocrine/Metabolic
- ALT increased [5]
- Appetite decreased [2]
- AST increased [5]
- Dehydration [2]
- Hypomagnesemia [6]
- Hyponatremia [2]

Genitourinary
- Hematuria (30%)

Renal
- Nephrotoxicity [5]
- Renal failure [2]

Hematologic
- Anemia (70%) [33]
- Febrile neutropenia [13]
- Hemolytic uremic syndrome [30]
- Hemotoxicity [6]
- Leukocytopenia [3]
- Leukopenia (62%) [23]
- Myelosuppression [7]
- Myelotoxicity [3]
- Neutropenia (61%) [73]
- Thrombocytopenia (30%) [58]
- Thrombosis [3]
- Thrombotic complications (microangiopathy) [2]

Local
- Injection-site reactions (4%)

Other
- Adverse effects [9]
- Allergic reactions (4%)
- Death [10]
- Infection (16%) [8]

GEMFIBROZIL

Trade name: Lopid (Pfizer)
Indications: Hyperlipidemia
Class: Fibrate, Lipid regulator
Half-life: 1.5 hours
Clinically important, potentially hazardous interactions with: atorvastatin, bexarotene, colchicine, cyclosporine, dicumarol, enzalutamide, ezetimibe, fluvastatin, interferon alfa, lovastatin, nicotinic acid, paclitaxel, pioglitazone, pitavastatin, pravastatin, repaglinide, rosiglitazone, rosuvastatin, roxithromycin, selexipag, simvastatin, treprostinil, warfarin
Pregnancy category: C
Important contra-indications noted in the prescribing guidelines for: nursing mothers; pediatric patients
Note: Contraindicated in patients with preexisting gallbladder disease.

Skin
- Eczema (2%)
- Exanthems (3%) [2]
- Psoriasis [3]
- Rash (2%)

Central Nervous System
- Headache [3]

Neuromuscular/Skeletal
- Asthenia (fatigue) (2%)
- Compartment syndrome [2]
- Myalgia/Myopathy [3]
- Rhabdomyolysis [35]

Gastrointestinal/Hepatic
- Abdominal pain (10%)
- Dyspepsia (20%)
- Hepatotoxicity [2]
- Pancreatitis [2]

Other
- Death [2]

GENTAMICIN

Trade names: Garamycin (Schering), Genoptic (Allergan)
Indications: Various infections caused by susceptible organisms
Class: Antibiotic, aminoglycoside
Half-life: 2–4 hours
Clinically important, potentially hazardous interactions with: adefovir, aldesleukin, aminoglycosides, atracurium, bumetanide, carbenicillin, cephalexin, cephalothin, doxacurium, ethacrynic acid, furosemide, methoxyflurane, non-polarizing muscle relaxants, pancuronium, pipecuronium, polypeptide antibiotics, rocuronium, succinylcholine, teicoplanin, torsemide, tubocurarine, vecuronium

Pregnancy category: C
Important contra-indications noted in the prescribing guidelines for: the elderly; nursing mothers
Note: Aminoglycosides may cause neurotoxicity and/or nephrotoxicity.

Skin
- Anaphylactoid reactions/Anaphylaxis [2]
- Dermatitis [8]
- Edema (<10%)
- Erythema (<10%)
- Exanthems [5]
- Photosensitivity [2]
- Pruritus (<10%)

Hair
- Alopecia [2]

Renal
- Fanconi syndrome [2]
- Nephrotoxicity [14]

Otic
- Ototoxicity [12]
- Tinnitus [4]

Local
- Injection-site necrosis [5]

GLATIRAMER

Synonym: copolymer-1
Trade names: Copaxone (Teva), Glatopa (Novartis)
Indications: Multiple sclerosis
Class: Immunomodulator
Half-life: N/A
Clinically important, potentially hazardous interactions with: Hemophilus B vaccine
Pregnancy category: B
Important contra-indications noted in the prescribing guidelines for: the elderly; nursing mothers; pediatric patients

---

Skin
- Acneform eruption (>2%)
- Anaphylactoid reactions/Anaphylaxis [3]
- Cyst (2%)
- Diaphoresis (15%)
- Ecchymoses (8%)
- Eczema (8%)
- Edema (8%)
- Erythema (4%)
- Facial edema (6%)
- Herpes simplex (4%)
- Hyperhidrosis (15%)
- Hypersensitivity (3%)
- Lipoatrophy [3]
- Nicolau syndrome [3]
- Nodular eruption (2%)
- Panniculitis [2]
- Peripheral edema (7%)
- Pruritus (4%)
- Purpura (8%)
- Rash (18%)

Hair
- Alopecia (>2%)

Nails
- Nail changes (>2%)

Mucosal
- Oral vesiculation (6%)
- Xerostomia (>2%)

Cardiovascular
- Chest pain (13%)
- Flushing [5]
- Palpitation (7%) [4]
- Vasodilation (20%)

Central Nervous System
- Anxiety (13%) [2]
- Chills (4%)
- Depression (>2%)
- Dysgeusia (taste perversion) (>2%)
- Fever (6%)
- Hyperesthesia (>2%)
- Migraine (4%)
- Pain (28%)
- Paresthesias (>2%)
- Tremor (7%)
- Vertigo (dizziness) (>2%)

Neuromuscular/Skeletal
- Arthralgia (24%)
- Asthenia (fatigue) (19%)
- Myalgia/Myopathy (>2%)

Gastrointestinal/Hepatic
- Hepatotoxicity [3]
- Nausea (15%)
- Vomiting (7%)

Respiratory
- Cough (>2%)
- Flu-like syndrome (26%)
- Sinusitis (>2%)

Endocrine/Metabolic
- Mastodynia (>2%)

Genitourinary
- Vaginitis (4%)

Otic
- Tinnitus (>2%)

Local
- Injection-site bleeding (5%)
- Injection-site ecchymoses (>2%)
- Injection-site erythema (66%) [3]
- Injection-site induration (13%) [3]
- Injection-site inflammation (49%)
- Injection-site lipoatrophy/lipohypertrophy [2]
- Injection-site pain (73%) [2]
- Injection-site pruritus (40%) [2]
- Injection-site reactions (6–67%) [12]
- Injection-site urticaria (5%)

Other
- Adverse effects [5]
- Infection (50%)

GLIMEPIRIDE

Trade names: Amaryl (Sanofi-Aventis), Avandaryl (GSK)
Indications: Non-insulin dependent diabetes Type II
Class: Sulfonylurea
Half-life: 5–9 hours
Clinically important, potentially hazardous interactions with: none known
Pregnancy category: C
Important contra-indications noted in the prescribing guidelines for: the elderly; nursing mothers; pediatric patients
Note: Glimepiride is a sulfonamide and can be absorbed systemically. Sulfonamides can produce severe, possibly fatal, reactions such as toxic epidermal necrolysis and Stevens-Johnson syndrome
Avandaryl is glimepiride and rosiglitazone.

Central Nervous System
- Headache [4]
- Vertigo (dizziness) [2]

Neuromuscular/Skeletal
- Arthralgia [2]

Gastrointestinal/Hepatic
- Diarrhea [5]
- Dyspepsia [2]
- Nausea [4]
- Pancreatitis [2]

Endocrine/Metabolic
- Hypoglycemia [8]
- Weight gain [3]

Genitourinary
- Genital mycotic infections [3]
- Urinary tract infection [3]

Other
- Adverse effects [5]

GLIPIZIDE

Trade names: Glucotrol (Pfizer), Metaglip (Bristol-Myers Squibb)
Indications: Non-insulin dependent diabetes Type II
Class: Sulfonylurea
Half-life: 2–4 hours
Clinically important, potentially hazardous interactions with: none known
Pregnancy category: C
Important contra-indications noted in the prescribing guidelines for: the elderly; nursing mothers; pediatric patients
Note: Glipizide is a sulfonamide and can be absorbed systemically. Sulfonamides can produce severe, possibly fatal, reactions such as toxic epidermal necrolysis and Stevens-Johnson syndrome.

Skin
- Photosensitivity (<10%)
- Pruritus (<3%)
- Rash (<10%)
- Urticaria (<10%)

Central Nervous System
- Hyperesthesia (<3%)
- Paresthesias (<3%)

Neuromuscular/Skeletal
- Myalgia/Myopathy (<3%)

Endocrine/Metabolic
- Hypoglycemia [3]

Other
- Adverse effects [2]

GLUCAGON

Trade name: Glucagon Emergency Kit (Lilly)
Indications: Hypoglycemic reactions
Class: Hormone, polypeptide
Half-life: 3–10 minutes
Clinically important, potentially hazardous interactions with: insulin degludec, insulin glargine, insulin glulisine, warfarin
Pregnancy category: B

Skin
- Erythema necrolyticum migrans [2]
- Exanthems [7]
- Folliculitis [2]
- Pyoderma gangrenosum [3]
- Rash [2]
- Sweet's syndrome [7]
- Urticaria (<10%) [2]
- Vasculitis [9]

Local
- Injection-site reactions [3]

GLYBURIDE

Synonyms: glibenclamide; glybenclamide
Trade names: Diabeta (Sanofi-Aventis), Glucovance (Bristol-Myers Squibb), Glynase (Pfizer), Micronase (Pfizer)
Indications: Non-insulin dependent diabetes Type II
Class: Sulfonylurea
Half-life: 5–16 hours
Clinically important, potentially hazardous interactions with: bosentan, colesevelam, norfloxacin
Pregnancy category: C
Note: Glyburide is a sulfonamide and can be absorbed systemically. Sulfonamides can produce severe, possibly fatal, reactions such as toxic epidermal necrolysis and Stevens-Johnson syndrome.
Glucovance is glyburide and metformin.

Skin
- Erythema (<5%)
- Exanthems (<5%) [3]
- Linear IgA bullous dermatosis [2]
- Pemphigus [2]
- Photosensitivity (<10%) [5]
- Pruritus (<10%) [3]
- Psoriasis [2]
- Purpura [2]
- Rash (<10%)
- Urticaria (<5%) [4]
- Vasculitis [5]

Cardiovascular
- Flushing [2]

Endocrine/Metabolic
- Hypoglycemia [2]
- Weight gain [2]

Other
- Adverse effects [2]

GLYCOPYRROLATE

Synonym: glycopyrronium bromide
Trade names: Cuvposa (Shionogi), Robinul (Forte), Seebri Neohaler (Novartis), Utibron Neohaler (Novartis)
Indications: Duodenal ulcer, irritable bowel syndrome, hyperhidrosis
Class: Anticholinergic, Muscarinic antagonist, Non-depolarizing muscle relaxant
Half-life: N/A
Clinically important, potentially hazardous interactions with: anticholinergics, arbutamine, belladonna alkaloids, digoxin, disopyramide, meperidine, phenothiazines, procainamide, quinidine, ritodrine, tricyclic antidepressants
Pregnancy category: C
Important contra-indications noted in the prescribing guidelines for: the elderly; nursing mothers; pediatric patients
Note: Utibron Neohaler is glycopyrrolate and indacaterol.

Skin
- Photosensitivity (<10%)
- Xerosis (>10%)

Mucosal
- Nasal congestion (30%)
- Xerostomia (40%) [7]

Cardiovascular
- Bradycardia [2]
- Flushing (30%)

Central Nervous System
- Headache (15%)

Gastrointestinal/Hepatic
- Constipation (35%)
- Vomiting (40%)

Respiratory
- Sinusitis (15%)
- Upper respiratory tract infection (15%)

Genitourinary
- Urinary retention (15%)

Local
- Injection-site irritation (>10%)

GOLIMUMAB

Trade name: Simponi (Centocor)
Indications: Rheumatoid arthritis, psoriatic arthritis, ankylosing spondylitis, ulcerative colitis
Class: Disease-modifying antirheumatic drug (DMARD), Monoclonal antibody, TNF inhibitor
Half-life: 2 weeks
Clinically important, potentially hazardous interactions with: abatacept, anakinra, live vaccines
Pregnancy category: B
Important contra-indications noted in the prescribing guidelines for: nursing mothers; pediatric patients
Note: TNF inhibitors should be used in patients with heart failure only after consideration of other treatment options. TNF inhibitors are contraindicated in patients with a personal or family history of multiple sclerosis or demyelinating disease. TNF inhibitors should not be administered to patients with moderate to severe heart failure (New York Heart Association Functional Class III/IV).
Black Box Warning: SERIOUS INFECTIONS AND MALIGNANCY

Skin
- Lupus erythematosus [3]
- Malignancies [5]
- Psoriasis [2]
- Rash [3]

Cardiovascular
- Hypertension [2]

Central Nervous System
- Headache [7]

Neuromuscular/Skeletal
- Arthralgia [3]
- Asthenia (fatigue) [2]

Gastrointestinal/Hepatic
- Colitis [2]
- Diarrhea [4]
- Nausea [5]

Respiratory
- Cough [2]
- Nasopharyngitis (6%) [7]
- Pneumonia [4]
- Pulmonary toxicity [2]
- Tuberculosis [2]
- Upper respiratory tract infection (7%) [7]

Endocrine/Metabolic
- ALT increased [4]
- AST increased [3]

Hematologic
- Sepsis [4]

Local
- Injection-site erythema [7]
- Injection-site reactions (6%) [5]

Other
- Adverse effects [12]
- Death [3]
- Infection (28%) [15]

GRISEOFULVIN

Trade names: Fulvicin (Schering), Grifulvin V (Ortho), Gris-PEG (Pedinol)
Indications: Fungal infections of the skin, hair and nails
Class: Antifungal
Half-life: 9–24 hours
Clinically important, potentially hazardous interactions with: alcohol, levonorgestrel, liraglutide, midazolam, thalidomide, ulipristal
Pregnancy category: C
Important contra-indications noted in the prescribing guidelines for: nursing mothers; pediatric patients

---

Skin
- Angioedema [3]
- Bullous dermatitis [2]
- Cold urticaria [2]
- Erythema multiforme [6]
- Exanthems [6]
- Exfoliative dermatitis [2]
- Fixed eruption [7]

Lichenoid eruption [2]
Lupus erythematosus [14]
Petechiae [2]
Photosensitivity (<10%) [18]
Pigmentation [2]
Pruritus [4]
Rash (>10%)
Serum sickness [3]
Stevens–Johnson syndrome [3]
Toxic epidermal necrolysis [4]
Urticaria (>10%) [5]
Vasculitis [2]

Mucosal

Oral candidiasis (<10%)

Central Nervous System

Dysgeusia (taste perversion) [3]

Endocrine/Metabolic

Gynecomastia [2]
Porphyria [12]

Other

Adverse effects [2]
Allergic reactions (<5%)

HALOPERIDOL

Trade name: Haldol (Ortho-McNeil)
Indications: Schizophrenia, Tourette's disorder
Class: Antiemetic, Antipsychotic, butyrophenone
Half-life: 20 hours
Clinically important, potentially hazardous interactions with: acemetacin, arsenic, benztropine, citalopram, clozapine, darifenacin, fluoxetine, itraconazole, lisdexamfetamine, lithium, meloxicam, methotrexate, moxifloxacin, nilotinib, oxybutynin, propranolol, quinine, sotalol, sulpiride, tetrabenazine, tiotropium, trospium, vandetanib, venlafaxine
Pregnancy category: C
Important contra-indications noted in the prescribing guidelines for: the elderly; pediatric patients
Black Box Warning: INCREASED MORTALITY IN ELDERLY PATIENTS WITH DEMENTIA-RELATED PSYCHOSIS

Skin
Cellulitis [2]
Diaphoresis [2]
Photosensitivity [3]
Seborrheic dermatitis [2]

Hair
Alopecia areata [2]

Mucosal
Xerostomia [3]

Cardiovascular
Arrhythmias [2]
QT prolongation [22]
Torsades de pointes [12]

Central Nervous System
Agitation [3]
Akathisia [7]
Delirium [2]
Extrapyramidal symptoms [8]
Insomnia [3]
Neuroleptic malignant syndrome [34]
Parkinsonism [5]
Sedation [2]
Somnolence (drowsiness) [3]
Tardive dyskinesia (<37%) [2]
Tremor [6]
Vertigo (dizziness) [2]

Neuromuscular/Skeletal
Dystonia [3]
Myoclonus [2]
Rhabdomyolysis [7]

Gastrointestinal/Hepatic
Pancreatitis [2]

Respiratory
Pneumonia [2]

Endocrine/Metabolic
Galactorrhea [3]
Hypoglycemia [2]
SIADH [3]
Weight gain [2]

Genitourinary
Priapism [3]
Urinary retention [3]

Local
Injection-site reactions [3]

Other
Adverse effects [4]
Death [7]

HEMOPHILUS B VACCINE

Trade names: ActHIB (Sanofi-Aventis), Comvax (Merck), HibTITER (Lederle), OmniHIB (GSK), PedivaxHIB (Merck), ProHIBIT (Connaught)
Indications: Hemophilus B immunization
Class: Vaccine
Half-life: N/A
Clinically important, potentially hazardous interactions with: azathioprine, basiliximab, corticosteroids, cyclosporine, daclizumab, glatiramer, mycophenolate, sirolimus, tacrolimus
Pregnancy category: C

Skin
Erythema [2]

HEPARIN

Trade names: Hep-Flush (Wyeth), Viaflex (Baxter)
Indications: Venous thrombosis, pulmonary embolism, intravascular coagulation, peripheral arterial embolism
Class: Anticoagulant, Heparinoid
Half-life: 1.5 hours
Clinically important, potentially hazardous interactions with: acenocoumarol, aliskiren, antihistamines, aspirin, balsalazide, bivalirudin, butabarbital, ceftobiprole, dabigatran, danaparoid, desvenlafaxine, iloprost, nandrolone, nicotine, nitroglycerin, palifermin, piperacillin/tazobactam, salicylates, tirofiban, warfarin
Pregnancy category: C
Important contra-indications noted in the prescribing guidelines for: the elderly
Note: A higher incidence of bleeding has been reported in patients over 60 years of age, especially women. Contraindicated in patients with severe thrombocyopenia.

Skin
Anaphylactoid reactions/Anaphylaxis [4]
Bullous dermatitis [3]
Dermatitis [6]
Ecchymoses [3]
Erythema [2]
Exanthems [2]
Hypersensitivity [17]
Lesions [2]
Livedo reticularis [2]
Necrosis [56]
Petechiae [2]
Purpura (>10%)
Toxic epidermal necrolysis [2]
Urticaria [6]
Vasculitis [6]

Hair
Alopecia [2]

Mucosal
Gingivitis (>10%)

Genitourinary
Priapism [6]

Hematologic
Bleeding [2]
Hemorrhage [6]
Thrombocytopenia [87]
Thrombosis [8]

Local
Injection-site eczematous eruption [5]
Injection-site induration [4]
Injection-site necrosis [4]
Injection-site plaques [2]

Other
Allergic reactions (<10%) [3]
Death [6]

HEPATITIS A VACCINE

Trade names: Avaxim (Sanofi Pasteur), Havrix (GSK), Vaqta (Merck)
Indications: Hepatitis A immunization
Class: Vaccine
Half-life: >2 years
Clinically important, potentially hazardous interactions with: none known
Pregnancy category: C

Skin
Rash (<10%)

Central Nervous System
Anorexia (<10%)
Chills (<10%)
Fever (>10%) [2]
Guillain–Barré syndrome [2]
Headache (>10%) [3]
Somnolence (drowsiness) (>10%)

Neuromuscular/Skeletal
Arm pain (<10%)
Asthenia (fatigue) (<10%)
Back pain (<10%)

Gastrointestinal/Hepatic
Constipation (<10%)
Diarrhea (<10%)
Nausea (<10%)
Vomiting (<10%)

Respiratory
Cough (<10%)
Nasopharyngitis (<10%)
Pharyngitis (<10%)
Rhinitis (<10%)
Upper respiratory tract infection (<10%)

Otic
Otitis media (<10%)

Ocular
Conjunctivitis (<10%)

Local
Injection-site erythema [2]
Injection-site pain (<10%) [7]
Injection-site reactions [5]

Other
Adverse effects [2]

HEPATITIS B VACCINE

Trade names: Comvax (Merck), Engerix B (GSK), Pediatrix (GSK), Recombivax HB (Merck), Twinrix (GSK)
Other common trade names: Heptavax-B
Indications: For immunization of infection caused by all known subtypes of hepatitis B virus
Class: Vaccine
Half-life: N/A
Clinically important, potentially hazardous interactions with: none known
Pregnancy category: C

Skin
Anaphylactoid reactions/Anaphylaxis [6]
Churg-Strauss syndrome [2]
Dermatomyositis [2]
Erythema multiforme [2]
Erythema nodosum [3]
Gianotti–Crosti syndrome [2]
Granuloma annulare [2]
Lichen planus [16]
Lichenoid eruption [3]
Lupus erythematosus [9]
Pemphigus [2]
Pseudolymphoma [2]
Purpura [6]
Urticaria [3]
Vasculitis [11]

Hair
Alopecia [2]

Cardiovascular
Polyarteritis nodosa [5]

Central Nervous System
Guillain–Barré syndrome [4]
Neurotoxicity [2]

Neuromuscular/Skeletal
Arthralgia [4]

Ocular
Optic neuropathy [3]
Uveitis [2]

Local
Injection-site edema [3]
Injection-site pain (22%) [3]

Other
Adverse effects [2]
Death [2]

HEROIN

Synonym: diacetylmorphine
Indications: Substance abuse drug
Class: Opiate agonist
Half-life: N/A
Clinically important, potentially hazardous interactions with: none known
Pregnancy category: B (category D if used for prolonged period or in high doses)

Skin
Abscess [7]
Acanthosis nigricans [2]
Burning (24%)
Candidiasis [3]
Cellulitis [3]
Edema [4]
Exanthems [2]
Fixed eruption [2]
Folliculitis (candidal) [4]
Necrosis [3]
Photosensitivity [2]
Pigmentation [4]
Pruritus [6]
Pustules [5]
Toxic epidermal necrolysis [2]
Ulcerations [5]
Urticaria [3]
Vasculitis [2]

Central Nervous System
Leukoencephalopathy [12]
Seizures (2%)

Neuromuscular/Skeletal
Myalgia/Myopathy [2]
Rhabdomyolysis [15]

Otic
Hearing loss [2]

Ocular
Diplopia [2]
Eyelid edema [2]

Local
Injection-site ulceration [3]

Other
Death [5]
Infection (13%)
Side effects (85%)
Teratogenicity [2]

HUMAN PAPILLOMA-VIRUS (HPV) VACCINE

Synonym: HPV4
Trade names: Gardasil (Merck), Silgard (Merck)
Indications: For prevention of HPV genital warts, cervical cancers and vulvar dysplasias (against Types 6, 11, 16 and 18 human papillomavirus)
Class: Vaccine
Half-life: N/A
Clinically important, potentially hazardous interactions with: immunosuppressants
Pregnancy category: B
Important contra-indications noted in the prescribing guidelines for: the elderly; nursing mothers; pediatric patients

---

Mucosal
Oropharyngeal pain (3%)

Central Nervous System
Fever (13%) [4]
Headache (28%) [5]
Myelitis [2]
Vertigo (dizziness) (<4%)

Neuromuscular/Skeletal
Asthenia (fatigue) [2]

Gastrointestinal/Hepatic
Diarrhea (3–4%)
Nausea (2–7%) [2]
Vomiting (<2%)

Respiratory
Cough (2%)
Nasopharyngitis (3%)
Upper respiratory tract infection (2%)

Local
Injection-site bruising (3%)
Injection-site edema (14–25%) [2]
Injection-site erythema (17–25%) [2]
Injection-site pain (61–84%) [3]
Injection-site pruritus (3%)
Injection-site reactions [4]

Other
Adverse effects [4]
Toothache (2%)

HUMAN PAPILLOMA-VIRUS VACCINE (BIVALENT)

Trade name: Cervarix (GSK)
Indications: Prevention of human papillomavirus (HPV) types 16 and 18 in females aged 10–25 years old
Class: Vaccine
Half-life: N/A
Clinically important, potentially hazardous interactions with: immunosuppressants
Pregnancy category: B
Important contra-indications noted in the prescribing guidelines for: the elderly; nursing mothers; pediatric patients

---

Skin
Anaphylactoid reactions/Anaphylaxis (3%) [2]
Erythema (<10%) [4]
Pruritus (<10%)
Rash (<10%)
Urticaria (7%)

Central Nervous System
Fever (13%) [3]
Headache (53%) [2]

Neuromuscular/Skeletal
Arthralgia (21%)
Asthenia (fatigue) (55%)
Myalgia/Myopathy (49%)

Gastrointestinal/Hepatic
Abdominal pain (28%)
Diarrhea (28%)
Nausea (28%)
Vomiting (28%)

Local
Injection-site edema (44%) [3]
Injection-site erythema (48%)
Injection-site pain (92%) [9]
Injection-site reactions [5]

Other
Adverse effects [2]

HYALURONIC ACID

Synonym: hyaluronidase
Trade names: Euflexxa (Ferring), Hyalgan (Sanofi-Aventis), Hylan G-F 20 (Synvisc), Juvederm (Allergan), Perlane (Q-Med AB), Restylane Fine Lines (Medicis), Vitrase (ISTA Pharma)
Indications: Oral: joint disorders **Injection**: adjunct in eye surgery, viscosupplementation in orthopedics, cosmetic surgery **Topical**: wounds, burns, skin ulcers, stomatitis
Class: Food supplement, Glycoaminoglycan
Half-life: 2.5–5.5 minutes
Clinically important, potentially hazardous interactions with: furosemide, local anesthetics, NSAIDs, oral anticoagulants
Pregnancy category: C
Important contra-indications noted in the prescribing guidelines for: nursing mothers; pediatric patients
Note: Most reported reactions relate to orthopedic use.

Skin
Acneform eruption (<29%)
Angioedema [6]
Churg-Strauss syndrome [12]
Dermatitis (24%)
Ecchymoses [3]
Edema [8]
Erythema [6]
Erythema multiforme [2]
Facial edema [2]
Hematoma [2]
Herpes simplex [2]
Hypersensitivity [6]
Induration [2]
Inflammation [7]
Necrosis [3]
Nodular eruption [2]
Pruritus [4]

Cardiovascular
Arterial occlusion [2]
Hypertension (4%)

Central Nervous System
Pain [3]

Neuromuscular/Skeletal
Arthralgia [7]
Back pain (5%)
Chondritis (<11%) [2]
Gouty tophi [3]
Tendinitis (2%)

Gastrointestinal/Hepatic
Nausea (2%)

Ocular
Orbital inflammation [2]

Local
Injection-site bruising [2]
Injection-site ecchymoses [2]
Injection-site edema (20%) [11]
Injection-site erythema (47%) [6]
Injection-site granuloma [2]
Injection-site nodules [3]
Injection-site pain (8–47%) [15]
Injection-site reactions (<11%) [12]

Other
Adverse effects [14]
Infection [2]

HYDRALAZINE

Trade names: Apresazide (Novartis), Apresoline (Novartis), Ser-Ap-Es (Novartis)
Indications: Hypertension
Class: Vasodilator
Half-life: 3–7 hours
Clinically important, potentially hazardous interactions with: acebutolol, alfuzosin, captopril, cilazapril, diclofenac, enalapril, fosinopril, levodopa, levomepromazine, lisinopril, meloxicam, olmesartan, quinapril, ramipril, trandolapril, triamcinolone, trifluoperazine, zuclopenthixol
Pregnancy category: C
Note: Apresazide is hydralazine and hydrochlorothiazide; Ser-Ap-Es is hydralazine, reserpine and hydrochlorothiazide.
Hydrochlorothiazide is a sulfonamide and can be absorbed systemically. Sulfonamides can produce severe, possibly fatal, reactions such as toxic epidermal necrolysis and Stevens-Johnson syndrome.

Skin
Edema [2]
Exanthems [4]
Lupus erythematosus (7%) [112]
Photosensitivity [2]
Purpura [3]
Sweet's syndrome [6]
Toxic epidermal necrolysis [2]
Ulcerations [2]
Vasculitis [13]

Mucosal
Oral ulceration [2]
Orogenital ulceration [2]

Cardiovascular
Flushing (>10%)

Respiratory
Alveolar hemorrhage (pulmonary) [2]

Renal
Glomerulonephritis [5]

HYDROCHLOROTHIAZIDE

Trade names: Accuretic (Pfizer), Aldactazide (Pfizer), Aldoril (Merck), Atacand HCT (AstraZeneca), Avalide (Bristol-Myers Squibb), Capozide (Par), Diovan HCT (Novartis), Dyazide (GSK), Hyzaar (Merck), Inderide (Wyeth), Lopressor (Novartis), Lotensin (Novartis), Lotensin HCT (Novartis), Micardis (Boehringer Ingelheim), Microzide (Watson), Moduretic (Merck), Prinzide (Merck), Tekturna HCT (Novartis), Teveten HCT (Biovail), Uniretic (Schwarz), Vaseretic (Biovail), Zestoretic (AstraZeneca), Ziac (Barr)
Indications: Edema
Class: Diuretic, thiazide
Half-life: 5.6–14.8 hours
Clinically important, potentially hazardous interactions with: digoxin, dofetilide, lithium, zinc
Pregnancy category: B
Important contra-indications noted in the prescribing guidelines for: nursing mothers; pediatric patients
Note: Hydrochlorothiazide is a sulfonamide and can be absorbed systemically. Sulfonamides can produce severe, possibly fatal, reactions such as toxic epidermal necrolysis and Stevens-Johnson syndrome.
Hydrochlorothiazide is often used in combination, e.g. with aliskiren (Tekturna HCT); amiloride (Moduretic); benazepril (Lotensin HCT); bisoprolol (Ziac); captopril (Capozide); enalapril (Vaseretic); irbesartan (Avalide); lisinopril (Prinzide and Zestoretic); losartan (Hyzaar); methyldopa (Aldoril); moexipril (Uniretic); spironolactone (Aldactazide); triamterene (Dyazide and Maxzide).

Skin
Dermatitis [2]
Diaphoresis [2]
Edema [2]
Erythema annulare centrifugum [2]
Lichenoid eruption [5]
Lupus erythematosus [15]
Peripheral edema [5]
Photosensitivity [18]
Phototoxicity [5]
Purpura [6]
Rash [2]
Toxic epidermal necrolysis [2]
Vasculitis [3]

Cardiovascular
Hypotension [5]

Central Nervous System
Headache [6]
Vertigo (dizziness) [7]

Neuromuscular/Skeletal
Asthenia (fatigue) [2]

Gastrointestinal/Hepatic
Pancreatitis [4]

Respiratory
Upper respiratory tract infection [2]

Endocrine/Metabolic
Hyponatremia [3]

SIADH [4]

Ocular

Glaucoma [2]

Other

Adverse effects [5]
Death [2]

HYDROCODONE

Trade names: Duratuss (UCB), Entex HC (Andrx), Hycotuss (Endo), Hydromet (Actavis), Hysingla ER (Purdue), Lortab (UCB), Maxidone (Watson), Norco (Watson), Tussionex (Celltech), Vicodin (AbbVie), Vicoprofen (AbbVie), Zohydro ER (Pernix), Zydone (Endo)
Indications: Acute pain, coughing
Class: Opiate agonist
Half-life: 3.8 hours
Clinically important, potentially hazardous interactions with: alcohol, buprenorphine, butorphanol, CYP3A4 inhibitors or inducers, MAO inhibitors, nalbuphine, pentazocine
Pregnancy category: C
Important contra-indications noted in the prescribing guidelines for: nursing mothers; pediatric patients
Note: Hydrocodone is included in many combination drugs. Other medications that can be included in these preparations include: phenylpropanolamine, phenylephrine, pyrilamine, pseudoephedrine, acetaminophen, ibuprofen, and others. Zohydro ER is the first extended-release, single-entity hydrocodone-containing drug product approved by the FDA and reflects the newly updated labeling requirements recently announced by the FDA.
Black Box Warning: ADDICTION, ABUSE, AND MISUSE; LIFE-THREATENING RESPIRATORY DEPRESSION; ACCIDENTAL INGESTION; NEONATAL OPIOID WITHDRAWAL SYNDROME; INTERACTION WITH ALCOHOL; and CYTOCHROME P450 3A4 INTERACTION

Skin

Hot flashes (<10%)
Hyperhidrosis (<10%)
Peripheral edema (<3%)
Pruritus (3%) [2]
Rash (<10%)

Mucosal

Xerostomia (3%)

Cardiovascular

Chest pain (<10%)

Central Nervous System

Fever (<10%)
Headache [2]
Migraine (<10%)
Paresthesias (<10%)
Somnolence (drowsiness) (<5%) [3]
Tremor (3%)
Vertigo (dizziness) (2–3%) [3]

Neuromuscular/Skeletal

Arthralgia (<10%)
Asthenia (fatigue) (<4%)
Back pain (<4%) [2]
Bone or joint pain (<10%)
Muscle spasm (<3%)
Myalgia/Myopathy (<10%)
Neck pain (<10%)
Pain in extremities (<10%)

Gastrointestinal/Hepatic

Abdominal pain (2–3%)
Constipation (8–11%) [6]
Gastroesophageal reflux (<10%)
Nausea (7–10%) [8]
Vomiting [7]

Respiratory

Cough (<10%)
Dyspnea (<10%)
Upper respiratory tract infection (<3%)

Endocrine/Metabolic

Dehydration (<10%)
GGT increased (<10%)
Hypokalemia (<10%)

Genitourinary

Urinary tract infection (<5%)

HYDROMORPHONE

Trade names: Dilaudid (AbbVie), Exalgo (Mallinckrodt), Jurnista (Janssen-Cilag), Palladone (Napp)
Indications: Pain
Class: Opiate agonist
Half-life: 1–3 hours; 2 hours (IV)
Clinically important, potentially hazardous interactions with: alcohol, alvimopan, ammonium chloride, amphetamines, anticholinergics, anxiolytics and hypnotics, buprenorphine, butorphanol, cimetidine, CNS depressants, desmopressin, domperidone, droperidol, linezolid, MAO inhibitors, metoclopramide, moclobemide, nalbuphine, pegvisomant, pentazocine, phenothiazines, sodium oxybate, SSRIs, St John's wort, succinylcholine, thiazide diuretics
Pregnancy category: C
Important contra-indications noted in the prescribing guidelines for: nursing mothers; pediatric patients
Note: OROS hydromorphone prolonged release (Jurnista) is a once-daily formulation of hydromorphone that utilizes OROS (osmotic-controlled release oral delivery system) technology to deliver the drug at a near constant rate.
Black Box Warning: ADDICTION, ABUSE, AND MISUSE; LIFE-THREATENING RESPIRATORY DEPRESSION; ACCIDENTAL INGESTION; NEONATAL OPIOID WITHDRAWAL SYNDROME; and INTERACTION WITH ALCOHOL

Skin

Pruritus (<11%) [12]

Mucosal

Xerostomia (<10%)

Cardiovascular

Bradycardia [2]
Flushing (<10%)
Hypotension [2]

Central Nervous System

Agitation [3]
Dysgeusia (taste perversion) [3]
Headache [5]
Hyperalgesia [3]
Somnolence (drowsiness) [4]
Tremor [2]
Vertigo (dizziness) [9]

Neuromuscular/Skeletal

Asthenia (fatigue) [4]
Myoclonus [3]

Gastrointestinal/Hepatic

Constipation [9]
Nausea [16]
Vomiting [9]

Other

Adverse effects [7]

HYDROQUINONE

Trade names: Ambi (Johnson & Johnson), Lustra (Taro)
Indications: Ultraviolet induced dyschromia and discoloration resulting from the use of oral contraceptives, pregnancy, hormone replacement therapy, or skin trauma
Class: Depigmentation agent
Half-life: N/A
Clinically important, potentially hazardous interactions with: none known
Pregnancy category: C
Important contra-indications noted in the prescribing guidelines for: nursing mothers; pediatric patients

---

Skin

Acneform eruption [2]
Burning [2]
Contact dermatitis (localized) [2]
Depigmentation [2]
Erythema [4]
Ochronosis [15]
Peeling [2]
Pigmentation [3]
Pruritus [2]
Scaling [2]
Striae [2]
Xerosis [2]

Other

Adverse effects [3]

HYDROXY-CHLOROQUINE

Trade name: Plaquenil (Sanofi-Aventis)
Indications: Malaria, lupus erythematosus, rheumatoid arthritis
Class: Antimalarial, Antiprotozoal, Disease-modifying antirheumatic drug (DMARD)
Half-life: 32–50 days
Clinically important, potentially hazardous interactions with: chloroquine, cholestyramine, dapsone, droperidol, ethosuximide, lacosamide, lanthanum, moxifloxacin, neostigmine, oxcarbazepine, penicillamine, tiagabine, typhoid vaccine, vigabatrin, yellow fever vaccine

Pregnancy category: C
Important contra-indications noted in the prescribing guidelines for: nursing mothers; pediatric patients

---

Skin
AGEP [22]
Bullous dermatitis [2]
DRESS syndrome [2]
Erythema annulare centrifugum [3]
Erythroderma [2]
Exanthems (<5%) [4]
Exfoliative dermatitis [3]
Lichenoid eruption [4]
Photosensitivity [6]
Phototoxicity [3]
Pigmentation (<10%) [17]
Pruritus (>10%) [12]
Psoriasis (exacerbation) [12]
Rash (<10%) [4]
Thrombocytopenic purpura [2]
Toxic epidermal necrolysis [3]
Urticaria [2]

Hair
Hair pigmentation (bleaching) (<10%) [7]

Nails
Nail pigmentation [3]

Mucosal
Oral pigmentation [7]
Stomatitis [2]

Cardiovascular
Cardiomyopathy [8]
Cardiotoxicity [3]
QT prolongation [3]

Central Nervous System
Anorexia [2]
Dysgeusia (taste perversion) [2]
Neurotoxicity [3]

Neuromuscular/Skeletal
Asthenia (fatigue) [3]
Myalgia/Myopathy [8]

Gastrointestinal/Hepatic
Diarrhea [4]
Dysphagia [2]
Nausea [5]
Vomiting [3]

Endocrine/Metabolic
Hypoglycemia [3]
Porphyria [7]
Weight loss [2]

Hematologic
Anemia [3]
Neutropenia [2]
Thrombocytopenia [4]

Otic
Hearing loss [2]

Ocular
Maculopathy [5]
Ocular adverse effects [2]
Ocular toxicity [8]
Reduced visual acuity [2]
Retinopathy [27]
Vision blurred [3]

Other
Adverse effects [6]
Death [3]

HYDROXYUREA

Synonym: hydroxycarbamide
Trade names: Droxia (Bristol-Myers Squibb), Hydrea (Bristol-Myers Squibb)
Indications: Leukemia, malignant tumors
Class: Antineoplastic, Antiretroviral
Half-life: 3–4 hours
Clinically important, potentially hazardous interactions with: adefovir, aldesleukin
Pregnancy category: D

Skin
Acral erythema [8]
Atrophy [4]
Dermatitis [3]
Dermatomyositis [28]
Exanthems (<10%)
Fixed eruption [4]
Ichthyosis [2]
Keratoses [2]
Leg ulceration (29%) [20]
Lichen planus [3]
Lichenoid eruption [3]
Lupus erythematosus [3]
Palmar–plantar desquamation [6]
Pigmentation (<58%) [17]
Poikiloderma [3]
Pruritus [3]
Purpura [2]
Radiation recall dermatitis [2]
Telangiectasia [2]
Tumors [5]
Ulcerations [26]
Vasculitis [6]
Xerosis (<10%) [7]

Hair
Alopecia (<10%) [8]

Nails
Atrophic nails [3]
Melanonychia [7]
Nail changes [4]
Nail dystrophy [2]
Nail pigmentation [18]
Onycholysis [2]

Mucosal
Oral lesions [2]
Oral pigmentation [2]
Oral squamous cell carcinoma [2]
Oral ulceration [8]
Stomatitis (>10%) [4]
Tongue pigmentation (<29%) [3]

Gastrointestinal/Hepatic
Pancreatitis [2]

Other
Adverse effects [2]
Death [2]
Side effects (7–35%) [3]

HYDROXYZINE

Trade names: Atarax (Pfizer), Vistaril (Pfizer)
Indications: Anxiety and tension, pruritus
Class: Histamine H1 receptor antagonist, Muscarinic antagonist
Half-life: 3–7 hours
Clinically important, potentially hazardous interactions with: alcohol, barbiturates, CNS depressants, efavirenz, lurasidone, narcotics, non-narcotic analgesics
Pregnancy category: C
Important contra-indications noted in the prescribing guidelines for: nursing mothers

---

Skin
AGEP [3]
Anaphylactoid reactions/Anaphylaxis [2]
Angioedema [3]
Erythema multiforme [2]
Exanthems [3]
Fixed eruption [3]
Urticaria [4]

Mucosal
Xerostomia (12%) [4]

Central Nervous System
Somnolence (drowsiness) [5]

Gastrointestinal/Hepatic
Vomiting [2]

HYOSCYAMINE

Trade names: IB-Stat (InKline), Levbid (Schwarz), Levsin (Schwarz), Levsin/SL (Schwarz), Levsinex (Schwarz), Nulev (Schwarz)
Indications: Treatment of gastrointestinal tract disorders caused by spasm, adjunctive therapy for peptic ulcers, cystitis, Parkinsonism, biliary and renal colic
Class: Anticholinergic, Muscarinic antagonist
Half-life: N/A
Clinically important, potentially hazardous interactions with: anticholinergics, arbutamine
Pregnancy category: C
Important contra-indications noted in the prescribing guidelines for: the elderly; nursing mothers; pediatric patients

---

Skin
Photosensitivity (<10%)
Xerosis (>10%)

Mucosal
Xerostomia (>10%)

Cardiovascular
Tachycardia [2]

Local
Injection-site inflammation (>10%)

IBANDRONATE

Synonym: ibandronic acid
Trade names: Bondronat (Roche), Boniva (Roche)
Indications: Postmenopausal osteoporosis
Class: Bisphosphonate
Half-life: 37–157 hours
Clinically important, potentially hazardous interactions with: alcohol, aminoglycosides, antacids, calcium salts, food, magnesium salts, NSAIDs, oral iron
Pregnancy category: C
Important contra-indications noted in the prescribing guidelines for: nursing mothers; pediatric patients

---

Skin
- Rash (<2%)

Cardiovascular
- Hypertension (6–7%)

Central Nervous System
- Fever (~9%) [4]
- Headache (3–7%)
- Vertigo (dizziness) (<4%)

Neuromuscular/Skeletal
- Arthralgia (3–6%) [2]
- Asthenia (fatigue) (4%) [3]
- Back pain (4–14%)
- Bone or joint pain [3]
- Cramps (2%)
- Joint disorder (4%)
- Myalgia/Myopathy (<6%)
- Osteonecrosis [13]
- Pain in extremities (<8%)

Gastrointestinal/Hepatic
- Abdominal pain (5–8%)
- Constipation (3–4%)
- Diarrhea (4–7%) [2]
- Dyspepsia (6–12%) [4]
- Gastritis (2%)
- Gastrointestinal disorder [3]
- Nausea (5%) [4]
- Vomiting (3%) [4]

Respiratory
- Bronchitis (3–10%)
- Flu-like syndrome (<4%) [7]
- Nasopharyngitis (4%)
- Pharyngitis (3%)
- Pneumonia (6%)
- Upper respiratory tract infection (2–34%)

Endocrine/Metabolic
- Hypercholesterolemia (5%)
- Hypocalcemia [3]
- Hypophosphatemia [2]

Genitourinary
- Urinary tract infection (2–6%)

Other
- Adverse effects [5]
- Allergic reactions (3%)
- Infection (4%)
- Tooth disorder (4%)

IBRUTINIB

Trade name: Imbruvica (Pharmacyclics)
Indications: Mantle cell lymphoma
Class: Bruton's tyrosine kinase (BTK) inhibitor
Half-life: 4–6 hours
Clinically important, potentially hazardous interactions with: carbamazepine, clarithromycin, grapefruit juice, itraconazole, ketoconazole, phenytoin, posaconazole, rifampin, St John's wort, strong or moderate CYP3A inhibitors or inducers, telithromycin, voriconazole
Pregnancy category: D
Important contra-indications noted in the prescribing guidelines for: nursing mothers; pediatric patients

---

Skin
- Cellulitis [3]
- Ecchymoses (30%) [3]
- Peripheral edema (35%) [2]
- Petechiae (11%)
- Rash (25%) [4]
- Toxicity (14%)
- Tumor lysis syndrome [2]

Mucosal
- Epistaxis (nosebleed) (11%)
- Stomatitis (17%)

Cardiovascular
- Atrial fibrillation [6]
- Hypertension [3]
- Hypotension [2]

Central Nervous System
- Fever (18%) [4]
- Headache (13%)
- Peripheral neuropathy [2]
- Vertigo (dizziness) (14%)

Neuromuscular/Skeletal
- Arthralgia (11%) [2]
- Asthenia (fatigue) (14–41%) [14]
- Bone or joint pain (37%)
- Muscle spasm (14%)

Gastrointestinal/Hepatic
- Abdominal pain (24%)
- Constipation (25%)
- Diarrhea (51%) [17]
- Dyspepsia (11%)
- Nausea (31%) [12]
- Vomiting (24%) [2]

Respiratory
- Cough (19%) [2]
- Dyspnea (27%)
- Pneumonia (14%) [3]
- Sinusitis (13%) [2]
- Upper respiratory tract infection (34%) [4]

Endocrine/Metabolic
- Appetite decreased (21%)
- Dehydration (12%)
- Hyperuricemia (15%)
- Hypokalemia [2]

Genitourinary
- Urinary tract infection (14%) [2]

Hematologic
- Anemia [7]
- Bleeding [5]
- Cytopenia [3]
- Febrile neutropenia [3]
- Hemorrhage [2]
- Lymphocytosis [2]
- Neutropenia [12]
- Sepsis [2]
- Thrombocytopenia [10]

Other
- Infection [7]

IBUPROFEN

Trade names: Advil (Wyeth), Motrin (McNeil), Vicoprofen (AbbVie)
Indications: Arthritis, pain
Class: Non-steroidal anti-inflammatory (NSAID)
Half-life: 2–4 hours
Clinically important, potentially hazardous interactions with: aspirin, ciprofibrate, diuretics, methotrexate, methyl salicylate, NSAIDs, oxycodone hydrochloride, salicylates, tacrine, tacrolimus, urokinase, voriconazole
Pregnancy category: D (category C prior to 30 weeks gestation; category D starting at 30 weeks gestation)
Note: NSAIDs may cause an increased risk of serious cardiovascular and gastrointestinal adverse events, which can be fatal. This risk may increase with duration of use.

Skin
- AGEP [5]
- Anaphylactoid reactions/Anaphylaxis [5]
- Angioedema [8]
- Bullous dermatitis [3]
- Bullous pemphigoid [2]
- Dermatitis [5]
- DRESS syndrome [4]
- Erythema multiforme [11]
- Erythema nodosum (<5%)
- Exanthems [9]
- Fixed eruption [14]
- Hypersensitivity [5]
- Lupus erythematosus [5]
- Nicolau syndrome [2]
- Peripheral edema [2]
- Photosensitivity [6]
- Pruritus (<5%) [5]
- Psoriasis (palms) [2]
- Rash (>10%) [2]
- Stevens–Johnson syndrome [10]
- Toxic epidermal necrolysis [8]
- Urticaria (>10%) [10]
- Vasculitis [8]
- Vesiculobullous eruption [2]

Hair
- Alopecia [2]

Cardiovascular
- Cardiotoxicity [2]
- Hypertension [4]

Central Nervous System
- Aseptic meningitis [16]
- Headache [3]

Neuromuscular/Skeletal
- Arthralgia [2]
- Back pain [2]
- Rhabdomyolysis [3]

Gastrointestinal/Hepatic
- Abdominal pain [6]

Constipation [4]
Diarrhea [4]
Dyspepsia [5]
Gastroesophageal reflux [2]
Gastrointestinal bleeding [2]
Gastrointestinal disorder [2]
Hepatotoxicity [2]
Nausea [7]
Pancreatitis [2]
Vanishing bile duct syndrome [2]
Vomiting [5]

Respiratory
Influenza [2]
Sinusitis [2]
Upper respiratory tract infection [2]

Endocrine/Metabolic
Pseudoporphyria [2]

Genitourinary
Urinary tract infection [2]

Renal
Nephrotoxicity [3]

Hematologic
Thrombocytopenia [5]

Otic
Hearing loss [2]
Tinnitus [2]

Ocular
Amblyopia [2]
Optic neuritis [2]
Periorbital edema [3]
Visual disturbances [2]

Other
Adverse effects [11]
Kounis syndrome [3]

IBUTILIDE

Trade name: Corvert (Pfizer)
Indications: Atrial fibrillation and flutter
Class: Antiarrhythmic, Antiarrhythmic class III
Half-life: 2–12 hours
Clinically important, potentially hazardous interactions with: degarelix
Pregnancy category: C
Important contra-indications noted in the prescribing guidelines for: nursing mothers; pediatric patients

---

Cardiovascular
Bradycardia [4]
Hypotension [2]
QT prolongation [5]
Tachycardia (3%)
Torsades de pointes [10]
Ventricular arrhythmia [4]
Ventricular tachycardia [5]

Central Nervous System
Headache (4%)

Gastrointestinal/Hepatic
Nausea (2%) [3]

IDARUBICIN

Synonyms: 4-demethoxydaunorubicin; 4-DMDR
Trade name: Idamycin (Pfizer)
Indications: Acute myeloid leukemia
Class: Antibiotic, anthracycline
Half-life: 14–35 hours (oral)
Clinically important, potentially hazardous interactions with: aldesleukin
Pregnancy category: D
Important contra-indications noted in the prescribing guidelines for: nursing mothers; pediatric patients

---

Skin
Rash (>10%) [2]
Urticaria (>10%)

Hair
Alopecia (77%) [8]

Mucosal
Mucositis (50%) [4]
Stomatitis (>10%)

Gastrointestinal/Hepatic
Diarrhea [2]
Nausea [2]
Vomiting [2]

Hematologic
Febrile neutropenia [2]

Other
Infection [2]

IDARUCIZUMAB *

Trade name: Praxbind (Boehringer Ingelheim)
Indications: Reversal of the anticoagulant effects of dabigatran in patients requiring emergency or urgent surgery or with life-threatening or uncontrolled bleeding
Class: Monoclonal antibody
Half-life: 10 hours
Clinically important, potentially hazardous interactions with: none known
Pregnancy category: N/A (No data available)
Important contra-indications noted in the prescribing guidelines for: nursing mothers; pediatric patients
Note: Risk of serious adverse reactions in patients with hereditary fructose intolerance due to sorbitol excipient.

Skin
Irritation [2]

Central Nervous System
Delirium (7%)
Fever (6%)
Headache [2]

Neuromuscular/Skeletal
Back pain [2]

Gastrointestinal/Hepatic
Constipation (7%)

Respiratory
Nasopharyngitis [2]
Pneumonia (6%)

Endocrine/Metabolic
Hypokalemia (7%)

IDELALISIB

Trade name: Zydelig (Gilead)
Indications: Relapsed chronic lymphocytic leukemia (with rituximab), follicular B-cell non-Hodgkin lymphoma, small lymphocytic lymphoma
Class: Phosphoinositide 3-kinase (PI3K) inhibitor
Half-life: 8 hours
Clinically important, potentially hazardous interactions with: carbamazepine, phenytoin, rifampin, St John's wort, strong CYP3A inducers and substrates
Pregnancy category: D
Important contra-indications noted in the prescribing guidelines for: nursing mothers; pediatric patients
Black Box Warning: FATAL AND SERIOUS TOXICITIES: HEPATIC, SEVERE DIARRHEA, COLITIS, PNEUMONITIS, and INTESTINAL PERFORATION

Skin
Diaphoresis (12%)
Peripheral edema (10%)
Rash (21%) [6]

Central Nervous System
Chills [5]
Fever [8]
Headache (11%)
Insomnia (12%)

Neuromuscular/Skeletal
Asthenia (fatigue) (30%) [7]

Gastrointestinal/Hepatic
Abdominal pain (26%)
Colitis [6]
Constipation [2]
Diarrhea (47%) [14]
Gastrointestinal perforation [2]
Hepatotoxicity [7]
Nausea (29%) [7]
Vomiting (15%) [2]

Respiratory
Cough (29%) [5]
Dyspnea (17%)
Pneumonia (25%) [8]
Pneumonitis [4]
Upper respiratory tract infection (12%) [2]

Endocrine/Metabolic
ALT increased (50%) [7]
Appetite decreased (16%) [2]
AST increased (41%) [7]

Hematologic
Anemia [5]
Febrile neutropenia [4]
Neutropenia [6]
Thrombocytopenia [5]

IFOSFAMIDE

Trade name: Ifex (Bristol-Myers Squibb)
Indications: Cancers, sarcomas, leukemias, lymphomas
Class: Alkylating agent
Half-life: 4–15 hours
Clinically important, potentially hazardous interactions with: aldesleukin, aprepitant
Pregnancy category: D

Skin
- Dermatitis (<10%)
- Pigmentation (<10%) [2]
- Toxicity [2]

Hair
- Alopecia (50–100%) [4]

Nails
- Ridging (<10%)

Cardiovascular
- Phlebitis (2%)

Central Nervous System
- Confusion [2]
- Delirium [2]
- Encephalopathy [8]
- Neurotoxicity [11]
- Seizures [2]

Neuromuscular/Skeletal
- Osteomalacia [2]

Gastrointestinal/Hepatic
- Hepatotoxicity [2]
- Nausea [6]
- Pancreatitis [2]
- Vomiting [6]

Endocrine/Metabolic
- SIADH [2]

Renal
- Fanconi syndrome [4]
- Nephrotoxicity [34]

Hematologic
- Anemia [3]
- Febrile neutropenia [2]
- Leukopenia [2]
- Myelosuppression [2]
- Neutropenia [4]
- Thrombocytopenia [4]

Other
- Allergic reactions (<10%)
- Death [2]
- Infection [2]

ILOPERIDONE

Trade name: Fanapt (Vanda)
Indications: Schizophrenia
Class: Antipsychotic
Half-life: 18–33 hours
Clinically important, potentially hazardous interactions with: alcohol, dextromethorphan, fluoxetine, itraconazole, ketoconazole, paroxetine hydrochloride, QT prolonging agents
Pregnancy category: C
Important contra-indications noted in the prescribing guidelines for: the elderly; nursing mothers; pediatric patients
Black Box Warning: INCREASED MORTALITY IN ELDERLY PATIENTS WITH DEMENTIA-RELATED PSYCHOSIS

Skin
- Rash (2%)

Mucosal
- Nasal congestion (8%) [2]
- Xerostomia (10%) [9]

Cardiovascular
- Hypotension (3%)
- Orthostatic hypotension (3%) [4]
- QT prolongation [8]
- Tachycardia (12%) [3]

Central Nervous System
- Akathisia (2%) [3]
- Anxiety [2]
- Headache [3]
- Insomnia (18%) [3]
- Sedation [3]
- Somnolence (drowsiness) (15%) [8]
- Tremor (3%)
- Vertigo (dizziness) (20%) [11]

Neuromuscular/Skeletal
- Arthralgia (3%)
- Asthenia (fatigue) (6%) [2]

Gastrointestinal/Hepatic
- Diarrhea (7%)
- Dyspepsia [3]
- Nausea (10%) [2]

Respiratory
- Dyspnea (2%)
- Nasopharyngitis (3%)
- Upper respiratory tract infection (3%)

Endocrine/Metabolic
- Weight gain (9%) [10]

Genitourinary
- Ejaculatory dysfunction (2%) [2]

IMATINIB

Trade name: Gleevec (Novartis)
Indications: Chronic myeloid leukemia
Class: Antineoplastic, Biologic, CYP3A4 inhibitor, Tyrosine kinase inhibitor
Half-life: 18 hours
Clinically important, potentially hazardous interactions with: acetaminophen, amlodipine, anisindione, anticoagulants, aprepitant, atorvastatin, barbiturates, benzodiazepines, butabarbital, carbamazepine, chlordiazepoxide, clarithromycin, clonazepam, clorazepate, corticosteroids, cyclosporine, dexamethasone, diazepam, dicumarol, efavirenz, erythromycin, ethotoin, felodipine, flurazepam, fluvastatin, fosphenytoin, isradipine, itraconazole, ketoconazole, lorazepam, lovastatin, mephenytoin, mephobarbital, midazolam, mifepristone, nicardipine, nifedipine, nimodipine, nisoldipine, oxazepam, oxcarbazepine, pentobarbital, phenobarbital, phenytoin, pimozide, pravastatin, primidone, quazepam, rifampin, rifapentine, secobarbital, simvastatin, St John's wort, temazepam, voriconazole, warfarin
Pregnancy category: D
Important contra-indications noted in the prescribing guidelines for: nursing mothers

---

Skin
- Acneform eruption [2]
- AGEP [6]
- Diaphoresis (13%)
- DRESS syndrome [3]
- Edema (<5%) [33]
- Erythema (<10%) [5]
- Erythroderma [3]
- Exanthems [8]
- Exfoliative dermatitis [3]
- Facial edema (<10%) [2]
- Hand–foot syndrome [3]
- Hypomelanosis [5]
- Lichen planus [5]
- Lichenoid eruption [8]
- Neutrophilic eccrine hidradenitis [2]
- Panniculitis [2]
- Peripheral edema (<10%) [5]
- Petechiae (<10%)
- Photosensitivity (<10%)
- Pigmentation [9]
- Pityriasis rosea [5]
- Pruritus (6–10%) [3]
- Pseudolymphoma [3]
- Psoriasis [2]
- Rash (32–39%) [23]
- Squamous cell carcinoma [2]
- Stevens–Johnson syndrome [11]
- Toxicity [8]
- Xerosis (<10%)

Hair
- Alopecia (10–15%)
- Follicular mucinosis [2]

Mucosal
- Mucositis [2]
- Oral lichenoid eruption [3]
- Oral pigmentation [3]
- Oral ulceration [3]

Cardiovascular
- Cardiotoxicity [2]
- Congestive heart failure [2]
- QT prolongation [2]

Central Nervous System
- Anorexia [4]
- Chills (11%)
- Depression (15%) [2]
- Fever (13–41%) [2]
- Headache (19–37%) [2]
- Hypoesthesia (<10%)
- Insomnia (10–19%)
- Subdural hemorrhage [2]
- Vertigo (dizziness) [2]

Neuromuscular/Skeletal
- Arthralgia (21–26%) [3]
- Asthenia (fatigue) (29–75%) [18]
- Bone or joint pain (11–31%) [11]
- Muscle spasm [7]
- Myalgia/Myopathy (16–62%) [10]
- Osteonecrosis [2]

Gastrointestinal/Hepatic
- Abdominal pain [4]
- Ascites [2]

Constipation (9–16%) [2]
Diarrhea (25–59%) [16]
Dyspepsia [2]
Gastrointestinal bleeding [5]
Hepatotoxicity (6–12%) [18]
Nausea (42–73%) [14]
Vomiting (23–58%) [12]

Respiratory
Cough (11–27%)
Dyspnea (21%)
Nasopharyngitis (10–31%)
Pharyngitis (10–15%)
Pleural effusion [3]
Pneumonitis (4–13%)
Pulmonary toxicity [2]
Rhinitis (17%)
Upper respiratory tract infection (3–21%)

Endocrine/Metabolic
Creatine phosphokinase increased [2]
Gynecomastia [4]
Hypophosphatemia [2]
Hypothyroidism [2]
Porphyria cutanea tarda [2]
Pseudoporphyria [4]
Weight gain (5–32%) [3]

Renal
Fanconi syndrome [2]
Nephrotoxicity [2]
Renal failure [2]

Hematologic
Anemia [10]
Febrile neutropenia [2]
Hemotoxicity [4]
Leukopenia [3]
Myelosuppression [2]
Neutropenia [13]
Thrombocytopenia [11]

Ocular
Epiphora (25%)
Eyelid edema [2]
Optic edema [2]
Periorbital edema (33%) [11]

Other
Adverse effects [14]
Death [3]
Side effects [2]

IMIPRAMINE

Trade name: Tofranil (Mallinckrodt)
Indications: Depression
Class: Antidepressant, tricyclic, Muscarinic antagonist
Half-life: 6–18 hours
Clinically important, potentially hazardous interactions with: amprenavir, arbutamine, artemether/lumefantrine, clonidine, cobicistat/elvitegravir/emtricitabine/tenofovir disoproxil, darifenacin, epinephrine, fluoxetine, formoterol, guanethidine, iobenguane, isocarboxazid, labetalol, linezolid, MAO inhibitors, phenelzine, propranolol, quinolones, ropivacaine, sparfloxacin, tranylcypromine, zaleplon, zolpidem
Pregnancy category: D
Black Box Warning: SUICIDALITY AND ANTIDEPRESSANT DRUGS

Skin
Diaphoresis (<25%) [8]
Exanthems (<6%) [6]
Exfoliative dermatitis [4]
Photosensitivity [3]
Pigmentation [13]
Pruritus (3%) [6]
Purpura [3]
Urticaria [6]

Hair
Alopecia [2]

Mucosal
Glossitis [2]
Oral lesions [3]
Stomatitis [2]
Xerostomia (>10%) [16]

Cardiovascular
QT prolongation [3]
Tachycardia [2]

Central Nervous System
Dysgeusia (taste perversion) (metallic taste) (>10%) [2]
Parkinsonism (<10%)

Neuromuscular/Skeletal
Asthenia (fatigue) [2]

Endocrine/Metabolic
SIADH [4]

Otic
Tinnitus [4]

IMIQUIMOD

Trade names: Aldara (3M), Zyclara (Graceway)
Indications: External genital and perianal warts, actinic keratoses
Class: Antiviral, Immunomodulator
Half-life: N/A
Clinically important, potentially hazardous interactions with: none known
Pregnancy category: C
Important contra-indications noted in the prescribing guidelines for: nursing mothers; pediatric patients

---

Skin
Angioedema [2]
Burning (9–31%) [7]
Crusting [3]
Depigmentation [3]
Eczema (<10%)
Edema (12–17%) [2]
Erosions (10–32%) [5]
Erythema (33–85%) [14]
Erythema multiforme [2]
Excoriations (18–25%) [2]
Flaking (18–67%) [3]
Fungal dermatitis (<10%)
Herpes simplex (<10%)
Hypomelanosis [2]
Induration (5%)
Lichen planus [3]
Lupus erythematosus [2]
Lymphadenopathy (2%)
Pemphigus [4]
Pemphigus foliaceus [3]
Pigmentation [3]
Pruritus (22–75%) [10]
Psoriasis [3]
Scabbing (4%)
Scar [3]
Seborrheic keratoses (<10%)
Tenderness (local) (12%) [2]
Ulcerations (5–10%) [5]
Vesiculation (2–3%)
Vitiligo [7]

Hair
Alopecia (<10%)
Poliosis [2]

Cardiovascular
Chest pain (<10%)

Central Nervous System
Anorexia (<10%)
Anxiety (<10%)
Fever (<10%) [2]
Headache (<10%) [3]
Neurotoxicity [2]
Pain (2–11%) [6]
Rigors (<10%)
Vertigo (dizziness) (<10%)

Neuromuscular/Skeletal
Asthenia (fatigue) (<10%) [2]
Back pain (<10%)
Myalgia/Myopathy (<10%)

Gastrointestinal/Hepatic
Nausea (<10%) [2]
Vomiting (<10%)

Respiratory
Cough (<10%)
Flu-like syndrome (<3%)
Pharyngitis (<10%)
Rhinitis (<10%)
Sinusitis (<10%)
Upper respiratory tract infection (<10%)

Genitourinary
Urinary tract infection (<10%)

Local
Application-site burning (<10%)
Application-site edema (<10%) [4]
Application-site erythema (<10%) [3]
Application-site pruritus (<10%) [4]
Application-site reactions [9]

Other
Adverse effects [5]

IMMUNE GLOBULIN IV

Synonyms: IGIV; IVIG
Trade names: Gamimune (Bayer), Gammagard (Baxter), Gammar PIV (ZLB Behring), Gamunex (Bayer), Iveegam (Baxter), Venoglobulin (Alpha Therapeutics)
Indications: Immunodeficiency in patients unable to produce sufficient amounts of IgG antibodies
Class: Immunomodulator
Half-life: N/A
Clinically important, potentially hazardous interactions with: live vaccines
Pregnancy category: C
Important contra-indications noted in the prescribing guidelines for: nursing mothers
Black Box Warning: THROMBOSIS, RENAL DYSFUNCTION and ACUTE RENAL FAILURE

Skin
Anaphylactoid reactions/Anaphylaxis [3]
Eczema [2]
Lichenoid eruption [2]
Pompholyx [3]
Rash [2]
Vasculitis [4]

Cardiovascular
Flushing [2]
Hypertension [2]
Myocardial infarction [2]
Palpitation [2]
Thromboembolism [3]

Central Nervous System
Aseptic meningitis [4]
Chills [2]
Fever [6]
Headache [10]

Gastrointestinal/Hepatic
Abdominal pain [2]
Diarrhea [2]
Nausea [4]
Vomiting [2]

Respiratory
Cough [2]
Dyspnea [2]
Pulmonary embolism [2]

Renal
Nephrotoxicity [6]
Renal failure [2]

Hematologic
Thrombosis [3]

Local
Application-site pain (16%)
Infusion-related reactions [4]
Injection-site edema [2]
Injection-site erythema [2]

Other
Adverse effects [8]

IMMUNE GLOBULIN SC *

Synonym: SCIG
Trade names: Cuvitru (Shire), Hizentra (CSL Behring), Vivaglobin (CSL Behring)
Indications: Primary immune deficiency
Class: Immunomodulator
Half-life: N/A
Clinically important, potentially hazardous interactions with: none known
Pregnancy category: C
Black Box Warning: THROMBOSIS

Skin
Pruritus [2]
Rash (<3%)

Mucosal
Oropharyngeal pain (17%)

Cardiovascular
Tachycardia (<3%)

Central Nervous System
Fever (<3%) [2]
Headache (2–32%) [2]

Neuromuscular/Skeletal
Asthenia (fatigue) (<5%)

Gastrointestinal/Hepatic
Gastrointestinal disorder (<5%)
Nausea (<11%)

Respiratory
Bronchitis [2]
Cough (10%)
Upper respiratory tract infection [2]

Local
Injection-site reactions (49–92%) [4]

Other
Allergic reactions (11%)

INDACATEROL

Trade names: Arcapta Neohaler (Novartis), Onbrez Breezhaler (Novartis), Utibron Neohaler (Novartis)
Indications: Long term, once-daily maintenance bronchodilator treatment of airflow obstruction in chronic obstructive pulmonary disease (COPD), including chronic bronchitis and/or emphysema
Class: Beta-2 adrenergic agonist, Bronchodilator
Half-life: 40–56 hours
Clinically important, potentially hazardous interactions with: acetazolamide, adrenergics, aminophylline, arsenic, corticosteroids, diuretics, erythromycin, ketoconazole, MAO inhibitors, pazopanib, QT prolonging agents, ritonavir, steroids, telavancin, theophylline, tricyclic antidepressants, verapamil, xanthine derivatives
Pregnancy category: C
Important contra-indications noted in the prescribing guidelines for: nursing mothers; pediatric patients
Note: Studies in asthma patients showed that long-acting beta$_2$-adrenergic agonists may increase the risk of asthma-related death. Contraindicated in patients with asthma without use of a long-term asthma control medication. Utibron Neohaler is indacaterol and glycopyrrolate.
Black Box Warning: ASTHMA-RELATED DEATH

Mucosal
Oropharyngeal pain [2]

Central Nervous System
Headache (5%) [3]
Pain (oropharyngeal) (2%)

Gastrointestinal/Hepatic
Nausea (2%)

Respiratory
COPD (exacerbation) [6]
Cough (7%) [8]
Influenza [2]
Nasopharyngitis (5%) [6]
Upper respiratory tract infection [3]

Other
Adverse effects [6]

INDAPAMIDE

Trade name: Lozol (Sanofi-Aventis)
Indications: Edema
Class: Diuretic, thiazide
Half-life: 14–18 hours
Clinically important, potentially hazardous interactions with: digoxin, lithium, zinc
Pregnancy category: B
Important contra-indications noted in the prescribing guidelines for: the elderly; nursing mothers; pediatric patients
Note: Indapamide is a sulfonamide and can be absorbed systemically. Sulfonamides can produce severe, possibly fatal, reactions such as toxic epidermal necrolysis and Stevens-Johnson syndrome.

Skin
Angioedema [3]
Erythema multiforme [2]
Pemphigus foliaceus [2]
Peripheral edema (<5%) [2]
Pruritus (<5%) [2]
Rash (<5%) [4]
Toxic epidermal necrolysis [3]
Urticaria (<5%)
Vasculitis (<5%)

Mucosal
Xerostomia (<5%) [2]

Cardiovascular
Flushing (<5%)
QT prolongation [5]

Central Nervous System
Paresthesias (<5%)
Vertigo (dizziness) [2]

Endocrine/Metabolic
Hypokalemia [2]
Hyponatremia [2]

INDINAVIR

Trade name: Crixivan (Merck)
Indications: HIV infection
Class: Antiretroviral, CYP3A4 inhibitor, HIV-1 protease inhibitor
Half-life: ~1.8 hours
Clinically important, potentially hazardous interactions with: abiraterone, alfuzosin, almotriptan, alosetron, alprazolam, amiodarone, amprenavir, antacids, antiarrhythmics, antifungal agents, artemether/lumefantrine, astemizole, atazanavir, atorvastatin, atovaquone, atovaquone/proguanil, avanafil, bepridil, bortezomib, bosentan, brinzolamide, cabazitaxel, cabozantinib, calcium channel blockers, carbamazepine, chlordiazepoxide, ciclesonide, cisapride, clarithromycin, clonazepam, clorazepate, colchicine, conivaptan, corticosteroids, crizotinib, cyclosporine, CYP3A4 inducers and substrates, darifenacin, darunavir, dasatinib, deferasirox, delavirdine, diazepam, didanosine, dienogest, digoxin, dihydroergotamine, dronedarone, dutasteride, efavirenz, enfuvirtide, eplerenone, ergot derivatives, ergotamine, estazolam, estrogens, etravirine, everolimus, felodipine, fentanyl, fesoterodine, flibanserin, flurazepam,

fluticasone propionate, food, fusidic acid, grapefruit juice, guanfacine, H_2-antagonists, halazepam, halofantrine, HMG-CoA reductase inhibitors, itraconazole, ixabepilone, ketoconazole, lapatinib, lidocaine, lomitapide, lopinavir, lovastatin, maraviroc, meperidine, methylergonovine, methylprednisolone, methysergide, midazolam, mifepristone, mometasone, nefazodone, nelfinavir, nevirapine, nicardipine, nifedipine, nilotinib, nisoldipine, P-glycoprotein inhibitors and inducers, paclitaxel, pantoprazole, paricalcitol, pazopanib, PEG-interferon, phenobarbital, phenytoin, pimecrolimus, pimozide, ponatinib, prasugrel, protease inhibitors, proton pump inhibitors, quazepam, quinidine, quinine, ranolazine, rifabutin, rifampin, rifapentine, rilpivirine, rivaroxaban, romidepsin, rosuvastatin, ruxolitinib, salmeterol, saxagliptin, sildenafil, silodosin, simeprevir, simvastatin, sirolimus, solifenacin, sorafenib, St John's wort, sunitinib, tacrolimus, tadalafil, tamsulosin, telithromycin, temsirolimus, tenofovir disoproxil, theophylline, ticagrelor, tolvaptan, trazodone, triazolam, tricyclic antidepressants, valproic acid, vardenafil, vemurafenib, venetoclax, venlafaxine, zidovudine
Pregnancy category: C
Important contra-indications noted in the prescribing guidelines for: nursing mothers; pediatric patients
Note: Protease inhibitors cause dyslipidemia which includes elevated triglycerides and cholesterol and redistribution of body fat centrally to produce the so-called 'protease paunch', breast enlargement, facial atrophy, and 'buffalo hump'.

Skin
Bromhidrosis (<2%)
Dermatitis (<2%)
Diaphoresis (<2%)
Folliculitis (<2%)
Herpes simplex (<2%)
Herpes zoster (<2%)
Jaundice (2%)
Lipodystrophy [8]
Lipomatosis [2]
Pruritus [2]
Rash [2]
Seborrhea (<2%)
Stevens–Johnson syndrome [2]
Xerosis [2]

Hair
Alopecia [5]

Nails
Onychocryptosis [2]
Paronychia [5]
Pyogenic granuloma [3]

Mucosal
Aphthous stomatitis (<2%)
Cheilitis [4]
Gingivitis (<2%)

Cardiovascular
Flushing (<2%)

Central Nervous System
Anorexia (3%)
Dysesthesia (<2%)
Dysgeusia (taste perversion) (3%)
Fever (2%)
Headache (5%)
Hyperesthesia (<2%)
Paresthesias (<2%)
Somnolence (drowsiness) (2%)
Vertigo (dizziness) (3%)

Neuromuscular/Skeletal
Asthenia (fatigue) (2%)
Back pain (8%)
Myalgia/Myopathy with lovastatin or simvastatin (<2%)

Gastrointestinal/Hepatic
Abdominal pain (17%) [2]
Diarrhea (3%)
Dyspepsia (2%)
Nausea (12%)
Vomiting (8%)

Respiratory
Cough (2%)

Endocrine/Metabolic
ALT increased (5%)
Appetite increased (2%)
AST increased (4%)
Creatine phosphokinase increased [2]
Diabetes mellitus [2]
Gynecomastia [4]
Porphyria (acute) [2]

Genitourinary
Crystalluria [2]
Dysuria (2%)

Renal
Nephrolithiasis (9%) [4]
Nephrotoxicity [13]

Ocular
Eyelid edema (<2%)

Other
Bruxism (<2%)

INDOMETHACIN

Synonym: indometacin
Indications: Arthritis
Class: Non-steroidal anti-inflammatory (NSAID)
Half-life: 4.5 hours
Clinically important, potentially hazardous interactions with: aldesleukin, aspirin, atenolol, cyclopenthiazide, diflunisal, diuretics, methotrexate, NSAIDs, prednisolone, prednisone, sermorelin, tiludronate, torsemide, triamterene, urokinase
Pregnancy category: C
Important contra-indications noted in the prescribing guidelines for: nursing mothers; pediatric patients
Note: NSAIDs may cause an increased risk of serious cardiovascular and gastrointestinal adverse events, which can be fatal. This risk may increase with duration of use.
Black Box Warning: RISK OF SERIOUS CARDIOVASCULAR AND GASTROINTESTINAL EVENTS

Skin
Angioedema [2]
Bullous dermatitis [2]
Dermatitis [5]
Dermatitis herpetiformis (exacerbation) [2]
Edema (3–9%)
Exanthems (<5%) [7]
Fixed eruption [2]
Pruritus (<10%) [3]
Psoriasis [7]
Purpura [5]
Rash (>10%)
Toxic epidermal necrolysis [6]
Urticaria [7]
Vasculitis [5]

Mucosal
Oral lesions (<7%) [2]
Oral ulceration [4]

Central Nervous System
Psychosis [3]

Gastrointestinal/Hepatic
Gastrointestinal bleeding [2]
Gastrointestinal perforation [3]
Gastrointestinal ulceration [3]
Pancreatitis [2]

Otic
Tinnitus [2]

Ocular
Periorbital edema [2]

Other
Adverse effects [8]

INFLIXIMAB

Trade names: Inflectra (Celltrion) ((Remsima)), Remicade (Centocor)
Indications: Crohn's disease, ulcerative colitis, rheumatoid arthritis, ankylosing spondylitis, psoriatic arthritis, plaque psoriasis
Class: Cytokine inhibitor, Disease-modifying antirheumatic drug (DMARD), Monoclonal antibody, TNF inhibitor
Half-life: 8–10 days
Clinically important, potentially hazardous interactions with: abatacept, anakinra, live vaccines, methotrexate, tocilizumab
Pregnancy category: B
Important contra-indications noted in the prescribing guidelines for: the elderly; nursing mothers
Note: TNF inhibitors should be used in patients with heart failure only after consideration of other treatment options.
Contraindicated in patients with a personal or family history of multiple sclerosis or demyelinating disease. TNF inhibitors should not be administered to patients with moderate to severe heart failure (New York Heart Association Functional Class III/IV).
Black Box Warning: SERIOUS INFECTIONS and MALIGNANCY

Skin
Abscess [4]
Acneform eruption [6]
AGEP [2]
Anaphylactoid reactions/Anaphylaxis [10]
Candidiasis (5%) [4]
Cellulitis [5]
Dermatitis [4]
Eczema [5]
Edema [3]

Erythema multiforme [2]
Exanthems [4]
Folliculitis [2]
Hand–foot syndrome [2]
Herpes simplex [4]
Herpes zoster [10]
Hypersensitivity [11]
Lichen planus [2]
Lichenoid eruption [3]
Lupus erythematosus [33]
Lupus syndrome [11]
Lymphoma [9]
Malignancies [2]
Molluscum contagiosum [2]
Neoplasms [2]
Nevi [2]
Palmar–plantar pustulosis [3]
Pityriasis lichenoides chronica [2]
Pruritus (7%) [8]
Pseudolymphoma [2]
Psoriasis [51]
Pustules [5]
Rash (10%) [13]
Sarcoidosis [3]
Serum sickness (<3%) [6]
Toxic epidermal necrolysis [2]
Toxicity [2]
Urticaria [6]
Vasculitis [16]
Vitiligo [4]

Hair
Alopecia [4]
Alopecia areata [3]

Cardiovascular
Cardiotoxicity [2]
Chest pain [3]
Hypertension (7%) [3]

Central Nervous System
Aseptic meningitis [2]
Chills (5–9%) [2]
Demyelination [2]
Fever (7%) [9]
Headache (18%) [10]
Leukoencephalopathy [2]
Neurotoxicity [6]
Pain (8%) [3]
Paresthesias (<4%) [2]
Peripheral neuropathy [5]
Seizures [2]
Vertigo (dizziness) [3]

Neuromuscular/Skeletal
Arthralgia (<8%) [13]
Asthenia (fatigue) (9%) [4]
Back pain (8%)
Myalgia/Myopathy (5%) [7]
Polymyositis [2]

Gastrointestinal/Hepatic
Abdominal pain (12%) [3]
Crohn's disease (26%)
Diarrhea (12%)
Dyspepsia (10%)
Hepatitis [10]
Hepatotoxicity [16]
Nausea (21%) [3]

Respiratory
Bronchitis (10%)
Cough (12%) [2]
Dyspnea (6%) [2]
Pharyngitis (12%)
Pneumonia [10]
Pulmonary toxicity [5]
Rhinitis (8%)
Sinusitis (14%) [2]
Tuberculosis [11]
Upper respiratory tract infection (32%) [4]

Endocrine/Metabolic
ALT increased [2]

Genitourinary
Cystitis [2]
Urinary tract infection (8%)

Renal
Nephrotoxicity [2]

Hematologic
Neutropenia [4]
Sepsis [2]
Thrombocytopenia [5]

Ocular
Optic neuritis [2]
Uveitis [2]

Local
Application-site reactions (mild) (<4%) [6]
Infusion-related reactions [14]
Infusion-site reactions (20%) [12]
Injection-site reactions (6%) [9]

Other
Adverse effects [42]
Allergic reactions [7]
Death [10]
Infection (36%) [51]
Nocardiosis [3]
Side effects [2]
Systemic reactions [2]

INFLUENZA VACCINE

Trade names: Afluria (Seqirus), Agrippal (Chiron), Comvax (Merck), Fluad (Novartis), Fluarix (GSK), FluMist (Medimmune) (Wyeth), Flurix (GSK), Fluviral (Shire), Inflexal V (Berna Biotech), Invivac (Solvay), Vaxigrip (Sanofi-Aventis)
Indications: Influenza prevention
Class: Vaccine
Half-life: N/A
Clinically important, potentially hazardous interactions with: aminophylline, carbamazepine, cyclosporine, mercaptopurine, phenobarbital, phenytoin, prednisone, vincristine, warfarin
Pregnancy category: C
Important contra-indications noted in the prescribing guidelines for: pediatric patients
Note: Inactivated influenza vaccine should not be given to persons with anaphylactic hypersensitivity to eggs or other components of the vaccine. For current data on influenza in the USA consult the Centers for Disease Control and Protection website (www.cdc.gov/flu).

Skin
Anaphylactoid reactions/Anaphylaxis (rare) [2]
Henoch–Schönlein purpura [2]
Linear IgA bullous dermatosis [2]
Purpura [2]
Rash [3]
Serum sickness [2]
Vasculitis [9]

Central Nervous System
Fever [12]
Guillain–Barré syndrome [11]
Headache [8]
Seizures [3]

Neuromuscular/Skeletal
Asthenia (fatigue) [6]
Myalgia/Myopathy [9]
Polymyositis [4]

Gastrointestinal/Hepatic
Abdominal pain [2]

Respiratory
Asthma [2]
Cough [2]

Hematologic
Thrombocytopenia [2]

Ocular
Oculorespiratory syndrome [15]
Optic neuritis [2]

Local
Injection-site edema [4]
Injection-site erythema [7]
Injection-site induration [5]
Injection-site inflammation [3]
Injection-site pain (20–28%) [14]
Injection-site reactions [2]

Other
Adverse effects [7]
Side effects [4]
Systemic reactions (injection site) [5]

INGENOL MEBUTATE

Trade name: Picato (Leo Pharma)
Indications: Actinic keratosis
Class: Cell death inducer
Half-life: N/A
Clinically important, potentially hazardous interactions with: none known
Pregnancy category: C
Important contra-indications noted in the prescribing guidelines for: pediatric patients

---

Skin
Crusting [4]
Erythema [4]
Flaking [4]
Scaling [3]

Central Nervous System
Headache (2%) [4]

Respiratory
Nasopharyngitis (2%) [2]

Ocular
Eyelid edema [2]
Periorbital edema (3%) [2]

Local
Application-site erythema [2]
Application-site infection (3%) [2]
Application-site pain (2–15%) [5]
Application-site pruritus (8%) [3]
Application-site reactions [3]

INSULIN ASPART

Trade names: NovoLog (Novo Nordisk), NovoRapid (Novo Nordisk), Ryzodeg (Novo Nordisk)
Indications: Diabetes mellitus
Class: Hormone, polypeptide
Half-life: 81 minutes
Clinically important, potentially hazardous interactions with: ACE inhibitors, alcohol, atypical antipsychotics, beta blockers, clonidine, corticosteroids, danazol, disopyramide, diuretics, epinephrine, estrogens, fibrates, fluoxetine, isoniazid, isoniazid, lithium salts, MAO inhibitors, niacin, octreotide, oral contraceptives, pentamidine, phenothiazine derivatives, pramlintide, propoxyphene, salbutamol, salicylates, somatropin, sulfonamide antibiotics, terbutaline, thyroid hormones
Pregnancy category: B
Important contra-indications noted in the prescribing guidelines for: the elderly; pediatric patients
Note: Ryzodeg is insulin aspart and insulin degludec; various forms of insulin are available - see other insulin profiles for reaction details.

Skin
Lipodystrophy (>5%)
Peripheral edema (>5%)

Nails
Onychomycosis (10%)

Cardiovascular
Chest pain (5%)

Central Nervous System
Headache (12%) [2]
Hyporeflexia (11%)

Gastrointestinal/Hepatic
Abdominal pain (5%)
Diarrhea (5%)
Nausea (7%)

Respiratory
Nasopharyngitis [2]
Sinusitis (5%)

Endocrine/Metabolic
Diabetic ketoacidosis [2]
Hypoglycemia (75%) [5]
Weight gain (>5%)

Genitourinary
Urinary tract infection (8%)

INSULIN DEGLUDEC

Trade names: Ryzodeg (Novo Nordisk), Tresiba (Novo Nordisk)
Indications: Diabetes mellitus
Class: Human insulin analog, long-acting
Half-life: 25 hours
Clinically important, potentially hazardous interactions with: ACE inhibitors, albuterol, alcohol, angiotensin II receptor blocking agents, beta blockers, clonidine, clozapine, corticosteroids, danazol, DDP-4-inhibitors, disopyramide, diuretics, epinephrine, estrogens, fibrates, fluoxetine, GLP-1 receptor agonists, glucagon, guanethidine, isoniazid, lithium, MAO inhibitors, niacin, octreotide, olanzapine, oral contraceptives, pentamidine, pentoxifylline, phenothiazines, pramlintide, propoxyphene, protease inhibitors, reserpine, salicylates, SGLT-2 inhibitors, somatropin, sulfonamide antibiotics, terbutaline, thyroid hormones
Pregnancy category: C
Important contra-indications noted in the prescribing guidelines for: the elderly; nursing mothers; pediatric patients
Note: Contraindicated during episodes of hypoglycemia. Ryzodeg is insulin degludec and insulin aspart; various forms of insulin are available - see other insulin profiles for reaction details.

Skin
Hypersensitivity [2]
Peripheral edema (<3%)

Central Nervous System
Headache (9–12%) [8]

Gastrointestinal/Hepatic
Diarrhea (6%) [5]
Gastroenteritis (5%)
Nausea [6]

Respiratory
Nasopharyngitis (13–24%) [9]
Sinusitis (5%)
Upper respiratory tract infection (8–12%) [2]

Endocrine/Metabolic
Diabetic ketoacidosis [2]
Hypoglycemia [9]

Ocular
Retinopathy [2]

Local
Injection-site reactions (4%) [6]

Other
Adverse effects [3]

INSULIN DETEMIR

Trade name: Levemir (Novo Nordisk)
Indications: Diabetes (Type I or II)
Class: Human insulin analog, long-acting
Half-life: 5–7 hours
Clinically important, potentially hazardous interactions with: albuterol, alcohol, antipsychotics, beta blockers, clonidine, clozapine, corticosteroids, danazol, diuretics, epinephrine, estrogens, guanethidine, isoniazid, lithium, niacin, olanzapine, oral antidiabetics, oral contraceptives, pentamidine, phenothiazines, propranolol, protease inhibitors, reserpine, somatropin, terbutaline, thiazolidinediones, thyroid hormones
Pregnancy category: B
Important contra-indications noted in the prescribing guidelines for: the elderly; nursing mothers; pediatric patients
Note: Various forms of insulin are available - see other insulin profiles for reaction details.

Central Nervous System
Fever (10%)
Headache (7–31%) [3]

Neuromuscular/Skeletal
Back pain (8%)

Gastrointestinal/Hepatic
Abdominal pain (6–13%)
Gastroenteritis (6–17%)
Nausea (7%)
Vomiting (7%)

Respiratory
Bronchitis (5%)
Cough (8%)
Flu-like syndrome (6–14%)
Pharyngitis (10–17%)
Rhinitis (7%)
Upper respiratory tract infection (13–36%)

Endocrine/Metabolic
Hyperglycemia [2]
Hypoglycemia [4]

Local
Injection-site reactions (3–4%) [4]

Other
Allergic reactions [3]
Infection (viral) (7%)

INSULIN GLARGINE

Trade names: Basaglar (Lilly), Lantus (Sanofi-Aventis)
Indications: Diabetes (Type I or II)
Class: Hormone analog, polypeptide
Half-life: N/A
Clinically important, potentially hazardous interactions with: ACE inhibitors, albuterol, alcohol, beta blockers, clonidine, clozapine, corticosteroids, danazol, disopyramide, diuretics, epinephrine, estrogens, fibrates, fluoxetine, glucagon, guanethidine, isoniazid, lithium, MAO inhibitors, niacin, olanzapine, oral antidiabetic products, oral contraceptives, pentamidine, pentoxifylline, phenothiazine derivatives, pramlintide, propoxyphene, propranolol, protease inhibitors, reserpine, salicylates, somatostain analogs, somatropin, sulfonamide antibiotics, terbutaline, thyroid hormones
Pregnancy category: C
Important contra-indications noted in the prescribing guidelines for: nursing mothers; pediatric patients
Note: Various forms of insulin are available - see other insulin profiles for reaction details.

Skin
Lipoatrophy [2]
Peripheral edema (20%)

Central Nervous System
Depression (11%)
Headache (6–10%) [4]

Neuromuscular/Skeletal
Arthralgia (14%)
Back pain (13%)
Pain in extremities (13%)

Gastrointestinal/Hepatic
Diarrhea (11%) [6]
Nausea [5]
Vomiting [4]

Respiratory
Bronchitis (15%)

Cough (12%)
Influenza (19%)
Nasopharyngitis [6]
Pharyngitis (8%)
Rhinitis (5%)
Sinusitis (19%)
Upper respiratory tract infection (11–29%) [3]

Endocrine/Metabolic
Hypoglycemia [4]

Genitourinary
Urinary tract infection (11%)

Ocular
Cataract (18%)
Retinopathy [2]

Local
Injection-site pain (3%)
Injection-site reactions [4]

Other
Adverse effects [5]
Infection (9–14%)

INSULIN GLULISINE

Trade name: Apidra (Sanofi-Aventis)
Indications: Diabetes
Class: Insulin analog
Half-life: 13–42 minutes
Clinically important, potentially hazardous interactions with: ACE inhibitors, albuterol, alcohol, anitpsychotics, beta blockers, clonidine, clozapine, corticosteroids, danazol, disopyramide, diuretics, epinephrine, fibrates, fluoxetine, glucagon, guanethidine, isoniazid, lithium, MAO inhibitors, niacin, oral antidiabetic agents, oral contraceptives, pentamidine, pentoxifylline, phenothiazine derivatives, pramlintide, propoxyphene, propranolol, protease inhibitors, reserpine, salicylates, somatostatin analogs, somatropin, sulfonamide antibiotics, terbutaline, thyroid hormones
Pregnancy category: C
Important contra-indications noted in the prescribing guidelines for: nursing mothers; pediatric patients
Note: Various forms of insulin are available - see other insulin profiles for reaction details.

Skin
Peripheral edema (8%)

Cardiovascular
Hypertension (4%)

Central Nervous System
Headache (7%)

Neuromuscular/Skeletal
Arthralgia (6%)

Respiratory
Influenza (4–6%)
Nasopharyngitis (8–11%)
Upper respiratory tract infection (7–11%)

Endocrine/Metabolic
Hypoglycemia (6–7%) [3]

Local
Injection-site reactions (10%) [2]

INTERFERON ALFA

Synonyms: IFN; INF
Trade names: Infergen (Intermune), Intron A (Schering), Rebetron (Schering), Roferon-A (Roche)
Indications: Chronic hepatitis C virus infection, hairy cell leukemia
Class: Biologic, Immunomodulator, Interferon
Half-life: 2 hours
Clinically important, potentially hazardous interactions with: aldesleukin, amitriptyline, captopril, gemfibrozil, metaxalone, methadone, ribavirin, telbivudine, theophylline, theophylline derivatives, zafirlukast, zidovudine
Pregnancy category: C (pregnancy category will be X when used in combination with ribavirin)
Important contra-indications noted in the prescribing guidelines for: nursing mothers; pediatric patients
Note: Many of the adverse reactions depend on the nature of the disease being treated. Either hairy cell leukemia [L] or AIDS-related Kaposi's sarcoma [K].

Skin
Angioedema [3]
Bullous dermatitis [4]
Dermatitis (6%)
Eczema [6]
Edema [L] (11%) [2]
Erythema [2]
Exanthems [3]
Herpes simplex [2]
Kaposi's sarcoma [2]
Lichen planus [8]
Linear IgA bullous dermatosis [3]
Livedo reticularis [2]
Lupus erythematosus [17]
Lupus syndrome [2]
Necrosis [6]
Pemphigus [2]
Photosensitivity [2]
Pigmentation [3]
Pruritus 13% [L] 5–7% [K] (13%) [4]
Psoriasis [22]
Purpura [2]
Rash 44% [L] 11% [K] [5]
Raynaud's phenomenon [11]
Sarcoidosis [47]
Seborrheic dermatitis [2]
Sjögren's syndrome [4]
Thrombocytopenic purpura [2]
Toxicity [4]
Urticaria [K] (<3%) [3]
Vasculitis [7]
Vitiligo [9]

Hair
Alopecia (23%) [16]
Hair pigmentation [3]
Hypertrichosis [3]
Straight hair [2]

Mucosal
Aphthous stomatitis [2]
Oral lichen planus [7]
Stomatitis (<10%)
Xerostomia (>10%) [4]

Cardiovascular
Cardiotoxicity [2]
Hypertension [3]
Hypotension [2]

Central Nervous System
Ageusia (taste loss) [2]
Anorexia [4]
Anosmia [4]
Anxiety [2]
Chills [4]
Depression (5–15%) [23]
Dysgeusia (taste perversion) [K] (25%) [2]
Fever (37%) [5]
Headache (54%) [4]
Insomnia (19%)
Irritability [2]
Neurotoxicity [4]
Paresthesias 8% [L] (12%)
Parkinsonism [3]
Restless legs syndrome [2]
Rigors (35%)
Seizures [2]
Suicidal ideation [6]
Tremor [2]
Vertigo (dizziness) (16%) [2]

Neuromuscular/Skeletal
Arthralgia (28%) [3]
Asthenia (fatigue) (56%) [10]
Back pain (9%)
Myalgia/Myopathy 69% [L] 71% [K] [10]
Myasthenia gravis [11]
Rhabdomyolysis [3]

Gastrointestinal/Hepatic
Abdominal pain (15%)
Constipation [2]
Diarrhea (24%) [5]
Nausea (24%) [6]
Pancreatitis [7]
Vomiting [5]

Respiratory
Cough [2]
Dyspnea (13%) [2]
Flu-like syndrome (>10%) [10]
Pulmonary hypertension [2]

Endocrine/Metabolic
ALT increased [2]
AST increased [2]
Hyperglycemia [2]
Hyperthyroidism [3]
Thyroid dysfunction [2]
Weight loss (16%) [5]

Genitourinary
Impotence [2]

Renal
Nephrotoxicity [3]
Proteinuria [2]

Hematologic
Anemia (11%) [7]
Febrile neutropenia [2]
Hemolytic uremic syndrome [6]
Leukopenia [5]
Lymphopenia (14%)
Neutropenia (21%) [4]
Thrombocytopenia [7]

Otic
Tinnitus [4]

Ocular
- Eyelashes – hypertrichosis [3]
- Optic neuropathy [4]
- Retinopathy [6]
- Vision blurred (4%)

Local
- Injection-site alopecia [2]
- Injection-site erythema [2]
- Injection-site induration [3]
- Injection-site necrosis [16]

Other
- Adverse effects [5]
- Infection [4]
- Vogt-Koyanagi-Harada syndrome [6]

INTERFERON BETA

Trade names: Avonex (Biogen), Betaferon (Bayer), Betaseron (Bayer), Plegridy (Biogen), Rebif (Merck)
Indications: Relapsing multiple sclerosis, cancers
Class: Immunomodulator, Interferon
Half-life: 10 hours
Clinically important, potentially hazardous interactions with: theophylline, theophylline derivatives, zidovudine
Pregnancy category: C
Important contra-indications noted in the prescribing guidelines for: nursing mothers; pediatric patients

---

Skin
- Cyst (4%)
- Diaphoresis (23%)
- Edema (generalized) (8%)
- Herpes simplex (2–3%)
- Herpes zoster (3)
- Hypersensitivity (3%)
- Lipoatrophy [2]
- Lupus erythematosus [8]
- Nevi (3%)
- Nicolau syndrome [2]
- Rash [2]
- Raynaud's phenomenon [2]
- Sarcoidosis [2]
- Thrombocytopenic purpura [4]
- Urticaria (5%)
- Vasculitis [4]

Hair
- Alopecia (4%)

Mucosal
- Mucosal bleeding (12–38%)

Cardiovascular
- Capillary leak syndrome [3]

Central Nervous System
- Chills (21%)
- Depression [8]
- Fever [3]
- Headache [4]
- Multiple sclerosis [2]
- Pain (52%)
- Paresthesias [2]
- Psychosis [2]
- Seizures (2%) [2]
- Vertigo (dizziness) (35%)

Neuromuscular/Skeletal
- Arthralgia [2]
- Asthenia (fatigue) [2]
- Myalgia/Myopathy (44%)
- Rhabdomyolysis [2]

Gastrointestinal/Hepatic
- Hepatotoxicity [5]

Respiratory
- Flu-like syndrome (61%) [12]
- Upper respiratory tract infection (31%)

Endocrine/Metabolic
- Mastodynia (7%)
- Thyroid dysfunction [4]

Genitourinary
- Vaginitis (4%)

Renal
- Nephrotoxicity [2]

Hematologic
- Hemolytic uremic syndrome [3]
- Thrombotic complications [2]

Ocular
- Retinopathy [3]

Local
- Injection-site ecchymoses (2%)
- Injection-site inflammation (3%)
- Injection-site necrosis [3]
- Injection-site purpura (2%)
- Injection-site reactions (4%) [8]

Other
- Adverse effects [4]
- Death [4]
- Infection (11%) [3]

IPILIMUMAB

Trade name: Yervoy (Bristol-Myers Squibb)
Indications: Melanoma
Class: Biologic, CTLA-4-blocking monoclonal antibody, Monoclonal antibody
Half-life: 15 days
Clinically important, potentially hazardous interactions with: none known
Pregnancy category: C
Important contra-indications noted in the prescribing guidelines for: nursing mothers; pediatric patients
Black Box Warning: IMMUNE-MEDIATED ADVERSE REACTIONS

Skin
- Dermatitis (12%) [11]
- Exanthems [5]
- Granulomas [3]
- Lymphadenopathy [2]
- Pruritus (21–31%) [18]
- Rash (19–29%) [25]
- Sarcoidosis [2]
- Toxicity [3]
- Urticaria (2%) [2]
- Vitiligo [3]

Cardiovascular
- Pericarditis [2]

Central Nervous System
- Anorexia [2]
- Encephalitis [2]
- Encephalopathy [3]
- Fever [3]
- Guillain–Barré syndrome [2]
- Headache (14%) [2]
- Neurotoxicity [3]

Neuromuscular/Skeletal
- Arthralgia [2]
- Asthenia (fatigue) (34–41%) [8]
- Myalgia/Myopathy [2]
- Myasthenia gravis [3]
- Rhabdomyolysis [2]

Gastrointestinal/Hepatic
- Abdominal pain [2]
- Colitis (5–8%) [38]
- Diarrhea (32–37%) [38]
- Enterocolitis (7%) [5]
- Gastrointestinal perforation [4]
- Hepatitis [12]
- Hepatotoxicity (<2%) [15]
- Nausea [3]
- Pancreatitis [2]

Respiratory
- Pneumonia [3]
- Pneumonitis [6]

Endocrine/Metabolic
- Adrenal insufficiency [2]
- ALT increased [9]
- AST increased [8]
- Hyperthyroidism [2]
- Hypophysitis [28]
- Hypopituitarism (<4%)
- Hypothyroidism [8]
- Thyroid dysfunction [3]
- Thyroiditis [11]

Renal
- Nephrotoxicity [6]
- Renal failure [3]

Hematologic
- Anemia [2]
- Neutropenia [4]
- Thrombocytopenia [4]

Ocular
- Iridocyclitis [2]
- Orbital inflammation [3]
- Retinitis [2]
- Uveitis [6]

Local
- Infusion-related reactions [3]

Other
- Adverse effects [19]
- Death [8]

IPRATROPIUM

Trade names: Atrovent (Boehringer Ingelheim), Combivent (Boehringer Ingelheim), Duoneb (Mylan Specialty), Ipratropium Steri-Neb (Ivax), Rinatec (Boehringer Ingelheim)
Indications: Bronchospasm
Class: Anticholinergic, Muscarinic antagonist
Half-life: 2 hours
Clinically important, potentially hazardous interactions with: anticholinergics
Pregnancy category: B
Important contra-indications noted in the prescribing guidelines for: nursing mothers
Note: Combivent is ipratropium and albuterol.

Mucosal
Oral lesions (<5%)
Oral ulceration [2]
Xerostomia (3%) [3]

Central Nervous System
Dysgeusia (taste perversion) [2]
Trembling (<10%)

Ocular
Mydriasis [2]

Other
Adverse effects [2]

IRBESARTAN

Trade names: Aprovel (Bristol-Myers Squibb), Avalide (Bristol-Myers Squibb), Avapro (Sanofi-Aventis)
Indications: Hypertension, diabetic nephropathy
Class: Angiotensin II receptor antagonist (blocker), Antihypertensive
Half-life: 11–15 hours
Clinically important, potentially hazardous interactions with: ACE inhibitors, adrenergic neurone blockers, alcohol, aldesleukin, aldosterone antagonists, aliskiren, alpha blockers, alprostadil, amifostine, antihypertensives, antipsychotics, anxiolytics and hypnotics, baclofen, beta blockers, calcium channel blockers, carvedilol, clonidine, corticosteroids, cyclosporine, CYP2C8 and CYP2C9 substrates, diazoxide, diuretics, eplerenone, fluconazole, general anesthetics, heparins, hypotensives, levodopa, lithium, MAO inhibitors, methyldopa, methylphenidate, moxisylyte, moxonidine, nitrates, NSAIDs, pentoxifylline, phosphodiesterase 5 inhibitors, potassium salts, prostacyclin analogues, rifamycin derivatives, rituximab, tacrolimus, tizanidine, tolvaptan, trimethoprim
Pregnancy category: D (category C in first trimester; category D in second and third trimesters)
Important contra-indications noted in the prescribing guidelines for: nursing mothers; pediatric patients
Note: Avalide is irbesartan and hydrochlorothiazide. Hydrochlorothiazide is a sulfonamide which can be absorbed systemically. Sulfonamides can produce severe, possibly fatal, reactions such as toxic epidermal necrolysis and Stevens-Johnson syndrome.
Black Box Warning: FETAL TOXICITY

Skin
Angioedema [3]
Edema (<10%)
Peripheral edema [2]
Rash (<10%)

Gastrointestinal/Hepatic
Pancreatitis [2]

Respiratory
Cough [2]

IRINOTECAN

Trade names: Camptosar (Pfizer), Onivyde (Merrimack)
Indications: Metastatic colorectal carcinoma (Camptosar), metastatic adenocarcinoma of the pancreas (Onivyde - in combination with fluorouracil and leucovorin)
Class: Antineoplastic, Topoisomerase I inhibitor
Half-life: 6–10 hours
Clinically important, potentially hazardous interactions with: aprepitant, atazanavir, bevacizumab, ketoconazole, lapatinib, sorafenib, St John's wort, strong CYP3A4 inhibitors, voriconazole
Pregnancy category: D
Important contra-indications noted in the prescribing guidelines for: the elderly; nursing mothers; pediatric patients
Black Box Warning: DIARRHEA and MYELOSUPPRESSION (Camptosar)
SEVERE NEUTROPENIA and SEVERE DIARRHEA (Onivyde)

Skin
Acneform eruption [4]
Exfoliative dermatitis (14%)
Hand–foot syndrome [6]
Pruritus [4]
Rash (46%) [7]

Hair
Alopecia (13–61%) [24]

Mucosal
Mucositis (30%) [2]
Stomatitis (<14%) [4]

Cardiovascular
Bradycardia [2]
Flushing (11%)
Hypertension [6]
Hypotension (5%)
Thrombophlebitis (<10%)
Vasodilation (6%)

Central Nervous System
Anorexia (44%) [15]
Chills (14%)
Confusion (3%)
Dysarthria [2]
Fever (44%) [3]
Insomnia [2]
Neurotoxicity [5]
Pain (23%)
Somnolence (drowsiness) (9%)
Vertigo (dizziness) (21%)

Neuromuscular/Skeletal
Asthenia (fatigue) (69%) [16]

Gastrointestinal/Hepatic
Abdominal pain (68%) [3]
Constipation (32%) [2]
Diarrhea (83%) [35]
Hepatotoxicity [4]
Nausea (82%) [16]
Vomiting (63%) [14]

Respiratory
Cough (20%)
Dyspnea (22%)
Pneumonia (4%) [4]

Endocrine/Metabolic
Dehydration [4]

Renal
Proteinuria [3]

Hematologic
Anemia (97%) [11]
Febrile neutropenia [7]
Leukopenia (96%) [10]
Lymphopenia [2]
Neutropenia (96%) [34]
Thrombocytopenia (96%) [7]

Other
Adverse effects [3]
Allergic reactions (9%)
Death [5]
Infection (14%) [2]

ISAVUCONAZONIUM SULFATE

Trade name: Cresemba (Astellas)
Indications: Invasive aspergillosis, mucormycosis
Class: Antifungal, azole
Half-life: 130 hours
Clinically important, potentially hazardous interactions with: carbamazepine, ketoconazole, rifampin, ritonavir, St John's wort, strong CYP3A4 inducers or inhibitors
Pregnancy category: C
Important contra-indications noted in the prescribing guidelines for: nursing mothers; pediatric patients
Note: Contraindicated in patients with familial short QT syndrome.

Skin
Dermatitis (<5%)
Erythema (<5%)
Exfoliative dermatitis (<5%)
Hypersensitivity (<5%)
Peripheral edema (15%)
Petechiae (<5%)
Pruritus (8%)
Rash (9%)
Urticaria (<5%)

Hair
Alopecia (<5%)

Mucosal
Gingivitis (<5%)
Stomatitis (<5%)

Cardiovascular
Atrial fibrillation (<5%)
Atrial flutter (<5%)
Bradycardia (<5%)
Cardiac arrest (<5%)
Chest pain (9%)
Extrasystoles (<5%)
Hypotension (8%)
Palpitation (<5%)
QT interval shortening (<5%)
Thrombophlebitis (<5%)

Central Nervous System
Anxiety (8%)
Chills (<5%)
Confusion (<5%)
Delirium (9%)

Depression (<5%)
Dysgeusia (taste perversion) (<5%)
Encephalopathy (<5%)
Gait instability (<5%)
Hallucinations (<5%)
Headache (17%)
Hypoesthesia (<5%)
Insomnia (11%)
Migraine (<5%)
Paresthesias (<5%)
Peripheral neuropathy (<5%)
Seizures (<5%)
Somnolence (drowsiness) (<5%)
Stupor (<5%)
Syncope (<5%)
Tremor (<5%)
Vertigo (dizziness) (<5%)

Neuromuscular/Skeletal
Asthenia (fatigue) (11%)
Back pain (10%)
Bone or joint pain (<5%)
Myalgia/Myopathy (<5%)
Neck pain (<5%)

Gastrointestinal/Hepatic
Abdominal distension (<5%)
Abdominal pain (17%)
Cholecystitis (<5%)
Cholelithiasis (gallstones) (<5%)
Constipation (14%)
Diarrhea (24%) [2]
Dyspepsia (6%)
Gastritis (<5%)
Hepatic failure (<5%)
Hepatomegaly (<5%)
Hepatotoxicity (17%)
Nausea (28%) [3]
Vomiting (25%)

Respiratory
Bronchospasm (<5%)
Dyspnea (17%)
Respiratory failure (7%)
Tachypnea (<5%)

Endocrine/Metabolic
Appetite decreased (9%)
Hypoalbuminemia (<5%)
Hypoglycemia (<5%)
Hypokalemia (19%)
Hypomagnesemia (5%)
Hyponatremia (<5%)

Genitourinary
Hematuria (<5%)

Renal
Proteinuria (<5%)
Renal failure (10%)

Hematologic
Agranulocytosis (<5%)
Leukopenia (<5%)
Pancytopenia (<5%)

Otic
Tinnitus (<5%)

Ocular
Optic neuropathy (<5%)

Local
Injection-site reactions (6%)

Other
Adverse effects [2]

ISONIAZID

Synonym: INH
Trade names: Rifamate (Sanofi-Aventis), Rifater (Sanofi-Aventis)
Indications: Tuberculosis
Class: Antibiotic, Antimycobacterial
Half-life: <4 hours
Clinically important, potentially hazardous interactions with: acetaminophen, betamethasone, ethosuximide, insulin aspart, insulin degludec, insulin detemir, insulin glargine, insulin glulisine, itraconazole, levodopa, metformin, phenytoin, prednisolone, propranolol, rifampin, rifapentine, triamcinolone
Pregnancy category: C

Skin
Acneform eruption [6]
AGEP [2]
Angioedema [2]
Bullous dermatitis [2]
Dermatitis [3]
DRESS syndrome [5]
Erythema multiforme [2]
Exanthems [4]
Exfoliative dermatitis [5]
Hypersensitivity [7]
Lichenoid eruption [2]
Lupus erythematosus [58]
Peripheral edema [21]
Photosensitivity [5]
Pruritus [2]
Purpura [7]
Pustules [2]
Stevens-Johnson syndrome [5]
Toxic epidermal necrolysis [9]
Toxicity [2]
Urticaria (<5%) [4]
Vasculitis [2]

Hair
Alopecia [3]

Mucosal
Oral lesions [2]

Central Nervous System
Fever [3]
Hallucinations [3]
Neurotoxicity [2]
Psychosis [2]
Seizures [9]

Neuromuscular/Skeletal
Arthralgia [2]
Rhabdomyolysis (3%) [3]

Gastrointestinal/Hepatic
Hepatotoxicity [31]
Pancreatitis [4]

Respiratory
Pleural effusion [2]

Endocrine/Metabolic
Gynecomastia [4]

Renal
Nephrotoxicity [2]

Ocular
Hallucinations, visual [2]
Optic neuritis [2]

Other
Adverse effects [5]
Death [2]
Side effects (2%) [2]

ISOSORBIDE

Indications: Acute angle-closure glaucoma
Class: Diuretic
Half-life: 5–9.5 hours
Clinically important, potentially hazardous interactions with: sildenafil
Pregnancy category: C
Note: Various forms of isosorbide are available – see other isosorbide profiles for reaction details.

Central Nervous System
Headache [10]

ISOSORBIDE DINITRATE

Trade names: Dilatrate-SR (Schwarz), Isordil (Wyeth), Sorbitrate (AstraZeneca)
Indications: Angina pectoris
Class: Nitrate, Vasodilator
Half-life: 4 hours (oral)
Clinically important, potentially hazardous interactions with: sildenafil
Pregnancy category: C
Important contra-indications noted in the prescribing guidelines for: the elderly; nursing mothers; pediatric patients
Note: Various forms of isosorbide are available – see other isosorbide profiles for reaction details.

Cardiovascular
Flushing (>10%)

Central Nervous System
Headache [3]

ISOSORBIDE MONO-NITRATE

Trade names: Imdur (Schering), Monoket (Schwarz)
Indications: Angina pectoris
Class: Nitrate, Vasodilator
Half-life: ~4 hours
Clinically important, potentially hazardous interactions with: sildenafil
Pregnancy category: B
Important contra-indications noted in the prescribing guidelines for: the elderly; nursing mothers; pediatric patients
Note: Various forms of isosorbide are available – see other isosorbide profiles for reaction details.

Cardiovascular
Flushing (>10%) [2]
Palpitation [2]

Central Nervous System
Headache [7]

Vertigo (dizziness) [2]

Other

Adverse effects [2]

ISOTRETINOIN

Synonym: 13-*cis*-retinoic acid
Trade names: Accutane (Roche), Amnesteem (Genpharm), Claravis (Barr), Roaccutane (Roche)
Indications: Cystic acne
Class: Retinoid
Half-life: 21–24 hours
Clinically important, potentially hazardous interactions with: acitretin, alcohol (ethyl), antacids, bexarotene, carbamazepine, cholestyramine, co-trimoxazole, corticosteroids, dairy products, minocycline, oral contraceptives, phenytoin, retinoids, St John's wort, tetracycline, tetracyclines, vitamin A
Pregnancy category: X
Important contra-indications noted in the prescribing guidelines for: nursing mothers; pediatric patients
Note: Oral retinoids can cause birth defects, and women should avoid isotretinoin when pregnant or trying to conceive.

Skin

Abscess [3]
Acneform eruption [19]
Angioedema [3]
Desquamation (palms and soles) (5%)
Diaphoresis [2]
Edema (subcutaneous, recurrent) [2]
Erythema nodosum [3]
Exfoliative dermatitis (<10%)
Facial edema (<10%)
Facial erythema [2]
Fragility [3]
Granulation tissue [4]
Keloid [5]
Pallor (<10%)
Photosensitivity (>10%) [7]
Pigmentation [2]
Pruritus (<5%) [5]
Pyoderma gangrenosum [2]
Rash [3]
Sweet's syndrome [2]
Urticaria [2]
Vasculitis [4]
Xanthomas [2]
Xerosis (>10%) [11]

Hair

Alopecia (16%) [3]
Curly hair [3]

Nails

Brittle nails [2]
Elkonyxis [2]
Median canaliform dystrophy [3]
Onycholysis [3]
Paronychia [4]
Pyogenic granuloma [8]

Mucosal

Cheilitis (>90%) [15]
Epistaxis (nosebleed) [2]
Mucositis [2]
Xerostomia (>10%) [5]

Central Nervous System

Depression [6]
Headache [7]
Pseudotumor cerebri [4]

Neuromuscular/Skeletal

Arthralgia [4]
Asthenia (fatigue) [2]
Myalgia/Myopathy [8]
Rhabdomyolysis [2]
Sacroiliitis [3]
Stiff person syndrome [2]

Gastrointestinal/Hepatic

Abdominal pain [3]
Hepatotoxicity [3]
Pancreatitis [3]

Endocrine/Metabolic

Amenorrhea [2]
Gynecomastia [2]
Hypercholesterolemia [2]
Hyperlipidemia [2]
Hypertriglyceridemia [5]

Hematologic

Neutropenia [2]

Ocular

Photophobia [2]
Xerophthalmia [2]

Other

Adverse effects [7]
Side effects [2]
Teratogenicity [8]

ISRADIPINE

Trade name: DynaCirc (Reliant)
Indications: Hypertension
Class: Calcium channel blocker
Half-life: 8 hours
Clinically important, potentially hazardous interactions with: amprenavir, delavirdine, epirubicin, imatinib, phenytoin
Pregnancy category: C

Skin

Edema (7%) [6]
Exanthems (2%) [2]
Pruritus (<6%)
Rash (2%)

Mucosal

Oral lesions (6%)

Cardiovascular

Flushing (2–9%) [9]
QT prolongation [2]

Central Nervous System

Headache (9%)
Vertigo (dizziness) (9%)

ITRACONAZOLE

Trade names: Onmel (Merz), Sporanox (Janssen)
Indications: Onychomycosis, deep mycoses, oropharyngeal candidiasis (oral solution only)
Class: Antibiotic, triazole, Antifungal, azole, CYP3A4 inhibitor
Half-life: 21 hours
Clinically important, potentially hazardous interactions with: abiraterone, afatinib, alfentanil, alfuzosin, aliskiren, alprazolam, amphotericin B, amprenavir, anisindione, antacids, aprepitant, aripiprazole, artemether/lumefantrine, astemizole, atazanavir, atorvastatin, avanafil, boceprevir, bosentan, budesonide, buspirone, busulfan, cabazitaxel, cabozantinib, calcium channel blockers, carbamazepine, cerivastatin, ciclesonide, cilostazol, cimetidine, cinacalcet, cisapride, clarithromycin, clopidogrel, clorazepate, cobicistat/elvitegravir/emtricitabine/tenofovir disoproxil, cobimetinib, colchicine, conivaptan, corticosteroids, coumarins, crizotinib, cyclophosphamide, cyclosporine, cyproterone, dabigatran, darifenacin, dasatinib, dexamethasone, diazepam, dicumarol, didanosine, digoxin, dihydroergotamine, dihydropyridines, disopyramide, docetaxel, dofetilide, dronedarone, efavirenz, eletriptan, enzalutamide, eplerenone, ergotamine, erlotinib, erythromycin, estradiol, ethotoin, everolimus, felodipine, fentanyl, fesoterodine, flibanserin, fluticasone propionate, fosamprenavir, fosphenytoin, gefitinib, grapefruit juice, halofantrine, haloperidol, histamine H_2-antagonists, HMG-CoA reductase inhibitors, iloperidone, imatinib, indinavir, irinotecan, isoniazid, ivabradine, ixabepilone, lapatinib, lercanidipine, levomethadyl, lomitapide, lopinavir, lovastatin, lurasidone, mephenytoin, methadone, methylergonovine, methylprednisolone, methysergide, micafungin, midazolam(oral), mifepristone, mizolastine, nevirapine, nilotinib, nisoldipine, omeprazole, oral hypoglycemics, osimertinib, paclitaxel, paliperidone, pantoprazole, pazopanib, phenobarbital, phenytoin, pimecrolimus, pimozide, ponatinib, prednisolone, prednisone, proton pump inhibitors, quetiapine, quinidine, ranolazine, reboxetine, regorafenib, repaglinide, rifabutin, rifampin, rilpivirine, rimonabant, ritonavir, rivaroxaban, romidepsin, ruxolitinib, saquinavir, sildenafil, silodosin, simeprevir, simvastatin, sirolimus, solifenacin, sunitinib, tacrolimus, tadalafil, telaprevir, telithromycin, temsirolimus, terfenadine, ticagrelor, tolterodine, tolvaptan, triamcinolone, triazolam, trimetrexate, ulipristal, vardenafil, vemurafenib, venetoclax, vinblastine, vincristine, vinflunine, vinorelbine, warfarin
Pregnancy category: C
Important contra-indications noted in the prescribing guidelines for: nursing mothers
Note: Contraindicated in patients with evidence of ventricular dysfunction such as congestive heart failure (CHF) or a history of CHF except for the treatment of life-threatening or other serious infections.

Black Box Warning: CONGESTIVE HEART FAILURE, CARDIAC EFFECTS AND DRUG INTERACTIONS

Skin
AGEP [3]
Angioedema [2]
Diaphoresis (3%)
Edema (<4%) [10]
Exanthems (<3%) [7]
Peripheral edema (4%)
Phototoxicity [2]
Pruritus (<3%) [8]
Rash (8%) [9]
Urticaria [3]

Hair
Alopecia [2]

Mucosal
Xerostomia [2]

Cardiovascular
Cardiac arrest [2]
Cardiac failure [3]
Congestive heart failure [3]
Hypertension (3%) [3]
QT prolongation [5]
Torsades de pointes [2]

Central Nervous System
Fever [2]
Headache (4%) [3]
Neurotoxicity [4]
Peripheral neuropathy [4]
Seizures [2]

Neuromuscular/Skeletal
Asthenia (fatigue) [2]
Back pain [2]
Rhabdomyolysis [6]

Gastrointestinal/Hepatic
Abdominal pain (2–6%) [4]
Diarrhea [3]
Hepatitis [2]
Hepatotoxicity [5]
Nausea (5–7%) [7]
Pancreatitis [2]
Vomiting [3]

Respiratory
Cough (4%)
Dyspnea (2%)
Flu-like syndrome [2]
Pneumonia (2%)

Endocrine/Metabolic
ALT increased [2]
AST increased [2]
Hyperbilirubinemia [2]
Hypertriglyceridemia [2]
Hypokalemia [6]

Hematologic
Leukopenia [2]
Thrombocytopenia [2]

Other
Adverse effects [8]
Death [3]
Side effects [2]

IVABRADINE

Trade names: Corlanor (Amgen), Procoralan (Servier)
Indications: Chronic stable angina pectoris
Class: Cardiotonic agent, HCN channel blocker
Half-life: 2 hours
Clinically important, potentially hazardous interactions with: azole antifungals, clarithromycin, CYP3A4 inducers, diltiazem, grapefruit juice, itraconazole, ketoconazole, macrolide antibiotics, nefazodone, nelfinavir, pentamidine, phenytoin, rifampin, ritonavir, sotalol, St John's wort, strong or moderate CYP3A4 inhibitors, telithromycin, verapamil
Pregnancy category: N/A
Important contra-indications noted in the prescribing guidelines for: nursing mothers; pediatric patients

---

Cardiovascular
Atrial fibrillation (8%) [2]
Atrioventricular block (<10%)
Bradycardia (10%) [5]
Hypertension (9%)

Central Nervous System
Headache (2–5%) [2]
Vertigo (dizziness) (<10%) [3]

Neuromuscular/Skeletal
Myalgia/Myopathy (<10%)

Gastrointestinal/Hepatic
Nausea [2]

Ocular
Luminous phenomena (14%) [5]
Vision blurred (<10%) [3]
Visual disturbances [2]

IVACAFTOR

Trade name: Kalydeco (Vertex)
Indications: Cystic fibrosis in patients aged 6 years and older who have a *G551D* mutation in the *CFTR* gene
Class: CFTR potentiator
Half-life: 12 hours
Clinically important, potentially hazardous interactions with: CYP3A inducers or inhibitors, fluconazole, grapefruit juice, ketoconazole, rifampin, St John's wort
Pregnancy category: B
Important contra-indications noted in the prescribing guidelines for: nursing mothers; pediatric patients
Note: See also separate profile for lumacaftor/ivacaftor.

Skin
Acneform eruption (4–7%)
Rash (13%) [6]

Mucosal
Nasal congestion (20%) [7]
Oropharyngeal pain (22%) [7]

Cardiovascular
Chest pain (4–7%)

Central Nervous System
Fever [2]
Headache (24%) [8]
Vertigo (dizziness) (9%) [4]

Neuromuscular/Skeletal
Arthralgia (4–7%)
Myalgia/Myopathy (4–7%)

Gastrointestinal/Hepatic
Abdominal pain (16%) [4]
Diarrhea (13%) [6]
Hepatotoxicity [3]
Nausea (12%) [3]
Vomiting [2]

Respiratory
Cough [5]
Hemoptysis [2]
Nasopharyngitis (15%) [4]
Rhinitis (4–7%)
Upper respiratory tract infection (22%) [7]
Wheezing (4–7%)

Endocrine/Metabolic
AST increased (4–7%)

Otic
Otitis media [2]

Other
Adverse effects [4]

IVERMECTIN

Trade names: Sklice (Sanofi Pasteur), Soolantra (Galderma), Stromectol (Merck)
Indications: Various infections caused by susceptible helmintic organisms
Class: Anthelmintic
Half-life: 16–35 hours
Clinically important, potentially hazardous interactions with: alprazolam, barbiturates, benzodiazepines, diazepam, midazolam, valproic acid
Pregnancy category: C
Important contra-indications noted in the prescribing guidelines for: nursing mothers; pediatric patients

---

Skin
Edema (10–53%) [7]
Exanthems (<34%) [3]
Facial edema [3]
Pruritus (38–71%) [14]
Rash (<93%) [6]
Urticaria (23%)

Cardiovascular
Tachycardia (4%)

Central Nervous System
Fever (23%) [2]
Headache [3]
Psychosis [2]
Vertigo (dizziness) (3%) [3]

Neuromuscular/Skeletal
Arthralgia (9%)
Myalgia/Myopathy (20%) [3]

Gastrointestinal/Hepatic
Abdominal pain [3]

Other
Adverse effects [4]
Side effects (mild) [3]

IXAZOMIB *

Trade name: Ninlaro (Millennium)
Indications: Multiple myeloma (in combination with lenalidomide and dexamethasone) in patients who have received at least one prior therapy
Class: Proteasome inhibitor
Half-life: 10 days
Clinically important, potentially hazardous interactions with: carbamazepine, phenytoin, rifampin, St John's wort, strong CYP3A inducers
Pregnancy category: N/A (Can cause fetal harm)
Important contra-indications noted in the prescribing guidelines for: nursing mothers; pediatric patients
Note: See separate profiles for dexamethasone and lenalidomide.

Skin
- Acneform eruption [3]
- Erythema [4]
- Erythema multiforme [2]
- Exanthems [6]
- Exfoliative dermatitis [4]
- Facial edema [2]
- Hyperhidrosis [4]
- Peripheral edema (25%) [2]
- Petechiae [3]
- Pigmentation [3]
- Pruritus [4]
- Rash (19%) [6]
- Urticaria [2]
- Xerosis [3]

Hair
- Alopecia [2]

Central Nervous System
- Chills [2]
- Fever [4]
- Insomnia [2]
- Peripheral neuropathy (28%) [7]

Neuromuscular/Skeletal
- Asthenia (fatigue) [8]
- Back pain (21%)

Gastrointestinal/Hepatic
- Abdominal pain [2]
- Constipation (34%) [2]
- Diarrhea (42%) [8]
- Nausea (26%) [7]
- Vomiting (22%) [7]

Respiratory
- Dyspnea [2]
- Upper respiratory tract infection (19%)

Endocrine/Metabolic
- Appetite decreased [4]
- Dehydration [3]
- Hypokalemia [2]

Hematologic
- Anemia [4]
- Leukopenia [3]
- Lymphopenia [5]
- Neutropenia (67%) [7]
- Platelets decreased [3]
- Thrombocytopenia (78%) [10]

Ocular
- Conjunctivitis (6%)
- Vision blurred (6%)
- Xerophthalmia (5%)

Other
- Adverse effects [3]

IXEKIZUMAB *

Trade name: Taltz (Lilly)
Indications: Plaque psoriasis
Class: Interleukin 17A (IL-17A) antagonist, Monoclonal antibody
Half-life: 13 days
Clinically important, potentially hazardous interactions with: live vaccines
Pregnancy category: N/A (Insufficient evidence to inform drug-associated risk)
Important contra-indications noted in the prescribing guidelines for: pediatric patients

---

Skin
- Hypersensitivity [4]
- Peripheral edema [2]
- Urticaria [2]

Central Nervous System
- Headache [6]

Gastrointestinal/Hepatic
- Crohn's disease [2]
- Nausea (2%)

Respiratory
- Nasopharyngitis [7]
- Upper respiratory tract infection (14%) [7]

Hematologic
- Neutropenia (11%) [2]
- Thrombocytopenia (3%)

Otic
- Ear infection (2%)

Local
- Injection-site reactions (17%) [6]

Other
- Infection [2]

JAPANESE ENCEPHALITIS VACCINE

Trade name: Ixiaro (Novartis)
Indications: Active immunization against Japanese encephalitis for adults
Class: Vaccine
Half-life: N/A
Clinically important, potentially hazardous interactions with: immunosuppressants

Pregnancy category: C
Important contra-indications noted in the prescribing guidelines for: nursing mothers; pediatric patients

---

Skin
Edema (4%)
Pruritus (4%)
Rash (<10%)

Central Nervous System
Fever [5]
Headache (28%) [5]
Seizures [2]

Neuromuscular/Skeletal
Asthenia (fatigue) (11%)
Myalgia/Myopathy (16%)

Gastrointestinal/Hepatic
Diarrhea (<10%)
Nausea (<10%)
Vomiting (<10%)

Respiratory
Flu-like syndrome (12%)

Local
Injection-site edema (<10%)
Injection-site erythema (<10%)
Injection-site induration (<10%)
Injection-site pain (33%) [3]
Injection-site pruritus (<10%)

Other
Adverse effects [5]

KANAMYCIN

Indications: Various infections caused by susceptible organisms
Class: Antibiotic, aminoglycoside
Half-life: 2–4 hours
Clinically important, potentially hazardous interactions with: aldesleukin, atracurium, bacitracin, bumetanide, doxacurium, ethacrynic acid, furosemide, methoxyflurane, neostigmine, non-depolarizing muscle relaxants, pancuronium, polypeptide antibiotics, rocuronium, succinylcholine, teicoplanin, torsemide, vecuronium
Pregnancy category: D
Important contra-indications noted in the prescribing guidelines for: nursing mothers
Note: Aminoglycosides may cause neurotoxicity and/or nephrotoxicity.

Skin
Edema (>10%)
Pruritus (<10%)
Rash (<10%)

Renal
Nephrotoxicity [2]

Otic
Ototoxicity [8]

KETAMINE

Trade name: Ketalar (Monarch)
Indications: Induction of anesthesia
Class: Anesthetic
Half-life: 2–3 hours
Clinically important, potentially hazardous interactions with: memantine, mivacurium
Pregnancy category: D

Skin
Pruritus [3]
Rash (<10%)

Mucosal
Sialorrhea [2]

Cardiovascular
Bradycardia [3]
Hypertension [3]
Hypotension [3]

Central Nervous System
Agitation [4]
Amnesia [2]
Hallucinations [13]
Headache [3]
Nightmares [2]
Sedation [2]
Tremor (>10%)
Vertigo (dizziness) [2]

Gastrointestinal/Hepatic
Hepatotoxicity [2]
Nausea [7]
Vomiting [8]

Respiratory
Apnea [2]
Hypoxia [2]
Laryngospasm [3]

Genitourinary
Cystitis [3]

Local
Injection-site pain (<10%)

Other
Adverse effects [2]

KETOCONAZOLE

Trade name: Nizoral (Janssen)
Indications: Fungal infections
Class: Antibiotic, imidazole, Antifungal, azole, CYP3A4 inhibitor
Half-life: initial: 2 hours; terminal: 8 hours
Clinically important, potentially hazardous interactions with: abiraterone, afatinib, alcohol, alfuzosin, aliskiren, alitretinoin, almotriptan, alprazolam, amphotericin B, amprenavir, anisindione, anticoagulants, aprepitant, aripiprazole, astemizole, atazanavir, avanafil, axitinib, beclomethasone, bedaquiline, benzodiazepines, boceprevir, bosentan, bosutinib, brentuximab vedotin, budesonide, buprenorphine, cabazitaxel, cabozantinib, caffeine, ceritinib, chlordiazepoxide, ciclesonide, cilostazol, cimetidine, cinacalcet, cisapride, clopidogrel, clorazepate, cobicistat/elvitegravir/emtricitabine/tenofovir disoproxil, colchicine, conivaptan, crizotinib, cyclosporine, cyproterone, dabigatran, darifenacin, darunavir, dasatinib, desvenlafaxine, dexlansoprazole, dicumarol, didanosine, disopyramide, docetaxel, dofetilide, domperidone, doxercalciferol, dronedarone, dutasteride, echinacea, eletriptan, eplerenone, erlotinib, erythromycin, estradiol, eszopiclone, everolimus, fentanyl, fesoterodine, fingolimod, flibanserin, flunisolide, fluticasone propionate, fosamprenavir, gastric alkanizers, halofantrine, HMG-CoA reductase inhibitors, ibrutinib, iloperidone, imatinib, indacaterol, indinavir, irinotecan, isavuconazonium sulfate, ivabradine, ivacaftor, ixabepilone, lanthanum, lapatinib, levomilnacipran, lomitapide, lopinavir, lurasidone, macitentan, maraviroc, mefloquine, methadone, methylergonovine, methylprednisolone, midazolam, mizolastine, mometasone, nevirapine, nilotinib, nisoldipine, non-sedating antihistamines, olaparib, omeprazole, ospemifene, oxybutynin, paclitaxel, palbociclib, pantoprazole, paricalcitol, pazopanib, pimecrolimus, pimozide, pomalidomide, ponatinib, prednisolone, prednisone, proton-pump inhibitors, quetiapine, quinidine, rabeprazole, ramelteon, ranolazine, reboxetine, regorafenib, rifampin, rilpivirine, rimonabant, ritonavir, rivaroxaban, roflumilast, romidepsin, ropivacaine, rupatadine, ruxolitinib, saquinavir, saxagliptin, sildenafil, silodosin, simeprevir, simvastatin, solifenacin, sonidegib, sucralfate, sunitinib, tacrolimus, tadalafil, tamsulosin, tasimelteon, telaprevir, telithromycin, temsirolimus, ticagrelor, tiotropium, tofacitinib, tolterodine, tolvaptan, trabectedin, tramadol, triamcinolone, triazolam, trospium, ulipristal, vardenafil, vemurafenib, venetoclax, venlafaxine, vilazodone, vinblastine, vincristine, vorapaxar, warfarin, zaleplon, ziprasidone, zolpidem, zotarolimus
Pregnancy category: C
Black Box Warning: HEPATOTXICITY, QT PROLONGATION AND DRUG INTERACTIONS LEADING TO QT PROLONGATION

Skin
Anaphylactoid reactions/Anaphylaxis [3]
Angioedema [3]
Dermatitis [3]
Exanthems (<9%) [7]
Exfoliative dermatitis [2]
Fixed eruption [2]
Hypersensitivity [3]
Pigmentation [3]
Pruritus (<9%) [5]
Purpura [2]
Rash (<3%) [3]
Urticaria (<3%) [2]
Xerosis [3]

Hair
Alopecia (<4%) [4]

Mucosal
Gingivitis [2]
Oral lesions (<5%) [3]
Oral lichenoid eruption [2]
Oral pigmentation [2]

Cardiovascular
QT prolongation [4]

Central Nervous System
Chills (<3%)
Fever [2]
Neurotoxicity [3]

Neuromuscular/Skeletal
Asthenia (fatigue) [3]
Rhabdomyolysis [3]

Gastrointestinal/Hepatic
Hepatotoxicity [18]
Nausea (3–10%) [4]
Vomiting (3–10%)

Endocrine/Metabolic
Gynecomastia (<3%) [8]

Hematologic
Eosinophilia [2]

Other
Adverse effects [5]
Death [5]

KETOPROFEN

Trade names: Orudis (Sanofi-Aventis), Oruvail (Wyeth)
Indications: Arthritis
Class: Non-steroidal anti-inflammatory (NSAID)
Half-life: 1.5–4 hours
Clinically important, potentially hazardous interactions with: aspirin, caffeine, methotrexate, probenecid
Pregnancy category: C
Important contra-indications noted in the prescribing guidelines for: nursing mothers; pediatric patients
Note: NSAIDs may cause an increased risk of serious cardiovascular and gastrointestinal adverse events, which can be fatal. This risk may increase with duration of use.

Skin
- Anaphylactoid reactions/Anaphylaxis [4]
- Contact dermatitis [5]
- Dermatitis [29]
- Eczema [3]
- Erythema [4]
- Exanthems [3]
- Peripheral edema (<3%)
- Photoallergic reaction [2]
- Photocontact dermatitis [5]
- Photosensitivity [34]
- Pruritus (<10%) [4]
- Rash (>10%)
- Urticaria [6]

Gastrointestinal/Hepatic
- Abdominal pain (3–9%) [2]
- Constipation [2]
- Diarrhea (3–9%)
- Dyspepsia (11%) [2]
- Gastrointestinal bleeding [2]
- Nausea (3–9%) [2]
- Pancreatitis [3]

Endocrine/Metabolic
- Pseudoporphyria [2]

Renal
- Renal function abnormal (3–9%)

Local
- Application-site reactions [2]

Other
- Adverse effects [9]
- Allergic reactions [2]

KETOROLAC

Trade names: Acular (Allergan), Toradol (Roche)
Indications: Pain, relief of inflammation following cataract surgery (ophthalmic solution)
Class: Analgesic, non-opioid, Non-steroidal anti-inflammatory (NSAID)
Half-life: 2–8 hours
Clinically important, potentially hazardous interactions with: aspirin, buprenorphine, dabigatran, diclofenac, enoxaparin, meloxicam, methotrexate, probenecid, rivaroxaban, salicylates, tiagabine, tinzaparin
Pregnancy category: C
Important contra-indications noted in the prescribing guidelines for: nursing mothers; pediatric patients
Black Box Warning: GASTROINTESTINAL, CARDIOVASCULAR, RENAL, AND BLEEDING RISK

Skin
- Anaphylactoid reactions/Anaphylaxis [3]
- Dermatitis (3–9%)
- Diaphoresis (<10%) [2]
- Edema (<10%)
- Exanthems (3–9%)
- Hematoma [2]
- Hypersensitivity [2]
- Pruritus (<10%)
- Purpura (<10%)
- Rash (<10%)

Mucosal
- Stomatitis (<10%)
- Xerostomia [2]

Cardiovascular
- Hypertension (<10%)

Central Nervous System
- Headache (>10%) [4]
- Somnolence (drowsiness) [3]
- Vertigo (dizziness) [4]

Gastrointestinal/Hepatic
- Abdominal pain (>10%)
- Constipation (<10%)
- Diarrhea (7%)
- Dyspepsia (>10%)
- Flatulence (<10%)
- Gastrointestinal bleeding [5]
- Gastrointestinal ulceration (<10%)
- Nausea (>10%) [11]
- Vomiting (<10%) [7]

Renal
- Renal function abnormal (<10%)

Hematologic
- Anemia (<10%)
- Prothrombin time increased (<10%)

Otic
- Tinnitus (<10%)

Ocular
- Corneal melting [4]
- Ocular burning [2]

Local
- Injection-site pain (<10%)

Other
- Adverse effects [9]
- Death [2]
- Side effects [2]

LABETALOL

Trade name: Trandate (Prometheus)
Indications: Hypertension
Class: Adrenergic beta-receptor antagonist, Antiarrhythmic class II
Half-life: 3–8 hours
Clinically important, potentially hazardous interactions with: cimetidine, halothane, imipramine, iobenguane, tricyclic antidepressants
Pregnancy category: C
Important contra-indications noted in the prescribing guidelines for: nursing mothers; pediatric patients
Note: Cutaneous side effects of beta-receptor blockers are clinically polymorphous. They apparently appear after several months of continuous therapy.

Skin
Anaphylactoid reactions/Anaphylaxis [2]
Edema (<2%)
Exanthems (<5%) [4]
Lichenoid eruption [4]
Lupus erythematosus [4]
Pityriasis rubra pilaris [2]
Pruritus (<10%) [3]
Psoriasis (exacerbation) [3]
Scalp tingling [3]

Cardiovascular
Flushing (19%)
Hypotension [4]

Central Nervous System
Dysgeusia (taste perversion) (<10%)
Paresthesias (7%) [2]

Neuromuscular/Skeletal
Myalgia/Myopathy [4]

Other
Side effects (6%) [2]

LACOSAMIDE

Trade name: Vimpat (UCB Pharma)
Indications: Partial-onset seizures
Class: Anticonvulsant, Antiepileptic
Half-life: 13 hours
Clinically important, potentially hazardous interactions with: alcohol, antipsychotics, carbamazepine, chloroquine, fosphenytoin, hydroxychloroquine, lamotrigine, MAO inhibitors, mefloquine, orlistat, phenobarbital, phenytoin, pregabalin, SSRIs, St John's wort, tricyclic antidepressants
Pregnancy category: C
Important contra-indications noted in the prescribing guidelines for: the elderly; nursing mothers; pediatric patients

---

Skin
Angioedema [2]
Pruritus (2%)
Rash [2]

Cardiovascular
Atrioventricular block [3]

Central Nervous System
Balance disorder (4%)
Depression (2%) [2]
Gait instability (2%) [3]
Headache (13%) [12]
Incoordination [2]
Memory loss (2%)
Sedation [3]
Seizures [4]
Somnolence (drowsiness) (7%) [8]
Tremor (7%) [2]
Vertigo (dizziness) (31%) [26]

Neuromuscular/Skeletal
Asthenia (fatigue) (2–9%) [5]
Ataxia (8%) [6]

Gastrointestinal/Hepatic
Diarrhea (4%)
Nausea (11%) [14]
Pancreatitis [2]
Vomiting (9%) [6]

Respiratory
Nasopharyngitis [2]
Upper respiratory tract infection [2]

Ocular
Diplopia (11%) [11]
Nystagmus (5%)
Vision blurred (8%) [3]

Local
Injection-site pain (2%)

Other
Adverse effects [6]

LAMIVUDINE

Synonym: 3TC
Trade names: Combivir (ViiV), Epivir (ViiV), Epzicom (ViiV), Triumeq (ViiV), Trizivir (ViiV)
Indications: HIV progression
Class: Antiretroviral, Nucleoside analog reverse transcriptase inhibitor
Half-life: 5–7 hours
Clinically important, potentially hazardous interactions with: cobicistat/elvitegravir/emtricitabine/tenofovir disoproxil, emtricitabine, trimethoprim
Pregnancy category: C
Note: Combivir is lamivudine and zidovudine; Epzicom is lamivudine and abacavir; Triumeq is abacavir, dolutegravir and lamivudine; Trizivir is lamivudine, abacavir and zidovudine,.

Skin
Angioedema [2]
Exanthems [2]
Hypersensitivity [4]
Jaundice [2]
Pigmentation [2]
Pruritus [3]
Rash (9%) [9]
Stevens–Johnson syndrome [2]
Toxic epidermal necrolysis [2]

Hair
Alopecia [3]

Central Nervous System
Abnormal dreams [2]
Chills (<10%)
Headache [5]
Insomnia [3]
Neurotoxicity [2]
Paresthesias (>10%)
Peripheral neuropathy [3]
Vertigo (dizziness) [4]

Neuromuscular/Skeletal
Asthenia (fatigue) [5]
Myalgia/Myopathy (8%)
Rhabdomyolysis [3]

Gastrointestinal/Hepatic
Abdominal pain [4]
Diarrhea [4]
Hepatotoxicity [2]
Nausea [5]
Pancreatitis [4]
Vomiting [2]

Respiratory
Upper respiratory tract infection [2]

Endocrine/Metabolic
Acidosis [3]

Hematologic
Anemia [2]

Other
Adverse effects [9]

LAMOTRIGINE

Trade name: Lamictal (GSK)
Indications: Epilepsy
Class: Anticonvulsant, Antiepileptic, Mood stabilizer
Half-life: 24 hours
Clinically important, potentially hazardous interactions with: eslicarbazepine, lacosamide, oral contraceptives, rufinamide
Pregnancy category: C
Important contra-indications noted in the prescribing guidelines for: the elderly; nursing mothers
Black Box Warning: SERIOUS SKIN RASHES

Skin
Angioedema (<10%)
Anticonvulsant hypersensitivity syndrome [17]
DRESS syndrome [14]
Erythema (<10%)
Erythema multiforme [4]
Exanthems (<10%) [18]
Hot flashes (<10%)
Hypersensitivity (<10%) [28]
Lupus erythematosus [4]
Photosensitivity [2]
Pruritus (3%)
Rash (10–20%) [49]
Stevens–Johnson syndrome (<10%) [45]
Toxic epidermal necrolysis [48]

Mucosal
Xerostomia (6%)

Central Nervous System
Agitation [2]
Aseptic meningitis [4]
Fever [2]
Hallucinations [3]
Headache [4]
Insomnia (5–10%)
Neuroleptic malignant syndrome [2]

Pain (5%)
Seizures [9]
Somnolence (drowsiness) (9%) [5]
Suicidal ideation [2]
Tic disorder [2]
Tremor [4]
Vertigo (dizziness) [6]

Neuromuscular/Skeletal
Asthenia (fatigue) (8%)
Ataxia (2–5%) [2]
Rhabdomyolysis [3]

Gastrointestinal/Hepatic
Abdominal pain (6%)
Hepatotoxicity [4]
Nausea [3]

Respiratory
Cough (5%)
Flu-like syndrome (7%)
Pharyngitis (5%)
Rhinitis (7%)

Endocrine/Metabolic
SIADH [2]

Genitourinary
Urinary frequency (<5%)
Vaginitis (4%)

Renal
Nephrotoxicity [2]

Hematologic
Agranulocytosis [3]

Ocular
Abnormal vision (2–5%)
Diplopia [4]
Hallucinations, visual [2]
Nystagmus (2–5%)

Other
Adverse effects [5]
Death [6]
Multiorgan failure [2]
Teratogenicity [6]

LANREOTIDE

Trade names: Somatuline Autogel (Ipsen), Somatuline Depot (Ipsen), Somatuline LA (Ipsen)
Indications: Acromegaly, carcinoid syndrome, thyrotrophic adenoma
Class: Somatostatin analog
Half-life: 2 hours (immediate release) 5 days (sustained release).
Clinically important, potentially hazardous interactions with: antidiabetics, bromocriptine, cyclosporine, insulin, metformin, repaglinide, sulfonylureas
Pregnancy category: C
Important contra-indications noted in the prescribing guidelines for: nursing mothers; pediatric patients

---

Hair
Alopecia [2]

Cardiovascular
Bradycardia (5–18%)
Hypertension (5%)

Central Nervous System
Headache (7%)
Pain (7%)

Neuromuscular/Skeletal
Arthralgia (7%)

Gastrointestinal/Hepatic
Abdominal pain (7–19%) [6]
Cholelithiasis (gallstones) (2–17%) [2]
Constipation (8%)
Diarrhea (31–65%) [6]
Flatulence (6–14%) [2]
Loose stools (6%)
Nausea (11%) [3]
Steatorrhea [2]
Vomiting (7%)

Endocrine/Metabolic
Diabetes mellitus (7%)
Hyperglycemia (7%)
Hypoglycemia (7%)
Weight loss (5–11%)

Hematologic
Anemia (5–14%)

Local
Injection-site induration [2]
Injection-site pain (4%) [4]
Injection-site reactions (6–22%) [2]

Other
Adverse effects [2]

LANSOPRAZOLE

Trade name: Prevacid (TAP)
Indications: Active duodenal ulcer
Class: Proton pump inhibitor (PPI)
Half-life: 2 hours
Clinically important, potentially hazardous interactions with: bosutinib, clopidogrel, delavirdine, eucalyptus, prednisone, rilpivirine, sucralfate
Pregnancy category: C
Important contra-indications noted in the prescribing guidelines for: nursing mothers

---

Skin
Anaphylactoid reactions/Anaphylaxis [6]
Erythema multiforme [2]
Facial edema [2]
Hypersensitivity [3]
Lupus erythematosus [3]
Peripheral edema [2]
Pruritus (3–10%)
Rash (3–10%)
Toxic epidermal necrolysis [4]
Urticaria [3]

Mucosal
Stomatitis [2]

Central Nervous System
Dysgeusia (taste perversion) [3]
Headache (3%) [3]

Gastrointestinal/Hepatic
Colitis [2]
Diarrhea (<5%) [5]
Hepatitis [2]

Endocrine/Metabolic
Gynecomastia [2]

Other
Death [2]

LAPATINIB

Trade name: Tykerb (Novartis)
Indications: Breast cancer
Class: Antineoplastic, Biologic, Epidermal growth factor receptor (EGFR) inhibitor, Tyrosine kinase inhibitor
Half-life: 24 hours
Clinically important, potentially hazardous interactions with: alfuzosin, artemether/lumefantrine, atazanavir, carbamazepine, chloroquine, ciprofloxacin, clarithromycin, clozapine, colchicine, conivaptan, CYP2C8 substrates, CYP3A4 inhibitors or inducers, dabigatran, deferasirox, dexamethasone, digoxin, docetaxel, dronedarone, efavirenz, eplerenone, everolimus, fentanyl, food, gadobutrol, grapefruit juice, histamine H_2-antagonists, indinavir, irinotecan, itraconazole, ketoconazole, nefazodone, nelfinavir, nilotinib, omeprazole, P-glycoprotein inducers, paclitaxel, pantoprazole, pazopanib, phenobarbital, phenytoin, pimecrolimus, pimozide, posaconazole, proton pump inhibitors, QT prolonging agents, quinine, repaglinide, rifabutin, rifampin, rifapentin, ritonavir, rivaroxaban, salmeterol, saquinavir, saxagliptin, silodosin, St John's wort, telithromycin, tetrabenazine, thioridazine, tolvaptan, topotecan, voriconazole, ziprasidone
Pregnancy category: D
Important contra-indications noted in the prescribing guidelines for: nursing mothers; pediatric patients
Note: Lapitinib is used in conjunction with capecitabine.
Black Box Warning: HEPATOXICITY

Skin
Acneform eruption (90%) [4]
Depigmentation (21%)
Hand-foot syndrome (53%) [8]
Inflammation (15%)
Pruritus [3]
Rash (28%) [24]
Toxicity [6]
Xerosis (10%)

Hair
Alopecia [2]

Nails
Paronychia [3]

Mucosal
Mucosal inflammation (15%)
Mucositis [2]
Stomatitis (14%)

Central Nervous System
Anorexia (24%) [2]
Insomnia (10%)

Neuromuscular/Skeletal
Asthenia (fatigue) (12%) [17]
Back pain (11%)
Bone or joint pain [2]
Pain in extremities (12%)

Gastrointestinal/Hepatic
Abdominal pain (15%)
Diarrhea (65%) [40]
Dyspepsia (11%)
Hepatotoxicity [11]
Nausea (44%) [8]

Vomiting (26%) [6]

Respiratory
Dyspnea (12%) [2]

Endocrine/Metabolic
ALT increased (37%) [5]
AST increased (49%) [4]
Hyperbilirubinemia [3]

Hematologic
Anemia [5]
Febrile neutropenia [2]
Leukopenia [4]
Neutropenia [8]

Otic
Tinnitus (14%)

Other
Adverse effects [10]

LATANOPROST

Trade name: Xalatan (Pfizer)
Indications: Reduction of elevated intraocular pressure in open angle glaucoma or ocular hypertension
Class: Prostaglandin analog
Half-life: 17 minutes
Clinically important, potentially hazardous interactions with: thimerosal
Pregnancy category: C
Important contra-indications noted in the prescribing guidelines for: nursing mothers; pediatric patients

---

Skin
Pigmentation [2]
Pruritus [2]
Rash (<10%)

Cardiovascular
Angina (<10%)
Chest pain (<10%)

Central Nervous System
Headache [3]
Vertigo (dizziness) [2]

Neuromuscular/Skeletal
Arthralgia (<10%)
Back pain (<10%)
Myalgia/Myopathy (<10%)

Respiratory
Flu-like syndrome (<10%)
Upper respiratory tract infection (<10%)

Ocular
Conjunctival hyperemia [19]
Deepening of upper lid sulcus [5]
Eyelashes – hypertrichosis [15]
Eyelashes – pigmentation [9]
Eyelid edema (<4%)
Eyelid erythema (<4%)
Eyelid pain (<10%)
Eyelid pigmentation [4]
Eyelid pruritus (2%)
Foreign body sensation [5]
Iris pigmentation [7]
Keratitis [3]
Macular edema [7]
Ocular adverse effects [7]
Ocular hyperemia [4]
Ocular itching [8]
Ocular pigmentation (5%) [12]
Periorbitopathy [2]
Uveitis [5]
Vision blurred [3]
Xerophthalmia (<10%)

Other
Allergic reactions (<10%)

LEDIPASVIR & SOFOSBUVIR

Trade name: Harvoni (Gilead)
Indications: Hepatitis C
Class: Hepatitis C virus NS5A inhibitor (ledipasvir), Hepatitis C virus nucleotide analog NS5B polymerase inhibitor (sofosbuvir)
Half-life: 47 hours (ledipasvir); <27 hours (sofosbuvir)
Clinically important, potentially hazardous interactions with: amiodarone, carbamazepine, cobicistat/elvitegravir/emtricitabine/tenofovir disoproxil, oxcarbazepine, phenobarbital, phenytoin, rifabutin, rifampin, rifapentine, ritonavir, rosuvastatin, simeprevir, St John's wort, tenofovir disoproxil
Pregnancy category: B
Important contra-indications noted in the prescribing guidelines for: nursing mothers; pediatric patients
Note: See also separate entry for sofosbuvir.

Skin
Pruritus [5]
Rash [4]

Cardiovascular
Bradycardia [2]

Central Nervous System
Headache (11–17%) [23]
Insomnia (3–6%) [8]
Irritability [4]
Vertigo (dizziness) [2]

Neuromuscular/Skeletal
Arthralgia [2]
Asthenia (fatigue) (7–18%) [24]
Muscle spasm [2]
Myalgia/Myopathy [2]

Gastrointestinal/Hepatic
Diarrhea (3–7%) [7]
Hepatotoxicity [2]
Nausea (6–9%) [14]

Respiratory
Cough [2]
Dyspnea [3]
Upper respiratory tract infection [6]

Renal
Nephrotoxicity [2]

Hematologic
Anemia [6]

Other
Adverse effects [4]

LENALIDOMIDE

Trade name: Revlimid (Celgene)
Indications: Transfusion-dependent anemia due to myeloplastic syndromes, multiple myeloma (in combination with dexamethasone)
Class: Biologic, Immunomodulator, Thalidomide analog
Half-life: 3–5 hours
Clinically important, potentially hazardous interactions with: abatacept, anakinra, canakinumab, certolizumab, denosumab, dexamethasone, digoxin, erythropoietin stimulating agents, estrogen containing therapies, leflunomide, natalizumab, pimecrolimus, rilonacept, sipuleucel-T, tacrolimus, trastuzumab, vaccines
Pregnancy category: X
Important contra-indications noted in the prescribing guidelines for: nursing mothers; pediatric patients
Black Box Warning: FETAL RISK, HEMATOLOGIC TOXICITY, and DEEP VEIN THOMBOSIS AND PULMONARY EMBOLISM

Skin
Cellulitis (5%)
DRESS syndrome [2]
Ecchymoses (5–8%)
Edema (10%)
Erythema (5%)
Exanthems [3]
Folliculitis [2]
Graft-versus-host reaction [2]
Hyperhidrosis (7%) [2]
Malignancies (secondary) [6]
Peripheral edema (26%) [3]
Pigmentation [2]
Pruritus (42%) [3]
Rash (36%) [15]
Stevens–Johnson syndrome [5]
Sweet's syndrome [3]
Toxicity [6]
Tumor lysis syndrome [3]
Tumors [5]
Xerosis (14%) [2]

Mucosal
Epistaxis (nosebleed) (15%)
Xerostomia (7%)

Cardiovascular
Chest pain (5%)
Hypertension (6%)
Palpitation (5%)
Thromboembolism [3]
Venous thromboembolism [13]

Central Nervous System
Anorexia (10%)
Depression (5%)
Dysgeusia (taste perversion) (6%)
Fever (21%) [3]
Headache (20%)
Hypoesthesia (7%)
Insomnia (10%) [4]
Neurotoxicity (7%) [8]
Pain (7%)
Peripheral neuropathy (5%) [9]
Rigors (6%)
Somnolence (drowsiness) [2]
Tremor (21%)

Vertigo (dizziness) (20%)

Neuromuscular/Skeletal
Arthralgia (21%) [4]
Asthenia (fatigue) (15–31%) [33]
Back pain (21%) [3]
Bone or joint pain (14%)
Cramps (33%)
Muscle spasm [4]
Myalgia/Myopathy (18%) [3]
Pain in extremities (12%)

Gastrointestinal/Hepatic
Abdominal pain (8–12%)
Constipation (24%) [7]
Diarrhea (49%) [12]
Gastrointestinal disorder [3]
Hepatotoxicity [3]
Loose stools (6%)
Nausea (24%) [8]
Vomiting (10%) [3]

Respiratory
Alveolar hemorrhage (pulmonary) [2]
Bronchitis (11%)
Cough (20%) [5]
Dyspnea (7–17%) [4]
Nasopharyngitis (23%)
Pharyngitis (16%)
Pneumonia (12%) [9]
Pneumonitis [6]
Pulmonary toxicity [3]
Rhinitis (7%)
Sinusitis (8%)
Upper respiratory tract infection (15%) [3]

Endocrine/Metabolic
ALT increased (8%) [3]
Appetite decreased (7%)
Hyperglycemia [2]
Hypocalcemia (9%)
Hypokalemia (11%) [4]
Hypomagnesemia (6%)
Hyponatremia [2]
Hypophosphatemia [3]
Hypothyroidism (7%)
Weight loss (20%)

Genitourinary
Urinary tract infection (11%)

Renal
Nephrotoxicity [3]

Hematologic
Anemia (31%) [22]
Cytopenia [3]
Febrile neutropenia (5%) [7]
Hemotoxicity [11]
Leukopenia (8%) [10]
Lymphopenia (5%) [8]
Myelosuppression [5]
Neutropenia (59%) [50]
Thrombocytopenia (62%) [45]
Thrombosis [4]

Ocular
Vision blurred (17%)

Local
Infusion-related reactions [2]
Injection-site reactions [2]

Other
Adverse effects [13]
Cancer [2]
Death [3]
Infection [16]
Teratogenicity [2]

LENVATINIB

Trade name: Lenvima (Eisai)
Indications: Differentiated thyroid cancer, renal cell cancer (in combination with everolimus)
Class: Tyrosine kinase inhibitor
Half-life: 28 hours
Clinically important, potentially hazardous interactions with: none known
Pregnancy category: N/A (Can cause fetal harm)
Important contra-indications noted in the prescribing guidelines for: nursing mothers; pediatric patients

---

Skin
Exanthems (21%)
Hand–foot syndrome (32%)
Hyperkeratosis (7%)
Peripheral edema (21%) [2]
Rash (21%)

Hair
Alopecia (12%)

Mucosal
Aphthous stomatitis (41%)
Epistaxis (nosebleed) (12%)
Gingivitis (10%)
Glossitis (41%)
Glossodynia (25%)
Mucosal inflammation (41%)
Oral ulceration (41%)
Oropharyngeal pain (25%)
Parotitis (10%)
Stomatitis (41%) [2]
Xerostomia (17%)

Cardiovascular
Hypertension (73%) [14]
Hypotension (9%)
QT prolongation (9%)

Central Nervous System
Anorexia [2]
Dysgeusia (taste perversion) (18%)
Headache (38%) [3]
Insomnia (12%)
Vertigo (dizziness) (15%)

Neuromuscular/Skeletal
Arthralgia (62%)
Asthenia (fatigue) (67%) [8]
Back pain (62%)
Bone or joint pain (62%)
Myalgia/Myopathy (62%)
Pain in extremities (62%)

Gastrointestinal/Hepatic
Abdominal pain (31%) [2]
Constipation (29%) [2]
Diarrhea (67%) [9]
Dyspepsia (13%)
Nausea (47%) [6]
Vomiting (36%) [4]

Respiratory
Cough (24%)
Dysphonia (31%)
Nasopharyngitis [2]

Endocrine/Metabolic
ALP increased (>5%)
ALT increased (4%)
Appetite decreased (54%) [5]
AST increased (5%)
Creatine phosphokinase increased (3%)
Dehydration (9%)
Hyperbilirubinemia (>5%)
Hypercalcemia (>5%)
Hypercholesterolemia (>5%)
Hyperkalemia (>5%)
Hypoalbuminemia (>5%)
Hypocalcemia (9%)
Hypoglycemia (>5%)
Hypokalemia (6%)
Hypomagnesemia (>5%)
Weight loss (51%) [4]

Genitourinary
Hematuria [2]
Urinary tract infection (11%)

Renal
Proteinuria (34%) [7]

Hematologic
Leukopenia [2]
Platelets decreased (2%)
Thrombocytopenia [3]

Other
Adverse effects [3]
Death [2]
Tooth disorder (10%)

LESINURAD *

Trade name: Zurampic (AstraZeneca)
Indications: Gout-associated hyperuricemia (in combination with a xanthine oxidase inhibitor)
Class: URAT1 inhibitor
Half-life: 5 hours
Clinically important, potentially hazardous interactions with: amiodarone, carbamazepine, CYP2C9 inducers or inhibitors, CYP3A substrates, fluconazole, rifampin, valproic acid
Pregnancy category: N/A (No available data)
Important contra-indications noted in the prescribing guidelines for: nursing mothers; pediatric patients
Note: Contraindicated in patients with severe renal impairment (including end stage renal disease, kidney transplant recipients or patients on dialysis), tumor lysis syndrome or Lesch-Nylan syndrome.
Black Box Warning: RISK OF ACUTE RENAL FAILURE, MORE COMMON WHEN USED WITHOUT A XANTHINE OXIDASE INHIBITOR

Cardiovascular
Cardiotoxicity (<2%)

Central Nervous System
Headache (5%) [2]
Vertigo (dizziness) [2]

Neuromuscular/Skeletal
Back pain [2]

Gastrointestinal/Hepatic
Diarrhea [2]
Gastroesophageal reflux (3%)

Respiratory
- Influenza (5%)
- Nasopharyngitis [2]

Endocrine/Metabolic
- Serum creatinine increased (4–8%)

Renal
- Nephrolithiasis (<3%)
- Renal failure (<4%)

LETROZOLE

Trade name: Femara (Novartis)
Indications: Breast cancer
Class: Aromatase inhibitor
Half-life: ~2 days
Clinically important, potentially hazardous interactions with: none known
Pregnancy category: X
Important contra-indications noted in the prescribing guidelines for: nursing mothers; pediatric patients

---

Skin
- Exanthems (5%)
- Hot flashes (6%) [7]
- Hyperhidrosis (<5%)
- Leukocytoclastic vasculitis [2]
- Pruritus (2%)
- Psoriasis (5%)
- Rash (<10%) [5]
- Vesiculation (5%)

Hair
- Alopecia (<5%) [3]

Cardiovascular
- Cardiac failure [2]
- Hypertension [2]
- Myocardial toxicity [2]

Central Nervous System
- Anorexia [3]
- Depression [2]
- Fever [2]
- Headache [3]
- Insomnia [2]
- Mood changes [2]
- Vertigo (dizziness) [2]

Neuromuscular/Skeletal
- Arthralgia [9]
- Asthenia (fatigue) [8]
- Back pain [3]
- Bone or joint pain [3]
- Myalgia/Myopathy [6]
- Osteoporosis [7]

Gastrointestinal/Hepatic
- Constipation [2]
- Diarrhea [7]
- Nausea [7]
- Vomiting [4]

Respiratory
- Dyspnea [2]

Endocrine/Metabolic
- Hypercholesterolemia [3]
- Hyperglycemia [3]

Genitourinary
- Vaginal dryness [4]

Hematologic
- Neutropenia [2]

Other
- Infection [2]

LEUCOVORIN

Synonyms: citrovorum factor; folinic acid
Indications: Overdose of methotrexate, in combination with fluorouracil in the palliative treatment of patients with colorectal cancer
Class: Adjuvant
Half-life: 15 minutes
Clinically important, potentially hazardous interactions with: capecitabine, glucarpidase, trimethoprim
Pregnancy category: C

Skin
- Rash [5]

Hair
- Alopecia [2]

Mucosal
- Mucositis [5]
- Stomatitis [2]

Cardiovascular
- Hypertension [5]

Central Nervous System
- Anorexia [4]
- Neurotoxicity [5]
- Peripheral neuropathy [3]

Neuromuscular/Skeletal
- Asthenia (fatigue) [6]

Gastrointestinal/Hepatic
- Abdominal pain [2]
- Diarrhea [16]
- Nausea [10]
- Vomiting [10]

Renal
- Proteinuria [2]

Hematologic
- Anemia [8]
- Febrile neutropenia [2]
- Leukopenia [5]
- Neutropenia [20]
- Thrombocytopenia [5]

Other
- Adverse effects [2]
- Infection [2]

LEUPROLIDE

Trade names: Eligard (Sanofi-Aventis), Lupron (TAP), Lupron Depot-Ped (AbbVie), Viadur (Bayer)
Indications: Prostate carcinoma, endometriosis
Class: Gonadotropin-releasing hormone (GnRH) agonist
Half-life: 3–4 hours
Clinically important, potentially hazardous interactions with: none known
Pregnancy category: X
Important contra-indications noted in the prescribing guidelines for: nursing mothers

---

Skin
- Anaphylactoid reactions/Anaphylaxis [3]
- Dermatitis (5%)
- Dermatitis herpetiformis [2]
- Ecchymoses (<5%)
- Edema (<10%)
- Granulomas [2]
- Hot flashes (12%) [6]
- Peripheral edema (4–12%)
- Pigmentation (<5%)
- Pruritus (<5%)
- Rash (<10%)
- Vasculitis [2]
- Xerosis (<5%)

Hair
- Alopecia (<5%)

Cardiovascular
- Flushing (61%) [2]
- Thrombophlebitis (2%)

Central Nervous System
- Dysgeusia (taste perversion) (<5%)
- Paresthesias (<5%)

Neuromuscular/Skeletal
- Myalgia/Myopathy [2]

Endocrine/Metabolic
- Gynecomastia (7%)
- Mastodynia (7%)

Ocular
- Diplopia [2]

Local
- Injection-site granuloma [6]
- Injection-site inflammation (2%)
- Injection-site pain [2]
- Injection-site reactions (24%)

LEVETIRACETAM

Trade names: Elepsia XR (Sun Pharma), Keppra (UCB)
Indications: Partial onset seizures
Class: Anticonvulsant
Half-life: 7 hours
Clinically important, potentially hazardous interactions with: carbamazepine, eslicarbazepine
Pregnancy category: C
Important contra-indications noted in the prescribing guidelines for: nursing mothers

---

Skin
- DRESS syndrome [7]
- Erythema [2]
- Erythema multiforme [2]
- Rash [4]
- Stevens–Johnson syndrome [3]
- Toxic epidermal necrolysis [2]
- Urticaria [2]

Central Nervous System
- Aggression [7]
- Agitation [4]
- Anorexia [2]
- Behavioral disturbances [4]

Compulsions [2]
Depression [7]
Encephalopathy [4]
Fever [2]
Headache (25%) [10]
Irritability [8]
Nervousness [2]
Neurotoxicity [2]
Paresthesias (2%)
Psychosis [3]
Seizures [4]
Sleep related disorder [2]
Somnolence (drowsiness) [15]
Suicidal ideation [4]
Vertigo (dizziness) (9–18%) [17]

Neuromuscular/Skeletal
Asthenia (fatigue) (<22%) [18]
Osteoporosis [2]
Rhabdomyolysis [2]

Gastrointestinal/Hepatic
Abdominal pain [2]
Nausea [3]
Vomiting [4]

Respiratory
Nasopharyngitis [4]

Endocrine/Metabolic
Creatine phosphokinase increased [2]
Libido decreased [2]
Weight gain [3]

Genitourinary
Sexual dysfunction [2]

Renal
Nephrotoxicity [2]

Hematologic
Hemotoxicity [2]
Pancytopenia [2]
Thrombocytopenia [2]

Other
Adverse effects [7]
Infection (13–26%) [7]

LEVOCETIRIZINE

Trade name: Xyzal (UCB Pharma)
Indications: Allergic rhinitis, chronic idiopathic urticaria
Class: Histamine H1 receptor antagonist
Half-life: 6–10 hours
Clinically important, potentially hazardous interactions with: none known
Pregnancy category: B
Important contra-indications noted in the prescribing guidelines for: the elderly; nursing mothers; pediatric patients

---

Skin
Fixed eruption [3]

Mucosal
Xerostomia (2–3%)

Central Nervous System
Headache [2]
Somnolence (drowsiness) (5–6%)

Neuromuscular/Skeletal
Asthenia (fatigue) (<4%)

Respiratory
Nasopharyngitis (4–6%)
Pharyngitis (<2%)

LEVODOPA

Synonyms: L-dopa; carbidopa
Trade names: Duopa (Abbvie), Rytary (Impax), Sinemet (Bristol-Myers Squibb), Stalevo (Orion)
Indications: Parkinsonism
Class: Dopamine precursor
Half-life: 1–3 hours
Clinically important, potentially hazardous interactions with: ACE inhibitors, acebutolol, alfuzosin, alpha blockers, amisulpride, ampicillin, angiotensin II receptor antagonists, antihypertensives, antimuscarinics, antipsychotics, baclofen, benzodiazepines, beta blockers, bupropion, calcium channel blockers, captopril, chloramphenicol, cholestyramine, cilazapril, clobazam, clonidine, darifenacin, diazoxide, diuretics, dopamine D_2 receptor antagonists, enalapril, erythromycin, fosinopril, hydralazine, irbesartan, iron salts, isoniazid, levomepromazine, linezolid, lisinopril, MAO inhibitors, memantine, methyldopa, metoclopramide, minoxidil, moclobemide, moxonidine, nitrates, olanzapine, olmesartan, oral iron, oxybutynin, paliperidone, papaverine, pericyazine, phenelzine, phenytoin, probenecid, pyridoxine, quetiapine, quinapril, ramipril, rifampin, risperidone, sapropterin, selegiline, sodium nitroprusside, sulpiride, tetrabenazine, tiotropium, trandolapril, tranylcypromine, tricyclic antidepressants, trospium, volatile liquid general anesthetics, ziprasidone, zuclopenthixol, zuclopenthixol acetate, zuclopenthixol decanoate, zuclopenthixol dihydrochloride
Pregnancy category: C
Important contra-indications noted in the prescribing guidelines for: nursing mothers; pediatric patients
Note: Levodopa is always used in conjuntion with carbidopa. Stalevo is levodopa, carbidopa and entacapone. Contraindicated in patients with narrow-angle glaucoma or those with a history of melanoma.

Skin
Chromhidrosis (<10%)
Edema [2]
Exanthems [2]
Lupus erythematosus [2]
Melanoma [28]
Rash [3]

Hair
Hair pigmentation [2]

Nails
Nail growth [2]

Mucosal
Xerostomia (<10%) [2]

Cardiovascular
Hypotension [2]
Orthostatic hypotension [3]

Central Nervous System
Agitation [2]
Anosmia [2]
Anxiety [2]
Confusion [3]
Delusions [2]
Depression [3]
Dyskinesia [41]
Gait instability [3]
Hallucinations [12]
Insomnia [6]
Narcolepsy [2]
Neuroleptic malignant syndrome [7]
Neurotoxicity [3]
Psychosis [5]
Restless legs syndrome [5]
Somnolence (drowsiness) [4]
Suicidal ideation [2]
Tardive dyskinesia [2]
Vertigo (dizziness) [4]

Neuromuscular/Skeletal
Arthralgia [2]
Asthenia (fatigue) [2]
Back pain [2]

Gastrointestinal/Hepatic
Abdominal pain [2]
Constipation [4]
Diarrhea [2]
Hepatotoxicity [2]
Nausea [9]
Vomiting [4]

Endocrine/Metabolic
Weight loss [2]

Ocular
Hallucinations, visual [2]
Ocular adverse effects [2]

Other
Adverse effects [2]
Hiccups [2]

LEVOFLOXACIN

Trade names: Iquix (Santen), Levaquin (Ortho-McNeil), Quixin (Johnson & Johnson), Tavanic (Sanofi-Aventis)
Indications: Various infections caused by susceptible organisms, inhalational anthrax (post exposure)
Class: Antibiotic, fluoroquinolone
Half-life: 6–8 hours
Clinically important, potentially hazardous interactions with: alfuzosin, aminophylline, amiodarone, antacids, antidiabetics, arsenic, artemether/lumefantrine, BCG vaccine, chloroquine, ciprofloxacin, corticosteroids, cyclosporine, didanosine, dronedarone, gadobutrol, insulin, lanthanum, mycophenolate, nilotinib, NSAIDs, oral iron, oral typhoid vaccine, phenindione, pimozide, probenecid, QT prolonging agents, quinine, strontium ranelate, sucralfate, sulfonylureas, tetrabenazine, thioridazine, vitamin K antagonists, warfarin, zinc, ziprasidone, zolmitriptan
Pregnancy category: C
Important contra-indications noted in the prescribing guidelines for: the elderly; nursing mothers
Note: Fluoroquinolones are associated with an increased risk of tendinitis and tendon rupture in all ages. This risk is further increased in older patients usually over 60 years of age, in patients

taking corticosteroid drugs, and in patients with kidney, heart or lung transplants.
Fluoroquinolones may exacerbate muscle weakness in persons with myasthenia gravis.
Black Box Warning: SERIOUS ADVERSE REACTIONS INCLUDING TENDINITIS, TENDON RUPTURE, PERIPHERAL NEUROPATHY, CENTRIAL NERVOUS SYSTEM EFFECTS and EXACERBATION OF MYASTHENIA GRAVIS

Skin
- Anaphylactoid reactions/Anaphylaxis [5]
- Erythema [2]
- Erythema nodosum (<3%)
- Exanthems [2]
- Hypersensitivity [5]
- Photosensitivity [3]
- Phototoxicity [5]
- Pruritus (2%) [2]
- Purpura [2]
- Radiation recall dermatitis [2]
- Rash (2%)
- Stevens–Johnson syndrome [2]
- Toxic epidermal necrolysis [5]
- Vasculitis [3]

Cardiovascular
- Myocardial infarction [2]
- QT prolongation [5]
- Torsades de pointes [6]

Central Nervous System
- Delirium [5]
- Headache (6%) [5]
- Insomnia (4%) [2]
- Seizures [8]
- Vertigo (dizziness) [5]

Neuromuscular/Skeletal
- Arthralgia [3]
- Myalgia/Myopathy [4]
- Myasthenia gravis (exacerbation) [3]
- Rhabdomyolysis [4]
- Tendinitis [2]
- Tendinopathy/Tendon rupture [35]

Gastrointestinal/Hepatic
- Abdominal pain [2]
- Constipation (3%)
- Diarrhea (5%) [3]
- Hepatotoxicity [4]
- Nausea (7%) [5]
- Vomiting [2]

Endocrine/Metabolic
- ALT increased [3]
- AST increased [3]
- Hypoglycemia [3]

Genitourinary
- Vaginitis (2%)

Renal
- Nephrotoxicity [5]

Hematologic
- Thrombocytopenia [4]

Other
- Adverse effects [12]
- Death [5]
- Side effects [2]

LEVOMILNACIPRAN

Trade name: Fetzima (Forest)
Indications: Major depressive disorder
Class: Antidepressant, Serotonin-norepinephrine reuptake inhibitor
Half-life: 12 hours
Clinically important, potentially hazardous interactions with: ketoconazole, MAO inhibitors, NSAIDs
Pregnancy category: C
Important contra-indications noted in the prescribing guidelines for: nursing mothers; pediatric patients
Black Box Warning: SUICIDAL THOUGHTS AND BEHAVIORS

Skin
- Hyperhidrosis (9%) [8]
- Pruritus (<2%)
- Rash (2%)
- Urticaria (<2%)
- Xerosis (<2%)

Mucosal
- Xerostomia [4]

Cardiovascular
- Angina (<2%)
- Extrasystoles (<2%)
- Hypertension (3%) [2]
- Hypotension (3%)
- Palpitation (5%) [4]
- Tachycardia (6%) [8]

Central Nervous System
- Aggression (<2%)
- Agitation (<2%)
- Extrapyramidal symptoms (<2%)
- Headache [5]
- Insomnia [3]
- Migraine (<2%)
- Panic attack (<2%)
- Paresthesias (<2%)
- Syncope (<2%)
- Vertigo (dizziness) [4]
- Yawning (<2%)

Gastrointestinal/Hepatic
- Abdominal pain (<2%)
- Constipation (9%) [8]
- Flatulence (<2%)
- Nausea (17%) [9]
- Vomiting (5%) [4]

Respiratory
- Upper respiratory tract infection [2]

Endocrine/Metabolic
- Appetite decreased (3%)

Genitourinary
- Ejaculatory dysfunction (5%) [3]
- Erectile dysfunction (6%) [6]
- Hematuria (<2%)
- Pollakiuria (<2%)
- Testicular pain (4%)
- Urinary hesitancy (4%) [3]

Renal
- Proteinuria (<2%)

Ocular
- Conjunctival hemorrhage (<2%)
- Vision blurred (<2%)
- Xerophthalmia (<2%)

Other
- Adverse effects [2]
- Bruxism (<2%)

LEVONORGESTREL

Trade names: Kyleena (Bayer), Mirena (Bayer), Plan B (Duramed)
Indications: Intrauterine contraception, treatment of heavy menstrual bleeding, emergency contraception
Class: Hormone, Progestogen
Half-life: 17 hours
Clinically important, potentially hazardous interactions with: barbiturates, bosentan, carbamazepine, CYP3A4 inducers and inhibitors, efavirenz, felbamate, griseofulvin, nevirapine, oxcarbazepine, phenytoin, rifabutin, rifampin, St John's wort, topiramate, ulipristal
Pregnancy category: X
Important contra-indications noted in the prescribing guidelines for: the elderly; nursing mothers; pediatric patients

---

Central Nervous System
- Headache (17%) [5]
- Vertigo (dizziness) (11%)

Neuromuscular/Skeletal
- Asthenia (fatigue) (17%)

Gastrointestinal/Hepatic
- Abdominal pain (18%)
- Diarrhea (5%)
- Nausea (23%) [6]
- Vomiting (6%) [3]

Endocrine/Metabolic
- Amenorrhea [3]
- Mastodynia (11%) [2]
- Menstrual irregularities (26%) [7]

Genitourinary
- Vaginal bleeding [3]

Other
- Adverse effects [2]

LEVOTHYROXINE

Synonyms: L-thyroxine sodium; T_4
Trade names: Levothyroid (Forest), Levoxyl (Monarch), Synthroid (AbbVie), Unithroid (Watson)
Indications: Hypothyroidism
Class: Thyroid hormone, synthetic
Half-life: 6–7 days
Clinically important, potentially hazardous interactions with: colesevelam, dicumarol, lanthanum, oral anticoagulants, orlistat, propranolol, raloxifene, red rice yeast, ritonavir, warfarin
Pregnancy category: A

Skin
- Angioedema [2]
- Urticaria [3]

Cardiovascular
- Circulatory collapse [2]

Central Nervous System
Restless legs syndrome [2]

Neuromuscular/Skeletal
Bone loss [2]
Fractures [2]

Endocrine/Metabolic
Thyrotoxicosis [3]

Other
Adverse effects [2]
Side effects [2]

LIDOCAINE

Synonyms: lignocaine; xylocaine
Trade names: Anamantle HC (Doak), ELA-Max (Ferndale), EMLA (AstraZeneca), Lidoderm (Endo), Xylocaine (AstraZeneca)
Indications: Ventricular arrhythmias, topical anesthesia
Class: Anesthetic, local, Antiarrhythmic, Antiarrhythmic class Ib
Half-life: terminal: 1.5–2 hours
Clinically important, potentially hazardous interactions with: amiodarone, amprenavir, antiarrhythmics, atazanavir, cimetidine, cobicistat/elvitegravir/emtricitabine/tenofovir disoproxil, darunavir, delavirdine, fosamprenavir, indinavir, lopinavir, mivacurium, nevirapine, nilutamide, oxprenolol, propranolol, telaprevir
Pregnancy category: B
Important contra-indications noted in the prescribing guidelines for: nursing mothers; pediatric patients

---

Skin
Anaphylactoid reactions/Anaphylaxis [7]
Angioedema [3]
Dermatitis [27]
Eczema [3]
Edema [2]
Erythema [3]
Erythema multiforme [2]
Exanthems [2]
Exfoliative dermatitis [2]
Fixed eruption [2]
Hypersensitivity [9]
Pruritus [3]
Toxicity [3]
Urticaria [5]

Cardiovascular
Bradycardia [2]

Central Nervous System
Hoigne's syndrome [2]
Seizures [14]
Shivering (<10%)

Hematologic
Methemoglobinemia [4]

Otic
Tinnitus [3]

Local
Application-site erythema [2]
Application-site reactions [2]
Injection-site pain [2]

Other
Adverse effects [3]
Death [3]

LIFITEGRAST *

Trade name: Xiidra (Shire)
Indications: Ophthalmic solution for dry eye disease
Class: Lymphocyte function-associated antigen-1 (LFA-1) antagonist
Half-life: N/A
Clinically important, potentially hazardous interactions with: none known
Pregnancy category: N/A (No data available)
Important contra-indications noted in the prescribing guidelines for: nursing mothers; pediatric patients

---

Central Nervous System
Dysgeusia (taste perversion) (5–25%) [2]
Headache (<5%)

Respiratory
Sinusitis (<5%)

Ocular
Conjunctival hyperemia (<5%)
Lacrimation (<5%)
Ocular adverse effects [2]
Ocular discharge (<5%)
Ocular pruritus (5–25%) [2]
Reduced visual acuity (5–25%)
Vision blurred (<5%)

Local
Application-site reactions [2]

LINACLOTIDE

Trade name: Linzess (Forest)
Indications: Irritable bowel syndrome with constipation and chronic idiopathic constipation
Class: Amino acid, Guanylate cyclase-C agonist
Half-life: N/A
Clinically important, potentially hazardous interactions with: none known
Pregnancy category: C
Important contra-indications noted in the prescribing guidelines for: nursing mothers; pediatric patients
Note: Contraindicated in patients with known or suspected mechanical gastrointestinal obstruction.
Black Box Warning: PEDIATRIC RISK

Central Nervous System
Headache (4%)

Neuromuscular/Skeletal
Asthenia (fatigue) (<2%)

Gastrointestinal/Hepatic
Abdominal distension (2–3%)
Abdominal pain (7%) [3]
Diarrhea (16–20%) [16]
Dyspepsia (<2%)
Flatulence (4–6%) [3]
Gastroenteritis (3%)
Gastroesophageal reflux (<2%)
Vomiting (<2%)

Respiratory
Sinusitis (3%)
Upper respiratory tract infection (5%)

LINAGLIPTIN

Trade names: Glyxambi (Boehringer Ingelheim), Tradjenta (Boehringer Ingelheim)
Indications: Type II diabetes mellitus
Class: Antidiabetic, Dipeptidyl peptidase-4 (DPP-4) inhibitor
Half-life: 12 hours
Clinically important, potentially hazardous interactions with: efavirenz, rifampin
Pregnancy category: B
Important contra-indications noted in the prescribing guidelines for: nursing mothers; pediatric patients
Note: Linagliptin should not be used in patients with Type I diabetes or for the treatment of diabetic ketoacidosis, and has not been studied in combination with insulin. Glyxambi is linagliptin and empagliflozin.

Cardiovascular
Cardiotoxicity [3]
Hypertension [2]

Central Nervous System
Headache [5]

Neuromuscular/Skeletal
Arthralgia [2]
Back pain [3]
Pain in extremities [2]

Gastrointestinal/Hepatic
Diarrhea [2]
Nausea [3]

Respiratory
Cough [4]
Nasopharyngitis [7]
Upper respiratory tract infection [5]

Endocrine/Metabolic
Hyperglycemia [2]
Hyperlipidemia [2]
Hypertriglyceridemia [2]
Hypoglycemia [15]

Genitourinary
Urinary tract infection [3]

Other
Adverse effects [16]
Infection [3]

LINCOMYCIN

Trade name: Lincocin (Pfizer)
Indications: Various infections caused by susceptible organisms
Class: Antibiotic, lincosamide
Half-life: 2–11.5 hours
Clinically important, potentially hazardous interactions with: mivacurium
Pregnancy category: C
Important contra-indications noted in the prescribing guidelines for: nursing mothers; pediatric patients

---

Skin
AGEP [3]
Dermatitis [2]

Other
- Allergic reactions (<5%)

LINDANE

Synonyms: hexachlorocyclohexane; gamma benzene hexachloride
Indications: Scabies, pediculosis capitis, pediculosis pubis
Class: Chemical, Scabicide
Half-life: 17–22 hours
Clinically important, potentially hazardous interactions with: oil-based hair dressings
Pregnancy category: C
Important contra-indications noted in the prescribing guidelines for: nursing mothers; pediatric patients

---

Skin
- Dermatitis [5]
- Erythema (2%) [2]
- Pruritus (2%) [5]
- Toxicity [2]
- Urticaria [2]

Central Nervous System
- Neurotoxicity [3]
- Pseudotumor cerebri [2]
- Seizures [11]

Neuromuscular/Skeletal
- Rhabdomyolysis [3]

Other
- Adverse effects [4]
- Death [19]

LINEZOLID

Trade name: Zyvox (Pfizer)
Indications: Various infections caused by susceptible organisms
Class: Antibiotic, oxazolidinone
Half-life: 4–5 hours
Clinically important, potentially hazardous interactions with: alcohol, alpha blockers, altretamine, amitriptyline, amoxapine, amphetamines, anilidopiperidine opioids, antihypertensives, atomoxetine, beta blockers, buprenorphine, bupropion, buspirone, caffeine, carbamazepine, clomipramine, cyclobenzaprine, desipramine, desvenlafaxine, dexmethylphenidate, dextromethorphan, diethylpropion, doxapram, doxepin, fluoxetine, fluvoxamine, hydromorphone, imipramine, levodopa, lithium, MAO inhibitors, maprotiline, meperidine, methadone, methyldopa, methylphenidate, mirtazapine, nortriptyline, oral typhoid vaccine, paroxetine hydrochloride, propoxyphene, protriptyline, reserpine, rifampin, serotonin 5-HT1D receptor agonists, serotonin/norepinephrine reuptake inhibitors, sertraline, sibutramine, SSRIs, tapentadol, tetrabenazine, tetrahydrozoline, tramadol, trazodone, tricyclic antidepressants, trimipramine, tryptophan, venlafaxine
Pregnancy category: C
Important contra-indications noted in the prescribing guidelines for: nursing mothers

---

Skin
- Edema (2%)
- Fungal dermatitis (2%)
- Rash (<7%) [2]

Central Nervous System
- Dysgeusia (taste perversion) (<2%)
- Fever (2–14%)
- Headache (<11%) [2]
- Insomnia (3%)
- Neurotoxicity [5]
- Peripheral neuropathy [11]
- Seizures (3%)
- Serotonin syndrome [24]
- Vertigo (dizziness) (2%)

Gastrointestinal/Hepatic
- Abdominal pain (<2%)
- Constipation (2%)
- Diarrhea (3–11%) [7]
- Gastrointestinal bleeding (2%)
- Gastrointestinal disorder [2]
- Loose stools (<2%)
- Nausea (3–10%) [7]
- Vomiting (<10%) [3]

Respiratory
- Apnea (2%)
- Cough (<2%)
- Dyspnea (3%)
- Pneumonia (3%)
- Upper respiratory tract infection (4%)

Endocrine/Metabolic
- Acidosis [4]
- ALP increased (<4%)
- ALT increased (2–10%)
- AST increased (2–5%)
- Hypoglycemia [2]
- Hypokalemia (3%)

Genitourinary
- Candidal vaginitis (<2%)

Renal
- Nephrotoxicity [2]

Hematologic
- Anemia (<6%) [5]
- Leukopenia [2]
- Myelosuppression [7]
- Pancytopenia [4]
- Sepsis (8%)
- Thrombocytopenia (<5%) [17]

Ocular
- Optic neuropathy [11]

Local
- Injection-site reactions (3%)

Other
- Adverse effects (4%) [15]
- Allergic reactions (4%)
- Death [2]

LIOTHYRONINE

Synonym: T_3 sodium
Trade names: Cytomel (Pfizer), Triostat (Par)
Indications: Hypothyroidism
Class: Thyroid hormone, synthetic
Half-life: 16–49 hours
Clinically important, potentially hazardous interactions with: anticoagulants, dicumarol, warfarin
Pregnancy category: A

Skin
- Urticaria [3]

LIRAGLUTIDE

Trade names: Saxenda (Novo Nordisk), Victoza (Novo Nordisk)
Indications: To improve glycemic control in adults with Type II diabetes mellitus (Victoza), adjunct to diet and exercise for chronic weight management (Saxenda)
Class: Glucagon-like peptide-1 (GLP-1) receptor agonist
Half-life: 13 hours
Clinically important, potentially hazardous interactions with: acetaminophen, atorvastatin, digoxin, griseofulvin, lisinopril, warfarin
Pregnancy category: C
Important contra-indications noted in the prescribing guidelines for: nursing mothers; pediatric patients
Note: Contraindicated in patients with a personal or family history of medullary thyroid carcinoma or in patients with multiple endocrine neoplasia syndrome Type 2.
Black Box Warning: RISK OF THYROID C-CELL TUMORS

Cardiovascular
- Cardiotoxicity [2]
- Hypertension (3%)

Central Nervous System
- Headache (~5%) [5]
- Vertigo (dizziness) (6%) [2]

Neuromuscular/Skeletal
- Asthenia (fatigue) [3]
- Back pain (5%) [2]

Gastrointestinal/Hepatic
- Abdominal pain [3]
- Cholelithiasis (gallstones) [3]
- Constipation (10%) [10]
- Diarrhea (17%) [27]
- Dyspepsia [3]
- Gastrointestinal disorder [3]
- Nausea (28%) [52]
- Pancreatitis [8]
- Vomiting (11%) [25]

Respiratory
- Influenza (7%)
- Nasopharyngitis (5%) [4]
- Sinusitis (6%)
- Upper respiratory tract infection (10%) [2]

Endocrine/Metabolic
- Appetite decreased [5]
- Hypoglycemia [10]
- Weight loss [6]

Genitourinary
- Urinary tract infection (6%)

Local
- Injection-site reactions (2%) [3]

Other
- Adverse effects [9]
- Malignant neoplasms (11%)

LISDEXAMFETAMINE

Trade name: Vyvanse (Shire)
Indications: Attention-deficit hyperactivity disorder (ADHD)
Class: CNS stimulant, Dextroamphetamine prodrug
Half-life: 1 hour
Clinically important, potentially hazardous interactions with: acetazolamide, ammonium chloride, analgesics, antacids, antihistamines, antihypertensives, antipsychotics, atomoxetine, cannabinoids, carbonic anhydrase inhibitors, chlorpromazine, epinephrine, ethosuximide, haloperidol, iobenguane, lithium, MAO inhibitors, meperidine, methenamine, phenobarbital, phenytoin, propoxyphene, sympathomimetics, tricyclic antidepressants, urinary alkalinizing agents
Pregnancy category: C
Important contra-indications noted in the prescribing guidelines for: nursing mothers; pediatric patients
Black Box Warning: ABUSE AND DEPENDENCE

Skin
Hyperhidrosis (3%)
Rash (3%)

Mucosal
Xerostomia (4–26%) [16]

Cardiovascular
Hypertension (3%)
Tachycardia [3]

Central Nervous System
Agitation (3%)
Anorexia (5%) [2]
Anxiety [6]
Fever (2%)
Headache [25]
Insomnia (13–23%) [23]
Irritability (10%) [15]
Restlessness (3%)
Somnolence (drowsiness) (2%)
Tic disorder (2%)
Vertigo (dizziness) (5%) [4]

Neuromuscular/Skeletal
Asthenia (fatigue) [2]

Gastrointestinal/Hepatic
Abdominal pain (12%) [9]
Constipation [2]
Diarrhea (7%)
Nausea (6–7%) [9]
Vomiting (9%) [2]

Respiratory
Dyspnea (2%)
Nasopharyngitis [3]
Upper respiratory tract infection [9]

Endocrine/Metabolic
Appetite decreased (27–39%) [23]
Libido decreased (<2%)
Weight loss (9%) [7]

Genitourinary
Erectile dysfunction (<2%)

Other
Adverse effects [6]

LISINOPRIL

Trade names: Prinivil (Merck), Prinzide (Merck), Zestoretic (AstraZeneca), Zestril (AstraZeneca)
Indications: Hypertension, as adjunctive therapy in the management of heart failure, short-term treatment following myocardial infarction in hemodynamically stable patients
Class: Angiotensin-converting enzyme (ACE) inhibitor
Half-life: 12 hours
Clinically important, potentially hazardous interactions with: alcohol, aldesleukin, allopurinol, alpha blockers, alprostadil, amifostine, amiloride, angiotensin II receptor antagonists, antacids, antidiabetics, antihypertensives, antipsychotics, anxiolytics and hypnotics, aprotinin, azathioprine, baclofen, beta blockers, calcium channel blockers, clonidine, corticosteroids, cyclosporine, diazoxide, diuretics, eplerenone, estrogens, everolimus, general anesthetics, gold & gold compounds, heparins, hydralazine, hypotensives, insulin, levodopa, liraglutide, lithium, MAO inhibitors, metformin, methyldopa, methylphenidate, minoxidil, moxisylyte, moxonidine, nitrates, nitroprusside, NSAIDs, pentoxifylline, phosphodiesterase 5 inhibitors, potassium salts, prostacyclin analogues, rituximab, salicylates, sirolimus, spironolactone, sulfonylureas, temsirolimus, tizanidine, tolvaptan, triamterene, trimethoprim, yohimbine
Pregnancy category: D (category C in first trimester; category D in second and third trimesters)
Important contra-indications noted in the prescribing guidelines for: nursing mothers; pediatric patients
Note: Prinzide and Zestoretic are lisinopril and hydrochlorothiazide. Hydrochlorothiazide is a sulfonamide and can be absorbed systemically. Sulfonamides can produce severe, possibly fatal, reactions such as toxic epidermal necrolysis and Stevens-Johnson syndrome.
Contraindicated in patients with a history of angioedema related to previous treatment with an ACE inhibitor and in patients with hereditary or idiopathic angioedema.
Black Box Warning: FETAL TOXICITY

Skin
Angioedema [41]
Edema of lip [2]
Exanthems (3%) [4]
Exfoliative dermatitis [2]
Kaposi's sarcoma [2]
Lichenoid eruption [2]
Pemphigus foliaceus [2]
Pityriasis rosea [2]
Purpura [2]
Rash (2%) [6]
Urticaria [2]

Mucosal
Tongue edema [2]

Cardiovascular
Flushing [2]
Hypotension (<4%) [3]

Central Nervous System
Headache (4–6%)
Vertigo (dizziness) (5–12%)

Neuromuscular/Skeletal
Asthenia (fatigue) (3%)

Gastrointestinal/Hepatic
Hepatotoxicity [2]
Intestinal angioedema [3]
Pancreatitis [10]

Respiratory
Cough (4–9%) [15]
Upper respiratory tract infection (<2%)

Endocrine/Metabolic
Hyperkalemia [3]

Other
Death [3]

LITHIUM

Trade names: Eskalith (GSK), Lithobid (Solvay)
Indications: Manic-depressive states
Class: Antipsychotic, Mood stabilizer
Half-life: 18–24 hours
Clinically important, potentially hazardous interactions with: aceclofenac, acemetacin, acetazolamide, acitretin, amitriptyline, arsenic, benazepril, bendroflumethiazide, benzthiazide, captopril, celecoxib, chlorothiazide, chlorthalidone, cilazapril, citalopram, clozapine, cyclopenthiazide, desvenlafaxine, dichlorphenamide, diclofenac, enalapril, ethoxzolamide, etoricoxib, fluoxetine, flurbiprofen, fosinopril, haloperidol, hydrochlorothiazide, hydroflumethiazide, indapamide, insulin degludec, insulin detemir, insulin glargine, insulin glulisine, irbesartan, levomepromazine, linezolid, lisdexamfetamine, lisinopril, lorcaserin, lurasidone, meloxicam, meperidine, mesoridazine, methyclothiazide, metolazone, metronidazole, milnacipran, neostigmine, olanzapine, olmesartan, paliperidone, paroxetine hydrochloride, pericyazine, phenylbutazone, piroxicam, polythiazide, quinapril, quinethazone, ramipril, rocuronium, rofecoxib, sibutramine, sulpiride, tenoxicam, tetrabenazine, thalidomide, thiazides, tinidazole, tolmetin, trandolapril, trichlormethiazide, trifluoperazine, valdecoxib, venlafaxine, xipamide, ziprasidone, zofenopril, zuclopenthixol
Pregnancy category: D

Skin
Acneform eruption [19]
Angioedema [2]
Atopic dermatitis (3%)
Darier's disease [3]
Dermatitis [4]
Dermatitis herpetiformis [3]
Edema [3]
Exanthems [10]
Exfoliative dermatitis [3]
Follicular keratosis [3]
Folliculitis [5]
Hidradenitis [3]
Ichthyosis [2]
Keratosis pilaris [2]
Linear IgA bullous dermatosis [4]
Lupus erythematosus [5]

Myxedema [10]
Papulo-nodular lesions (elbows) [2]
Pruritus [8]
Psoriasis (2%) [58]
Purpura [2]
Pustules [2]
Rash (<10%)
Seborrheic dermatitis [3]
Ulcerations (lower extremities) [5]
Urticaria [3]
Vasculitis [4]

Hair
Alopecia (10–19%) [17]
Alopecia areata (2%) [3]

Nails
Nail dystrophy [2]

Mucosal
Lichenoid stomatitis [3]
Oral ulceration [4]
Sialorrhea [4]
Stomatitis [2]
Xerostomia [5]

Cardiovascular
Brugada syndrome [5]
QT prolongation [4]

Central Nervous System
Amnesia [2]
Coma [2]
Dysgeusia (taste perversion) (>10%)
Hallucinations [2]
Neuroleptic malignant syndrome [7]
Neurotoxicity [3]
Parkinsonism [8]
Pseudohallucinations [2]
Restless legs syndrome [4]
Serotonin syndrome [5]
Somnambulism [3]
Tremor [3]

Neuromuscular/Skeletal
Myasthenia gravis [2]
Rhabdomyolysis [3]

Endocrine/Metabolic
Diabetes insipidus [4]
Hypercalcemia [3]
Hyperparathyroidism [5]
Hyperthyroidism [2]
Hypothyroidism [3]
Thyrotoxicosis [2]
Weight gain [3]

Genitourinary
Polyuria [2]
Priapism [5]

Renal
Nephrogenic diabetes insipidus [2]
Nephrotoxicity [13]

Other
Adverse effects [4]
Side effects (23–33%) [4]
Teratogenicity [3]

LIXISENATIDE *

Trade names: Adlyxin (Sanofi-Aventis), Lyxumia (Sanofi-Aventis)
Indications: To improve glycemic control in adults with Type II diabetes mellitus
Class: Glucagon-like peptide-1 (GLP-1) receptor agonist
Half-life: 3 hours
Clinically important, potentially hazardous interactions with: none known
Pregnancy category: N/A (Use during pregnancy only if the potential benefit justifies the potential risk to the fetus)
Important contra-indications noted in the prescribing guidelines for: nursing mothers; pediatric patients

---

Central Nervous System
Headache (9%) [2]
Vertigo (dizziness) (7%) [2]

Gastrointestinal/Hepatic
Abdominal distension (2%)
Abdominal pain (2%)
Constipation (3%)
Diarrhea (8%) [6]
Dyspepsia (3%)
Nausea (25%) [16]
Vomiting (10%) [15]

Endocrine/Metabolic
Hypoglycemia (3%) [7]

Local
Injection-site reactions (4%) [2]

Other
Adverse effects [3]
Allergic reactions [2]

LOMITAPIDE

Trade name: Juxtapid (Aegerion)
Indications: Homozygous familial hypercholesterolemia
Class: Lipid regulator
Half-life: 39.7 hours
Clinically important, potentially hazardous interactions with: bile acid sequestrants, boceprevir, clarithromycin, conivaptan, grapefruit juice, indinavir, itraconazole, ketoconazole, lopinavir, lovastatin, mibefradil, nefazodone, nelfinavir, oral contraceptives, P-glycoprotein substrates, posaconazole, ritonavir, saquinavir, simvastatin, strong or moderate CYP3A4 inhibitors, telaprevir, telithromycin, voriconazole, warfarin
Pregnancy category: X
Important contra-indications noted in the prescribing guidelines for: nursing mothers; pediatric patients
Black Box Warning: RISK OF HEPATOTOXICITY

Mucosal
Nasal congestion (10%)

Cardiovascular
Angina (10%)
Chest pain (24%)
Palpitation (10%)

Central Nervous System
Fever (10%)
Headache (10%)
Vertigo (dizziness) (10%)

Neuromuscular/Skeletal
Asthenia (fatigue) (17%)
Back pain (14%)

Gastrointestinal/Hepatic
Abdominal pain (21–34%)
Constipation (21%)
Defecation (urgency) (10%)
Diarrhea (79%) [3]
Dyspepsia (38%) [3]
Flatulence (21%)
Gastroenteritis (14%)
Gastroesophageal reflux (10%)
Hepatotoxicity [5]
Nausea (65%) [2]
Tenesmus (10%)
Vomiting (34%) [3]

Respiratory
Influenza (21%)
Nasopharyngitis (17%)
Pharyngolaryngeal pain (14%)

Endocrine/Metabolic
ALT increased (17%) [3]
Weight loss (24%)

Other
Adverse effects [5]

LOPERAMIDE

Trade names: Imodium (McNeil), Maalox (Novartis)
Indications: Diarrhea
Class: Opiate agonist
Half-life: 9–14 hours
Clinically important, potentially hazardous interactions with: St John's wort
Pregnancy category: B
Important contra-indications noted in the prescribing guidelines for: nursing mothers; pediatric patients

---

Gastrointestinal/Hepatic
Abdominal pain [2]
Constipation [3]
Nausea [2]

LOPINAVIR

Trade name: Kaletra (AbbVie)
Indications: HIV-1 infected children above the age of 2 years and adults, in combination with other antiretroviral agents
Class: Antiretroviral, HIV-1 protease inhibitor
Half-life: 5–6 hours
Clinically important, potentially hazardous interactions with: abacavir, alfuzosin, amiodarone, amprenavir, aripiprazole, artemether/lumefantrine, atazanavir, atorvastatin, atovaquone, bepridil, bosentan, bupropion, cabozantinib, carbamazepine, chlorpheniramine, cisapride, clarithromycin, colchicine, cyclosporine, darifenacin, darunavir, dasatinib,

delavirdine, dexamethasone, didanosine, digoxin, disulfiram, efavirenz, eltrombopag, ergotamine, estradiol, felodipine, fentanyl, flecainide, fluticasone propionate, fosamprenavir, indinavir, itraconazole, ketoconazole, lidocaine, lidocaine, lomitapide, lovastatin, maraviroc, methadone, methylergonovine, metronidazole, midazolam, mifepristone, nelfinavir, nevirapine, nicardipine, nifedipine, nilotinib, ombitasvir/paritaprevir/ritonavir, phenobarbital, phenytoin, pimozide, pitavastatin, ponatinib, primidone, quinidine, ranolazine, rifabutin, rifampin, rilpivirine, rivaroxaban, rosuvastatin, ruxolitinib, salmeterol, saquinavir, sildenafil, simeprevir, simvastatin, sirolimus, St John's wort, tacrolimus, tadalafil, telithromycin, tenofovir disoproxil, tipranavir, tolterodine, trazodone, triazolam, vardenafil, venetoclax, vinblastine, vincristine, voriconazole, warfarin, zidovudine
Pregnancy category: C
Important contra-indications noted in the prescribing guidelines for: nursing mothers
Note: Kaletra is lopinavir and ritonavir.

Skin
Acneform eruption (<10%)
Lipodystrophy (<10%)
Rash (<10%) [5]

Hair
Alopecia [3]

Central Nervous System
Vertigo (dizziness) [2]

Neuromuscular/Skeletal
Asthenia (fatigue) (<10%) [2]

Gastrointestinal/Hepatic
Diarrhea (>10%) [5]
Flatulence (<10%)
Nausea (<10%) [4]
Pancreatitis [2]
Vomiting (<10%) [3]

Renal
Nephrolithiasis [2]

LORATADINE

Trade names: Alavert (Wyeth), Claritin (Schering), Claritin-D (Schering)
Indications: Allergic rhinitis, urticaria
Class: Histamine H1 receptor antagonist
Half-life: 3–20 hours
Clinically important, potentially hazardous interactions with: amiodarone
Pregnancy category: B

Skin
Anaphylactoid reactions/Anaphylaxis (>2%)
Angioedema (>2%)
Dermatitis (>2%)
Diaphoresis (>2%)
Erythema multiforme (>2%)
Fixed eruption [3]
Peripheral edema (>2%)
Photosensitivity (>2%)
Pruritus (>2%)
Purpura (>2%)
Rash (>2%)
Urticaria (>2%) [4]
Xerosis (>2%)

Hair
Alopecia (>2%)
Dry hair (>2%)

Mucosal
Sialorrhea (>2%)
Stomatitis (>2%)
Xerostomia (>10%) [9]

Cardiovascular
Flushing (>2%)
QT prolongation [2]
Torsades de pointes [4]

Central Nervous System
Dysgeusia (taste perversion) (>2%)
Headache (12%) [2]
Hyperesthesia (>2%)
Paresthesias (>2%)
Somnolence (drowsiness) [2]

Neuromuscular/Skeletal
Asthenia (fatigue) (4%) [2]
Myalgia/Myopathy (>2%)

Endocrine/Metabolic
Gynecomastia (>2%)
Mastodynia (<10%)

Genitourinary
Vaginitis (>2%)

LORAZEPAM

Trade name: Ativan (Valeant)
Indications: Anxiety, depression
Class: Benzodiazepine
Half-life: 10–20 hours
Clinically important, potentially hazardous interactions with: alcohol, amprenavir, barbiturates, chlorpheniramine, clarithromycin, clozapine, CNS depressants, efavirenz, erythromycin, esomeprazole, eszopiclone, imatinib, MAO inhibitors, narcotics, nelfinavir, phenothiazines, valproate
Pregnancy category: D

Skin
Dermatitis (<10%)
Diaphoresis (>10%)
Pseudolymphoma [2]
Rash (>10%)

Mucosal
Nasal congestion (<10%)
Sialopenia (>10%)
Xerostomia (>10%)

Cardiovascular
Hypotension [2]

Central Nervous System
Agitation [2]
Akathisia (<10%)
Amnesia (<10%) [18]
Catatonia [2]
Confusion (<10%)
Delirium [2]
Depression (<10%)
Hallucinations [2]
Headache (<10%)
Somnolence (drowsiness) (<10%) [2]
Tremor (<10%)
Vertigo (dizziness) (<10%)

Respiratory
Apnea (<10%)
Hyperventilation (<10%)

Ocular
Visual disturbances (<10%)

Local
Injection-site pain (>10%)
Injection-site phlebitis (>10%)

Other
Adverse effects [2]

LORCASERIN

Trade name: Belviq (Arena)
Indications: Obesity in adults who have at least one weight-related health condition, such as high blood pressure, Type II diabetes, or high cholesterol
Class: Serotonin receptor agonist
Half-life: ~11 hours
Clinically important, potentially hazardous interactions with: antipsychotics, bupropion, dextromethorphan, lithium, MAO inhibitors, SNRIs, SSRIs, St John's wort, tramadol, tricyclic antidepressants, triptans
Pregnancy category: X
Important contra-indications noted in the prescribing guidelines for: nursing mothers; pediatric patients

---

Skin
Peripheral edema (5%)
Rash (2%)

Mucosal
Nasal congestion (3%)
Oropharyngeal pain (4%)
Xerostomia (5%) [2]

Cardiovascular
Hypertension (5%)
Valvulopathy (2–3%) [5]

Central Nervous System
Anxiety (4%)
Cognitive impairment (2%) [2]
Depression (2%) [2]
Euphoria [2]
Headache (15–17%) [11]
Insomnia (4%)
Vertigo (dizziness) (7–9%) [9]

Neuromuscular/Skeletal
Asthenia (fatigue) (7%) [3]
Back pain (6–12%) [2]
Bone or joint pain (2%)
Muscle spasm (5%)

Gastrointestinal/Hepatic
Constipation (6%)
Diarrhea (7%)
Gastroenteritis (3%)
Nausea (8–9%) [9]
Vomiting (4%)

Respiratory
Cough (4%)
Nasopharyngitis (11–13%) [2]
Upper respiratory tract infection (14%)

Endocrine/Metabolic
Appetite decreased (2%)
Diabetes mellitus (exacerbation) (3%)

Hypoglycemia (29%) [3]

Genitourinary
Urinary tract infection (7–9%)

Other
Toothache (3%)

LOSARTAN

Trade names: Cozaar (Merck), Hyzaar (Merck)
Indications: Hypertension
Class: Angiotensin II receptor antagonist (blocker), Antihypertensive
Half-life: 2 hours
Clinically important, potentially hazardous interactions with: aliskiren, rifampin, voriconazole
Pregnancy category: D (category C in first trimester; category D in second and third trimesters)
Important contra-indications noted in the prescribing guidelines for: nursing mothers
Note: Hyzaar is losartan and hydrochlorothiazide. Hydrochlorothiazide is a sulfonamide and can be absorbed systemically. Sulfonamides can produce severe, possibly fatal, reactions such as toxic epidermal necrolysis and Stevens-Johnson syndrome.
Black Box Warning: USE IN PREGNANCY

Skin
Anaphylactoid reactions/Anaphylaxis [2]
Angioedema [11]
Purpura [2]

Mucosal
Nasal congestion (2%)

Central Nervous System
Ageusia (taste loss) [2]
Vertigo (dizziness) (3%)

Neuromuscular/Skeletal
Back pain (2%)

Respiratory
Upper respiratory tract infection (8%)

Endocrine/Metabolic
Hyperkalemia [7]

Other
Adverse effects [7]

LOVASTATIN

Trade names: Advicor (Kos), Altoprev (Shionogi), Mevacor (Merck)
Indications: Hypercholesterolemia
Class: HMG-CoA reductase inhibitor, Statin
Half-life: 1–2 hours
Clinically important, potentially hazardous interactions with: amprenavir, atazanavir, azithromycin, boceprevir, bosentan, cholestyramine, clarithromycin, cyclosporine, darunavir, delavirdine, efavirenz, erythromycin, exenatide, fenofibrate, fosamprenavir, gemfibrozil, grapefruit juice, imatinib, indinavir, itraconazole, lomitapide, lopinavir, mifepristone, nelfinavir, ombitasvir/paritaprevir/ritonavir, paclitaxel, posaconazole, red rice yeast, tacrolimus, telaprevir, telithromycin, ticagrelor, tipranavir, tolvaptan, verapamil
Pregnancy category: X
Important contra-indications noted in the prescribing guidelines for: nursing mothers

---

Skin
Exanthems (<5%) [3]
Lupus erythematosus [4]
Pruritus (5%) [2]
Rash (5%) [3]

Central Nervous System
Parkinsonism [2]

Neuromuscular/Skeletal
Asthenia (fatigue) [2]
Myalgia/Myopathy (<10%) [6]
Rhabdomyolysis [41]

Gastrointestinal/Hepatic
Hepatotoxicity [2]
Pancreatitis [2]

Endocrine/Metabolic
Gynecomastia (<10%)

LOXAPINE

Trade names: Adasuve (Teva), Loxitane (Watson)
Indications: Psychoses
Class: Antipsychotic, tricyclic
Half-life: 12–19 hours (terminal)
Clinically important, potentially hazardous interactions with: none known
Pregnancy category: C
Important contra-indications noted in the prescribing guidelines for: the elderly; nursing mothers; pediatric patients
Black Box Warning: BRONCHOSPASM and INCREASED MORTALITY IN ELDERLY PATIENTS WITH DEMENTIA-RELATED PSYCHOSIS

Skin
Rash (<10%)

Mucosal
Xerostomia (>10%)

Central Nervous System
Dysgeusia (taste perversion) (14%) [7]
Neuroleptic malignant syndrome [2]
Sedation (12%) [3]
Somnolence (drowsiness) [2]
Vertigo (dizziness) [2]

Neuromuscular/Skeletal
Rhabdomyolysis [3]

Respiratory
Bronchospasm [3]
Pulmonary toxicity [3]

Endocrine/Metabolic
Gynecomastia (<10%)

LUBIPROSTONE

Trade name: Amitiza (Takeda)
Indications: Constipation, irritable bowel syndrome
Class: Chloride channel activator
Half-life: 0–1.4 hours
Clinically important, potentially hazardous interactions with: none known
Pregnancy category: C
Important contra-indications noted in the prescribing guidelines for: nursing mothers; pediatric patients
Note: Contraindicated in patients with known or suspected mechanical gastrointestinal obstruction.

Skin
Peripheral edema (4%)

Central Nervous System
Headache (13%) [7]

Neuromuscular/Skeletal
Arthralgia (3%)
Asthenia (fatigue) (2%)
Back pain (2%)

Gastrointestinal/Hepatic
Abdominal distension [5]
Abdominal pain (7%) [8]
Diarrhea [16]
Flatulence [3]
Nausea [16]
Vomiting [7]

Respiratory
Dyspnea [3]
Flu-like syndrome (2%)
Sinusitis (5%)
Upper respiratory tract infection (4%)

Other
Adverse effects [2]

LULICONAZOLE

Trade name: Luzu (Medicis)
Indications: Interdigital tinea pedis, tinea cruris, and tinea corporis caused by the organisms *Trichophyton rubrum* and *Epidermophyton floccosum*
Class: Antifungal, azole
Half-life: N/A
Clinically important, potentially hazardous interactions with: none known
Pregnancy category: C
Important contra-indications noted in the prescribing guidelines for: nursing mothers; pediatric patients

---

Skin
Contact dermatitis [2]

LUMACAFTOR/IVACAFTOR

Trade name: Orkambi (Vertex)
Indications: Cystic fibrosis in patients aged 12 years and older who are homozygous for the *F508del* mutation in the *CFTR* gene
Class: CFTR potentiator, CYP3A4 inducer
Half-life: 26 hours
Clinically important, potentially hazardous interactions with: rifampin, St John's wort
Pregnancy category: B
Important contra-indications noted in the prescribing guidelines for: nursing mothers; pediatric patients
Note: See also separate profile for ivacaftor.

Skin
Rash (7%) [2]

Mucosal
Rhinorrhea (6%)

Neuromuscular/Skeletal
Asthenia (fatigue) (9%)

Gastrointestinal/Hepatic
Diarrhea (12%)
Flatulence (7%)
Nausea (13%)

Respiratory
Dyspnea (13%) [2]
Influenza (5%)
Nasopharyngitis (13%)
Upper respiratory tract infection (10%)

Endocrine/Metabolic
Creatine phosphokinase increased (7%)
Menstrual irregularities (10%)

Other
Adverse effects [2]

LURASIDONE

Trade name: Latuda (Sunovion)
Indications: Schizophrenia, depressive epidodes associated with bipolar I disorder
Class: Antipsychotic
Half-life: 18 hours
Clinically important, potentially hazardous interactions with: alcohol, amphetamines, CNS depressants, dasatinib, deferasirox, diltiazem, disopyramide, dopamine, dopamine agonists, droperidol, efavirenz, epinephrine, hydroxyzine, ketoconazole, levomepromazine, lithium, MAO inhibitors, methylphenidate, metoclopramide, ombitasvir/paritaprevir/ritonavir, pimozide, procainamide, quinagolide, quinidine, rifampin, strong CYP3A4 inducers or inhibitors, tetrabenazine, tocilizumab
Pregnancy category: B
Important contra-indications noted in the prescribing guidelines for: the elderly; nursing mothers; pediatric patients
Black Box Warning: INCREASED MORTALITY IN ELDERLY PATIENTS WITH DEMENTIA-RELATED PSYCHOSIS

Mucosal
Sialorrhea (2%)

Central Nervous System
Agitation (5%)
Akathisia (13%) [18]
Anxiety (5%)
Extrapyramidal symptoms [2]
Insomnia (10%) [2]
Parkinsonism (10%) [5]
Restlessness (2%)
Sedation [7]
Somnolence (drowsiness) (17%) [11]
Vertigo (dizziness) (4%) [3]

Neuromuscular/Skeletal
Dystonia (5%)

Gastrointestinal/Hepatic
Dyspepsia (6%)
Nausea (10%) [10]
Vomiting (8%) [2]

Endocrine/Metabolic
Weight gain (5%) [3]

Other
Adverse effects [3]

MACITENTAN

Trade name: Opsumit (Actelion)
Indications: Pulmonary arterial hypertension
Class: Endothelin receptor (ETR) antagonist
Half-life: 16 hours
Clinically important, potentially hazardous interactions with: ketoconazole, rifampin, ritonavir, strong CYP3A4 inducers or inhibitors
Pregnancy category: X
Important contra-indications noted in the prescribing guidelines for: nursing mothers; pediatric patients
Note: Contraindicated in pregnancy.
Black Box Warning: EMBRYO-FETAL TOXICITY

Skin
Peripheral edema [2]

Central Nervous System
Headache (14%) [6]

Gastrointestinal/Hepatic
Hepatotoxicity [5]

Respiratory
Bronchitis (12%) [2]
Influenza (6%)
Nasopharyngitis (20%) [6]
Pharyngitis (20%)
Upper respiratory tract infection [2]

Genitourinary
Urinary tract infection (9%)

Hematologic
Anemia (13%) [7]

MARAVIROC

Trade names: Celsentri (ViiV), Selzentry (ViiV)
Indications: HIV infection
Class: Antiretroviral
Half-life: 14–18 hours
Clinically important, potentially hazardous interactions with: atazanavir, clarithromycin, conivaptan, CYP3A4 inhibitors or inducers, darunavir, dasatinib, deferasirox, delavirdine, efavirenz, etravirine, indinavir, ketoconazole, lopinavir, nelfinavir, oxcarbazepine, rifampin, rifapentine, ritonavir, saquinavir, St John's wort, telithromycin, voriconazole
Pregnancy category: B
Important contra-indications noted in the prescribing guidelines for: the elderly; nursing mothers; pediatric patients
Black Box Warning: HEPATOTOXICITY

Skin
Dermatitis (5%)
Folliculitis (5%)
Lipodystrophy (5%)
Pruritus (6%) [2]
Rash (17%) [2]

Mucosal
Stomatitis (4%)

Cardiovascular
Postural hypotension [2]

Central Nervous System
Depression (6%)
Fever (21%) [2]
Headache [3]
Pain (8%)
Paresthesias (8%)
Peripheral neuropathy (5%)
Sleep disturbances (12%)
Vertigo (dizziness) (14%)

Neuromuscular/Skeletal
Asthenia (fatigue) [2]
Myalgia/Myopathy (5%)

Gastrointestinal/Hepatic
Abdominal pain (14%)
Diarrhea [2]
Hepatotoxicity [2]

Respiratory
Cough (22%) [2]
Flu-like syndrome (3%)
Nasopharyngitis [2]
Pneumonia (4%)
Upper respiratory tract infection (37%) [2]

Genitourinary
Urinary tract infection (4%)

Other
Adverse effects [6]

MARIHUANA

Synonyms: marijuana; grass; hashish; pot; cannabis
Indications: Nausea and vomiting, substance abuse drug
Class: Antiemetic, Cannabinoid, Hallucinogen
Half-life: N/A
Clinically important, potentially hazardous interactions with: atazanavir
Pregnancy category: N/A
Note: Marihuana is the popular name for the dried flowering leaves of the hemp plant, *cannabis sativa*. It contains tetrahydrocannabinols.

Cardiovascular
Cardiotoxicity [4]
Myocardial infarction [2]

Central Nervous System
Amnesia [2]
Hallucinations [2]
Schizophrenia [3]
Seizures [2]
Stroke [2]

Gastrointestinal/Hepatic
Pancreatitis [2]

Genitourinary
Priapism [2]

Ocular
Hallucinations, visual [2]

Other
Adverse effects [2]

MDMA

Synonyms: 3,4-methylenedioxymethamphetamine; ecstasy; E; X; molly; club drug
Indications: N/A
Class: Amphetamine
Half-life: N/A
Clinically important, potentially hazardous interactions with: none known

---

Skin
Diaphoresis [4]

Mucosal
Xerostomia [5]

Cardiovascular
Cardiotoxicity [2]
Myocardial infarction [2]

Central Nervous System
Amnesia [2]
Confusion [2]
Depression (37%) [14]
Hallucinations [4]
Headache [2]
Hyperthermia [2]
Memory loss [3]
Neuroleptic malignant syndrome [4]
Neurotoxicity [5]
Parkinsonism [4]
Psychosis [4]
Seizures [3]
Serotonin syndrome [6]

Neuromuscular/Skeletal
Myalgia/Myopathy [2]
Rhabdomyolysis [33]

Gastrointestinal/Hepatic
Hepatitis [2]
Hepatotoxicity [4]
Nausea [2]

Endocrine/Metabolic
Hyponatremia [4]
SIADH [8]

Genitourinary
Priapism [2]

Ocular
Hallucinations, visual [2]

Other
Bruxism [8]
Death [47]
Dipsia (thirst) [2]
Multiorgan failure [2]

MEASLES, MUMPS & RUBELLA (MMR) VIRUS VACCINE

Trade name: M-M-R II (Merck)
Indications: Protection against measles (rubeola), mumps and rubella (German measles)
Class: Vaccine
Half-life: N/A
Clinically important, potentially hazardous interactions with: none known

Pregnancy category: C
Important contra-indications noted in the prescribing guidelines for: nursing mothers; pediatric patients
Note: Contraindicated for pregnant females; patients who have had anaphylactic or anaphylactoid reactions to neomycin; febrile respiratory illness or other active febrile infection; patients receiving immunosuppressive therapy or with blood dyscrasias, leukemia, lymphomas of any type, or other malignant neoplasms affecting the bone marrow or lymphatic systems; primary and acquired immunodeficiency states, or individuals with a family history of congenital or hereditary immunodeficiency, until the immune competence of the potential vaccine recipient is demonstrated.

Skin
Henoch–Schönlein purpura [2]
Rash [4]

Central Nervous System
Fever [7]
Seizures [3]

Neuromuscular/Skeletal
Asthenia (fatigue) [2]

Gastrointestinal/Hepatic
Vomiting [2]

Local
Injection-site erythema [2]
Injection-site pain [2]
Injection-site reactions [3]

Other
Adverse effects [4]
Infection [2]

MEBENDAZOLE

Trade name: Vermox (Janssen)
Indications: Parasitic worm infestations
Class: Anthelmintic, Antibiotic, imidazole
Half-life: 1–12 hours
Clinically important, potentially hazardous interactions with: aminophylline
Pregnancy category: C

Skin
Stevens–Johnson syndrome [2]

Hair
Alopecia [3]

Central Nervous System
Headache [2]
Vertigo (dizziness) [2]

Gastrointestinal/Hepatic
Abdominal pain [4]

MECHLORETHAMINE

Synonyms: mustine; nitrogen mustard
Indications: Hodgkin's disease, mycosis fungoides
Class: Alkylating agent
Half-life: <1 minute
Clinically important, potentially hazardous interactions with: aldesleukin, vaccines
Pregnancy category: D

Skin
Anaphylactoid reactions/Anaphylaxis (<10%) [4]
Bullous dermatitis [3]
Dermatitis [26]
Herpes zoster (>10%)
Hypersensitivity (<10%)
Pigmentation [8]
Pruritus [2]
Squamous cell carcinoma [3]
Urticaria [3]

Hair
Alopecia (<10%)

Central Nervous System
Dysgeusia (taste perversion) (<10%)

Local
Injection-site extravasation (<10%)
Injection-site thrombophlebitis (<10%) [2]

MEDROXY-PROGESTERONE

Trade names: Depo-Provera (Pfizer), Lunelle (Pfizer), Premphase (Wyeth), Prempro (Wyeth), Provera (Pfizer)
Indications: Secondary amenorrhea, renal or endometrial carcinoma
Class: Progestogen
Half-life: 30 days
Clinically important, potentially hazardous interactions with: acitretin, dofetilide
Pregnancy category: X

Skin
Acneform eruption (<5%)
Chloasma (<10%)
Diaphoresis (<31%)
Edema (>10%)
Melasma (<10%)
Pruritus (<10%)
Rash (<5%)

Hair
Alopecia (<5%)

Cardiovascular
Flushing (12%)
Thrombophlebitis (<10%)

Neuromuscular/Skeletal
Osteoporosis [2]

Endocrine/Metabolic
Amenorrhea [3]
Galactorrhea [2]
Mastodynia (<5%)
Weight gain [3]

Genitourinary
Vaginitis (<5%)

Local
Injection-site pain (>10%)

MEFENAMIC ACID

Trade name: Ponstel (First Horizon)
Indications: Pain, dysmenorrhea
Class: Non-steroidal anti-inflammatory (NSAID)
Half-life: 3.5 hours
Clinically important, potentially hazardous interactions with: methotrexate
Pregnancy category: C
Important contra-indications noted in the prescribing guidelines for: nursing mothers; pediatric patients
Note: NSAIDs may cause an increased risk of serious cardiovascular and gastrointestinal adverse events, which can be fatal. This risk may increase with duration of use.
Black Box Warning: CARDIOVASCULAR AND GASTROINTESTINAL RISK

Skin
Anaphylactoid reactions/Anaphylaxis [2]
Erythema multiforme [2]
Fixed eruption [11]
Pruritus (<10%)
Rash (>10%)
Toxic epidermal necrolysis [2]

Cardiovascular
Myocardial infarction [2]

Central Nervous System
Seizures [2]

Gastrointestinal/Hepatic
Hepatotoxicity [2]

Renal
Renal failure [2]

Ocular
Glaucoma [2]

MEFLOQUINE

Trade name: Lariam (Roche)
Indications: Malaria
Class: Antimalarial, Antiprotozoal
Half-life: 21–22 days
Clinically important, potentially hazardous interactions with: acebutolol, artemether/lumefantrine, ethosuximide, halofantrine, ketoconazole, lacosamide, moxifloxacin, oxcarbazepine, quinine, tiagabine, typhoid vaccine, vigabatrin
Pregnancy category: C
Important contra-indications noted in the prescribing guidelines for: nursing mothers
Black Box Warning: NEUROPSYCHIATRIC ADVERSE REACTIONS

Skin
Anaphylactoid reactions/Anaphylaxis [2]
Erythema [2]
Exanthems (30%)
Pruritus (4–10%) [2]
Psoriasis [2]
Rash (<10%)
Stevens–Johnson syndrome [2]
Toxic epidermal necrolysis [2]
Vasculitis [3]

Cardiovascular
- Palpitation [3]
- Tachycardia [2]

Central Nervous System
- Abnormal dreams [2]
- Aggression [2]
- Anorexia [2]
- Anxiety [4]
- Chills (<10%)
- Delusions [2]
- Depression [6]
- Fever (<10%) [2]
- Hallucinations [3]
- Headache (<10%) [5]
- Insomnia [3]
- Mania [4]
- Neurotoxicity [8]
- Psychosis [8]
- Seizures [5]
- Suicidal ideation [2]
- Vertigo (dizziness) (<10%) [19]

Neuromuscular/Skeletal
- Arthralgia [2]
- Asthenia (fatigue) (<10%) [2]
- Myalgia/Myopathy (<10%) [2]

Gastrointestinal/Hepatic
- Abdominal pain [4]
- Diarrhea [4]
- Nausea [8]
- Vomiting [14]

Otic
- Tinnitus (<10%)

Ocular
- Maculopathy [2]

Other
- Adverse effects [2]
- Death [3]

MELOXICAM

Trade name: Mobic (Boehringer Ingelheim)
Indications: Osteoarthritis
Class: COX-2 inhibitor, Non-steroidal anti-inflammatory (NSAID)
Half-life: 15–20 hours
Clinically important, potentially hazardous interactions with: ACE inhibitors, adrenergic neurone blockers, alcohol, aliskiren, alpha blockers, angiotensin II receptor antagonists, anticoagulants, antidepressants, antiplatelet agents, aspirin, baclofen, beta blockers, bile acid sequestrants, calcium channel blockers, cardiac glycosides, cholestyramine, clonidine, clopidogrel, collagenase, conivaptan, corticosteroids, coumarins, cyclosporine, dabigatran, dasatinib, desmopressin, diazoxide, digoxin, diuretics, drotrecogin alfa, eplerenone, erlotinib, glucosamine, haloperidol, heparins, hydralazine, ibritumomab, iloprost, ketorolac, lithium, methotrexate, methyldopa, mifamurtide, minoxidil, moxonidine, nitrates, nitroprusside, NSAIDs, pemetrexed, penicillamine, pentosan, pentoxifylline, phenindione, pralatrexate, prasugrel, probenecid, prostacyclin analogues, quinolones, ritonavir, serotonin/norepinephrine reuptake inhibitors, SSRIs, sulfonylureas, tacrolimus, thrombolytic agents, tositumomab & iodine[131], treprostinil, vancomycin, venlafaxine, vitamin K antagonists, voriconazole, zidovudine
Pregnancy category: C (category D from 30 weeks gestation)
Important contra-indications noted in the prescribing guidelines for: the elderly; nursing mothers
Note: NSAIDs may cause an increased risk of serious cardiovascular and gastrointestinal adverse events, which can be fatal. This risk may increase with duration of use.
Black Box Warning: CARDIOVASCULAR AND GASTROINTESTINAL RISKS

Skin
- Anaphylactoid reactions/Anaphylaxis (<2%)
- Angioedema (<2%) [3]
- Bullous dermatitis (<2%)
- Edema (2–5%)
- Erythema [2]
- Erythema multiforme (<2%)
- Exanthems (<2%)
- Facial edema (<2%)
- Hematoma [3]
- Hot flashes (<2%)
- Hyperhidrosis (<2%)
- Hypersensitivity [2]
- Photosensitivity (<2%)
- Pruritus (<2%) [3]
- Purpura (<2%)
- Rash (<3%) [3]
- Stevens–Johnson syndrome (<2%)
- Toxic epidermal necrolysis (<2%)
- Urticaria (<2%) [4]
- Vasculitis (<2%)

Hair
- Alopecia (<2%)

Mucosal
- Ulcerative stomatitis (<2%)
- Xerostomia (<2%)

Cardiovascular
- Angina (<2%)
- Arrhythmias (<2%)
- Cardiac failure (<2%)
- Hypertension (<2%)
- Hypotension (<2%)
- Myocardial infarction (<2%)
- Palpitation (<2%)
- Tachycardia (<2%)

Central Nervous System
- Abnormal dreams (<2%)
- Anxiety (<2%)
- Confusion (<2%)
- Depression (<2%)
- Dysgeusia (taste perversion) (<2%)
- Fever (<2%)
- Headache (2–6%) [2]
- Insomnia (<4%)
- Nervousness (<2%)
- Pain (4%)
- Paresthesias (<2%)
- Seizures (<2%)
- Somnolence (drowsiness) (<2%)
- Syncope (<2%)
- Tremor (<2%)
- Vertigo (dizziness) (<3%)

Neuromuscular/Skeletal
- Arthralgia (<5%)
- Asthenia (fatigue) [2]
- Back pain (<3%)
- Bone or joint pain (2%)

Gastrointestinal/Hepatic
- Abdominal pain (2–5%) [2]
- Black stools (<2%)
- Colitis (<2%)
- Constipation (<3%) [2]
- Diarrhea (2–6%) [2]
- Dyspepsia (4–10%) [2]
- Eructation (belching) (<2%)
- Esophagitis (<2%)
- Flatulence (<3%)
- Gastritis (<2%)
- Gastroesophageal reflux (<2%)
- Gastrointestinal bleeding [2]
- Gastrointestinal perforation (<2%) [2]
- Gastrointestinal ulceration (<2%) [3]
- Hematemesis (<2%)
- Hepatitis (<2%)
- Hepatotoxicity [5]
- Nausea (3–7%) [4]
- Pancreatitis (<2%)
- Vomiting (<3%)

Respiratory
- Asthma (<2%)
- Bronchospasm (<2%)
- Cough (<2%)
- Dyspnea (<2%)
- Flu-like syndrome (2–3%)
- Upper respiratory tract infection (<8%)

Endocrine/Metabolic
- ALT increased (<2%)
- Appetite increased (<2%)
- AST increased (<2%)
- Dehydration (<2%)
- GGT increased (<2%)
- Weight gain (<2%)
- Weight loss (<2%)

Genitourinary
- Albuminuria (<2%)
- Hematuria (<2%)
- Urinary frequency (<2%)
- Urinary tract infection (<7%)

Renal
- Nephrotoxicity [2]
- Renal failure (<2%)

Hematologic
- Anemia (<4%)
- Leukopenia (<2%)

Otic
- Tinnitus (<2%)

Ocular
- Abnormal vision (<2%)
- Conjunctivitis (<2%)

Other
- Adverse effects (18%) [6]
- Allergic reactions (<2%)

MELPHALAN

Trade names: Alkeran (GSK), Evomela (Spectrum)
Indications: Multiple myeloma, carcinomas
Class: Alkylating agent
Half-life: 90 minutes
Clinically important, potentially hazardous interactions with: aldesleukin, PEG-interferon, tasonermin
Pregnancy category: D
Important contra-indications noted in the prescribing guidelines for: the elderly; nursing mothers; pediatric patients
Black Box Warning: SEVERE BONE MARROW SUPPRESSION, HYPERSENSITIVITY, and LEUKEMOGENICITY

Skin
Anaphylactoid reactions/Anaphylaxis [2]
Angioedema [2]
Exanthems (4%) [4]
Hypersensitivity (<10%)
Pruritus (<10%)
Rash (<10%)
Toxicity [3]
Urticaria [3]
Vasculitis (<10%)
Vesiculation (<10%)

Hair
Alopecia (<10%) [2]

Nails
Beau's lines (transverse nail bands) [4]

Mucosal
Mucositis [7]
Oral mucositis [4]
Stomatitis (<10%) [2]

Central Nervous System
Peripheral neuropathy [3]

Neuromuscular/Skeletal
Rhabdomyolysis [2]

Gastrointestinal/Hepatic
Diarrhea [2]
Nausea [2]

Hematologic
Febrile neutropenia [2]
Neutropenia [4]
Thrombocytopenia [5]

MEMANTINE

Trade names: Ebixa (Lundbeck), Namenda (Forest)
Indications: Alzheimer's disease, vascular dementia
Class: Adamantane, NMDA receptor antagonist
Half-life: 60–80 hours
Clinically important, potentially hazardous interactions with: amantadine, bromocriptine, darifenacin, dextromethorphan, ketamine, levodopa, levomepromazine, oxybutynin, risperidone, rotigotine, tiotropium, trimethoprim, trospium, zuclopenthixol
Pregnancy category: B
Important contra-indications noted in the prescribing guidelines for: nursing mothers; pediatric patients

---

Skin
Peripheral edema (>2%)

Central Nervous System
Agitation [2]
Confusion [3]
Depression (>2%)
Gait instability [3]
Headache (6%) [3]
Vertigo (dizziness) (7%) [6]

Neuromuscular/Skeletal
Arthralgia (>2%)
Asthenia (fatigue) (2%)
Back pain (3%)
Myoclonus [2]

Gastrointestinal/Hepatic
Constipation [2]
Diarrhea [2]
Vomiting [2]

Respiratory
Cough (4%)
Flu-like syndrome (>2%)
Nasopharyngitis [2]

Genitourinary
Urinary tract infection [2]

Ocular
Hallucinations, visual [2]

Other
Adverse effects [3]

MENINGOCOCCAL GROUP B VACCINE

Trade names: Bexsero (Novartis), Trumenba (Wyeth)
Indications: Immunization to prevent invasive disease caused by *Neisseria meningitidis* serogroup B
Class: Vaccine
Half-life: N/A
Clinically important, potentially hazardous interactions with: none known
Pregnancy category: B
Important contra-indications noted in the prescribing guidelines for: the elderly; nursing mothers; pediatric patients

---

Central Nervous System
Chills (18–30%)
Fever (2–8%) [3]
Headache (41–57%)

Neuromuscular/Skeletal
Arthralgia (16–22%)
Asthenia (fatigue) (44–65%)
Myalgia/Myopathy (35–41%)

Gastrointestinal/Hepatic
Diarrhea (9–15%)
Vomiting (2–8%)

Respiratory
Upper respiratory tract infection [2]

Local
Injection-site edema (18–22%)
Injection-site erythema (15–20%)
Injection-site pain (85–93%) [2]

MENINGOCOCCAL GROUPS C & Y & HAEMOPHILUS B TETANUS TOXOID CONJUGATE VACCINE

Synonym: HibMenCY
Trade name: Menhibrix (GSK)
Indications: Immunization to prevent invasive disease caused by *Neisseria meningitidis* serogroups C and Y and *Haemophilus influenzae* Type B
Class: Vaccine
Half-life: N/A
Clinically important, potentially hazardous interactions with: immunosuppressants
Pregnancy category: C
Important contra-indications noted in the prescribing guidelines for: pediatric patients

---

Central Nervous System
Fever (11–26%)
Irritability (62–71%)
Sedation (49–63%)

Endocrine/Metabolic
Appetite decreased (30–34%)

Local
Injection-site edema (15–25%) [2]
Injection-site erythema (21–36%)
Injection-site pain (42–46%) [2]

MEPERIDINE

Synonym: pethidine
Trade name: Demerol (Sanofi-Aventis)
Indications: Pain
Class: Opiate agonist
Half-life: 3–4 hours
Clinically important, potentially hazardous interactions with: acyclovir, alcohol, amphetamines, barbiturates, CNS depressants, darunavir, duloxetine, fluoxetine, furazolidone, general anesthetics, glycopyrrolate, glycopyrronium, indinavir, isocarboxazid, linezolid, lisdexamfetamine, lithium, MAO inhibitors, moclobemide, phenelzine, phenobarbital, phenothiazines, phenytoin, rasagiline, ritonavir, selegiline, sibutramine, SSRIs, tipranavir, tranquilizers, tranylcypromine, tricyclic antidepressants, valacyclovir
Pregnancy category: C
Important contra-indications noted in the prescribing guidelines for: the elderly; nursing mothers; pediatric patients

---

Skin
Pruritus [3]

Mucosal
Xerostomia (<10%)

Central Nervous System
Catatonia [2]
Seizures [2]
Serotonin syndrome [6]

Local
Injection-site erythema [2]
Injection-site pain (<10%)

MEPOLIZUMAB *

Trade name: Nucala (GSK)
Indications: Adjunctive treatment for severe eosinophilic asthma
Class: Interleukin-5 antagonist, Monoclonal antibody
Half-life: 16–22 days
Clinically important, potentially hazardous interactions with: none known
Pregnancy category: N/A (Insufficent evidence to inform drug-associated risk)
Important contra-indications noted in the prescribing guidelines for: nursing mothers; pediatric patients

---

Skin
Eczema (3%)
Pruritus (3%)
Rash (>3%)

Mucosal
Nasal congestion (>3%)

Central Nervous System
Fever (>3%)
Headache (19%) [2]
Vertigo (dizziness) (>3%)

Neuromuscular/Skeletal
Asthenia (fatigue) (5%) [2]
Back pain (5%)
Bone or joint pain (>3%)
Muscle spasm (3%)

Gastrointestinal/Hepatic
Abdominal pain (3%)
Gastroenteritis (>3%)
Nausea (>3%) [2]
Vomiting (>3%)

Respiratory
Bronchitis (>3%) [2]
Dyspnea (>3%)
Influenza (3%)
Nasopharyngitis (>3%)
Pharyngitis (>3%)
Rhinitis (>3%)
Sinusitis [2]
Upper respiratory tract infection [2]

Genitourinary
Cystitis (>3%)
Urinary tract infection (3%)

Otic
Ear infection (>3%)

Local
Injection-site reactions (8%)

Other
Infection (>3%)
Toothache (>3%)

MERCAPTOPURINE

Synonyms: 6-mercaptopurine; 6-MP
Trade name: Purinethol (Gate)
Indications: Leukemias
Class: Antimetabolite, Antineoplastic
Half-life: triphasic: 45 minutes; 2.5 hours; 10 hours
Clinically important, potentially hazardous interactions with: aldesleukin, allopurinol, balsalazide, febuxostat, influenza vaccine, mycophenolate, natalizumab, olsalazine, trimethoprim, typhoid vaccine, vaccines, yellow fever vaccine
Pregnancy category: D

Skin
Dermatitis (2%)
Hand–foot syndrome [2]
Hypersensitivity [2]
Neoplasms [2]
Peripheral edema [2]
Photosensitivity [2]
Pigmentation (<10%)
Rash (<10%) [2]

Hair
Alopecia [2]

Mucosal
Mucositis (<10%)
Oral lesions (<5%) [2]
Stomatitis (<10%)

Central Nervous System
Fever [3]

Gastrointestinal/Hepatic
Hepatotoxicity [5]
Nausea [2]
Pancreatitis [9]

Hematologic
Leukopenia [2]
Myelosuppression [2]
Myelotoxicity [3]

Other
Death [2]

MEROPENEM

Trade name: Meronem (AstraZeneca)
Indications: Aerobic and anaerobic infections, febrile neutropenia
Class: Antibiotic, carbapenem, Thienamycin
Half-life: 4–6 hours
Clinically important, potentially hazardous interactions with: oral contraceptives, probenecid, valproic acid
Pregnancy category: B

Skin
AGEP [2]
Hypersensitivity [2]
Rash (2%) [5]

Central Nervous System
Headache (2%)
Seizures [7]

Gastrointestinal/Hepatic
Diarrhea [3]
Hepatotoxicity [3]
Nausea [2]

Endocrine/Metabolic
ALT increased [3]
AST increased [3]

Local
Injection-site pain [3]

Other
Adverse effects [14]
Death [2]

MESALAMINE

Synonyms: 5-aminosalicylic acid; 5-ASA; fisalamine; mesalazine
Trade names: Asacol (Procter & Gamble), Canasa (Aptalis), Lialda (Shire), Pentasa (Shire), Rowasa (Solvay)
Indications: Ulcerative colitis
Class: Aminosalicylate
Half-life: 0.5–1.5 hours
Clinically important, potentially hazardous interactions with: azathioprine, NSAIDs, pantoprazole
Pregnancy category: B
Important contra-indications noted in the prescribing guidelines for: the elderly; nursing mothers

---

Skin
Diaphoresis (3%)
Exanthems [3]
Hypersensitivity [8]
Lupus erythematosus [2]
Photosensitivity [3]
Psoriasis [2]
Rash (3%) [6]

Hair
Alopecia [6]

Cardiovascular
Cardiotoxicity [2]
Myocarditis [6]
Pericarditis [5]

Central Nervous System
Fever (<6%) [6]
Headache (2–25%) [5]
Pain (14%)
Vertigo (dizziness) (2–8%)

Neuromuscular/Skeletal
Myalgia/Myopathy (3%)

Gastrointestinal/Hepatic
Abdominal pain (<18%) [6]
Colitis (ulcerative / exacerbation) [3]
Diarrhea (2–8%) [4]
Eructation (belching) (16%)
Flatulence (<6%) [2]
Nausea (3–13%) [3]
Pancreatitis [20]
Vomiting (<5%) [2]

Respiratory
Eosinophilic pneumonia [3]
Pharyngitis (11%)
Pneumonia [5]
Pneumonitis [2]
Pulmonary toxicity [9]

Renal
Nephrotoxicity [6]

Hematologic
Anemia [2]
Eosinophilia [3]

Otic
Tinnitus (<3%)

Other
Adverse effects [11]
Allergic reactions [2]
Kounis syndrome [2]

METAXALONE

Trade name: Skelaxin (Elan)
Indications: Muscle spasm
Class: Central muscle relaxant
Half-life: 4–14 hours
Clinically important, potentially hazardous interactions with: alcohol, barbiturates, conivaptan, droperidol, interferon alfa, levomepromazine, St John's wort, tricyclic antidepressants
Pregnancy category: B
Important contra-indications noted in the prescribing guidelines for: nursing mothers; pediatric patients
Note: Contraindicated in patients with known tendency to drug induced, hemolytic, or other anemias, or significantly impaired renal or hepatic function.

Cardiovascular
Tachycardia [2]

Central Nervous System
Agitation [2]
Serotonin syndrome [2]
Somnolence (drowsiness) [3]
Vertigo (dizziness) [3]

Gastrointestinal/Hepatic
Nausea [2]
Vomiting [2]

METFORMIN

Trade names: Avandamet (GSK), Fortamet (Andrx), Glucophage (Merck Serono), Glucovance (Merck Serono), Invokamet (Janssen), Janumet (Merck Sharpe & Dohme), Synjardy (Boehringer Ingelheim), Xigduo XR (AstraZeneca)
Indications: Diabetes
Class: Antidiabetic, Biguanide
Half-life: 6 hours
Clinically important, potentially hazardous interactions with: ACE inhibitors, acetazolamide, alcohol, amiloride, anabolic steroids, beta blockers, calcium channel blockers, captopril, cephalexin, cilazapril, cimetidine, corticosteroids, diazoxide, dichlorphenamide, digoxin, disopyramide, diuretics, enalapril, estrogens, fosinopril, iodinated contrast agents, isoniazid, ketotifen, lanreotide, lisinopril, luteinizing hormone releasing hormone analogs, MAO inhibitors, morphine, nicotinic acid, octreotide, oral contraceptives, pegvisomant, phenothiazines, phenytoin, procainamide, progestogens, quinapril, quinidine, quinine, ramipril, ranitidine, somatropin, sympathomimetics, testosterone, thiazides, thyroid products, topiramate, trandolapril, triamterene, trimethoprim, trospium, vancomycin, zonisamide
Pregnancy category: B
Important contra-indications noted in the prescribing guidelines for: the elderly; nursing mothers; pediatric patients
Note: Lactic acidosis is a rare, but serious, metabolic complication that can occur due to metformin accumulation.
Avandamet is metformin and rosiglitazone; Glucovance is metformin and glyburide; Invokamet is metformin and canagliflozin; Janumet is metformin and sitagliptin; Synjardy is metformin and empagliflozin; Xigduo XR is metformin and dapagliflozin.
Black Box Warning: LACTIC ACIDOSIS

Skin
Angioedema [2]
Bullous pemphigoid [2]
Erythema (transient) [3]
Lichenoid eruption [2]
Peripheral edema [5]
Photosensitivity (<10%)
Rash (<10%) [4]
Urticaria (<10%) [4]
Vasculitis [2]

Cardiovascular
Flushing (<10%)
Hypertension [3]
Palpitation (<10%)

Central Nervous System
Chills (<10%)
Dysgeusia (taste perversion) (3%)
Headache (6%) [10]
Vertigo (dizziness) (<10%) [6]

Neuromuscular/Skeletal
Arthralgia [5]
Asthenia (fatigue) (9%)
Back pain [5]
Myalgia/Myopathy (<10%)

Gastrointestinal/Hepatic
Abdominal pain (6%) [3]
Constipation [3]
Diarrhea (10–35%) [28]
Dyspepsia [4]
Gastroenteritis [2]
Hepatotoxicity [6]
Nausea (7–26%) [22]
Pancreatitis [5]
Vomiting (7–26%) [10]

Respiratory
Bronchitis [3]
Dyspnea (<10%)
Influenza [2]
Nasopharyngitis [6]
Respiratory tract infection (<10%)
Sinusitis [2]
Upper respiratory tract infection [5]

Endocrine/Metabolic
Acidosis [19]
Appetite decreased [4]
Hypoglycemia [15]
Weight gain [2]
Weight loss [5]

Genitourinary
Genital mycotic infections [8]
Pollakiuria [3]
Urinary tract infection [11]

Renal
Nephrotoxicity [5]

Other
Adverse effects [24]
Death [2]
Vitamin B-12 deficiency [4]

METHADONE

Trade names: Dolophine (Roxane), Methadose (Mallinckrodt)
Indications: Pain, narcotic addiction
Class: Opiate agonist
Half-life: 15–25 hours
Clinically important, potentially hazardous interactions with: abacavir, amprenavir, boceprevir, citalopram, darunavir, delavirdine, diazepam, efavirenz, erythromycin, fluconazole, fluvoxamine, interferon alfa, ketoconazole, linezolid, lopinavir, nelfinavir, nilotinib, paroxetine hydrochloride, PEG-interferon, quetiapine, rifapentine, rilpivirine, St John's wort, tipranavir, vandetanib, voriconazole, zidovudine, zuclopenthixol
Pregnancy category: C
Important contra-indications noted in the prescribing guidelines for: pediatric patients
Note: Methadone is not licensed for use in children though it can be employed for the management of neonatal opiate withdrawal syndrome.

Skin
Diaphoresis (<48%) [4]
Pruritus [2]

Mucosal
Xerostomia (<10%)

Cardiovascular
QT prolongation [35]
Torsades de pointes [27]
Ventricular arrhythmia [2]

Central Nervous System
Hallucinations [2]
Hyperalgesia [2]
Syncope [2]

Neuromuscular/Skeletal
Rhabdomyolysis [4]

Respiratory
Respiratory depression [3]

Genitourinary
Sexual dysfunction [2]

Local
Injection-site pain (<10%)

Other
Adverse effects [2]
Death [14]

METHAMPHETAMINE

Trade name: Desoxyn (Recordati)
Indications: Attention deficit disorder, obesity
Class: Amphetamine
Half-life: 4–5 hours
Clinically important, potentially hazardous interactions with: fluoxetine, fluvoxamine, MAO inhibitors, paroxetine hydrochloride, phenelzine, sertraline, tranylcypromine
Pregnancy category: C
Important contra-indications noted in the prescribing guidelines for: nursing mothers; pediatric patients
Black Box Warning: POTENTIAL FOR ABUSE

Skin
Diaphoresis (<10%)

Mucosal
Xerostomia (<10%) [5]

Cardiovascular
Polyarteritis nodosa [2]

Central Nervous System
Depression [2]
Hallucinations [4]
Insomnia [2]
Neurotoxicity [6]
Paranoia [2]
Parkinsonism [2]
Psychosis [11]

Neuromuscular/Skeletal
Rhabdomyolysis (43%) [5]

Other
Bruxism [4]
Death [3]
Dental disease [2]

METHIMAZOLE

Synonym: thiamazole
Trade name: Tapazole (Paladin)
Indications: Hyperthyroidism
Class: Antithyroid, hormone modifier
Half-life: 4–13 hours
Clinically important, potentially hazardous interactions with: anticoagulants, dicumarol, warfarin
Pregnancy category: D

Skin
Aplasia cutis congenita [4]
Exanthems (<15%) [5]
Hypersensitivity [2]
Lupus erythematosus (<10%) [10]
Pruritus (<5%) [4]
Rash (>10%)
Urticaria (>5%) [2]
Vasculitis [6]

Central Nervous System
Ageusia (taste loss) (<10%)

Neuromuscular/Skeletal
Arthralgia [4]

Gastrointestinal/Hepatic
Hepatotoxicity [11]
Pancreatitis [3]

Respiratory
Pulmonary toxicity [2]

Hematologic
Agranulocytosis [10]
Neutropenia [2]

Other
Side effects (in high dosages) (28%) [2]
Teratogenicity [2]

METHOTREXATE

Synonyms: amethopterin; MTX
Trade names: Rasuvo (Medac), Rheumatrex (Stada)
Indications: Carcinomas, leukemias, lymphomas, psoriasis, rheumatoid arthritis
Class: Antimetabolite, Disease-modifying antirheumatic drug (DMARD), Folic acid antagonist
Half-life: 3–10 hours
Clinically important, potentially hazardous interactions with: acemetacin, acitretin, aldesleukin, aminoglycosides, amiodarone, amoxicillin, ampicillin, aspirin, bacampicillin, bismuth, carbenicillin, chloroquine, ciprofloxacin, cisplatin, cloxacillin, co-trimoxazole, cyclopenthiazide, dapsone, demeclocycline, dexamethasone, diclofenac, dicloxacillin, doxycycline, echinacea, etodolac, etoricoxib, etretinate, fenoprofen, flurbiprofen, folic acid antagonists, gadobenate, haloperidol, hydrocortisone, ibuprofen, indomethacin, infliximab, ketoprofen, ketorolac, leflunomide, magnesium trisalicylate, meclofenamate, mefenamic acid, meloxicam, methicillin, mezlocillin, minocycline, nabumetone, nafcillin, naproxen, natalizumab, NSAIDs, omeprazole, oxacillin, oxaprozin, oxtriphylline, oxytetracycline, pantoprazole, paromomycin, penicillin G, penicillin V, penicillins, phenylbutazone, piperacillin, piperacillin/tazobactam, piroxicam, polypeptide antibiotics, prednisolone, prednisone, pristinamycin, probenecid, procarbazine, rofecoxib, salicylates, salsalate, sapropterin, sulfadiazine, sulfamethoxazole, sulfapyridine, sulfasalazine, sulfisoxazole, sulindac, taxobactam, tenoxicam, tetracycline, ticarcillin, tolmetin, trimethoprim, vaccines
Pregnancy category: X
Important contra-indications noted in the prescribing guidelines for: the elderly; nursing mothers; pediatric patients
Black Box Warning: SEVERE TOXIC REACTIONS, INCLUDING EMBRYOFETAL TOXICITY AND DEATH

Skin
Abscess (peritoneal) [2]
Acral erythema [13]
Anaphylactoid reactions/Anaphylaxis (<10%) [9]
Bullous acral erythema [2]
Bullous dermatitis [4]
Capillaritis [2]
Carcinoma [2]
Dermatitis [2]
Edema [2]
Erosion of psoriatic plaques [8]
Erythema (>10%)
Erythema multiforme [4]
Erythroderma [2]
Exanthems (15%) [5]
Folliculitis [2]
Herpes simplex [2]
Herpes zoster [7]
Hypersensitivity [2]
Lymphoma [5]
Malignant lymphoma [4]
Molluscum contagiosum [2]
Necrosis [4]
Neoplasms [2]
Nodular eruption [15]
Non-Hodgkin's lymphoma [2]
Photosensitivity (5%) [9]
Pigmentation (<10%)
Pruritus (<5%)
Pseudolymphoma [10]
Radiation recall dermatitis [7]
Rash (<3%) [11]
Squamous cell carcinoma [2]
Stevens–Johnson syndrome [4]
Sunburn (reactivation) [6]
Toxic epidermal necrolysis [8]
Toxicity [6]
Ulceration of psoriatic plaques [4]
Ulcerations [11]
Urticaria [4]
Vasculitis (>10%) [9]

Hair
Alopecia (<6%) [25]

Nails
Nail pigmentation [2]
Paronychia [2]

Mucosal
Aphthous stomatitis [2]
Gingivitis (>10%)
Glossitis (>10%)
Mucocutaneous reactions [2]
Mucositis [10]
Nasal septal perforation [2]
Oral mucositis [6]
Oral ulceration [10]
Stomatitis (3–10%) [17]

Cardiovascular
Hypertension [2]
Pericardial effusion [2]
Pericarditis [3]

Central Nervous System
Encephalopathy [2]
Fever [4]
Headache [15]
Leukoencephalopathy [60]
Migraine [2]
Neurotoxicity [8]
Vertigo (dizziness) [2]

Neuromuscular/Skeletal
Arthralgia [5]
Asthenia (fatigue) [13]
Back pain [2]
Bone or joint pain [2]

Gastrointestinal/Hepatic
Abdominal pain [9]
Diarrhea [11]
Dyspepsia [3]
Gastroenteritis [2]
Hepatic steatosis [2]

Hepatitis [3]
Hepatotoxicity [54]
Nausea [26]
Vomiting [10]

Respiratory
Cough [3]
Nasopharyngitis [6]
Pharyngitis [2]
Pneumonia [6]
Pneumonitis [6]
Pulmonary toxicity [8]
Upper respiratory tract infection [7]

Endocrine/Metabolic
ALT increased [6]
AST increased [3]
Diabetes mellitus [2]
Gynecomastia [8]
Hypoalbuminemia [2]
Weight gain [2]

Genitourinary
Urinary tract infection [4]

Renal
Nephrotoxicity [24]
Renal failure [2]

Hematologic
Anemia [8]
Febrile neutropenia [3]
Hemotoxicity [2]
Leukopenia [9]
Myelosuppression [6]
Myelotoxicity [4]
Neutropenia [8]
Pancytopenia [8]
Thrombocytopenia [8]

Ocular
Cotton wool spots [2]
Optic neuropathy [2]

Local
Injection-site reactions [2]

Other
Adverse effects [37]
Death [12]
Hodgkin's disease (nodular sclerosing) [2]
Infection [20]
Side effects [3]
Teratogenicity [3]

METHOXSALEN

Trade name: Oxsoralen (Valeant)
Indications: Psoriasis, vitiligo
Class: CYP1A2 inhibitor, Psoralen, Repigmenting agent
Half-life: 1.1 hours
Clinically important, potentially hazardous interactions with: caffeine, chloroquine, cyclosporine, fluoroquinolones, phenothiazines, sulfonamides
Pregnancy category: C
Important contra-indications noted in the prescribing guidelines for: pediatric patients
Note: Potential hazards of long-term therapy include the possibilities of carcinogenicity and cataractogenicity.

Skin
Anaphylactoid reactions/Anaphylaxis [2]
Basal cell carcinoma [3]
Bullous dermatitis (with UVA) [4]
Burning (<10%) [3]
Carcinoma [5]
Dermatitis [4]
Edema (<10%)
Ephelides (<10%) [5]
Erythema (<10%)
Exanthems [2]
Herpes zoster [2]
Hypomelanosis (<10%)
Lupus erythematosus [3]
Photosensitivity [9]
Phototoxicity [7]
Pigmentation [3]
Porokeratosis (actinic) [3]
Pruritus (>10%)
Rash (<10%)
Squamous cell carcinoma [4]
Tumors [2]
Vitiligo [2]

Hair
Hypertrichosis [3]

Nails
Nail pigmentation [5]
Photo-onycholysis [5]

Mucosal
Cheilitis (<10%)

Central Nervous System
Pain [2]

METHYLDOPA

Trade name: Aldoclor (Merck)
Indications: Hypertension
Class: Adrenergic alpha-receptor agonist
Half-life: 1.7 hours
Clinically important, potentially hazardous interactions with: acebutolol, alfuzosin, bromocriptine, captopril, cilazapril, cyclopenthiazide, diclofenac, enalapril, ephedrine, fosinopril, irbesartan, levodopa, levomepromazine, linezolid, lisinopril, meloxicam, olmesartan, quinapril, ramipril, risperidone, rotigotine, trandolapril, triamcinolone, zuclopenthixol
Pregnancy category: B
Important contra-indications noted in the prescribing guidelines for: nursing mothers
Note: Aldoril is methyldopa and hydrochlorothiazide. Hydrochlorothiazide is a sulfonamide and can be absorbed systemically. Sulfonamides can produce severe, possibly fatal, reactions such as toxic epidermal necrolysis and Stevens-Johnson syndrome.

Skin
Eczema [3]
Erythema multiforme [2]
Exanthems (3%) [3]
Lichen planus [3]
Lichenoid eruption [9]
Lupus erythematosus [14]
Peripheral edema (>10%)
Photosensitivity [2]
Pigmentation [3]
Seborrheic dermatitis [3]
Urticaria [2]

Mucosal
Oral lichenoid eruption [3]
Oral ulceration [6]
Xerostomia (<10%)

Central Nervous System
Anxiety (<10%)
Depression (<10%)
Dyskinesia [2]
Fever (<10%)
Headache (<10%)
Nightmares (<10%)
Parkinsonism [2]

Gastrointestinal/Hepatic
Hepatitis [2]
Hepatotoxicity [7]

Endocrine/Metabolic
Amenorrhea [2]
Galactorrhea [4]

Hematologic
Hemolytic anemia [2]

METHYLPHENIDATE

Trade names: Metadate CD (Celltech), Methylin (Mallinckrodt), Ritalin (Novartis)
Indications: Attention deficit disorder, narcolepsy
Class: Amphetamine
Half-life: 2–4 hours
Clinically important, potentially hazardous interactions with: amitriptyline, benazepril, bupropion, captopril, citalopram, clevidipine, cyclosporine, enalapril, escitalopram, irbesartan, linezolid, lisinopril, lurasidone, MAO inhibitors, olmesartan, paliperidone, pantoprazole, paroxetine hydrochloride, phenylbutazone, pimozide, quinapril, ziprasidone
Pregnancy category: C
Important contra-indications noted in the prescribing guidelines for: the elderly; nursing mothers
Black Box Warning: DRUG DEPENDENCE

Skin
Angioedema [2]
Exanthems [2]
Exfoliative dermatitis [2]
Hypersensitivity (<10%)
Leukoderma [2]

Mucosal
Xerostomia [5]

Cardiovascular
Cardiotoxicity [3]
Palpitation [4]
QT prolongation [2]
Tachycardia [3]

Central Nervous System
Anorexia [6]
Anxiety [5]
Compulsions [2]
Hallucinations [6]
Headache [10]
Insomnia [10]
Irritability [4]

Neurotoxicity [3]
Seizures [3]
Somnolence (drowsiness) [2]
Suicidal ideation [2]
Tic disorder [5]
Tremor [2]
Vertigo (dizziness) [4]

Gastrointestinal/Hepatic
Abdominal pain [9]
Nausea [6]
Vomiting [4]

Respiratory
Cough [2]
Nasopharyngitis [2]
Upper respiratory tract infection [2]

Endocrine/Metabolic
Appetite decreased [11]
Weight loss [6]

Genitourinary
Priapism [5]

Ocular
Hallucinations, visual [5]

Other
Adverse effects [6]
Bruxism [2]

METHYL-PREDNISOLONE

Trade names: Advantan (Intendis), Medrol (Pharmacia), Solu-Medrol (Pharmacia)
Indications: Arthralgias, asthma, dermatoses, inflammatory ocular conditions, rhinitis
Class: Corticosteroid, systemic
Half-life: 12–36 hours; 2–4 hours (plasma)
Clinically important, potentially hazardous interactions with: aminophylline, aprepitant, aspirin, carbamazepine, clarithromycin, conivaptan, cyclosporine, daclizumab, darunavir, delavirdine, erythromycin, indinavir, itraconazole, ketoconazole, live vaccines, oral contraceptives, phenobarbital, phenytoin, rifampin, telaprevir, telithromycin, troleandomycin, voriconazole, warfarin
Pregnancy category: C
Important contra-indications noted in the prescribing guidelines for: nursing mothers; pediatric patients

---

Skin
Anaphylactoid reactions/Anaphylaxis [15]
Dermatitis [5]
Hypersensitivity [3]
Pruritus [2]
Rash [2]
Urticaria [5]

Cardiovascular
Arrhythmias [2]
Bradycardia [6]
Flushing [2]
Hypertension [6]
Myocardial infarction [2]
Myocardial toxicity [2]

Central Nervous System
Depression [5]
Dysgeusia (taste perversion) [4]
Neurotoxicity [2]
Psychosis [3]
Seizures [3]
Vertigo (dizziness) [2]

Neuromuscular/Skeletal
Arthralgia [2]
Myalgia/Myopathy [4]
Osteonecrosis [9]
Osteoporosis [2]
Tendinopathy/Tendon rupture [2]

Gastrointestinal/Hepatic
Abdominal pain [3]
Gastrointestinal bleeding [2]
Hepatotoxicity [8]

Respiratory
Dysphonia [2]

Endocrine/Metabolic
Hyperglycemia [4]

Ocular
Cataract [3]
Glaucoma [2]

Other
Adverse effects [6]
Allergic reactions [3]
Death [2]
Hiccups [2]
Infection [7]

METHYL-TESTOSTERONE

Trade names: Android (Valeant), Estratest (Solvay), Testred (Valeant)
Indications: Hypogonadism, impotence, metastatic breast cancer
Class: Androgen
Half-life: 2.5–3.5 hours
Clinically important, potentially hazardous interactions with: anticoagulants, cyclosporine, warfarin
Pregnancy category: X
Important contra-indications noted in the prescribing guidelines for: nursing mothers; pediatric patients

---

Skin
Acneform eruption (>10%) [12]
Edema (>10%)

Hair
Alopecia [2]
Hirsutism (in females) (<10%) [9]

Cardiovascular
Flushing (<5%)

Endocrine/Metabolic
Mastodynia (>10%)

Genitourinary
Priapism (>10%)

METHYSERGIDE

Trade name: Sansert (Novartis)
Indications: Vascular (migraine) headaches
Class: Hallucinogen, Psychotomimetic
Half-life: 10 hours
Clinically important, potentially hazardous interactions with: acebutolol, almotriptan, amprenavir, azithromycin, chlortetracycline, clarithromycin, delavirdine, demeclocycline, doxycycline, efavirenz, eletriptan, erythromycin, frovatriptan, indinavir, itraconazole, lymecycline, minocycline, naratriptan, nelfinavir, oxytetracycline, ritonavir, rizatriptan, saquinavir, sibutramine, sumatriptan, telithromycin, tetracycline, tigecycline, troleandomycin, voriconazole, zolmitriptan
Pregnancy category: X
Important contra-indications noted in the prescribing guidelines for: nursing mothers; pediatric patients

---

Skin
Lupus erythematosus [2]
Peripheral edema (<10%)
Rash (<10%)
Scleroderma [4]

Hair
Alopecia [4]

Cardiovascular
Valvulopathy [3]

METOPROLOL

Trade names: Lopressor (Novartis), Toprol XL (AstraZeneca)
Indications: Hypertension, angina pectoris
Class: Adrenergic beta-receptor agonist, Antiarrhythmic class II
Half-life: 3–4 hours
Clinically important, potentially hazardous interactions with: cinacalcet, clonidine, cobicistat/elvitegravir/emtricitabine/tenofovir disoproxil, dronedarone, epinephrine, mirabegron, paroxetine hydrochloride, propoxyphene, tadalafil, telithromycin, tipranavir, venlafaxine, verapamil
Pregnancy category: C
Important contra-indications noted in the prescribing guidelines for: the elderly; pediatric patients
Note: Cutaneous side effects of beta-receptor blockers are clinically polymorphous. They apparently appear after several months of continuous therapy.

Skin
Eczema [2]
Erythroderma [2]
Lichenoid eruption [4]
Pruritus (<5%)
Psoriasis (induction and aggravation of) [8]
Rash (<5%) [3]
Raynaud's phenomenon [3]

Cardiovascular
Arrhythmias [2]
Bradycardia [8]

Hypotension [4]

Central Nervous System
- Delirium [3]
- Hallucinations [2]
- Sleep disturbances [2]

Neuromuscular/Skeletal
- Asthenia (fatigue) [2]

Gastrointestinal/Hepatic
- Gastrointestinal disorder [2]

Genitourinary
- Peyronie's disease [5]

Ocular
- Hallucinations, visual [3]

METRONIDAZOLE

Trade names: Flagyl (Pfizer), Metrocream (Galderma), MetroGel (Galderma), Metrolotion (Galderma), Noritate (Dermik), Vandazole (Upsher-Smith)
Indications: Various infections caused by susceptible organisms, rosacea
Class: Antibacterial, Antibiotic, nitroimidazole
Half-life: 6–12 hours
Clinically important, potentially hazardous interactions with: alcohol, anisindione, anticoagulants, astemizole, barbiturates, busulfan, cimetidine, dicumarol, disulfiram, dronabinol, fluorouracil, lithium, lopinavir, mycophenolate, phenytoin, primidone, thalidomide, tipranavir, uracil/tegafur, warfarin
Pregnancy category: B (in patients with trichomoniasis, metronidazole is contraindicated during the first trimester of pregnancy)
Important contra-indications noted in the prescribing guidelines for: nursing mothers

---

Skin
- AGEP [2]
- Dermatitis [2]
- Exanthems (<5%) [2]
- Fixed eruption [13]
- Pruritus (<10%) [6]
- Serum sickness [2]
- Stevens–Johnson syndrome [4]
- Toxic epidermal necrolysis [2]
- Urticaria [3]

Mucosal
- Glossitis [2]
- Tongue furry [2]

Cardiovascular
- Flushing [2]
- Hypertension [2]
- Torsades de pointes [2]

Central Nervous System
- Cerebellar syndrome [6]
- Dysgeusia (taste perversion) [7]
- Encephalopathy [23]
- Fever [7]
- Headache (7%) [6]
- Neurotoxicity [12]
- Peripheral neuropathy [2]
- Psychosis [3]

Neuromuscular/Skeletal
- Ataxia [2]

Gastrointestinal/Hepatic
- Abdominal pain (5%) [7]
- Diarrhea [14]
- Hepatotoxicity [5]
- Nausea [18]
- Pancreatitis [6]
- Vomiting [13]

Endocrine/Metabolic
- ALT increased [2]
- AST increased [2]

Genitourinary
- Vulvovaginal candidiasis [2]

Hematologic
- Anemia [2]
- Bleeding [2]

Otic
- Hearing loss [2]

Ocular
- Vision loss [2]

Other
- Adverse effects [10]
- Death [3]
- Infection (fungal) (12%)

MICAFUNGIN

Trade name: Mycamine (Astellas)
Indications: Invasive candidiasis, esophageal candidiasis
Class: Antifungal
Half-life: 11–21 hours
Clinically important, potentially hazardous interactions with: amphotericin B, conivaptan, cyclosporine, itraconazole, nifedipine, sirolimus
Pregnancy category: C
Important contra-indications noted in the prescribing guidelines for: nursing mothers; pediatric patients

---

Skin
- Anaphylactoid reactions/Anaphylaxis [2]
- Peripheral edema (7%)
- Pruritus (6%)
- Rash (9%) [6]
- Ulcerations (5%)

Mucosal
- Epistaxis (nosebleed) (6%) [2]
- Mucosal inflammation (14%)

Cardiovascular
- Bradycardia (3%)
- Hypertension (7%) [2]
- Hypotension (9%)
- Phlebitis (6%)
- Tachycardia (8%)

Central Nervous System
- Anorexia (6%)
- Anxiety (6%)
- Fever (20%) [6]
- Headache (16%) [3]
- Insomnia (10%)
- Rigors (9%)
- Shock (8%)

Neuromuscular/Skeletal
- Asthenia (fatigue) (6%)
- Back pain (5%)

Gastrointestinal/Hepatic
- Abdominal pain (10%) [3]
- Constipation (11%)
- Diarrhea (23%) [8]
- Dyspepsia (6%)
- Hepatotoxicity [6]
- Nausea (22%) [6]
- Vomiting (22%) [5]

Respiratory
- Cough (8%)
- Dyspnea (6%)
- Pneumonia (2%)

Endocrine/Metabolic
- ALP increased (5%) [2]
- ALT increased (5%) [6]
- AST increased (6%) [4]
- Hyperbilirubinemia [3]
- Hyperglycemia (6%)
- Hyperkalemia (5%)
- Hypernatremia (5%)
- Hypocalcemia (7%)
- Hypoglycemia (6%)
- Hypokalemia (18%) [3]
- Hypomagnesemia (13%)

Hematologic
- Anemia (10%) [3]
- Febrile neutropenia (6%)
- Hemolysis [3]
- Neutropenia (14%)
- Sepsis (5%)
- Thrombocytopenia (15%) [2]

Other
- Adverse effects [5]
- Infection (40%)

MICONAZOLE

Trade names: Monistat (Janssen), Oravig (Dara)
Indications: Fungal infections, oropharyngeal candidiasis
Class: Antibiotic, imidazole, Antifungal, azole
Half-life: initial: 40 minutes; terminal: 24 hours
Clinically important, potentially hazardous interactions with: anisindione, anticoagulants, astemizole, clopidogrel, dicumarol, gliclazide, simvastatin, thioridazine, tolvaptan, vinblastine, vincristine, warfarin
Pregnancy category: C
Important contra-indications noted in the prescribing guidelines for: nursing mothers; pediatric patients

---

Skin
- Angioedema (2%)
- Contact dermatitis [2]
- Dermatitis [11]
- Exanthems (2–87%) [5]
- Pruritus (2–36%) [3]
- Purpura (3–8%)
- Rash (9%)
- Urticaria (2%)

Cardiovascular
- Flushing (<2%) [2]
- Phlebitis (5–79%) [3]

Central Nervous System
- Chills (>5%)

Gastrointestinal/Hepatic
Nausea [2]

Local
Injection-site pain (10%)

Other
Adverse effects [2]

MIDAZOLAM

Trade name: Versed (Roche)
Indications: Preoperative sedation
Class: Benzodiazepine
Half-life: 1–4 hours
Clinically important, potentially hazardous interactions with: amprenavir, aprepitant, atazanavir, atorvastatin, boceprevir, carbamazepine, chlorpheniramine, cimetidine, clarithromycin, clorazepate, CNS depressants, cobicistat/elvitegravir/emtricitabine/tenofovir disoproxil, conivaptan, darunavir, delavirdine, dexamethasone, efavirenz, enzalutamide, erythromycin, esomeprazole, fluconazole, fluoxetine, fosamprenavir, grapefruit juice, griseofulvin, imatinib, indinavir, itraconazole, ivermectin, ketoconazole, lopinavir, nelfinavir, nevirapine, nilotinib, ombitasvir/paritaprevir/ritonavir, phenobarbital, phenytoin, posaconazole, primidone, rifabutin, rifampin, ritonavir, roxithromycin, saquinavir, St John's wort, telaprevir, telithromycin, tibolone, tipranavir, voriconazole
Pregnancy category: D

Skin
Edema [2]
Pruritus [3]

Cardiovascular
Hypotension [9]

Central Nervous System
Agitation [3]
Amnesia [38]
Sedation [2]

Gastrointestinal/Hepatic
Vomiting [2]

Local
Injection-site pain (>10%)
Injection-site reactions (>10%)

Other
Adverse effects [6]
Hiccups [3]

MIFEPRISTONE

Trade names: Korlym (Corcept), Mifeprex (Danco)
Indications: Medical termination of intrauterine pregnancy (Mifeprex), Cushing's syndrome in patients with Type II diabetes (Korlym)
Class: Corticosteroid antagonist, CYP3A4 inhibitor, Progestogen antagonist
Half-life: 85 hours
Clinically important, potentially hazardous interactions with: amprenavir, aprepitant, atazanavir, boceprevir, bupropion, carbamazepine, ciclesonide, ciprofloxacin, clarithromycin, conivaptan, cyclosporine, darunavir, dihydroergotamine, diltiazem, efavirenz, ergotamine, erythromycin, fentanyl, fluconazole, fluvastatin, fosamprenavir, grapefruit juice, imatinib, indinavir, itraconazole, lopinavir, lovastatin, mibefradil, nefazodone, nelfinavir, NSAIDs, oral contraceptives, phenobarbital, phenytoin, pimozide, posaconazole, quinidine, repaglinide, rifabutin, rifampin, rifapentine, ritonavir, ritonavir, saquinavir, simvastatin, sirolimus, St John's wort, tacrolimus, telaprevir, telithromycin, tenoxicam, triamcinolone, verapamil, voriconazole, warfarin
Pregnancy category: X
Important contra-indications noted in the prescribing guidelines for: nursing mothers; pediatric patients
Note: Contraindicated in pregnancy, with concurrent use of simvastatin or lovastatin and CYP3A substrates with narrow therapeutic range or long-term corticosteroid use, and in women with a history of unexplained vaginal bleeding or with endometrial hyperplasia with atypia or endometrial carcinoma.
Black Box Warning: TERMINATION OF PREGNANCY

Skin
Edema (5–10%)
Peripheral edema (26%)
Pruritus (4%)
Rash (4%)

Mucosal
Xerostomia (18%)

Cardiovascular
Chest pain (5–10%)
Hypertension (24%)

Central Nervous System
Anorexia (10%)
Anxiety (10%)
Chills (3–38%)
Fever (4%)
Headache (2–44%)
Insomnia (5–10%)
Pain (14%)
Somnolence (drowsiness) (10%)
Vertigo (dizziness) (<22%)

Neuromuscular/Skeletal
Arthralgia (30%)
Asthenia (fatigue) (<48%)
Back pain (9–16%)
Myalgia/Myopathy (14%)
Pain in extremities (12%)

Gastrointestinal/Hepatic
Abdominal pain (5–89%) [2]
Constipation (10%)
Diarrhea (12–20%)
Gastroesophageal reflux (5–10%)
Nausea (43–61%)
Vomiting (16–26%)

Respiratory
Dyspnea (16%)
Nasopharyngitis (12%)
Sinusitis (14%)

Endocrine/Metabolic
Adrenal insufficiency (4%)
Appetite decreased (20%)
Hypoglycemia (5–10%)
Hypokalemia (44%) [2]
Menstrual irregularities [2]

Genitourinary
Metrorrhagia (5–10%)
Uterine pain (83%)
Vaginal bleeding (5–10%)
Vaginitis (3%)

Other
Dipsia (thirst) (5–10%)
Infection [2]

MILNACIPRAN

Trade name: Savella (Forest)
Indications: Fibromyalgia
Class: Antidepressant, Selective norepinepherine reuptake inhibitor
Half-life: 6–8 hours
Clinically important, potentially hazardous interactions with: alcohol, alpha / beta argonists, antipsychotics, aspirin, clomipramine, clonidine, CNS-active drugs, digoxin, droperidol, epinephrine, levomepromazine, lithium, MAO inhibitors, norepinephrine, NSAIDs, serotonergic drugs, sibutramine, St John's wort, tryptophan, vitamin K antagonists
Pregnancy category: C
Important contra-indications noted in the prescribing guidelines for: the elderly; nursing mothers; pediatric patients
Note: Contraindicated in patients with uncontrolled narrow-angle glaucoma.
Black Box Warning: SUICIDALITY AND ANTIDEPRESSANT DRUGS

Skin
Hot flashes (12%)
Hyperhidrosis (9%) [5]
Pruritus (2%)
Rash (4%)

Mucosal
Xerostomia (5%)

Cardiovascular
Chest pain (2%)
Flushing (4%)
Hypertension (4%) [3]
Palpitation (7%)
Tachycardia (2%)

Central Nervous System
Anxiety (3%)
Chills (2%)
Headache (17%) [6]
Hypoesthesia (2%)
Insomnia (12%)
Migraine (4%)
Paresthesias (3%)
Serotonin syndrome [2]
Tremor (2%)
Vertigo (dizziness) (10%) [2]

Gastrointestinal/Hepatic
Abdominal pain (3%)
Constipation (15%) [5]
Nausea (39%) [16]
Vomiting (7%)

Respiratory
Dyspnea (2%)
Upper respiratory tract infection (6%)

Endocrine/Metabolic
Appetite decreased (2%)

Genitourinary
Dysuria (>2%) [2]
Ejaculatory dysfunction (>2%) [2]

Ocular
Vision blurred (2%)

Other
Adverse effects [3]

MILRINONE

Trade name: Primacor (Sanofi-Aventis)
Indications: Severe congestive heart failure unresponsive to conventional maintenance therapy, acute heart failure, including low output states following cardiac surgery
Class: Phosphodiesterase inhibitor
Half-life: 2.3 hours
Clinically important, potentially hazardous interactions with: anagrelide
Pregnancy category: C
Important contra-indications noted in the prescribing guidelines for: nursing mothers; pediatric patients

---

Cardiovascular
Hypotension (<10%) [5]
Supraventricular arrhythmias (<10%)
Vasodilation [2]
Ventricular tachycardia (<10%)

Central Nervous System
Headache (<10%)

MINOCYCLINE

Trade names: Dynacin (Medicis), Minocin (Wyeth), Solodyn (Medicis)
Indications: Various infections caused by susceptible organisms
Class: Antibiotic, tetracycline, Disease-modifying antirheumatic drug (DMARD)
Half-life: 11–23 hours
Clinically important, potentially hazardous interactions with: acitretin, aluminum, amoxicillin, ampicillin, antacids, bacampicillin, BCG vaccine, bismuth, carbenicillin, cloxacillin, coumarins, digoxin, ergotamine, estradiol, estrogens, isotretinoin, kaolin, magnesium salts, methotrexate, methoxyflurane, methysergide, mezlocillin, nafcillin, oral iron, oral typhoid vaccine, oxacillin, penicillin G, penicillin V, penicillins, phenindione, piperacillin, quinapril, retinoids, St John's wort, strontium ranelate, sucralfate, sulfonylureas, ticarcillin, tripotassium dicitratobismuthate, vitamin A, zinc
Pregnancy category: D
Important contra-indications noted in the prescribing guidelines for: nursing mothers; pediatric patients

---

Skin
Anaphylactoid reactions/Anaphylaxis [3]
Angioedema [2]
Candidiasis [2]
Cellulitis [2]
DRESS syndrome [13]
Erythema multiforme [2]
Erythema nodosum [2]
Exanthems [5]
Exfoliative dermatitis [3]
Fixed eruption [8]
Folliculitis [2]
Hypersensitivity [25]
Livedo reticularis [3]
Lupus erythematosus [50]
Photosensitivity (<10%) [9]
Pigmentation [112]
Pruritus [7]
Purpura [4]
Rash [8]
Raynaud's phenomenon [2]
Serum sickness (3–5%) [10]
Stevens-Johnson syndrome [2]
Sweet's syndrome [4]
Urticaria [9]
Vasculitis [13]

Hair
Alopecia [2]

Nails
Nail pigmentation (<5%) [18]
Photo-onycholysis [2]

Mucosal
Black tongue [2]
Gingival pigmentation (8%) [2]
Oral pigmentation (7%) [22]

Cardiovascular
Polyarteritis nodosa [12]

Central Nervous System
Fever [2]
Headache [6]
Intracranial pressure increased [4]
Pseudotumor cerebri [14]
Vertigo (dizziness) [7]

Neuromuscular/Skeletal
Arthralgia [6]
Asthenia (fatigue) [4]
Black bone disease [6]
Myalgia/Myopathy [7]

Gastrointestinal/Hepatic
Abdominal pain [2]
Diarrhea [2]
Hepatitis [10]
Hepatotoxicity [19]
Nausea [5]
Pancreatitis [2]
Vomiting [3]

Respiratory
Eosinophilic pneumonia [5]
Pneumonitis [2]

Endocrine/Metabolic
Black thyroid syndrome [4]
Galactorrhea (black) [2]
Thyroid dysfunction [2]

Otic
Tinnitus [2]

Ocular
Conjunctival pigmentation [2]
Diplopia [2]
Papilledema [2]
Scleral pigmentation [4]

Other
Adverse effects [4]
Tooth pigmentation (primarily in children) (>10%) [21]

MINOXIDIL

Trade names: Loniten (Par), Rogaine (Pfizer) (topical)
Indications: Hypertension, androgenetic alopecia
Class: Vasodilator
Half-life: 4.2 hours
Clinically important, potentially hazardous interactions with: acebutolol, alcohol, alfuzosin, captopril, cilazapril, diclofenac, enalapril, fosinopril, guanethidine, levodopa, levomepromazine, lisinopril, meloxicam, olmesartan, quinapril, ramipril, trandolapril, triamcinolone, trifluoperazine
Pregnancy category: C
Note: Topical [T].

Skin
Bullous dermatitis [2]
Dermatitis [T] (7%) [17]
Eczema [2]
Edema [T] (>10%) [2]
Exanthems [4]
Lupus erythematosus [3]
Peripheral edema (7%)
Pruritus [T] [10]
Stevens-Johnson syndrome [2]

Hair
Alopecia [T] [2]
Hair pigmentation [2]
Hirsutism (in women) (100%) [4]
Hypertrichosis (80–100%) [21]

Cardiovascular
Palpitation [3]
Pericardial effusion [2]

Central Nervous System
Headache [2]
Vertigo (dizziness) [2]

Respiratory
Pleural effusion [2]

MIRABEGRON

Trade name: Myrbetriq (Astellas)
Indications: Overactive bladder
Class: Beta-3 adrenergic agonist
Half-life: 50 hours
Clinically important, potentially hazardous interactions with: antimuscarinics, desipramine, digoxin, flecainide, metoprolol, propafenone, thioridazine
Pregnancy category: C
Important contra-indications noted in the prescribing guidelines for: nursing mothers; pediatric patients

---

Mucosal
Xerostomia (3%) [3]

Cardiovascular
Hypertension (8–11%) [5]

Tachycardia (<2%) [2]

Central Nervous System
Headache (2–4%) [3]
Vertigo (dizziness) (3%)

Neuromuscular/Skeletal
Arthralgia (<2%)
Back pain (3%)

Gastrointestinal/Hepatic
Constipation (2–3%) [2]
Diarrhea (<2%)

Respiratory
Influenza (3%)
Nasopharyngitis (4%) [2]
Sinusitis (<3%)
Upper respiratory tract infection (2%)

Genitourinary
Cystitis (2%)
Urinary tract infection (3–6%) [3]

Other
Adverse effects [3]

MIRTAZAPINE

Trade name: Remeron (Organon)
Indications: Depression
Class: Adrenergic alpha-receptor agonist, Antidepressant, tetracyclic
Half-life: 20–40 hours
Clinically important, potentially hazardous interactions with: linezolid, tapentadol, venlafaxine
Pregnancy category: C
Black Box Warning: SUICIDALITY AND ANTIDEPRESSANT DRUGS

Skin
Diaphoresis [2]
Edema (<10%) [2]
Peripheral edema (<10%)
Pigmentation [2]
Rash (<10%)

Mucosal
Glossitis (<10%)
Xerostomia (25%) [3]

Central Nervous System
Abnormal dreams (4%)
Anorexia (<10%)
Headache [2]
Mania [2]
Neurotoxicity [3]
Nightmares [2]
Restless legs syndrome [9]
Sedation [2]
Seizures [3]
Serotonin syndrome [7]
Somnolence (drowsiness) (54%) [8]
Tremor (<10%) [2]
Vertigo (dizziness) (7%)

Neuromuscular/Skeletal
Arthralgia [4]
Asthenia (fatigue) [6]
Myalgia/Myopathy (<10%)
Rhabdomyolysis [4]

Gastrointestinal/Hepatic
Abdominal pain (<10%)
Constipation (<10%)
Hepatotoxicity [3]
Pancreatitis [2]
Vomiting (<10%)

Respiratory
Flu-like syndrome (<10%)

Endocrine/Metabolic
ALT increased (2%)
Appetite increased (12%)
Galactorrhea [2]
Gynecomastia [2]
Weight gain (12%) [8]

Other
Adverse effects [2]

MISOPROSTOL

Trade names: Arthrotec (Pfizer), Cytotec (Pfizer)
Indications: Prevention of NSAID-induced ulcer
Class: Corticosteroid antagonist, Progestogen antagonist
Half-life: 20–40 minutes
Clinically important, potentially hazardous interactions with: none known
Pregnancy category: X
Important contra-indications noted in the prescribing guidelines for: nursing mothers; pediatric patients
Note: Arthrotec is diclofenac and misoprostol.

Skin
Anaphylactoid reactions/Anaphylaxis [2]

Central Nervous System
Chills [6]
Dysgeusia (taste perversion) [2]
Fever [12]
Headache (2%)
Shivering (17%) [8]

Gastrointestinal/Hepatic
Abdominal pain (7%) [6]
Diarrhea (13%)
Dyspepsia (2%)
Flatulence (3%)
Nausea (3%) [3]
Vomiting [3]

Other
Adverse effects [6]

MITOMYCIN

Synonyms: mitomycin-C; MTC
Trade name: Mutamycin (Bristol-Myers Squibb)
Indications: Carcinomas
Class: Alkylating agent, Antibiotic, anthracycline
Half-life: 23–78 minutes
Clinically important, potentially hazardous interactions with: aldesleukin
Pregnancy category: D
Important contra-indications noted in the prescribing guidelines for: nursing mothers; pediatric patients

---

Skin
Dermatitis [9]
Erythema multiforme [2]
Exanthems [2]
Exfoliative dermatitis [2]
Hand–foot syndrome [2]
Thrombocytopenic purpura [2]

Hair
Alopecia (<10%)

Nails
Nail pigmentation (purple) (<10%)

Mucosal
Oral lesions (2–8%) [4]
Oral ulceration (<10%)
Stomatitis (>10%)

Cardiovascular
Congestive heart failure (3–15%)

Central Nervous System
Anorexia (14%)
Fever (14%)
Paresthesias (<10%)

Neuromuscular/Skeletal
Asthenia (fatigue) [2]

Gastrointestinal/Hepatic
Nausea (14%)
Vomiting (14%)

Respiratory
Cough (7%)

Renal
Nephrotoxicity [2]

Hematologic
Anemia (19–24%)
Hemolytic uremic syndrome [41]
Neutropenia [2]

Ocular
Epiphora [2]
Keratitis [2]
Ocular toxicity [3]

Local
Injection-site cellulitis (>10%)
Injection-site necrosis (>10%) [3]

MITOXANTRONE

Trade name: Novantrone (OSI)
Indications: Acute myelogenous leukemia, multiple sclerosis, prostate cancer
Class: Antibiotic, anthracycline, Antineoplastic
Half-life: median terminal: 75 hours
Clinically important, potentially hazardous interactions with: aldesleukin
Pregnancy category: D
Important contra-indications noted in the prescribing guidelines for: nursing mothers; pediatric patients

---

Skin
Diaphoresis (<10%)
Ecchymoses (7%)
Edema (>10%)
Fungal dermatitis (>15%)
Peripheral edema [2]
Petechiae (>10%)
Purpura (>10%)

Hair
Alopecia (20–60%) [4]

Cardiovascular
Cardiac failure [2]
Cardiotoxicity [3]
Congestive heart failure [3]

Central Nervous System
Chills (<10%)

Gastrointestinal/Hepatic
Diarrhea [2]
Nausea [4]
Vomiting [3]

Endocrine/Metabolic
Amenorrhea [3]

Hematologic
Anemia [2]
Leukemia [4]
Leukopenia [3]
Neutropenia [5]

Other
Infection (>66%) [2]

MODAFINIL

Trade name: Provigil (Cephalon)
Indications: Narcolepsy
Class: Analeptic, CNS stimulant, CYP1A2 inducer, CYP3A4 inducer
Half-life: ~15 hours
Clinically important, potentially hazardous interactions with: enzalutamide, oral contraceptives, thalidomide
Pregnancy category: C
Important contra-indications noted in the prescribing guidelines for: the elderly; nursing mothers; pediatric patients

---

Skin
Fixed eruption [2]

Mucosal
Xerostomia (5%)

Cardiovascular
Hypertension [2]
Palpitation [2]

Central Nervous System
Agitation [2]
Chills (2%)
Hallucinations [2]
Headache (28%) [13]
Insomnia (5%) [6]
Nervousness [2]
Paresthesias (3%)
Vertigo (dizziness) (5%) [3]

Neuromuscular/Skeletal
Back pain (6%)

Gastrointestinal/Hepatic
Abdominal pain [2]
Diarrhea (6%) [3]
Nausea (11%) [6]

Respiratory
Rhinitis (7%)

Ocular
Hallucinations, visual [2]

Other
Adverse effects [3]

MONTELUKAST

Trade name: Singulair (Merck)
Indications: Asthma
Class: Leukotriene receptor antagonist
Half-life: 2.7–5.5 hours
Clinically important, potentially hazardous interactions with: prednisone
Pregnancy category: B
Important contra-indications noted in the prescribing guidelines for: nursing mothers

---

Skin
Angioedema [3]
Churg-Strauss syndrome [27]
Rash (2%) [2]
Urticaria (2%)

Central Nervous System
Aggression [2]
Anxiety [2]
Depression [2]
Hallucinations [2]
Headache [4]
Neurotoxicity [5]
Nightmares [2]
Sleep disturbances [2]
Suicidal ideation [2]

Gastrointestinal/Hepatic
Hepatotoxicity [3]

Respiratory
Cough [2]
Flu-like syndrome (<10%)

Other
Adverse effects [3]

MORPHINE

Trade names: Avinza (Ligand), Duramorph (Baxter) (Elkins-Sinn), Infumorph (Baxter), Kadian (aaiPharma), Morphabond (Inspirion), MS Contin (Purdue), MSIR Oral (Purdue), Roxanol (aaiPharma)
Indications: Severe pain, acute myocardial infarction
Class: Opiate agonist
Half-life: 2–4 hours
Clinically important, potentially hazardous interactions with: buprenorphine, cimetidine, furazolidone, MAO inhibitors, metformin, mianserin, pentazocine, rifapentine, trospium
Pregnancy category: C
Important contra-indications noted in the prescribing guidelines for: nursing mothers; pediatric patients
Black Box Warning: ADDICTION, ABUSE, AND MISUSE; LIFETHREATENING RESPIRATORY DEPRESSION; ACCIDENTAL INGESTION; NEONATAL OPIOID WITHDRAWAL SYNDROME; and INTERACTION WITH ALCOHOL

Skin
AGEP [3]
Edema [2]
Pruritus (5–65%) [34]

Mucosal
Xerostomia (>10%) [6]

Cardiovascular
Cardiotoxicity [3]
Hypotension [5]

Central Nervous System
Allodynia [4]
Confusion [2]
Hallucinations [4]
Hyperalgesia [10]
Sedation [2]
Somnolence (drowsiness) [4]
Trembling (<10%)
Vertigo (dizziness) [5]

Neuromuscular/Skeletal
Myoclonus [5]
Rhabdomyolysis [2]

Gastrointestinal/Hepatic
Constipation [7]
Nausea [14]
Vomiting [11]

Respiratory
Respiratory depression [5]

Endocrine/Metabolic
Amenorrhea [2]

Genitourinary
Urinary retention [2]

Local
Injection-site pain (>10%)

Other
Death [3]
Hiccups [3]

MOXIFLOXACIN

Trade names: Avelox (Bayer), Moxeza (Alcon)
Indications: Various infections caused by susceptible organisms
Class: Antibiotic, fluoroquinolone
Half-life: 12 hours
Clinically important, potentially hazardous interactions with: alfuzosin, aminophylline, amiodarone, amitriptyline, antacids, arsenic, artemether/lumefantrine, asenapine, atomoxetine, BCG vaccine, benperidol, bepridil, bretylium, chloroquine, ciprofloxacin, corticosteroids, cyclosporine, degarelix, didanosine, disopyramide, dronedarone, droperidol, erythromycin, gadobutrol, haloperidol, hydroxychloroquine, insulin, lanthanum, levomepromazine, magnesium salts, mefloquine, mizolastine, mycophenolate, nilotinib, NSAIDs, oral iron, oral typhoid vaccine, pentamidine, phenothiazines, pimozide, probenecid, procainamide, QT prolonging agents, quinapril, quinidine, quinine, sevelamer, sotalol, strontium ranelate, sucralfate, sulfonylureas, tetrabenazine, thioridazine, tricyclic antidepressants, vandetanib, vitamin K antagonists, warfarin, zinc, ziprasidone, zolmitriptan, zuclopenthixol

Pregnancy category: C
Important contra-indications noted in the prescribing guidelines for: the elderly; nursing mothers; pediatric patients
Note: Fluoroquinolones are associated with an increased risk of tendinitis and tendon rupture in all ages. This risk is further increased in older patients usually over 60 years of age, in patients taking corticosteroid drugs, and in patients with kidney, heart or lung transplants.
Fluoroquinolones may exacerbate muscle weakness in persons with myasthenia gravis.
Moxeza is for topical ophthalmic use only.
Black Box Warning: SERIOUS ADVERSE REACTIONS INCLUDING TENDINITIS, TENDON RUPTURE, PERIPHERAL NEUROPATHY, CENTRAL NERVOUS SYSTEM EFFECTS and EXACERBATION OF MYASTHENIA GRAVIS

Skin
- Anaphylactoid reactions/Anaphylaxis [5]
- Bullous dermatitis [2]
- Hypersensitivity [6]
- Photosensitivity [5]
- Pruritus [2]
- Rash [3]
- Thrombocytopenic purpura [2]
- Toxic epidermal necrolysis [2]
- Urticaria [3]

Cardiovascular
- Phlebitis [2]
- QT prolongation [13]
- Torsades de pointes [7]

Central Nervous System
- Dysgeusia (taste perversion) [3]
- Hallucinations [2]
- Headache (4%) [5]
- Somnolence (drowsiness) [2]
- Vertigo (dizziness) (3%) [6]

Neuromuscular/Skeletal
- Myasthenia gravis (exacerbation) [2]
- Tendinopathy/Tendon rupture [3]

Gastrointestinal/Hepatic
- Abdominal pain [5]
- Diarrhea (6%) [6]
- Gastrointestinal disorder [2]
- Hepatotoxicity [3]
- Nausea (7%) [8]
- Vomiting [5]

Local
- Injection-site reactions [2]

Other
- Adverse effects [6]

MYCOPHENOLATE

Synonyms: mycophenolate mofetil, mycophenolate sodium
Trade names: CellCept (Roche), Myfortic (Novartis)
Indications: Prophylaxis of organ rejection
Class: Immunosuppressant
Half-life: 18 hours
Clinically important, potentially hazardous interactions with: antacids, azathioprine, basiliximab, belatacept, cholestyramine, ciprofloxacin, corticosteroids, cyclophosphamide, cyclosporine, daclizumab, gemifloxacin, Hemophilus B vaccine, levofloxacin, mercaptopurine, metronidazole, moxifloxacin, norfloxacin, ofloxacin, pantoprazole, rifapentine, sevelamer, tacrolimus, vaccines
Pregnancy category: D
Important contra-indications noted in the prescribing guidelines for: the elderly; nursing mothers; pediatric patients
Black Box Warning: EMBRYOFETAL TOXICITY, MALIGNANCIES AND SERIOUS INFECTIONS

Skin
- Acneform eruption (>10%) [3]
- Carcinoma (non-melanoma) (4%)
- Edema (12%)
- Herpes simplex [3]
- Herpes zoster [6]
- Peripheral edema (29%)
- Rash (8%) [2]
- Warts [2]

Hair
- Alopecia [3]

Mucosal
- Oral candidiasis (10%)
- Oral ulceration [5]

Cardiovascular
- Hypertension [4]
- Thrombophlebitis (<10%)

Central Nervous System
- Fever [2]
- Headache (>20%) [5]
- Insomnia [2]
- Leukoencephalopathy [4]
- Neurotoxicity [2]
- Pain (>20%)
- Tremor (11%)

Neuromuscular/Skeletal
- Arthralgia [4]
- Asthenia (fatigue) [6]
- Back pain (6%)
- Myalgia/Myopathy [4]

Gastrointestinal/Hepatic
- Abdominal distension [2]
- Abdominal pain [6]
- Colitis [3]
- Diarrhea [13]
- Hepatotoxicity [4]
- Nausea [5]
- Vomiting [5]

Respiratory
- Bronchitis [2]
- Cough [2]
- Upper respiratory tract infection [3]

Endocrine/Metabolic
- Hyperglycemia [4]
- Hyperlipidemia [3]

Genitourinary
- Urinary tract infection [2]

Renal
- Nephrotoxicity [3]

Hematologic
- Anemia (>20%)
- Bone marrow suppression [2]
- Dyslipidemia [2]
- Leukopenia [4]
- Lymphopenia [3]
- Myelotoxicity [2]
- Neutropenia [4]
- Thrombocytopenia [4]

Other
- Adverse effects [18]
- Infection (12–20%) [17]
- Teratogenicity [4]

NABILONE

Trade name: Cesamet (Valeant)
Indications: Nausea and vomiting
Class: Antiemetic, Cannabinoid
Half-life: 2 hours
Clinically important, potentially hazardous interactions with: CNS depressants
Pregnancy category: C

Mucosal
Xerostomia [6]

Cardiovascular
Hypotension [7]

Central Nervous System
Dyskinesia [3]
Somnolence (drowsiness) [2]
Vertigo (dizziness) [14]

Neuromuscular/Skeletal
Asthenia (fatigue) [5]

NABUMETONE

Trade name: Relafen (GSK)
Indications: Arthritis
Class: Non-steroidal anti-inflammatory (NSAID)
Half-life: 22.5–30 hours
Clinically important, potentially hazardous interactions with: methotrexate
Pregnancy category: C
Important contra-indications noted in the prescribing guidelines for: nursing mothers; pediatric patients
Note: NSAIDs may cause an increased risk of serious cardiovascular and gastrointestinal adverse events, which can be fatal. This risk may increase with duration of use.
Black Box Warning: CARDIOVASCULAR AND GASTROINTESTINAL RISKS

Skin
Diaphoresis (<3%)
Edema (3–9%)
Erythema [2]
Hypersensitivity [2]
Photosensitivity [2]
Pruritus (3–9%) [2]
Rash (3–9%) [4]

Mucosal
Stomatitis (<3%)
Xerostomia (<3%)

Central Nervous System
Headache (3–9%) [2]
Insomnia (3–9%)
Nervousness (3–9%)
Somnolence (drowsiness) (3–9%)
Vertigo (dizziness) (3–9%)

Gastrointestinal/Hepatic
Abdominal pain (12%) [5]
Constipation (3–9%)
Diarrhea (14%) [5]
Dyspepsia (13%) [4]
Flatulence (3–9%)
Gastrointestinal ulceration [3]
Hepatotoxicity [2]
Nausea (3–9%) [2]
Vomiting (3–9%)

Endocrine/Metabolic
Pseudoporphyria [8]

Renal
Nephrotoxicity [2]

Otic
Tinnitus (<10%)

Other
Adverse effects [6]

NADOLOL

Trade name: Corzide (Monarch)
Indications: Hypertension, angina pectoris
Class: Adrenergic beta-receptor antagonist, Antiarrhythmic class II
Half-life: 10–24 hours
Clinically important, potentially hazardous interactions with: clonidine, epinephrine, verapamil
Pregnancy category: C
Important contra-indications noted in the prescribing guidelines for: nursing mothers; pediatric patients
Note: Corzide is nadolol and bendroflumethiazide. Cutaneous side effects of beta-receptor blockers are clinically polymorphous. They apparently appear after several months of continuous therapy. Contraindicated in patients with bronchial asthma, sinus bradycardia and greater than first degree conduction block, cardiogenic shock, and overt cardiac failure.

Skin
Edema (<5%)
Psoriasis [4]
Raynaud's phenomenon (2%) [2]

Cardiovascular
Bradycardia (2%)

Central Nervous System
Hypoesthesia (fingers and toes) (>5%)
Paresthesias (>5%)
Vertigo (dizziness) (2%)

Neuromuscular/Skeletal
Asthenia (fatigue) (2%)

Other
Adverse effects [4]

NALBUPHINE

Trade name: Nubain (Endo)
Indications: Moderate to severe pain
Class: Opiate agonist
Half-life: 5 hours
Clinically important, potentially hazardous interactions with: CNS depressants, diazepam, hydrocodone, hydromorphone, oxymorphone, pentobarbital, promethazine, tapentadol
Pregnancy category: B
Note: Nalbuphine contains sulfites.

Skin
Clammy skin (9%)
Diaphoresis (9%)

Mucosal
Xerostomia (4%)

Central Nervous System
Vertigo (dizziness) (5%)

Local
Injection-site pain [4]

NALOXEGOL

Trade name: Movantik (AstraZeneca)
Indications: Opioid-induced constipation
Class: Opioid receptor antagonist
Half-life: 6–11 hours
Clinically important, potentially hazardous interactions with: diltiazem, erythromycin, grapefruit juice, verapamil
Pregnancy category: C
Important contra-indications noted in the prescribing guidelines for: nursing mothers; pediatric patients
Note: Contraindicated in patients with known or suspected gastrointestinal obstruction, patients at increased risk of recurrent gastrointestinal obstruction, and patients concomitantly using strong CYP3A4 inhibitors.

Skin
Hyperhidrosis (<3%)

Central Nervous System
Headache (4%) [3]

Gastrointestinal/Hepatic
Abdominal pain (12–21%) [4]
Diarrhea (6–9%) [4]
Flatulence (3–6%) [2]
Nausea (7–8%) [5]
Vomiting (3–5%)

Other
Adverse effects [2]

NALOXONE

Trade names: Suboxone (Reckitt Benckiser), Talwin-NX (Sanofi-Aventis), Targiniq (Purdue)
Indications: Narcotic overdose
Class: Opioid antagonist
Half-life: <1.5 hours
Clinically important, potentially hazardous interactions with: cobicistat/elvitegravir/emtricitabine/tenofovir disoproxil, thioridazine
Pregnancy category: C
Important contra-indications noted in the prescribing guidelines for: nursing mothers
Note: Subuxone contains buprenorphine; Targiniq is naloxone and oxycodone.

Skin
Diaphoresis (<10%)
Pruritus [2]
Rash (<10%)

Mucosal
Xerostomia [2]

Cardiovascular
Arrhythmias [2]
Bradycardia [2]
Hypertension [8]

Hypotension [2]
Pulmonary edema [2]

Central Nervous System
Headache [3]
Seizures [5]
Somnolence (drowsiness) [3]

Neuromuscular/Skeletal
Asthenia (fatigue) [3]
Myoclonus [2]

Gastrointestinal/Hepatic
Constipation [5]
Nausea [3]
Vomiting [2]

Other
Adverse effects [3]
Death [2]

NALTREXONE

Trade names: Contrave (Takeda), Depade (Mallinckrodt), Nalorex (Bristol-Myers Squibb), Opizone (Genus), ReVia (Meda), Troxyca (Pfizer), Vivitrex (Alkermes), Vivitrol (Alkermes)
Indications: Substance abuse, opioid dependence, alcohol dependence
Class: Opioid antagonist
Half-life: 4 hours
Clinically important, potentially hazardous interactions with: opioid analgesics, opioid containing medications
Pregnancy category: C
Important contra-indications noted in the prescribing guidelines for: nursing mothers; pediatric patients
Note: Naltrexone has the capacity to cause hepatocellular injury when given in excessive doses.
Troxyca is naltrexone and oxycodone. Contraindicated in acute hepatitis or liver failure; patients receiving opioid analgesics, with current physiologic opioid dependence, or in acute opioid withdrawal.

Skin
Pruritus [2]
Rash (<10%)

Cardiovascular
Hypertension [3]

Central Nervous System
Chills (<10%)
Compulsions [2]
Depression [2]
Headache [3]
Insomnia [3]
Seizures [2]
Vertigo (dizziness) [4]

Neuromuscular/Skeletal
Arthralgia (>10%)
Asthenia (fatigue) [3]

Gastrointestinal/Hepatic
Constipation [5]
Hepatotoxicity [5]
Nausea [7]
Vomiting [5]

Respiratory
Influenza [2]
Nasopharyngitis [2]

Local
Injection-site pain [2]
Injection-site reactions [3]

Other
Adverse effects [3]

NANDROLONE

Trade name: Deca-Durabolin (Organon)
Indications: Anemia of renal insufficiency, control of metastatic breast cancer, osteoporosis in post-menopausal women
Class: Anabolic steroid
Half-life: 6–14 days
Clinically important, potentially hazardous interactions with: acenocoumarol, anisindione, anticoagulants, dabigatran, danaparoid, fondaparinux, heparin, warfarin
Pregnancy category: X
Important contra-indications noted in the prescribing guidelines for: nursing mothers; pediatric patients
Note: Deca Durabolin contains Arachis oil (peanut oil) and should not be taken / applied by patients known to be allergic to peanut.

Hair
Hirsutism [3]

Other
Adverse effects [2]

NAPROXEN

Trade names: Aleve (Bayer), Naprosyn (Roche), Synflex (Roche)
Indications: Pain, arthritis
Class: Non-steroidal anti-inflammatory (NSAID)
Half-life: 15 hours
Clinically important, potentially hazardous interactions with: methotrexate, methyl salicylate, prednisolone
Pregnancy category: C
Important contra-indications noted in the prescribing guidelines for: the elderly; nursing mothers; pediatric patients
Note: NSAIDs may cause an increased risk of serious cardiovascular and gastrointestinal adverse events, which can be fatal. This risk may increase with duration of use.

Skin
Anaphylactoid reactions/Anaphylaxis [2]
Angioedema [5]
Bullous dermatitis [5]
Diaphoresis (<3%) [3]
DRESS syndrome [4]
Ecchymoses (3–9%)
Edema (<9%)
Erythema multiforme [2]
Exanthems (<14%) [9]
Fixed eruption [24]
Hypersensitivity [2]
Lichen planus [3]
Lichenoid eruption [3]
Lupus erythematosus [2]
Photosensitivity [16]
Pruritus (3–17%) [5]
Purpura (<3%) [4]
Pustules [2]
Rash (3–9%) [2]
Toxic epidermal necrolysis [5]
Urticaria (<5%) [6]
Vasculitis [9]

Hair
Alopecia [3]

Mucosal
Stomatitis (<3%)
Xerostomia [2]

Cardiovascular
Chest pain [2]
Myocardial infarction [2]

Central Nervous System
Somnolence (drowsiness) [2]
Vertigo (dizziness) [6]

Neuromuscular/Skeletal
Leg cramps [2]

Gastrointestinal/Hepatic
Abdominal pain [4]
Constipation [2]
Diarrhea [3]
Dyspepsia [9]
Hepatotoxicity [3]
Nausea [10]

Respiratory
Nasopharyngitis [2]

Endocrine/Metabolic
Pseudoporphyria [29]

Renal
Nephrotoxicity [3]

Hematologic
Thrombocytopenia [2]

Otic
Tinnitus [2]

Other
Adverse effects [9]
Death [2]
Side effects (5–9%) [3]

NATALIZUMAB

Synonym: antegren
Trade name: Tysabri (Biogen)
Indications: Multiple sclerosis, Crohn's disease
Class: Immunomodulator, Monoclonal antibody
Half-life: 11 days
Clinically important, potentially hazardous interactions with: abatacept, alefacept, azacitidine, azathioprine, betamethasone, cabazitaxel, certolizumab, cortocosteroids, cyclosporine, denileukin, docetaxel, fingolimod, gefitinib, leflunomide, lenalidomide, mercaptopurine, methotrexate, oxaliplatin, pazopanib, pemetrexed, rilonacept, temsirolimus, triamcinolone, vedolizumab

Pregnancy category: C
Important contra-indications noted in the prescribing guidelines for: nursing mothers; pediatric patients
Note: Contraindicated in patients who have or have had progressive multifocal leukoencephalopathy.
Black Box Warning: PROGRESSIVE MULTIFOCAL LEUKOENCEPHALOPATHY

Skin
Dermatitis (6%)
Herpes simplex [2]
Hypersensitivity [5]
Pruritus (4%)
Rash (9%)

Central Nervous System
Depression (17%)
Headache (35%) [2]
Leukoencephalopathy [72]
Tremor (3%)

Neuromuscular/Skeletal
Asthenia (fatigue) (24%) [3]

Gastrointestinal/Hepatic
Hepatotoxicity [3]

Genitourinary
Vaginitis (8%)

Local
Application-site reactions (22%)
Infusion-site reactions [2]

Other
Adverse effects [2]
Allergic reactions (7%) [3]
Death [5]
Infection (2%)

NATEGLINIDE

Trade name: Starlix (Novartis)
Indications: Diabetes Type II
Class: Meglitinide
Half-life: 1.5 hours
Clinically important, potentially hazardous interactions with: none known
Pregnancy category: C
Important contra-indications noted in the prescribing guidelines for: nursing mothers; pediatric patients

---

Respiratory
Flu-like syndrome (4%)

NEBIVOLOL

Trade names: Bystolic (Forest), Byvalson (Forest), Nebilet (Menarini)
Indications: Hypertension
Class: Adrenergic beta-receptor antagonist, Beta blocker
Half-life: 8 hours
Clinically important, potentially hazardous interactions with: beta blockers, cinacalcet, clonidine, CYP2D6 inhibitors, delavirdine, digitalis glycosides, duloxetine, terbinafine, tipranavir
Pregnancy category: C
Important contra-indications noted in the prescribing guidelines for: nursing mothers; pediatric patients
Note: Byvalson is nebivolol and valsartan.
Black Box Warning: Byvalson: FETAL TOXICITY

Cardiovascular
Bradycardia [3]

Central Nervous System
Headache (6–9%) [9]
Vertigo (dizziness) (2–4%) [5]

Neuromuscular/Skeletal
Asthenia (fatigue) (2–5%) [4]

Gastrointestinal/Hepatic
Diarrhea (<2%)
Nausea (<3%)

Respiratory
Nasopharyngitis [3]
Upper respiratory tract infection [3]

Other
Adverse effects [3]

NECITUMUMAB *

Trade name: Portrazza (Lilly)
Indications: Metastatic squamous non-small cell lung cancer (in combination with cisplatin and gemcitabine)
Class: Epidermal growth factor receptor (EGFR) inhibitor, Monoclonal antibody
Half-life: 14 days
Clinically important, potentially hazardous interactions with: none known
Pregnancy category: N/A (Can cause fetal harm)
Important contra-indications noted in the prescribing guidelines for: nursing mothers; pediatric patients
Note: See separate entries for cisplatin and gemcitabine.
Black Box Warning: CARDIOPULMONARY ARREST and HYPOMAGNESEMIA

Skin
Acneform eruption (9–15%)
Fissures (5%)
Hypersensitivity (2%)
Pruritus (7%) [2]
Rash (44%) [7]
Toxicity (8%)
Xerosis (7%) [2]

Mucosal
Stomatitis (11%)

Cardiovascular
Cardiac arrest (3%)
Phlebitis (2%)
Venous thromboembolism (9%) [3]

Central Nervous System
Headache (11%) [2]

Neuromuscular/Skeletal
Asthenia (fatigue) [2]
Muscle spasm (2%)

Gastrointestinal/Hepatic
Diarrhea (16%)
Dysphagia (3%)
Vomiting (29%)

Respiratory
Hemoptysis (10%)
Pulmonary embolism (5%)

Endocrine/Metabolic
Hypocalcemia (45%)
Hypokalemia (28%)
Hypomagnesemia (83%) [5]
Hypophosphatemia (31%)
Weight loss (13%)

Hematologic
Neutropenia [3]
Thrombocytopenia [2]

Ocular
Conjunctivitis (7%)

Local
Infusion-related reactions (2%)

Other
Adverse effects [2]
Death [2]

NELFINAVIR

Trade name: Viracept (ViiV)
Indications: HIV infection
Class: Antiretroviral, CYP3A4 inhibitor, HIV-1 protease inhibitor
Half-life: 3.5–5 hours
Clinically important, potentially hazardous interactions with: abiraterone, afatinib, alfuzosin, amiodarone, amprenavir, aripiprazole, artemether/lumefantrine, atorvastatin, avanafil, barbiturates, benzodiazepines, cabazitaxel, cabozantinib, carbamazepine, chlordiazepoxide, ciclesonide, cisapride, clonazepam, clorazepate, crizotinib, cyclosporine, darifenacin, dasatinib, delavirdine, diazepam, dihydroergotamine, eletriptan, eplerenone, ergot alkaloids, ergotamine, erlotinib, estrogens, eszopiclone, etravirine, eucalyptus, everolimus, fentanyl, fesoterodine, flibanserin, flurazepam, fluticasone propionate, indinavir, ivabradine, ixabepilone, lapatinib, lomitapide, lopinavir, lorazepam, lovastatin, maraviroc, methadone, methylergonovine, methysergide, midazolam, mifepristone, olaparib, omeprazole, oral contraceptives, oxazepam, paclitaxel, palbociclib, pantoprazole, pazopanib, phenytoin, pimozide, ponatinib, primidone, progestogens, quazepam, quinidine, quinine, ranolazine, rifabutin, rifampin, rilpivirine, ritonavir, rivaroxaban, romidepsin, rosuvastatin, ruxolitinib, saquinavir, sildenafil, simeprevir, simvastatin, solifenacin, St John's wort, sunitinib, tacrolimus, tadalafil, telithromycin, temazepam, temsirolimus, ticagrelor, tolterodine, tolvaptan, triazolam, vardenafil, vemurafenib, vorapaxar
Pregnancy category: B
Important contra-indications noted in the prescribing guidelines for: nursing mothers
Note: Protease inhibitors cause dyslipidemia which includes elevated triglycerides and cholesterol and redistribution of body fat centrally to produce the so-called 'protease paunch',

breast enlargement, facial atrophy, and 'buffalo hump'.

Skin
Rash (<10%) [4]

Gastrointestinal/Hepatic
Diarrhea [3]
Hepatotoxicity [3]

Genitourinary
Urolithiasis [2]

Hematologic
Lymphopenia [2]

NEOMYCIN

Trade names: Maxitrol (Falcon), Neosporin (Monarch)
Indications: Various infections caused by susceptible organisms
Class: Antibiotic, aminoglycoside
Half-life: 3 hours
Clinically important, potentially hazardous interactions with: acarbose, aldesleukin, aminoglycosides, atracurium, bacitracin, bumetanide, doxacurium, ethacrynic acid, furosemide, methoxyflurane, neostigmine, pancuronium, penicillin V, polypeptide antibiotics, rocuronium, sorafenib, succinylcholine, teicoplanin, torsemide, vecuronium
Pregnancy category: D
Important contra-indications noted in the prescribing guidelines for: nursing mothers; pediatric patients
Note: Aminoglycosides may cause neurotoxicity and/or nephrotoxicity.

Skin
Anaphylactoid reactions/Anaphylaxis [2]
Contact dermatitis (<10%) [72]
Eczema [2]
Exanthems [2]
Rash (<10%)
Toxic epidermal necrolysis [2]
Urticaria (<10%)

Otic
Hearing loss [3]

NEOSTIGMINE

Trade name: Prostigmin (Valeant)
Indications: Myasthenia gravis
Class: Acetylcholinesterase inhibitor, Cholinesterase inhibitor, Parasympathomimetic
Half-life: 52 minutes
Clinically important, potentially hazardous interactions with: aminoglycosides, antiarrhythmics, anticholinergics, chloroquine, clindamycin, hydroxychloroquine, kanamycin, lithium, local and general anesthetics, neomycin, non-depolarising muscle relaxants, polymixins, propafenone, propranolol, streptomycin, succinylcholine
Pregnancy category: C (anticholinesterase drugs may cause uterine irritability and induce premature labor when given intravenously to pregnant women near term)
Important contra-indications noted in the prescribing guidelines for: nursing mothers; pediatric patients
Note: Neostigmine bromide is given orally; neostigmine methylsulfate is given parenterally. Contraindicated in patients with a previous history of reaction to bromides, or those with peritonitis or mechanical obstruction of the intestinal or urinary tract.

Skin
Anaphylactoid reactions/Anaphylaxis [3]

Cardiovascular
Atrioventricular block [3]
Bradycardia [3]
Cardiac arrest [3]

Central Nervous System
Anxiety [2]
Sedation [2]

Gastrointestinal/Hepatic
Abdominal pain [3]
Diarrhea [2]
Nausea [12]
Vomiting [10]

Respiratory
Bronchospasm [3]

NETUPITANT & PALONOSETRON

Synonym: NEPA
Trade name: Akynzeo (Helsinn)
Indications: Acute and delayed nausea and vomiting associated with cancer chemotherapy
Class: Neurokinin 1 receptor antagonist (netupitant), Serotonin type 3 receptor antagonist (palonosetron)
Half-life: 40 hours
Clinically important, potentially hazardous interactions with: rifampin
Pregnancy category: C
Important contra-indications noted in the prescribing guidelines for: nursing mothers; pediatric patients

---

Skin
Erythema (3%)

Central Nervous System
Headache (9%) [7]

Neuromuscular/Skeletal
Asthenia (fatigue) (4–8%)

Gastrointestinal/Hepatic
Constipation (3%) [6]
Dyspepsia (4%) [2]

Other
Adverse effects [2]
Hiccups [2]

NEVIRAPINE

Trade name: Viramune (Boehringer Ingelheim)
Indications: HIV infection
Class: Antiretroviral, CYP3A4 inducer, Non-nucleoside reverse transcriptase inhibitor
Half-life: 45 hours
Clinically important, potentially hazardous interactions with: amiodarone, amprenavir, atazanavir, carbamazepine, caspofungin, clarithromycin, clonazepam, cyclosporine, diltiazem, disopyramide, efavirenz, ethosuximide, etravirine, fentanyl, fluconazole, fosamprenavir, indinavir, itraconazole, ketoconazole, levonorgestrel, lidocaine, lopinavir, midazolam, nifedipine, rifampin, rilpivirine, simeprevir, St John's wort, verapamil
Pregnancy category: B
Important contra-indications noted in the prescribing guidelines for: nursing mothers
Black Box Warning: LIFE-THREATENING (INCLUDING FATAL) HEPATOTOXICITY and SKIN REACTIONS

Skin
Angioedema [2]
DRESS syndrome [12]
Exanthems [6]
Hypersensitivity [15]
Lipodystrophy [2]
Rash (<48%) [30]
Stevens-Johnson syndrome [32]
Toxic epidermal necrolysis [15]
Toxicity [3]

Mucosal
Gingivitis (<3%)
Ulcerative stomatitis (4%)

Central Nervous System
Fever [2]
Paresthesias (2%)
Peripheral neuropathy [2]

Neuromuscular/Skeletal
Myalgia/Myopathy (<10%)

Gastrointestinal/Hepatic
Hepatic failure [2]
Hepatotoxicity [28]

Endocrine/Metabolic
Acidosis [2]

Other
Adverse effects [7]
Death [3]

NIACIN

Synonyms: nicotinic acid; vitamin B_3
Trade names: Advicor (Kos), Niacor (Upsher-Smith), Niaspan (Merck), Simcor (AbbVie), Slo-Niacin (Upsher-Smith)
Indications: Hyperlipidemia
Class: Vitamin
Half-life: 45 minutes
Clinically important, potentially hazardous interactions with: antihypertensives, atorvastatin, bile acid sequestrants, insulin aspart,

insulin degludec, insulin detemir, insulin glargine, insulin glulisine, pitavastatin, rosuvastatin, selenium
Pregnancy category: C (where niacin is co-administered with a statin, refer to the pregnancy category for the statin)
Important contra-indications noted in the prescribing guidelines for: nursing mothers; pediatric patients
Note: Contraindicated in patients with active liver or peptic ulcer disease, or arterial bleeding. Simcor is niacin and simvastatin.

Skin
Acanthosis nigricans (8%) [14]
Exanthems (<3%)
Pruritus (<5%) [9]
Rash [5]

Cardiovascular
Flushing (<30%) [30]

Central Nervous System
Paresthesias (<10%) [2]

Neuromuscular/Skeletal
Myalgia/Myopathy [4]

Gastrointestinal/Hepatic
Hepatotoxicity [3]

Endocrine/Metabolic
Hyperglycemia [2]

Ocular
Maculopathy [3]

NIACINAMIDE

Synonyms: nicotinamide; vitamin B_3
Indications: Prophylaxis and treatment of pellagra
Class: Vitamin
Half-life: 45 minutes
Clinically important, potentially hazardous interactions with: atorvastatin, primidone, rosuvastatin
Pregnancy category: A (the pregnancy category will be C if used in doses above the RDA)

Skin
Pruritus (<5%) [2]

Central Nervous System
Paresthesias (<10%)

Hematologic
Thrombocytopenia [2]

NICARDIPINE

Trade name: Cardene (Roche)
Indications: Angina, hypertension
Class: Calcium channel blocker
Half-life: 2–4 hours
Clinically important, potentially hazardous interactions with: amprenavir, atazanavir, boceprevir, cobicistat/elvitegravir/emtricitabine/tenofovir disoproxil, delavirdine, epirubicin, imatinib, indinavir, lopinavir, posaconazole, propranolol, telaprevir
Pregnancy category: C
Important contra-indications noted in the prescribing guidelines for: the elderly; pediatric patients

---

Skin
Peripheral edema (7%) [2]
Rash [3]
Urticaria [3]

Mucosal
Gingival hyperplasia/hypertrophy [2]

Cardiovascular
Erythromelalgia [2]
Flushing (6%) [2]
Pulmonary edema [5]

Endocrine/Metabolic
Gynecomastia [2]

Other
Adverse effects [2]
Side effects [2]

NICOTINE

Trade names: Habitrol Patch (Novartis), Nicoderm (GSK), Nicorette (GSK), Nicotrol (Pfizer)
Indications: Aid to smoking cessation
Class: Alkaloid
Half-life: varies with the delivery system
Clinically important, potentially hazardous interactions with: adenosine, bendamustine, heparin, horsetail
Pregnancy category: D
Important contra-indications noted in the prescribing guidelines for: nursing mothers; pediatric patients
Note: Smoking cessation therapy has various delivery systems. These include: transdermal patches, chewing gum, nasal spray, inhaler, and oral forms.

Skin
Acneform eruption (3%)
Diaphoresis (<3%)
Erythema (>10%)
Pigmentation [3]
Pruritus (>10%)

Mucosal
Sialorrhea (>10%)
Stomatitis (>10%)
Xerostomia (<3%)

Central Nervous System
Headache (18–26%)

Neuromuscular/Skeletal
Arthralgia (5%)
Back pain (6%)
Myalgia/Myopathy (<10%)

Gastrointestinal/Hepatic
Dyspepsia (18%)
Flatulence (4%)
Pancreatitis [2]
Throat irritation/pain (66%)

Respiratory
Cough (32%) [2]
Rhinitis (23%)

Other
Death [2]
Hiccups [2]

NIFEDIPINE

Trade names: Adalat (Bayer), Coracten (UCB), Procardia (Pfizer), Tenif (AstraZeneca), Tensipine MR (Genus), Valni XL (Winthrop)
Indications: Angina, hypertension
Class: Calcium channel blocker
Half-life: 2–5 hours (immediate release products)
Clinically important, potentially hazardous interactions with: acebutolol, amprenavir, atazanavir, beta blockers, boceprevir, carbamazepine, cobicistat/elvitegravir/emtricitabine/tenofovir disoproxil, cyclosporine, delavirdine, digoxin, diltiazem, dronedarone, efavirenz, epirubicin, fentanyl, fluoxetine, grapefruit juice, imatinib, indinavir, insulin, lopinavir, micafungin, mizolastine, nevirapine, oxcarbazepine, parenteral magnesium, phenytoin, posaconazole, propranolol, rifampin, ritonavir, St John's wort, tacrolimus, vardenafil, vincristine
Pregnancy category: C
Important contra-indications noted in the prescribing guidelines for: the elderly; nursing mothers; pediatric patients
Note: Tenif is atenolol and nifedipine.

Skin
AGEP [3]
Angioedema [2]
Bullous dermatitis [2]
Dermatitis (<2%)
Diaphoresis (<2%) [2]
Edema [3]
Erysipelas [2]
Erythema [2]
Erythema multiforme [5]
Erythema nodosum [2]
Exanthems [9]
Exfoliative dermatitis [5]
Fixed eruption [2]
Lichenoid eruption [3]
Lupus erythematosus [3]
Peripheral edema [12]
Photosensitivity [5]
Pruritus (<2%) [3]
Purpura (<2%) [3]
Rash (<3%) [2]
Stevens–Johnson syndrome [3]
Telangiectasia [2]
Toxic epidermal necrolysis [2]
Urticaria [7]
Vasculitis [4]

Hair
Alopecia [4]

Mucosal
Gingival hyperplasia/hypertrophy (6–10%) [74]
Xerostomia (<3%)

Cardiovascular
Erythromelalgia [4]
Flushing (3–25%) [9]
Hypotension [8]
Pulmonary edema [3]
Tachycardia [4]

Central Nervous System
Chills (2%)
Headache (19%) [7]
Paresthesias (<3%)
Tremor (2–8%)
Vertigo (dizziness) [5]

Neuromuscular/Skeletal
Asthenia (fatigue) (4%)

Gastrointestinal/Hepatic
Hepatotoxicity [3]
Nausea (2%) [2]

Endocrine/Metabolic
Gynecomastia [6]

Other
Adverse effects [4]
Side effects [3]

NILOTINIB

Trade name: Tasigna (Novartis)
Indications: Chronic myelogenous leukemia (CML)
Class: Antineoplastic, Epidermal growth factor receptor (EGFR) inhibitor, Tyrosine kinase inhibitor
Half-life: 17 hours
Clinically important, potentially hazardous interactions with: amiodarone, amitriptyline, amoxapine, arsenic, astemizole, bepridil, carbamazepine, chloroquine, cisapride, citalopram, clarithromycin, clozapine, conivaptan, darunavir, dasatinib, degarelix, delavirdine, digoxin, dihydroergotamine, disopyramide, dolasetron, efavirenz, ergotamine, grapefruit juice, halofantrine, haloperidol, indinavir, itraconazole, ketoconazole, lapatinib, levofloxacin, lopinavir, methadone, midazolam, moxifloxacin, oxcarbazepine, pazopanib, phenobarbital, phenytoin, pimozide, procainamide, quinidine, rifampin, rifapentine, ritonavir, sotalol, St John's wort, telavancin, telithromycin, terfenadine, voriconazole, vorinostat, ziprasidone
Pregnancy category: D
Important contra-indications noted in the prescribing guidelines for: nursing mothers; pediatric patients
Note: Contraindicated in patients with hypokalemia, hypomagnesemia, or long QT syndrome.
Black Box Warning: QT PROLONGATION AND SUDDEN DEATHS

Skin
Acneform eruption (<10%)
Dermatitis (<10%)
Eczema (<10%)
Edema [2]
Erythema (<10%) [2]
Folliculitis (<10%)
Hematoma (<10%)
Hyperhidrosis (<10%)
Peripheral edema (<10%)
Pruritus (<10%) [8]
Rash (<10%) [10]
Toxicity [6]
Urticaria (<10%)

Hair
Alopecia (<10%) [2]

Cardiovascular
Angina (<10%)
Arrhythmias (<10%) [2]
Arterial occlusion [4]
Atrial fibrillation (<10%)
Atrioventricular block (<10%)
Bradycardia (<10%)
Cardiotoxicity [3]
Chest pain (<10%)
Extrasystoles (<10%)
Flushing (<10%)
Hypertension (<10%)
Myocardial infarction [2]
Palpitation (<10%)
QT prolongation (<10%) [8]

Central Nervous System
Anorexia (<10%)
Depression (<10%) [2]
Fever (<10%) [2]
Headache (~10%) [10]
Hypoesthesia (<10%)
Insomnia (<10%)
Pain [2]
Paresthesias (<10%)
Vertigo (dizziness) (<10%)

Neuromuscular/Skeletal
Arthralgia (<10%) [2]
Asthenia (fatigue) (<10%) [6]
Bone or joint pain (<10%)
Muscle spasm [3]
Myalgia/Myopathy (<10%) [4]
Neck pain (<10%)

Gastrointestinal/Hepatic
Abdominal distension (<10%)
Abdominal pain (<10%) [2]
Constipation (~10%)
Diarrhea (~10%) [4]
Dyspepsia (<10%)
Flatulence (<10%)
Hepatotoxicity [5]
Nausea (~10%) [4]
Pancreatitis (<10%) [2]
Vomiting (~10%)

Respiratory
Cough (<10%)
Dysphonia (<10%)
Dyspnea (<10%)
Pleural effusion [2]
Pulmonary hypertension [2]
Pulmonary toxicity [2]

Endocrine/Metabolic
ALT increased (4%) [2]
AST increased (<3%)
Diabetes mellitus (<10%)
Hyperamylasemia [2]
Hyperbilirubinemia [5]
Hypercalcemia (<10%)
Hypercholesterolemia (<10%)
Hyperglycemia (6–12%) [5]
Hyperkalemia (2–6%)
Hyperlipidemia (<10%)
Hypocalcemia (<10%)
Hypokalemia (<10%) [2]
Hypomagnesemia (<10%)
Hyponatremia (<10%)
Hypophosphatemia (5–17%) [2]
Hypothyroidism [2]
Weight gain (<10%)
Weight loss (<10%)

Genitourinary
Pollakiuria (<10%)

Hematologic
Anemia (4–27%) [7]
Febrile neutropenia (<10%)
Hyperlipasemia [3]
Lymphopenia (<10%)
Neutropenia (12–42%) [8]
Pancytopenia (<10%)
Thrombocytopenia (10–42%) [8]

Ocular
Conjunctivitis (<10%)
Ocular hemorrhage (<10%)
Periorbital edema (<10%)
Xerophthalmia (<10%)

Other
Adverse effects [3]
Death [3]
Side effects [3]

NINTEDANIB

Trade name: Ofev (Boehringer Ingelheim)
Indications: Idiopathic pulmonary fibrosis
Class: Tyrosine kinase inhibitor
Half-life: 9.5 hours
Clinically important, potentially hazardous interactions with: anticoagulants, carbamazepine, erythromycin, phenytoin, St John's wort
Pregnancy category: D
Important contra-indications noted in the prescribing guidelines for: nursing mothers; pediatric patients

---

Skin
Hand–foot syndrome [2]
Rash [4]

Hair
Alopecia [2]

Cardiovascular
Hypertension (5%) [7]
Myocardial infarction (2%)

Central Nervous System
Anorexia [5]
Headache (8%)
Peripheral neuropathy [2]

Neuromuscular/Skeletal
Asthenia (fatigue) [13]

Gastrointestinal/Hepatic
Abdominal pain (15%) [5]
Diarrhea (62%) [25]
Gastrointestinal disorder [4]
Hepatotoxicity (14%) [8]
Nausea (24%) [18]
Vomiting (12%) [15]

Respiratory
Bronchitis [2]
Cough [2]
Dyspnea [3]
Nasopharyngitis [2]
Pneumonia [2]

Endocrine/Metabolic
ALT increased [11]
Appetite decreased (11%) [5]
AST increased [9]
Weight loss (10%)

Hematologic
Anemia [3]
Bleeding (10%) [2]
Leukopenia [2]
Neutropenia [4]
Thrombocytopenia [2]

Other
Adverse effects [5]
Death [3]

NISOLDIPINE

Trade name: Sular (First Horizon)
Indications: Hypertension
Class: Calcium channel blocker
Half-life: 7–12 hours
Clinically important, potentially hazardous interactions with: amprenavir, conivaptan, cyclosporine, darunavir, delavirdine, efavirenz, epirubicin, grapefruit juice, imatinib, indinavir, itraconazole, ketoconazole, oxcarbazepine, propranolol, telaprevir, telithromycin, voriconazole
Pregnancy category: C

Skin
Peripheral edema (22%) [6]
Rash (2%)

Central Nervous System
Headache [4]

Endocrine/Metabolic
Gynecomastia [2]

NITAZOXANIDE

Trade name: Alinia (Romark)
Indications: Diarrhea caused by *Cryptosporidium parvum* or *Giardia lamblia* (in children)
Class: Antiprotozoal
Half-life: N/A
Clinically important, potentially hazardous interactions with: none known
Pregnancy category: B

Central Nervous System
Headache [2]

Gastrointestinal/Hepatic
Abdominal pain [3]
Diarrhea [2]

NITROFURANTOIN

Trade names: Furadantin (First Horizon), Macrobid (Procter & Gamble), Macrodantin (Procter & Gamble)
Indications: Various urinary tract infections caused by susceptible organisms
Class: Antibiotic
Half-life: 1–2 minutes
Clinically important, potentially hazardous interactions with: norfloxacin
Pregnancy category: B
Important contra-indications noted in the prescribing guidelines for: nursing mothers; pediatric patients

---

Skin
Anaphylactoid reactions/Anaphylaxis [2]
Angioedema [4]
Dermatitis [3]
DRESS syndrome [4]
Eczema [2]
Erythema multiforme [3]
Exanthems (<5%) [9]
Exfoliative dermatitis [3]
Lupus erythematosus [8]
Purpura [2]
Rash [2]
Stevens–Johnson syndrome [2]
Toxic epidermal necrolysis [5]
Urticaria [8]

Hair
Alopecia [5]

Central Nervous System
Neurotoxicity [2]
Paresthesias (<10%)

Gastrointestinal/Hepatic
Hepatitis [2]
Hepatotoxicity [11]

Respiratory
Pneumonitis [3]
Pulmonary toxicity [7]

Other
Adverse effects [3]
Death [3]

NITROGLYCERIN

Synonyms: glyceryl trinitrate; nitroglycerol; NTG
Trade names: Minitran (3M), Nitrodur (Schering) (Key), Nitrolingual (First Horizon), Nitrostat (Pfizer)
Indications: Acute angina
Class: Nitrate, Vasodilator
Half-life: 1–4 minutes
Clinically important, potentially hazardous interactions with: acetylcysteine, alteplase, heparin, sildenafil, tadalafil, vardenafil
Pregnancy category: C
Important contra-indications noted in the prescribing guidelines for: nursing mothers; pediatric patients

---

Skin
Dermatitis (to topical systems) [25]
Eczema [2]
Erythema (to transdermal delivery system) [2]
Exfoliative dermatitis (<10%)
Purpura [2]
Rash (<10%)
Urticaria [2]

Cardiovascular
Bradycardia [2]
Flushing (>10%)
Hypotension [4]

Central Nervous System
Headache [14]
Migraine [2]

NIVOLUMAB

Trade name: Opdivo (Bristol-Myers Squibb)
Indications: Metastatic squamous non-small cell lung cancer with progression on or after platinum-based chemotherapy, unresectable or metastatic melanoma and disease progression following ipilimumab and, if BRAF V600 mutation positive, a BRAF inhibitor, advanced renal cell carcinoma with prior anti-angiogenic therapy, Hodgkin lymphoma that has relapsed or progressed after autologous hematopoietic stem cell transplantation and post-transplantation brentuximab vedotin
Class: Monoclonal antibody, Programmed death receptor-1 (PD-1) inhibitor
Half-life: 27 days
Clinically important, potentially hazardous interactions with: none known
Pregnancy category: N/A (can cause fetal harm)
Important contra-indications noted in the prescribing guidelines for: nursing mothers; pediatric patients

---

Skin
Edema (17%)
Erythema multiforme (<10%)
Exanthems [2]
Exfoliative dermatitis (<10%)
Pruritus (11–19%) [16]
Psoriasis (<10%)
Rash (16–21%) [20]
Toxicity [2]
Vitiligo (<10%) [7]

Mucosal
Stomatitis (<10%)
Xerostomia [2]

Cardiovascular
Chest pain (13%)
Myocarditis [4]
Ventricular arrhythmia (<10%)

Central Nervous System
Fever (17%) [5]
Neurotoxicity [2]
Pain (10%)
Peripheral neuropathy (<10%)
Vertigo (dizziness) (<10%)

Neuromuscular/Skeletal
Arthralgia (13%) [2]
Asthenia (fatigue) (19–50%) [18]
Bone or joint pain (36%)
Myalgia/Myopathy [4]
Myasthenia gravis [4]

Gastrointestinal/Hepatic
- Abdominal pain (16%)
- Colitis [9]
- Constipation (24%)
- Diarrhea (18%) [17]
- Hepatotoxicity [7]
- Nausea (29%) [9]
- Pancreatitis [3]
- Vomiting (19%) [2]

Respiratory
- Bronchitis (<10%)
- Cough (17–32%)
- Dyspnea (38%) [2]
- Pneumonia (10%) [2]
- Pneumonitis [13]
- Upper respiratory tract infection (11%)

Endocrine/Metabolic
- ALP increased (14–22%)
- ALT increased (12–16%) [4]
- Appetite decreased (35%) [5]
- AST increased (16–28%) [3]
- Creatine phosphokinase increased (22%)
- Diabetes mellitus [4]
- Hypercalcemia (20%)
- Hyperkalemia (15–18%)
- Hyperthyroidism [6]
- Hypocalcemia (18%)
- Hypokalemia (20%)
- Hypomagnesemia (20%)
- Hyponatremia (25–38%)
- Hypophosphatemia [2]
- Hypophysitis [6]
- Hypothyroidism [7]
- Thyroid dysfunction [4]
- Thyroiditis [4]
- Weight loss (13%)

Renal
- Nephrotoxicity [6]
- Renal failure [2]

Hematologic
- Anemia (28%)
- Hyperlipasemia [2]
- Lymphopenia (47%) [2]
- Neutropenia [2]
- Thrombocytopenia (14%) [3]

Ocular
- Iridocyclitis (<10%)

Local
- Infusion-related reactions (<10%) [3]

Other
- Adverse effects [18]
- Death [5]
- Side effects [2]

NORFLOXACIN

Trade names: Chibroxin (Merck), Noroxin (Merck)
Indications: Various urinary tract infections caused by susceptible organisms, conjunctivitis
Class: Antibiotic, fluoroquinolone, CYP3A4 inhibitor
Half-life: 3–4 hours
Clinically important, potentially hazardous interactions with: aminophylline, amiodarone, antacids, arsenic, artemether/lumefantrine, bepridil, bretylium, caffeine, ciprofibrate, clozapine, cyclosporine, dairy products, didanosine, disopyramide, erythromycin, glyburide, lanthanum, mycophenolate, nitrofurantoin, NSAIDs, oral iron, oral typhoid vaccine, oxtriphylline, phenothiazines, probenecid, procainamide, quinidine, ropinirole, sotalol, strontium ranelate, sucralfate, tacrine, tamoxifen, tizanidine, tricyclic antidepressants, warfarin, zinc, zolmitriptan
Pregnancy category: C
Important contra-indications noted in the prescribing guidelines for: the elderly; nursing mothers; pediatric patients
Note: Fluoroquinolones are associated with an increased risk of tendinitis and tendon rupture in all ages. This risk is further increased in older patients usually over 60 years of age, in patients taking corticosteroid drugs, and in patients with kidney, heart or lung transplants.
Fluoroquinolones may exacerbate muscle weakness in persons with myasthenia gravis.

Skin
- Exanthems [2]
- Fixed eruption [2]
- Phototoxicity [4]
- Toxic epidermal necrolysis [2]

Nails
- Photo-onycholysis [2]

Neuromuscular/Skeletal
- Rhabdomyolysis [2]
- Tendinopathy/Tendon rupture [4]

NORTRIPTYLINE

Trade names: Aventyl (Ranbaxy), Pamelor (Mallinckrodt)
Indications: Depression
Class: Antidepressant, tricyclic
Half-life: 28–31 hours
Clinically important, potentially hazardous interactions with: amprenavir, arbutamine, clonidine, cobicistat/elvitegravir/emtricitabine/tenofovir disoproxil, epinephrine, fluoxetine, formoterol, guanethidine, isocarboxazid, linezolid, MAO inhibitors, phenelzine, quinolones, sparfloxacin, tranylcypromine
Pregnancy category: D
Important contra-indications noted in the prescribing guidelines for: pediatric patients
Black Box Warning: SUICIDALITY AND ANTIDEPRESSANT DRUGS

Skin
- Diaphoresis (<10%)
- Photosensitivity [2]

Mucosal
- Xerostomia (>10%) [9]

Central Nervous System
- Dysgeusia (taste perversion) (>10%)
- Parkinsonism (<10%)
- Vertigo (dizziness) [2]

Other
- Adverse effects [2]

NYSTATIN

Trade names: Mycology-II (Bristol-Myers Squibb), Mycostatin (Bristol-Myers Squibb)
Indications: Candidiasis
Class: Antifungal
Half-life: ~2–3 hours
Clinically important, potentially hazardous interactions with: none known
Pregnancy category: C
Important contra-indications noted in the prescribing guidelines for: nursing mothers

---

Skin
- AGEP [5]
- Dermatitis [12]
- Eczema [2]
- Fixed eruption [2]

OBETICHOLIC ACID *

Trade name: Ocaliva (Intercept)
Indications: Primary biliary cholangitis
Class: Farnesoid X receptor (FXR) agonist
Half-life: N/A
Clinically important, potentially hazardous interactions with: aminophylline, tizanidine, warfarin
Pregnancy category: N/A (Insufficient evidence to inform drug-associated risk)
Important contra-indications noted in the prescribing guidelines for: nursing mothers; pediatric patients
Note: Contraindicated in patients with complete biliary obstruction.

Skin
Eczema (3–6%)
Peripheral edema (3–7%)
Pruritus (56–70%) [3]
Rash (7–10%)
Urticaria (<10%)

Mucosal
Oropharyngeal pain (7–8%)

Cardiovascular
Palpitation (3–7%)

Central Nervous System
Fever (<7%)
Syncope (<7%)
Vertigo (dizziness) (7%)

Neuromuscular/Skeletal
Arthralgia (6–10%)
Asthenia (fatigue) (19–25%)

Gastrointestinal/Hepatic
Abdominal pain (10–19%)
Constipation (7%)

Endocrine/Metabolic
Thyroid dysfunction (4–6%)

OBINUTUZUMAB

Trade name: Gazyva (Genentech)
Indications: Chronic lymphocytic leukemia (in combination with chlorambucil), follicular lymphoma (firstly with bendamustine then as monotherapy)
Class: Monoclonal antibody
Half-life: 28 days
Clinically important, potentially hazardous interactions with: live vaccines
Pregnancy category: N/A (Insufficient evidence to inform drug-associated risk)
Important contra-indications noted in the prescribing guidelines for: nursing mothers; pediatric patients
Black Box Warning: HEPATITIS B VIRUS REACTIVATION AND PROGRESSIVE MULTIFOCAL LEUKOENCEPHALOPATHY

Skin
Tumor lysis syndrome [4]

Central Nervous System
Fever (10%) [4]
Headache [2]
Leukoencephalopathy [2]

Gastrointestinal/Hepatic
Nausea [2]

Respiratory
Cough (10%) [2]

Endocrine/Metabolic
ALP increased (16%)
AST increased (25%)
Hyperkalemia (31%)
Hypoalbuminemia (22%)
Hypocalcemia (32%)
Hypokalemia (13%)

Hematologic
Anemia (12%) [3]
Leukopenia (7%)
Neutropenia (40%) [11]
Thrombocytopenia (15%) [6]

Local
Infusion-related reactions (69%) [14]

Other
Infection (38%) [7]

OCRIPLASMIN

Trade name: Jetrea (ThromboGenics)
Indications: Symptomatic vitreomacular adhesion
Class: Enzyme
Half-life: N/A
Clinically important, potentially hazardous interactions with: none known
Pregnancy category: C
Important contra-indications noted in the prescribing guidelines for: nursing mothers; pediatric patients

---

Ocular
Cataract (2–4%)
Conjunctival hemorrhage (5–20%)
Conjunctival hyperemia (2–4%)
Dyschromatopsia (2%)
Intraocular inflammation (7%)
Intraocular pressure increased (4%)
Iritis (2–4%)
Macular edema (2–4%)
Macular hole (5–20%)
Ocular adverse effects [2]
Ocular hemorrhage (2%)
Ocular pain (5–20%) [2]
Photophobia (2–4%)
Photopsia (5–20%) [4]
Reduced visual acuity (5–20%) [2]
Retinal edema (5–20%)
Vision blurred (5–20%)
Vision impaired (5–20%)
Vision loss [3]
Vitreous detachment (2–4%)
Vitreous floaters (5–20%) [4]
Xerophthalmia (2–4%)

OCTREOTIDE

Trade name: Sandostatin (Novartis)
Indications: Diarrhea, sulfonylurea poisoning
Class: Somatostatin analog
Half-life: 1.5 hours
Clinically important, potentially hazardous interactions with: bromocriptine, insulin aspart, insulin degludec, metformin
Pregnancy category: B
Important contra-indications noted in the prescribing guidelines for: the elderly; nursing mothers; pediatric patients

---

Skin
Cellulitis (<4%)
Diaphoresis (5–15%)
Edema (<10%)
Petechiae (<4%)
Pruritus (18%)
Purpura (<4%)
Rash (5–15%)
Raynaud's phenomenon (<4%)
Urticaria (<4%)

Hair
Alopecia (~13%) [4]

Cardiovascular
Arrhythmias (3–9%)
Bradycardia (19–25%) [4]
Chest pain (20%)
Flushing (<4%)
Hypertension (13%) [2]
QT prolongation [2]
Thrombophlebitis (<4%)

Central Nervous System
Anorexia (4–6%)
Headache [3]
Pain (4–6%)
Rigors (5–15%)
Vertigo (dizziness) [2]

Neuromuscular/Skeletal
Arthralgia (5–15%)
Asthenia (fatigue) [3]
Myalgia/Myopathy (5–15%) [2]

Gastrointestinal/Hepatic
Abdominal pain (5–61%) [3]
Diarrhea (34–58%) [4]
Flatulence (38%)
Hepatotoxicity [3]
Nausea (5–61%) [3]
Pancreatitis [2]
Vomiting (4–21%)

Respiratory
Cough (5–15%)
Pharyngitis (5–15%)
Rhinitis (5–15%)
Sinusitis (5–15%)

Endocrine/Metabolic
Galactorrhea (<4%)
Gynecomastia (<4%)
Hyperglycemia [5]
Hypothyroidism (12%)

Genitourinary
Vaginitis (<4%)

Hematologic
Anemia (15%)
Thrombocytopenia [3]

Otic
Ear pain (5–15%)

Local
Injection-site granuloma [2]
Injection-site pain (8%)

OFATUMUMAB

Trade name: Arzerra (Novartis)
Indications: Chronic lymphocytic leukemia
Class: CD20-directed cytolytic monoclonal antibody, Monoclonal antibody
Half-life: 14 days
Clinically important, potentially hazardous interactions with: live vaccines
Pregnancy category: N/A (May cause fetal B-cell depletion)
Important contra-indications noted in the prescribing guidelines for: nursing mothers; pediatric patients
Black Box Warning: HEPATITIS B VIRUS REACTIVATION AND PROGRESSIVE MULTIFOCAL LEUKOENCEPHALOPATHY

Skin
Herpes (6%)
Hyperhidrosis (5%)
Peripheral edema (9%)
Rash (14%) [2]
Urticaria (8%)

Cardiovascular
Hypertension (5%)
Hypotension (5%)
Tachycardia (5%)

Central Nervous System
Chills (8%)
Fever (20%)
Headache (6%)
Insomnia (7%)
Peripheral neuropathy [2]

Neuromuscular/Skeletal
Asthenia (fatigue) (15%) [3]
Back pain (8%)

Gastrointestinal/Hepatic
Diarrhea (18%)
Nausea (11%) [2]

Respiratory
Bronchitis (11%)
Cough (19%)
Dyspnea (14%)
Nasopharyngitis (8%)
Pneumonia (23%)
Pulmonary toxicity [2]
Upper respiratory tract infection (11%)

Hematologic
Anemia (16%) [3]
Leukopenia [2]
Lymphopenia [2]
Neutropenia (>10%) [9]
Sepsis (8%)
Thrombocytopenia [4]

Local
Infusion-related reactions [7]
Infusion-site reactions [2]

Other
Adverse effects [2]
Infection (70%) [7]

OFLOXACIN

Trade names: Floxin (Ortho-McNeil), Ocuflox (Allergan), Taravid (Sanofi-Aventis)
Indications: Various infections caused by susceptible organisms
Class: Antibiotic, fluoroquinolone
Half-life: 4–8 hours
Clinically important, potentially hazardous interactions with: aminophylline, amiodarone, antacids, arsenic, artemether/lumefantrine, BCG vaccine, bendamustine, bepridil, bretylium, calcium salts, clozapine, corticosteroids, cyclosporine, CYP1A2 substrates, didanosine, disopyramide, erythromycin, insulin, lanthanum, magnesiuim salts, mycophenolate, NSAIDs, oral iron, oral typhoid vaccine, oxtriphylline, phenothiazines, probenecid, procainamide, quinapril, quinidine, sevelamer, sotalol, St John's wort, strontium ranelate, sucralfate, sulfonylureas, tricyclic antidepressants, vitamin K antagonists, warfarin, zinc, zolmitriptan
Pregnancy category: C
Important contra-indications noted in the prescribing guidelines for: the elderly; nursing mothers; pediatric patients
Note: Fluoroquinolones are associated with an increased risk of tendinitis and tendon rupture in all ages. This risk is further increased in older patients usually over 60 years of age, in patients taking corticosteroid drugs, and in patients with kidney, heart or lung transplants.
Fluoroquinolones may exacerbate muscle weakness in persons with myasthenia gravis.
Black Box Warning: SERIOUS ADVERSE REACTIONS INCLUDING TENDINITIS, TENDON RUPTURE, PERIPHERAL NEUROPATHY, CENTRIAL NERVOUS SYSTEM EFFECTS and EXACERBATION OF MYASTHENIA GRAVIS

Skin
Anaphylactoid reactions/Anaphylaxis [4]
Angioedema [2]
Exanthems [3]
Fixed eruption [4]
Hypersensitivity [2]
Photosensitivity [8]
Phototoxicity [3]
Pruritus (<3%) [4]
Pruritus ani et vulvae (<3%)
Rash (<10%) [5]
Stevens–Johnson syndrome [3]
Toxic epidermal necrolysis [3]
Urticaria [3]
Vasculitis [4]

Nails
Photo-onycholysis [2]

Mucosal
Oral mucosal eruption [3]
Xerostomia (<3%)

Cardiovascular
QT prolongation [3]

Central Nervous System
Dysgeusia (taste perversion) (<3%) [2]
Hallucinations [2]
Headache [2]
Psychosis [2]
Seizures [2]
Vertigo (dizziness) [2]

Neuromuscular/Skeletal
Arthralgia [2]
Arthropathy [2]
Rhabdomyolysis [2]
Tendinopathy/Tendon rupture [7]

Gastrointestinal/Hepatic
Abdominal pain [2]
Diarrhea [2]
Nausea [3]
Vomiting [2]

Genitourinary
Vaginitis (<10%)

Local
Injection-site pain (<10%)

Other
Adverse effects [8]
Death [2]
Side effects [2]

OLANZAPINE

Trade names: Symbyax (Lilly), Zyprexa (Lilly), Zyprexa Relprevv (Lilly)
Indications: Schizophrenia, bipolar I disorder
Class: Antipsychotic, Muscarinic antagonist
Half-life: 21–54 hours
Clinically important, potentially hazardous interactions with: alcohol, antihypertensive agents, carbamazepine, ciprofloxacin, CNS acting drugs, diazepam, dopamine agonists, eszopiclone, fluoxetine, fluvoxamine, insulin degludec, insulin detemir, insulin glargine, levodopa, lithium, tetrabenazine, valproic acid
Pregnancy category: C
Important contra-indications noted in the prescribing guidelines for: the elderly; nursing mothers; pediatric patients
Note: Can cause DRESS and other serious skin reactions.
Symbyax is olanzapine and fluoxetine; Zypraxa Relprevv is olanzapine pamoate.
Black Box Warning: INCREASED MORTALITY IN ELDERLY PATIENTS WITH DEMENTIA-RELATED PSYCHOSIS
POST-INJECTION DELIRIUM/SEDATION SYNDROME (Zyprexa Relprevv)

Skin
Angioedema [2]
Edema [3]
Hypersensitivity [2]
Peripheral edema (<10%) [5]
Psoriasis [2]
Purpura (<10%)
Rash (>2%) [2]
Vesiculobullous eruption (2%)
Xanthomas [2]

Hair
Alopecia [3]

Mucosal
- Epistaxis (nosebleed) (<10%)
- Sialorrhea [3]
- Xerostomia (13%) [9]

Cardiovascular
- Hypertension (<10%)
- Hypotension (<10%) [4]
- Orthostatic hypotension [2]
- QT prolongation [6]
- Tachycardia (<10%)
- Torsades de pointes [3]
- Venous thromboembolism [4]

Central Nervous System
- Akathisia (<10%) [7]
- Amnesia [2]
- Compulsions [2]
- Delirium [5]
- Extrapyramidal symptoms [3]
- Hallucinations [2]
- Headache (17%) [3]
- Insomnia (12%) [3]
- Neuroleptic malignant syndrome [33]
- Parkinsonism (<10%) [4]
- Restless legs syndrome [7]
- Sedation [13]
- Seizures [8]
- Serotonin syndrome [2]
- Somnolence (drowsiness) (20–39%) [10]
- Tardive dyskinesia [3]
- Tremor (<10%) [5]
- Twitching (2%)
- Vertigo (dizziness) [4]

Neuromuscular/Skeletal
- Asthenia (fatigue) (8–20%) [4]
- Back pain (<10%)
- Dystonia [5]
- Myalgia/Myopathy [2]
- Rhabdomyolysis [9]

Gastrointestinal/Hepatic
- Abdominal pain (<10%)
- Constipation (9–11%)
- Diarrhea (<10%) [2]
- Dyspepsia (7–11%)
- Flatulence (<10%)
- Hepatotoxicity [3]
- Nausea (<10%)
- Pancreatitis [6]
- Vomiting (<10%)

Respiratory
- Cough (<10%)
- Nasopharyngitis [2]
- Pharyngitis (<10%)
- Pulmonary embolism [3]
- Rhinitis (<10%)
- Sinusitis (<10%)

Endocrine/Metabolic
- Appetite increased [2]
- Diabetes mellitus [6]
- Diabetic ketoacidosis [2]
- Galactorrhea [2]
- Glucose dysregulation [3]
- Hypercholesterolemia [2]
- Hyperglycemia [6]
- Metabolic syndrome [9]
- Weight gain (5–40%) [57]

Genitourinary
- Priapism [19]
- Sexual dysfunction [2]
- Urinary incontinence (<10%)
- Urinary tract infection (<10%)

Hematologic
- Agranulocytosis [2]
- Dyslipidemia [4]
- Eosinophilia [2]
- Neutropenia [4]

Ocular
- Amblyopia (<10%)
- Oculogyric crisis [2]

Other
- Adverse effects [7]
- Death [7]

OLAPARIB

Trade name: Lynparza (AstraZeneca)
Indications: BRCA-mutated ovarian cancer
Class: Poly (ADP-ribose) polymerase (PARP) inhibitor
Half-life: 7–17 hours
Clinically important, potentially hazardous interactions with: amprenavir, aprepitant, atazanavir, boceprevir, bosentan, carbamazepine, ciprofloxacin, clarithromycin, crizotinib, darunavir, diltiazem, efavirenz, erythromycin, etravirine, fluconazole, fosamprenavir, grapefruit juice, imatinib, indinavir, itraconazole, ketoconazole, lopinavir, modafinil, nafcillin, nefazodone, nelfinavir, phenytoin, posaconazole, rifampin, ritonavir, saquinavir, St John's wort, strong and moderate CYP3A inhibitors, telaprevir, telithromycin, verapamil, voriconazole
Pregnancy category: D
Important contra-indications noted in the prescribing guidelines for: nursing mothers; pediatric patients

---

Skin
- Eczema (<10%)
- Hot flashes (<10%)
- Peripheral edema (10–20%)
- Pruritus (<10%)
- Rash (25%) [2]
- Xerosis (<10%)

Hair
- Alopecia [2]

Mucosal
- Stomatitis (<10%)

Cardiovascular
- Hypertension (<10%) [2]
- Venous thromboembolism (<10%)

Central Nervous System
- Anxiety (<10%)
- Depression (<10%)
- Dysgeusia (taste perversion) (21%) [2]
- Fever (<10%)
- Headache (25%) [3]
- Insomnia (<10%)
- Peripheral neuropathy (<10%) [2]

Neuromuscular/Skeletal
- Arthralgia (21–32%)
- Asthenia (fatigue) (66–68%) [15]
- Back pain (25%)
- Myalgia/Myopathy (22–25%)

Gastrointestinal/Hepatic
- Abdominal pain (43–47%) [2]
- Constipation (10–20%) [2]
- Diarrhea (28–31%) [7]
- Dyspepsia (25%) [3]
- Nausea (64–75%) [12]
- Vomiting (32–43%) [8]

Respiratory
- Cough (21%)
- Dyspnea (10–20%)
- Nasopharyngitis (26–43%)
- Pharyngitis (43%)
- Pulmonary embolism (<10%)
- Upper respiratory tract infection (26–43%)

Endocrine/Metabolic
- Appetite decreased (22–25%) [3]
- Creatine phosphokinase increased (26–30%)
- Hyperglycemia (<10%)
- Hypomagnesemia (<10%)

Genitourinary
- Dysuria (<10%)
- Urinary incontinence (<10%)
- Urinary tract infection (10–20%)

Hematologic
- Anemia (25–34%) [13]
- Febrile neutropenia [2]
- Leukopenia (<10%) [2]
- Lymphopenia (56%)
- Myelodysplastic syndrome [2]
- Neutropenia (25–32%) [9]
- Thrombocytopenia (26–30%) [7]

Other
- Adverse effects [5]
- Death [2]

OLARATUMAB *

Trade name: Lartruvo (Lilly)
Indications: Treatment of adult patients with soft tissue sarcoma (with doxorubicin) with a histologic subtype for which an anthracycline-containing regimen is appropriate and which is not amenable to curative treatment with radiotherapy or surgery
Class: Monoclonal antibody, Platelet-derived growth factor receptor alpha blocking antibody
Half-life: ~11 days
Clinically important, potentially hazardous interactions with: none known
Pregnancy category: N/A (Can cause fetal harm)
Important contra-indications noted in the prescribing guidelines for: the elderly; nursing mothers; pediatric patients
Note: See separate entry for doxorubicin.

Hair
- Alopecia (52%)

Mucosal
- Mucositis (53%)

Central Nervous System
- Anxiety (11%)
- Headache (20%)
- Neurotoxicity (22%)

Neuromuscular/Skeletal
- Asthenia (fatigue) (64%)

Bone or joint pain (64%)

Gastrointestinal/Hepatic
Abdominal pain (23%)
Diarrhea (34%) [2]
Nausea (73%)
Vomiting (45%)

Endocrine/Metabolic
ALP increased (16%)
Appetite decreased (31%)
Hyperglycemia (52%)
Hypokalemia (21%)
Hypomagnesemia (16%)

Hematologic
Lymphopenia (77%)
Neutropenia (65%)
Prothrombin time increased (33%)
Thrombocytopenia (63%)

Ocular
Xerophthalmia (11%)

Local
Infusion-related reactions (13%)

OLMESARTAN

Trade names: Benicar (Sankyo), Olmetec (Daiichi Sankyo)
Indications: Hypertension
Class: Angiotensin II receptor antagonist (blocker), Antihypertensive
Half-life: ~13 hours
Clinically important, potentially hazardous interactions with: ACE inhibitors, adrenergic neurone blockers, aldesleukin, aliskiren, alprostadil, amifostine, antihypertensives, antipsychotics, anxiolytics and hypnotics, baclofen, beta blockers, calcium channel blockers, clonidine, colesevelam, corticosteroids, cyclosporine, diazoxide, diuretics, eltrombopag, eplerenone, estrogens, general anesthetics, heparins, hydralazine, levodopa, lithium, MAO inhibitors, methyldopa, methylphenidate, minoxidil, moxisylyte, moxonidine, nitrates, nitroprusside, NSAIDs, pentoxifylline, phosphodiesterase 5 inhibitors, potassium salts, quinine, rituximab, tacrolimus, tizanidine, tolvaptan, trimethoprim
Pregnancy category: D (category C in first trimester; category D in second and third trimesters)
Important contra-indications noted in the prescribing guidelines for: nursing mothers; pediatric patients
Note: Contraindicated in patients with diabetes.
Black Box Warning: FETAL TOXICITY

Skin
Angioedema [3]
Edema [2]
Peripheral edema [2]

Cardiovascular
Hypotension [2]

Central Nervous System
Vertigo (dizziness) (3%) [7]

Gastrointestinal/Hepatic
Diarrhea [3]
Enteropathy [16]
Gastrointestinal disorder [6]

Endocrine/Metabolic
Hyperkalemia [3]

Other
Adverse effects [6]

OLODATEROL

Trade names: Stiolto Respimat (Boehringer Ingelheim), Striverdi Respimat (Boehringer Ingelheim)
Indications: Chronic obstructive pulmonary disease including chronic bronchitis and emphysema
Class: Beta-2 adrenergic agonist
Half-life: 8 hours
Clinically important, potentially hazardous interactions with: adrenergics, beta blockers, diuretics, MAO inhibitors, QT interval prolonging agents, steroids, tricyclic antidepressants, xanthine derivatives
Pregnancy category: C
Important contra-indications noted in the prescribing guidelines for: nursing mothers; pediatric patients
Note: Stiolto Respimat is olodaterol and tiotropium.
Black Box Warning: ASTHMA-RELATED DEATH

Skin
Rash (2%)

Cardiovascular
Hypertension [2]

Central Nervous System
Fever (>2%)
Headache [3]
Vertigo (dizziness) (2%) [2]

Neuromuscular/Skeletal
Arthralgia (2%) [2]
Back pain (4%) [4]

Gastrointestinal/Hepatic
Constipation (>2%)
Diarrhea (3%) [3]

Respiratory
Bronchitis (5%) [4]
COPD [2]
Cough (4%) [3]
Dyspnea [3]
Nasopharyngitis (11%) [4]
Pneumonia (>2%) [3]
Upper respiratory tract infection (8%) [4]

Genitourinary
Urinary tract infection (3%) [3]

OLOPATADINE

Trade names: Pataday (Alcon), Patanol (Alcon)
Indications: Pruritus due to allergic conjunctivitis, rhinitis
Class: Histamine H1 receptor antagonist
Half-life: 3 hours
Clinically important, potentially hazardous interactions with: none known
Pregnancy category: C
Important contra-indications noted in the prescribing guidelines for: nursing mothers; pediatric patients

---

Central Nervous System
Headache (7%) [2]

Ocular
Eyelid burning (<5%)
Eyelid edema (<5%)
Eyelid stinging (<5%)

OMACETAXINE

Trade name: Synribo (Ivax)
Indications: Chronic myeloid leukemia (CML) in patients with resistance and/or intolerance to two or more tyrosine kinase inhibitors
Class: Protein synthesis inhibitor
Half-life: ~6 hours
Clinically important, potentially hazardous interactions with: none known
Pregnancy category: D
Important contra-indications noted in the prescribing guidelines for: the elderly; nursing mothers; pediatric patients

---

Skin
Burning (<10%)
Ecchymoses (<10%)
Edema (<10%)
Erythema (<10%)
Exfoliative dermatitis (<10%)
Hematoma (<10%)
Hot flashes (<10%)
Hyperhidrosis (<10%)
Hypersensitivity (<10%)
Lesions (<10%)
Peripheral edema (13%)
Petechiae (<10%)
Pigmentation (<10%)
Pruritus (<10%)
Purpura (<10%)
Rash (10%)
Ulcerations (<10%)
Xerosis (<10%)

Hair
Alopecia (15%)

Mucosal
Aphthous stomatitis (<10%)
Epistaxis (nosebleed) (11–15%)
Gingival bleeding (<10%)
Nasal congestion (<10%)
Oral bleeding (<10%)
Oral ulceration (<10%)
Rhinorrhea (<10%)
Stomatitis (<10%)
Xerostomia (<10%)

Cardiovascular
Acute coronary syndrome (<10%)
Angina (<10%)
Arrhythmias (<10%)
Bradycardia (<10%)
Extrasystoles (<10%)
Hypertension (<10%)
Hypotension (<10%)
Palpitation (<10%)

Tachycardia (<10%)

Central Nervous System
Agitation (<10%)
Anorexia (13%)
Anxiety (<10%)
Cerebral hemorrhage (<10%)
Chills (13%)
Confusion (<10%)
Depression (<10%)
Dysgeusia (taste perversion) (<10%)
Fever (24–29%) [4]
Headache (13%) [4]
Hypoesthesia (<10%)
Insomnia (10%)
Mood changes (<10%)
Paresthesias (<10%)
Seizures (<10%)
Tremor (<10%)
Vertigo (dizziness) (<10%)

Neuromuscular/Skeletal
Arthralgia (19%)
Asthenia (fatigue) (23–31%) [5]
Back pain (11%)
Bone or joint pain (<10%)
Gouty tophi (<10%)
Muscle spasm (<10%)
Myalgia/Myopathy (<10%)
Pain in extremities (11–13%)

Gastrointestinal/Hepatic
Abdominal distension (<10%)
Abdominal pain (13–14%)
Black stools (<10%)
Constipation (15%)
Diarrhea (35–42%) [6]
Dyspepsia (<10%)
Gastritis (<10%)
Gastroesophageal reflux (<10%)
Gastrointestinal bleeding (<10%)
Hemorrhoids (<10%)
Nausea (32%) [6]
Vomiting (12–15%)

Respiratory
Cough (15–16%)
Dysphonia (<10%)
Dyspnea (11%)
Hemoptysis (<10%)
Pharyngolaryngeal pain (<10%)

Endocrine/Metabolic
ALT increased (2–6%)
Appetite decreased (<10%)
Creatine phosphokinase increased (9–16%)
Dehydration (<10%)
Diabetes mellitus (<10%)

Genitourinary
Dysuria (<10%)

Hematologic
Anemia (51–61%) [6]
Bone marrow suppression (10%)
Febrile neutropenia (10–20%)
Hemoglobin decreased (62–80%)
Leukocytosis (6%)
Myelosuppression [2]
Neutropenia (50%) [7]
Platelets decreased (85–88%)
Thrombocytopenia (56–74%) [8]

Otic
Ear pain (<10%)
Ototoxicity (<10%)
Tinnitus (<10%)

Ocular
Cataract (<10%)
Conjunctival hemorrhage (<10%)
Conjunctivitis (<10%)
Diplopia (<10%)
Eyelid edema (<10%)
Lacrimation (<10%)
Ocular pain (<10%)
Vision blurred (<10%)
Xerophthalmia (<10%)

Local
Infusion-site reactions (22–34%)
Injection-site reactions (22–34%)

Other
Infection (46–56%) [3]

OMALIZUMAB

Trade name: Xolair (Genentech)
Indications: Asthma
Class: IgE-targeting monoclonal antibody, Monoclonal antibody
Half-life: 26 days
Clinically important, potentially hazardous interactions with: none known
Pregnancy category: B
Important contra-indications noted in the prescribing guidelines for: nursing mothers
Black Box Warning: ANAPHYLAXIS

Skin
Anaphylactoid reactions/Anaphylaxis [9]
Angioedema [2]
Churg-Strauss syndrome [11]
Dermatitis (2%)
Pruritus (2%)
Rash [2]
Serum sickness [3]
Urticaria (7%) [2]

Central Nervous System
Headache (15%) [7]
Pain (7%)
Vertigo (dizziness) (3%)

Neuromuscular/Skeletal
Arthralgia (8%) [2]
Asthenia (fatigue) (3%) [2]
Myalgia/Myopathy [2]

Gastrointestinal/Hepatic
Abdominal pain [3]
Diarrhea [2]
Nausea [3]

Respiratory
Nasopharyngitis [2]
Sinusitis (16%) [3]
Upper respiratory tract infection (20%) [4]

Local
Injection-site pain [2]
Injection-site reactions (45%) [7]

Other
Adverse effects [5]

OMBITASVIR/ PARITAPREVIR/ RITONAVIR

Trade names: Technivie (AbbVie), Viekira Pak (AbbVie), Viekirax (AbbVie)
Indications: Genotype 4 chronic hepatitis C virus infection in patients without cirrhosis (in combination with ribavirin)
Class: CYP3A4 inhibitor (ritonavir), Hepatitis C virus NS3/4A protease inhibitor (paritaprevir), Hepatitis C virus NS5A inhibitor (ombitasvir)
Half-life: 21–25 hours (ombitasvir); 6 hours (paritaprevir); 4 hours (ritonavir)
Clinically important, potentially hazardous interactions with: atazanavir, carbamazepine, cisapride, colchicine, dihydroergotamine, dronedarone, efavirenz, ergotamine, ethinyl estradiol-containing medications, lopinavir, lovastatin, lurasidone, methylergonovine, midazolam, phenobarbital, phenytoin, pimozide, ranolazine, rifampin, rilpivirine, salmeterol, sildenafil, simvastatin, St John's wort, triazolam, voriconazole
Pregnancy category: B (pregnancy category will be X when administered with ribavirin)
Important contra-indications noted in the prescribing guidelines for: nursing mothers; pediatric patients
Note: Contraindicated in patients with moderate or severe hepatic impairment or with known hypersensitivity to ritonavir (see separate entry). See also separate entry for ribavirin. Viekira Pak is ombitasvir/paritaprevir/ritonavir co-packaged with dasabuvir.

Skin
Dermatitis (<5%)
Eczema (<5%)
Erythema (<5%)
Exfoliative dermatitis (<5%)
Photosensitivity (<5%)
Pruritus (5%) [5]
Psoriasis (<5%)
Rash (<5%) [4]
Ulcerations (<5%)
Urticaria (<5%)

Central Nervous System
Headache [14]
Insomnia (5%) [10]
Irritability [2]

Neuromuscular/Skeletal
Arthralgia [2]
Asthenia (fatigue) (7–25%) [13]

Gastrointestinal/Hepatic
Diarrhea [9]
Nausea (9%) [11]
Vomiting [2]

Respiratory
Cough [3]
Dyspnea [2]
Nasopharyngitis [2]

Endocrine/Metabolic
ALT increased [3]
AST increased [3]

Hematologic
Anemia [4]
Hemoglobin decreased [2]

OMEPRAZOLE

Trade names: Prilosec (AstraZeneca), Yosprala (Aralez)
Indications: Duodenal ulcer, gastric ulcer, gastroesophageal reflux disease (GERD), erosive esophagitis
Class: CYP1A2 inducer, Proton pump inhibitor (PPI)
Half-life: 0.5–1 hour
Clinically important, potentially hazardous interactions with: amoxicillin, atazanavir, bendamustine, benzodiazepines, cilostazol, clarithromycin, clobazam, clopidogrel, clozapine, coumarins, cyclosporine, dasatinib, delavirdine, diazepam, digoxin, disulfiram, enzalutamide, erlotinib, escitalopram, itraconazole, ketoconazole, lapatinib, methotrexate, nelfinavir, phenytoin, posaconazole, prednisone, raltegravir, rilpivirine, saquinavir, St John's wort, tacrolimus, tipranavir, ulipristal, voriconazole, warfarin
Pregnancy category: C
Important contra-indications noted in the prescribing guidelines for: nursing mothers; pediatric patients
Note: Yosprala is omeprazole and aspirin.

Skin
AGEP [2]
Anaphylactoid reactions/Anaphylaxis [7]
Angioedema [5]
Baboon syndrome (SDRIFE) [2]
Bullous pemphigoid [2]
Contact dermatitis [2]
Edema (<10%) [2]
Erythroderma [2]
Exfoliative dermatitis [3]
Hypersensitivity [2]
Lichen planus [2]
Lichen spinulosus [2]
Lichenoid eruption [2]
Lupus erythematosus [5]
Pemphigus (exacerbation) [2]
Peripheral edema [2]
Pruritus (<10%) [8]
Rash (2%) [6]
Toxic epidermal necrolysis [5]
Urticaria (<10%) [8]
Vasculitis [2]
Xerosis [2]

Hair
Alopecia [2]

Mucosal
Oral candidiasis [3]
Xerostomia (<10%) [2]

Central Nervous System
Anorexia [3]
Dysgeusia (taste perversion) (<10%) [3]
Headache (7%)
Paresthesias [2]
Vertigo (dizziness) (2%)

Neuromuscular/Skeletal
Asthenia (fatigue) [2]
Myalgia/Myopathy (<10%)
Rhabdomyolysis [2]

Gastrointestinal/Hepatic
Abdominal distension [2]
Abdominal pain (5%) [3]
Constipation [2]
Diarrhea (4%) [7]
Flatulence (3%)
Hepatitis [4]
Hepatotoxicity [3]
Nausea (4%) [5]
Pancreatitis [2]
Vomiting (3%) [5]

Respiratory
Cough [2]
Upper respiratory tract infection (2%)

Endocrine/Metabolic
Gynecomastia [11]
Hypomagnesemia [7]

Renal
Nephrotoxicity [9]

Hematologic
Agranulocytosis [3]
Hemolytic anemia [2]
Leukopenia [3]
Neutropenia [3]

Ocular
Visual disturbances [2]

Other
Adverse effects [8]

ONDANSETRON

Trade names: Zofran (GSK), Zuplenz (Par)
Indications: Nausea and vomiting
Class: 5-HT3 antagonist, Antiemetic, Serotonin type 3 receptor antagonist
Half-life: 3–6 hours
Clinically important, potentially hazardous interactions with: apomorphine, carbamazepine, phenytoin, rifampin, tramadol
Pregnancy category: B
Important contra-indications noted in the prescribing guidelines for: nursing mothers; pediatric patients

---

Skin
Anaphylactoid reactions/Anaphylaxis [5]
Fixed eruption [2]
Pruritus (5%)

Mucosal
Sialopenia (<5%)
Xerostomia (<10%) [3]

Cardiovascular
Bradycardia [2]
Flushing [2]
Hypotension [3]
Myocardial ischemia [2]
QT prolongation [11]
Torsades de pointes [3]
Ventricular tachycardia [2]

Central Nervous System
Anxiety (6%)
Chills (5–10%)
Fever (2–8%)
Headache (17–25%) [13]
Paresthesias (2%)
Seizures [3]
Somnolence (drowsiness) (8%) [4]
Vertigo (dizziness) (4–7%) [8]

Neuromuscular/Skeletal
Asthenia (fatigue) (9–13%)

Gastrointestinal/Hepatic
Abdominal pain [2]
Constipation (6–11%) [6]
Diarrhea (8–16%) [3]

Respiratory
Hypoxia (9%)

Endocrine/Metabolic
ALT increased [2]

Local
Injection-site reactions (4%)

Other
Adverse effects [3]
Death [2]
Hiccups [2]

ORAL CONTRACEPTIVES

Trade names: Alesse (Wyeth), Aviane (Barr), Brevicon (Watson), Demulen (Pfizer), Desogen (Organon), Estrostep (Pfizer), Evra (Johnson & Johnson), Levlen (Bayer), Levlite (Bayer), Levora (Watson), Lo/Ovral (Wyeth), Loestrin (Barr), Lunelle (Pfizer), Mircette (Organon), Modicon (Ortho), Necon (Watson), Nordette (Monarch), Norinyl (Watson), Ortho Tri-Cyclen (Ortho-McNeil), Ortho-Cept (Ortho-McNeil), Ortho-Cyclen (Ortho-McNeil), Ortho-Novum (Ortho-McNeil), Ovcon (Warner Chilcott), Ovral (Wyeth), Tri-Levlen (Bayer), Tri-Norinyl (Watson), Triphasil (Wyeth), Trivora (Watson), Yasmin (Bayer), Yaz (Bayer), Zovia (Watson)
Indications: Prevention of pregnancy
Class: Hormone
Half-life: N/A
Clinically important, potentially hazardous interactions with: aminophylline, amprenavir, anticonvulsants, aprepitant, atazanavir, atorvastatin, beclomethasone, bexarotene, bosentan, budesonide, cigarette smoking, danazol, doxycycline, efavirenz, eslicarbazepine, exenatide, flucloxacillin, flunisolide, fluticasone propionate, hydrocortisone, insulin aspart, insulin degludec, insulin detemir, insulin glargine, insulin glulisine, isotretinoin, lamotrigine, lomitapide, lymecycline, metformin, methylprednisolone, mifepristone, modafinil, naratriptan, nelfinavir, oxcarbazepine, perampanel, prednisolone, prednisone, rifabutin, rifampin, ritonavir, roflumilast, selegiline, St John's wort, teriflunomide, tigecycline, triamcinolone, troleandomycin, tuberculostatics, ursodiol, zolmitriptan
Black Box Warning: CIGARETTE SMOKING AND SERIOUS CARDIOVASCULAR EVENTS

Skin
Acneform eruption [17]
Angioedema [4]
Candidiasis [9]
Chloasma [13]

Erythema multiforme [2]
Erythema nodosum [18]
Exanthems [2]
Herpes gestationis [3]
Lupus erythematosus [29]
Melanoma [5]
Melasma [8]
Perioral dermatitis [8]
Photosensitivity [12]
Pigmentation [18]
Pruritus [5]
Purpura [3]
Seborrhea [3]
Spider angioma [2]
Sweet's syndrome [2]
Telangiectasia [6]
Urticaria [2]

Hair
Alopecia [19]
Alopecia areata [4]
Hirsutism [12]

Mucosal
Gingival hyperplasia/hypertrophy [2]

Cardiovascular
Thrombophlebitis [2]
Venous thromboembolism [6]

Central Nervous System
Chorea [2]
Depression [2]
Headache [3]

Gastrointestinal/Hepatic
Colitis [3]
Nausea [4]

Endocrine/Metabolic
Acute intermittent porphyria [5]
Galactorrhea [2]
Mastodynia [3]
Porphyria cutanea tarda [28]
Porphyria variegata [2]

Genitourinary
Vaginal bleeding [4]

Local
Application-site reactions (92%) [2]

Other
Adverse effects [3]

ORITAVANCIN

Trade name: Orbactiv (Medicines Co)
Indications: Acute bacterial skin and skin structure infections caused or suspected to be caused by susceptible isolates of designated Gram-positive microorganisms
Class: Antibiotic, lipoglycopeptide
Half-life: 245 hours
Clinically important, potentially hazardous interactions with: warfarin
Pregnancy category: C
Important contra-indications noted in the prescribing guidelines for: nursing mothers; pediatric patients

---

Skin
Abscess (4%) [2]
Angioedema (<2%)
Cellulitis [3]
Erythema multiforme (<2%)
Hypersensitivity (<2%)
Leukocytoclastic vasculitis (<2%)
Pruritus (<2%) [3]
Rash (<2%)
Urticaria (<2%)

Cardiovascular
Phlebitis [2]
Tachycardia (3%)

Central Nervous System
Fever [4]
Headache (7%) [5]
Vertigo (dizziness) (3%) [3]

Neuromuscular/Skeletal
Myalgia/Myopathy (<2%)
Osteomyelitis (<2%)

Gastrointestinal/Hepatic
Constipation [5]
Diarrhea (4%) [5]
Nausea (10%) [6]
Vomiting (5%) [4]

Respiratory
Bronchospasm (<2%)
Wheezing (<2%)

Endocrine/Metabolic
ALT increased (3%) [3]
AST increased (2%)
Hyperuricemia (<2%)
Hypoglycemia (<2%)

Hematologic
Anemia (<2%)
Eosinophilia (<2%)

Local
Infusion-site reactions (2%) [2]
Injection-site extravasation [3]
Injection-site phlebitis [2]
Injection-site reactions [2]

ORLISTAT

Trade names: Alli (GSK), Xenical (Roche)
Indications: Obesity, weight reduction
Class: Lipase inhibitor
Half-life: 1–2 hours
Clinically important, potentially hazardous interactions with: acarbose, amiodarone, antiepileptics, coumarins, cyclosporine, ergocalciferol, ethosuximide, lacosamide, levothyroxine, oxcarbazepine, paricalcitol, phytonadione, tiagabine, vigabatrin, vitamin A, vitamin E, warfarin
Pregnancy category: B
Important contra-indications noted in the prescribing guidelines for: nursing mothers; pediatric patients
Note: Contraindicated in organ transplant recipients. Orlistat interferes with the medicines used to prevent transplant rejection.

Skin
Lichenoid eruption [2]
Peripheral edema (3%)
Rash (4%)
Xerosis (2%)

Mucosal
Gingivitis (2–4%)

Central Nervous System
Anxiety (3–5%)
Depression (3%)
Headache (31%) [2]
Sleep related disorder (4%)
Vertigo (dizziness) (5%)

Neuromuscular/Skeletal
Arthralgia (5%)
Asthenia (fatigue) (3–7%)
Back pain (14%)
Bone or joint pain (2%)
Myalgia/Myopathy (4%)
Tendinitis (2%)

Gastrointestinal/Hepatic
Abdominal pain (26%) [4]
Cholelithiasis (gallstones) (3%)
Defecation (increased) (3–11%) [2]
Fecal incontinence (2–8%)
Fecal urgency (3–23%) [2]
Flatulence (with discharge) (2–24%) [2]
Hepatic failure [2]
Hepatitis [3]
Hepatotoxicity [4]
Nausea (4–8%)
Pancreatitis [5]
Vomiting (4%)

Respiratory
Influenza (40%)
Upper respiratory tract infection (26–38%) [2]

Endocrine/Metabolic
Hypoglycemia (in diabetic patients) [2]
Menstrual irregularities (10%)

Genitourinary
Urinary tract infection (6–8%)
Vaginitis (3–4%)

Renal
Nephrotoxicity [9]
Renal failure [2]

Otic
Otitis media (3–4%)

Other
Adverse effects [7]
Tooth disorder (3–4%)

OSELTAMIVIR

Trade name: Tamiflu (Roche)
Indications: Influenza infection
Class: Antiviral, Neuraminidase inhibitor
Half-life: 6–10 hours
Clinically important, potentially hazardous interactions with: none known
Pregnancy category: C

Skin
Rash [5]
Toxic epidermal necrolysis [2]

Central Nervous System
Delirium [5]
Hallucinations [3]
Headache [2]
Insomnia [2]
Neuropsychiatric disturbances [3]
Neurotoxicity [5]
Seizures [2]

Suicidal ideation [2]

Gastrointestinal/Hepatic
Abdominal pain (2–5%)
Diarrhea (<3%) [4]
Hemorrhagic colitis [5]
Nausea (4–10%) [13]
Vomiting (2–15%) [13]

Respiratory
Upper respiratory tract infection [2]

Hematologic
Thrombocytopenia [2]

Other
Adverse effects [7]

OSIMERTINIB *

Trade name: Tagrisso (AstraZeneca)
Indications: Metastatic epidermal growth factor receptor T790M mutation-positive non-small cell lung cancer
Class: Kinase inhibitor
Half-life: 48 hours
Clinically important, potentially hazardous interactions with: carbamazepine, cyclosporine, ergot alkaloids, fentanyl, itraconazole, nefazodone, phenytoin, quinidine, rifampin, ritonavir, St John's wort, strong CYP3A inhibitors or inducers, telithromycin
Pregnancy category: N/A (Can cause fetal harm)
Important contra-indications noted in the prescribing guidelines for: nursing mothers; pediatric patients

---

Skin
Rash (41%) [3]
Xerosis (31%)

Nails
Nail toxicity (25%)

Mucosal
Stomatitis (12%)

Cardiovascular
QT prolongation (3%)
Venous thromboembolism (7%)

Central Nervous System
Cerebrovascular accident (3%)
Headache (10%)

Neuromuscular/Skeletal
Asthenia (fatigue) (14%)
Back pain (13%)

Gastrointestinal/Hepatic
Constipation (15%)
Diarrhea (42%) [3]
Nausea (17%) [2]

Respiratory
Cough (14%)
Pneumonia (4%)
Pneumonitis (3%)
Pulmonary toxicity [2]

Endocrine/Metabolic
Appetite decreased (16%) [2]
Hypermagnesemia (20%)
Hyponatremia (26%)

Hematologic
Anemia (44%)
Lymphopenia (63%)
Neutropenia (33%)
Thrombocytopenia (54%)

Ocular
Ocular adverse effects (18%)

OSPEMIFENE

Trade name: Osphena (Shionogi)
Indications: Dyspareunia due to menopausal vulvar and vaginal atrophy
Class: Estrogen agonist, Estrogen antagonist, Selective estrogen receptor modulator (SERM)
Half-life: 26 hours
Clinically important, potentially hazardous interactions with: fluconazole, ketoconazole, other estrogen agonists or antagonists, rifampin
Pregnancy category: X
Important contra-indications noted in the prescribing guidelines for: nursing mothers; pediatric patients
Note: Contraindicated in patients with undiagnosed abnormal genital bleeding, known or suspected estrogen-dependent neoplasia, active DVT or pulmonary embolism, or active arterial thromboembolic disease.
Black Box Warning: ENDOMETRIAL CANCER AND CARDIOVASCULAR DISORDERS

Skin
Hot flashes (8%) [7]
Hyperhidrosis (2%)

Neuromuscular/Skeletal
Muscle spasm (3%)

Genitourinary
Urinary tract infection [2]
Vaginal discharge (4%)

OXACILLIN

Indications: Various infections caused by susceptible organisms
Class: Antibiotic, penicillin
Half-life: 23–60 minutes
Clinically important, potentially hazardous interactions with: anticoagulants, cyclosporine, demeclocycline, doxycycline, imipenem/cilastatin, methotrexate, minocycline, oxytetracycline, tetracycline
Pregnancy category: B
Important contra-indications noted in the prescribing guidelines for: the elderly; nursing mothers; pediatric patients

---

Skin
Exanthems [2]
Rash (<22%)

Other
Adverse effects [2]

OXALIPLATIN

Trade name: Eloxatin (Sanofi-Aventis)
Indications: Metastatic carcinoma of the colon or rectum (in combination with fluorouracil/leucovorin (FOLFOX))
Class: Alkylating agent, Antineoplastic
Half-life: 391 hours
Clinically important, potentially hazardous interactions with: aminoglycosides, BCG vaccine, capreomycin, cardiac glycosides, clozapine, denosumab, diuretics, leflunomide, natalizumab, pimecrolimus, polymyxins, sipuleucel-T, tacrolimus, taxanes, topotecan, trastuzumab, vaccines, vitamin K antagonists
Pregnancy category: D
Important contra-indications noted in the prescribing guidelines for: nursing mothers; pediatric patients
Black Box Warning: ANAPHYLACTIC REACTIONS

Skin
Anaphylactoid reactions/Anaphylaxis [11]
Diaphoresis (5%) [2]
Edema (13–15%) [2]
Erythema [4]
Exanthems (2–5%)
Hand–foot syndrome (7–13%) [9]
Hot flashes (2–5%)
Hypersensitivity (12%) [29]
Peripheral edema (11%)
Pruritus (6%) [5]
Purpura (2–5%)
Radiation recall dermatitis [3]
Rash (5–11%) [11]
Thrombocytopenic purpura [2]
Toxicity [2]
Urticaria [2]
Xerosis (6%)

Hair
Alopecia (3–38%) [2]

Mucosal
Epistaxis (nosebleed) (<16%)
Gingivitis (2–5%)
Mucositis (10%) [4]
Stomatitis (32–42%) [3]
Xerostomia (5%)

Cardiovascular
Chest pain (4%) [2]
Flushing (2–7%) [2]
Hypertension [5]
Hypotension (5%) [2]
Tachycardia [3]
Thromboembolism (4%)

Central Nervous System
Anorexia (13–35%) [3]
Anxiety (5%)
Chills [3]
Depression (9%)
Dysesthesia (often cold-induced or cold-exacerbated) (38%) [7]
Dysgeusia (taste perversion) (<14%)
Dysphasia (5%)
Fever (16–27%) [9]
Headache (7–13%)
Hyperalgesia [2]
Hypoesthesia [2]

Insomnia (4–13%)
Leukoencephalopathy [4]
Neurotoxicity (48%) [34]
Pain (5–9%)
Paresthesias (77%) [7]
Peripheral neuropathy (92%) [32]
Rigors (8%)
Sensory disturbances (8%)
Vertigo (dizziness) (7–8%)

Neuromuscular/Skeletal
Arthralgia (5–10%)
Asthenia (fatigue) (44–70%) [17]
Ataxia [2]
Back pain (11–16%)
Myalgia/Myopathy (14%)

Gastrointestinal/Hepatic
Abdominal pain (18–31%) [4]
Constipation (22–32%) [2]
Diarrhea (44–56%) [34]
Dyspepsia (8–12%)
Flatulence (6–9%)
Gastroesophageal reflux (3%)
Hepatotoxicity [8]
Nausea (59–74%) [18]
Vomiting (27–47%) [16]

Respiratory
Cough (9–35%)
Dyspnea (5–18%) [2]
Pharyngitis (10%)
Pneumonia [2]
Pulmonary embolism [2]
Pulmonary fibrosis [2]
Pulmonary toxicity [2]
Rhinitis (4–10%)
Upper respiratory tract infection (4%)

Endocrine/Metabolic
ALP increased (42%)
ALT increased (57%)
Creatine phosphokinase increased (4%)
Dehydration (9%)
Hyperglycemia (14%)
Hypoalbuminemia (8%)
Hypocalcemia (7%)
Hypokalemia (11%)
Hyponatremia (8%) [2]
Weight gain (10%)
Weight loss (11%)

Genitourinary
Urinary frequency (5%)

Renal
Nephrotoxicity [3]

Hematologic
Anemia (27–76%) [21]
Febrile neutropenia (<4%) [5]
Hemolytic anemia [4]
Leukocytopenia [2]
Leukopenia (34–85%) [9]
Lymphopenia (6%)
Myelosuppression [4]
Neutropenia (25–81%) [45]
Thrombocytopenia (20–77%) [34]
Thrombosis (6%)

Ocular
Abnormal vision (5%)
Conjunctivitis (9%)
Epiphora [3]
Lacrimation (4–9%)
Vision blurred [2]

Local
Injection-site reactions (5–11%) [2]

Other
Adverse effects [2]
Allergic reactions (3%) [4]
Death [3]
Hiccups (5%)
Infection (8–25%) [2]

OXAPROZIN

Trade name: Daypro (Pfizer)
Indications: Arthritis
Class: Non-steroidal anti-inflammatory (NSAID)
Half-life: 42–50 hours
Clinically important, potentially hazardous interactions with: methotrexate
Pregnancy category: C
Important contra-indications noted in the prescribing guidelines for: nursing mothers; pediatric patients
Note: NSAIDs may cause an increased risk of serious cardiovascular and gastrointestinal adverse events, which can be fatal. This risk may increase with duration of use.

Skin
Pruritus (<10%)
Rash (>10%) [2]
Stevens–Johnson syndrome [2]
Toxic epidermal necrolysis [4]

Gastrointestinal/Hepatic
Hepatotoxicity [2]

Endocrine/Metabolic
Pseudoporphyria [3]

Renal
Nephrotoxicity [2]

Other
Adverse effects [3]

OXAZEPAM

Trade name: Serax (Mayne)
Indications: Anxiety, depression
Class: Benzodiazepine
Half-life: 3–6 hours
Clinically important, potentially hazardous interactions with: amprenavir, chlorpheniramine, clarithromycin, efavirenz, esomeprazole, imatinib, nelfinavir
Pregnancy category: D
Important contra-indications noted in the prescribing guidelines for: pediatric patients

---

Skin
Dermatitis (<10%)
Diaphoresis (>10%)
Rash (>10%)

Mucosal
Sialopenia (>10%)
Sialorrhea (<10%)
Xerostomia (>10%)

OXCARBAZEPINE

Trade names: Oxtellar XR (Supernus), Trileptal (Novartis)
Indications: Partial epileptic seizures
Class: Anticonvulsant, CYP3A4 inducer, Mood stabilizer
Half-life: 1–2.5 hours
Clinically important, potentially hazardous interactions with: alcohol, antipsychotics, carbamazepine, chloroquine, clopidogrel, cobicistat/elvitegravir/emtricitabine/tenofovir disoproxil, cyclosporine, CYP3A4 substrates, dronedarone, emtricitabine/rilpivirine/tenofovir alafenamide, eslicarbazepine, everolimus, exemestane, guanfacine, hydroxychloroquine, imatinib, ixabepilone, ledipasvir & sofosbuvir, levomepromazine, levonorgestrel, MAO inhibitors, maraviroc, mefloquine, nifedipine, nilotinib, nisoldipine, oral contraceptives, orlistat, pazopanib, perampanel, phenobarbital, phenytoin, praziquantel, ranolazine, rilpivirine, risperidone, romidepsin, saxagliptin, selegiline, simeprevir, sofosbuvir, sorafenib, SSRIs, St John's wort, tadalafil, thiazide diuretics, tolvaptan, tricyclic antidepressants, ulipristal, valproic acid, zuclopenthixol
Pregnancy category: C
Important contra-indications noted in the prescribing guidelines for: nursing mothers; pediatric patients

---

Skin
Acneform eruption (<2%)
Diaphoresis (3%)
DRESS syndrome [6]
Ecchymoses (4%)
Edema (<2%)
Exanthems [4]
Hot flashes (<2%)
Hyperhidrosis (3%)
Hypersensitivity [6]
Lymphadenopathy (2%)
Purpura (2%)
Rash (<6%) [10]
Stevens–Johnson syndrome [7]
Toxic epidermal necrolysis [4]

Mucosal
Epistaxis (nosebleed) (4%)
Rectal hemorrhage (2%)
Xerostomia (3%)

Cardiovascular
Chest pain (2%)
Hypotension (<3%)

Central Nervous System
Agitation (<2%)
Amnesia (4%)
Anorexia (3–5%)
Anxiety (5–7%)
Coma [2]
Confusion (<7%)
Dysgeusia (taste perversion) (5%)
Emotional lability (2–3%)
Fever (3%)
Gait instability (5–17%)
Headache (13–32%) [8]
Hyperesthesia (3%)
Hypoesthesia (<3%)
Incoordination (<4%)

Insomnia (2–6%)
Nervousness (2–4%)
Seizures (2–5%) [5]
Somnolence (drowsiness) (5–36%) [4]
Speech disorder (<3%)
Tremor (3–16%)
Vertigo (dizziness) (3–49%) [12]

Neuromuscular/Skeletal
Asthenia (fatigue) (3–15%) [5]
Ataxia (<31%) [2]
Back pain (4%)
Myoclonus [3]
Osteoporosis [2]

Gastrointestinal/Hepatic
Abdominal pain (3–13%)
Constipation (2–6%)
Diarrhea (5–7%)
Dyspepsia (5–6%)
Gastritis (<2%)
Nausea (15–29%) [8]
Vomiting (13–36%) [4]

Respiratory
Cough (5%)
Pharyngitis (3%)
Pneumonia (2%)
Rhinitis (2–5%)
Sinusitis (4%)
Upper respiratory tract infection (5–10%)

Endocrine/Metabolic
Hyponatremia (<5%) [15]
SIADH [3]
Weight gain (<2%)

Genitourinary
Ejaculatory dysfunction [3]
Urinary frequency (<2%)
Urinary tract infection (<5%)
Vaginitis (2%)

Hematologic
Leukopenia [3]
Thrombocytopenia [2]

Otic
Ear pain (<2%)

Ocular
Abnormal vision (2–14%)
Accommodation disorder (<3%)
Diplopia (<40%) [9]
Nystagmus (2–26%)

Other
Adverse effects [7]
Allergic reactions (2%) [3]
Dipsia (thirst) (2%)
Infection (2–7%)
Teratogenicity [3]
Toothache (2%)

OXYBUTYNIN

Trade names: Cystrin (Sanofi-Aventis), Ditropan (Ortho-McNeil), Lyrinel (Janssen-Cilag)
Indications: Neurogenic bladder, urinary incontinence, palmar and axillary hyperhidrosis
Class: Anticholinergic, Antimuscarinic, Muscarinic antagonist
Half-life: 2–3 hours
Clinically important, potentially hazardous interactions with: alcohol, anticholinergics, antihistamines, arbutamine, cannabinoids, clozapine, conivaptan, diphenoxylate, disopyramide, domperidone, haloperidol, ketoconazole, levodopa, MAO inhibitors, memantine, metoclopramide, nefopam, nitrates, parasympathomimetics, pramlintide, secretin, tricyclic antidepressants
Pregnancy category: B
Important contra-indications noted in the prescribing guidelines for: nursing mothers
Note: Contraindicated in patients with urinary retention, gastric retention and other severe decreased gastrointestinal motility conditions, uncontrolled narrow-angle glaucoma and in patients who are at risk for these conditions.

Skin
Hot flashes (<10%)
Pruritus [2]
Rash (<10%)

Mucosal
Sialopenia [2]
Xerostomia (71%) [28]

Central Nervous System
Cognitive impairment [4]
Headache (8%)
Insomnia (6%)
Nervousness (7%)
Somnolence (drowsiness) (14%)
Vertigo (dizziness) (17%) [2]

Gastrointestinal/Hepatic
Constipation (15%) [3]
Dyspepsia (6%)
Nausea [2]

Genitourinary
Urinary retention (6%)
Urinary tract infection (7%)

Ocular
Vision blurred (10%)

Other
Adverse effects [4]
Allergic reactions [2]

OXYCODONE

Trade names: OxyContin (Purdue), OxyIR (Purdue), Percocet (Endo), Roxicodone (aaiPharma), Targiniq (Purdue), Troxyca (Pfizer), Tylox (Ortho-McNeil), Xtampza ER (Collegium)
Indications: Pain
Class: Opiate agonist
Half-life: 4.6 hours
Clinically important, potentially hazardous interactions with: cimetidine, clonazepam, telithromycin, voriconazole
Pregnancy category: B
Important contra-indications noted in the prescribing guidelines for: the elderly; nursing mothers; pediatric patients
Note: Oxycodone is often combined with acetaminophen (Percocet, Roxicet, Tylox) or aspirin (Percodan, Roxiprin); Targiniq is oxycodone and naloxone; Troxyca is oxycodone and naltrexone. Contraindicated in patients with significant respiratory depression, acute or severe bronchial asthma, or with known or suspected gastrointestinal obstruction, including paralytic ileus.
Black Box Warning: ADDICTION, ABUSE and MISUSE; LIFETHREATENING RESPIRATORY DEPRESSION; ACCIDENTAL INGESTION; NEONATAL OPIOID WITHDRAWAL SYNDROME; and CYTOCHROME P450 3A4 INTERACTION

Skin
Pruritus [7]

Mucosal
Xerostomia [2]

Central Nervous System
Headache [6]
Insomnia [3]
Sedation [2]
Serotonin syndrome [2]
Somnolence (drowsiness) [12]
Vertigo (dizziness) [7]

Neuromuscular/Skeletal
Asthenia (fatigue) [7]

Gastrointestinal/Hepatic
Abdominal pain [3]
Constipation [11]
Nausea [19]
Vomiting [16]

Ocular
Hallucinations, visual [2]

Local
Injection-site pain (<10%)

Other
Adverse effects [6]
Death [3]
Tooth disorder [2]

OXYMORPHONE

Trade name: Opana (Endo)
Indications: Pain (moderate to severe)
Class: Analgesic, Opiate agonist
Half-life: 7–9 hours
Clinically important, potentially hazardous interactions with: anticholinergics, buprenorphine, butorphanol, cimetidine, CNS depressants, MAO inhibitors, nalbuphine, pentazocine
Pregnancy category: C
Important contra-indications noted in the prescribing guidelines for: the elderly; nursing mothers; pediatric patients
Note: Contraindicated in patients with a known hypersensitivity to morphine analogs such as codeine; in patients with respiratory depression, except in monitored settings and in the presence of resuscitative equipment; in patients with acute

or severe bronchial asthma or hypercarbia; in any patient who has or is suspected of having paralytic ileus; and in patients with moderate or severe hepatic impairment.

Skin
Hyperhidrosis (<10%)
Pruritus (8%) [2]

Mucosal
Xerostomia (<10%)

Cardiovascular
Hypotension (<10%)
Tachycardia (<10%)

Central Nervous System
Anxiety (<10%)
Confusion (3%)
Fever (14%)
Headache (7%)
Sedation (<10%)
Somnolence (drowsiness) (9%) [2]
Vertigo (dizziness) (7%)

Gastrointestinal/Hepatic
Abdominal distension (<10%)
Constipation (4%) [3]
Flatulence (<10%)
Nausea (19%) [4]
Vomiting (9%) [2]

Respiratory
Hypoxia (<10%)

Local
Injection-site reactions (<10%)

OXYTOCIN

Trade name: Pitocin (Par)
Indications: Induction of labor
Class: Oxytocic
Half-life: N/A
Clinically important, potentially hazardous interactions with: cyclopropane, gemeprost, halothane, prostaglandins

Pregnancy category: X

Skin
Anaphylactoid reactions/Anaphylaxis [7]

Mucosal
Xerostomia [3]

Cardiovascular
Bradycardia [2]

Respiratory
Hypoxia [2]

Genitourinary
Urinary frequency [3]
Uterine hyperstimulation [2]

PACLITAXEL

Trade name: Taxol (Bristol-Myers Squibb)
Indications: Breast cancer and metastatic carcinoma of the ovary
Class: Antineoplastic, Taxane
Half-life: 5–17 hours
Clinically important, potentially hazardous interactions with: atazanavir, bexarotene, buspirone, carbamazepine, cisplatin, clarithromycin, delavirdine, doxorubicin, efavirenz, eletriptan, felodipine, gadobenate, gemfibrozil, indinavir, itraconazole, ketoconazole, lapatinib, lovastatin, nefazodone, nelfinavir, repaglinide, rifampin, ritonavir, rosiglitazone, saquinavir, sildenafil, simvastatin, telithromycin, teriflunomide, thalidomide, trastuzumab, triazolam
Pregnancy category: D
Important contra-indications noted in the prescribing guidelines for: the elderly; nursing mothers; pediatric patients
Note: Studies have shown that elderly patients have an increased risk of severe myelosuppression, severe neuropathy and a higher incidence of cardiovascular events.

Skin
- Acneform eruption [5]
- Acral erythema [4]
- Anaphylactoid reactions/Anaphylaxis [3]
- Dermatitis [2]
- Desquamation (7%)
- Edema (21%) [2]
- Erythema [6]
- Exanthems [2]
- Fixed eruption [2]
- Folliculitis [2]
- Hand–foot syndrome [15]
- Hypersensitivity (31–45%) [24]
- Lupus erythematosus [5]
- Photosensitivity [4]
- Pigmentation [2]
- Pruritus [6]
- Pustules [2]
- Radiation recall dermatitis [10]
- Rash (12%) [15]
- Recall reaction [2]
- Scleroderma [6]
- Toxicity [6]
- Tumor lysis syndrome [2]
- Urticaria (2–4%) [4]

Hair
- Alopecia (87–100%) [42]

Nails
- Leukonychia (Mees' lines) [2]
- Nail changes (2%) [6]
- Nail pigmentation (2%) [2]
- Onycholysis [9]
- Pyogenic granuloma [2]

Mucosal
- Epistaxis (nosebleed) [2]
- Mucosal inflammation [2]
- Mucositis (17–35%) [11]
- Oral lesions (3–8%)
- Stomatitis (2–39%) [8]

Cardiovascular
- Atrial fibrillation [2]
- Bradycardia (3%)
- Cardiotoxicity [3]
- Congestive heart failure [3]
- Flushing (28%) [3]
- Hypertension [9]
- Hypotension (4–12%)
- Tachycardia (2%)

Central Nervous System
- Anorexia [5]
- Dysgeusia (taste perversion) [3]
- Fever [4]
- Headache [2]
- Insomnia [2]
- Neurotoxicity [33]
- Pain [8]
- Paresthesias (>10%) [4]
- Peripheral neuropathy (42–70%) [29]
- Vertigo (dizziness) [7]

Neuromuscular/Skeletal
- Arthralgia (60%) [15]
- Asthenia (fatigue) (17%) [47]
- Bone or joint pain [3]
- Myalgia/Myopathy (19–60%) [22]

Gastrointestinal/Hepatic
- Abdominal pain (>10%) [2]
- Constipation [5]
- Diarrhea (38%) [33]
- Dyspepsia [2]
- Gastrointestinal bleeding [2]
- Gastrointestinal disorder [2]
- Gastrointestinal perforation [3]
- Hepatotoxicity [5]
- Nausea (52%) [30]
- Pancreatitis [4]
- Vomiting [25]

Respiratory
- Cough [3]
- Dyspnea (2%) [4]
- Pneumonia [4]
- Pneumonitis [3]
- Pulmonary toxicity [3]

Endocrine/Metabolic
- ALP increased [2]
- ALT increased [9]
- Appetite decreased [3]
- AST increased [6]
- Hyperglycemia [4]
- SIADH [3]

Renal
- Proteinuria [2]

Hematologic
- Anemia (47%) [27]
- Bleeding [2]
- Febrile neutropenia [14]
- Hemotoxicity [4]
- Leukopenia (90%) [22]
- Lymphopenia [2]
- Myelosuppression [2]
- Myelotoxicity [3]
- Neutropenia (78–98%) [65]
- Thrombocytopenia (4–20%) [26]

Ocular
- Macular edema [9]
- Maculopathy [2]

Local
- Injection-site cellulitis (>10%)
- Injection-site extravasation (>10%) [4]
- Injection-site pain (>10%)
- Injection-site reactions (13%) [2]

Other
- Adverse effects [5]
- Allergic reactions (15%) [8]
- Death [11]
- Infection (3–22%) [11]
- Kounis syndrome [2]

PALBOCICLIB

Trade name: Ibrance (Pfizer)
Indications: Treatment of postmenopausal women with estrogen receptor (ER)-positive, human epidermal growth factor receptor 2 (HER2)-negative advanced breast cancer (in combination with letrozole)
Class: Kinase inhibitor
Half-life: 29 hours
Clinically important, potentially hazardous interactions with: bosentan, carbamazepine, clarithromycin, efavirenz, etravirine, grapefruit juice, indinavir, itraconazole, ketoconazole, lopinavir, modafinil, nafcillin, nefazodone, nelfinavir, phenytoin, posaconazole, rifampin, ritonavir, saquinavir, St John's wort, telaprevir, telithromycin, verapamil, voriconazole
Pregnancy category: N/A (Can cause fetal harm)
Important contra-indications noted in the prescribing guidelines for: nursing mothers; pediatric patients

---

Skin
- Peripheral edema [2]
- Rash [3]

Hair
- Alopecia (22%)

Mucosal
- Epistaxis (nosebleed) (11%) [2]
- Stomatitis (25%)

Central Nervous System
- Fever [2]
- Headache [2]
- Peripheral neuropathy (13%)

Neuromuscular/Skeletal
- Asthenia (fatigue) (13–41%) [8]

Gastrointestinal/Hepatic
- Constipation [2]
- Diarrhea (21%) [6]
- Nausea (25%) [6]
- Vomiting (15%) [2]

Respiratory
- Dyspnea [2]
- Upper respiratory tract infection (31%)

Endocrine/Metabolic
- Appetite decreased (16%)

Hematologic
- Anemia (35%) [9]
- Febrile neutropenia [4]
- Leukopenia (43%) [8]
- Lymphopenia [2]
- Neutropenia (75%) [14]
- Thrombocytopenia (17%) [6]

Other
- Adverse effects [2]

PALIFERMIN

Trade name: Kepivance (Amgen)
Indications: Severe oral mucositis in cancer patients
Class: Keratinocyte growth factor
Half-life: 4.5 hours
Clinically important, potentially hazardous interactions with: heparin
Pregnancy category: C
Important contra-indications noted in the prescribing guidelines for: nursing mothers

Skin
Acanthosis nigricans [2]
Edema (28%) [2]
Erythema (32%) [2]
Hand–foot syndrome [3]
Pruritus (35%) [3]
Rash (62%) [7]

Mucosal
Tongue edema (17%) [3]
Tongue pigmentation (17%)

Cardiovascular
Hypertension (~12%)

Central Nervous System
Dysesthesia (12%)
Dysgeusia (taste perversion) (16%) [4]
Fever (39%)
Pain (16%)
Paresthesias (12%)

Neuromuscular/Skeletal
Arthralgia (10%)

PALIPERIDONE

Trade name: Invega (Janssen)
Indications: Schizophrenia
Class: Antipsychotic
Half-life: ~23 hours
Clinically important, potentially hazardous interactions with: ACE inhibitors, alcohol, alpha blockers, amphetamines, angiotensin II receptor antagonists, carbamazepine, CNS depressants, dopamine agonists, droperidol, general anesthetics, itraconazole, levodopa, levomepromazine, lithium, methylphenidate, metoclopramide, myleosuppressives, P-glycoprotein inhibitors or inducers, quinagolide, risperidone, tetrabenazine, valproic acid
Pregnancy category: C
Important contra-indications noted in the prescribing guidelines for: the elderly; nursing mothers; pediatric patients
Note: Invega is not recommended for patients with creatinine clearance below 10 mL/min. Paliperidone is the active metabolite of risperidone (see separate entry).
Black Box Warning: INCREASED MORTALITY IN ELDERLY PATIENTS WITH DEMENTIA-RELATED PSYCHOSIS

Skin
Anaphylactoid reactions/Anaphylaxis (<2%)
Edema (<2%)
Peripheral edema [2]
Pruritus (<2%)
Rash (<2%)

Mucosal
Nasal congestion (<2%)
Sialorrhea (<6%) [2]
Tongue edema (3%)
Xerostomia (<4%)

Cardiovascular
Arrhythmias (<2%)
Atrioventricular block (<2%)
Bradycardia (<2%)
Bundle branch block (<3%)
Hypertension (<2%)
Palpitation (<2%)
Tachycardia (<14%) [6]

Central Nervous System
Agitation (<2%) [6]
Akathisia (3–17%) [18]
Anxiety (2–9%) [8]
Depression [2]
Dysarthria (<4%) [2]
Extrapyramidal symptoms (4–23%) [11]
Headache (4–14%) [14]
Insomnia (<2%) [20]
Neuroleptic malignant syndrome [5]
Nightmares (<2%)
Psychosis [3]
Schizophrenia [6]
Sleep related disorder (2–3%)
Somnolence (drowsiness) (6–26%) [13]
Tardive dyskinesia [3]
Tremor [5]
Vertigo (dizziness) (2–6%) [3]

Neuromuscular/Skeletal
Asthenia (fatigue) (<4%) [3]
Dystonia [5]
Rhabdomyolysis [2]

Gastrointestinal/Hepatic
Abdominal pain (<3%)
Constipation (4–5%) [3]
Dyspepsia (5–6%)
Flatulence (<2%)
Nausea [3]
Vomiting (3–11%)

Respiratory
Cough (<3%)
Nasopharyngitis (2–5%) [5]
Pharyngolaryngeal pain (<2%)
Pulmonary embolism [2]
Rhinitis (<3%)

Endocrine/Metabolic
ALT increased (<2%)
Amenorrhea (6%) [3]
Appetite decreased (<2%)
Appetite increased (2–3%)
AST increased (<2%)
Galactorrhea (4%) [4]
Gynecomastia (3%)
Hyperprolactinemia [7]
Menstrual irregularities (<2%)
Weight gain (2–7%) [18]

Genitourinary
Ejaculatory dysfunction (<2%)
Erectile dysfunction [2]
Sexual dysfunction [2]
Urinary tract infection (<2%)

Ocular
Vision blurred (3%)

Local
Injection-site pain [7]

Other
Adverse effects [7]
Death [2]

PALIVIZUMAB

Trade name: Synagis (Medimmune)
Indications: Prophylaxis of serious lower respiratory tract disease caused by respiratory syncytial virus in pediatric patients
Class: Immunomodulator, Monoclonal antibody
Half-life: 18 days
Clinically important, potentially hazardous interactions with: none known
Pregnancy category: C

Skin
Anaphylactoid reactions/Anaphylaxis [3]
Rash (26%)

Central Nervous System
Fever [2]

Local
Injection-site bruising (<3%)
Injection-site edema (<3%)
Injection-site erythema [3]
Injection-site induration (<3%)
Injection-site pain (<9%) [2]
Injection-site reactions [2]

PALONOSETRON

Trade name: Aloxi (MGI)
Indications: Antiemetic (for cancer chemotherapy)
Class: 5-HT3 antagonist, Antiemetic, Serotonin type 3 receptor antagonist
Half-life: 40 hours
Clinically important, potentially hazardous interactions with: none known
Pregnancy category: B
Note: See also the fixed drug combination Netupitant & Palonosetron (separate entry).

Skin
Hot flashes (<15)
Pruritus (8–22%)
Rash (6%)

Central Nervous System
Anorexia [2]
Fever [2]
Headache (9%) [12]
Vertigo (dizziness) [4]

Neuromuscular/Skeletal
Asthenia (fatigue) [3]
Osteonecrosis (jaw) [13]

Gastrointestinal/Hepatic
Abdominal pain [2]
Constipation [9]
Diarrhea [2]

Endocrine/Metabolic
AST increased [2]

Renal
Nephrotoxicity [3]

Other
Hiccups [3]

PAMIDRONATE

Trade name: Aredia (Novartis)
Indications: Hypercalcemia, Paget's disease, osteogenesis imperfecta
Class: Bisphosphonate
Half-life: 1.6 hours
Clinically important, potentially hazardous interactions with: none known
Pregnancy category: D
Important contra-indications noted in the prescribing guidelines for: nursing mothers; pediatric patients

---

Skin
Candidiasis (6%)

Cardiovascular
Atrial fibrillation (6%)
Hypertension (6%)
Tachycardia (6%)

Central Nervous System
Anorexia (26%)
Fever (18–39%) [8]
Headache (26%)
Insomnia (22%)
Somnolence (drowsiness) (6%)

Neuromuscular/Skeletal
Arthralgia (14%) [2]
Asthenia (fatigue) (37%) [2]
Bone or joint pain [3]
Fractures [3]
Myalgia/Myopathy [3]
Osteonecrosis [19]

Gastrointestinal/Hepatic
Abdominal pain (23%)
Constipation (6%)
Dyspepsia (23%)
Nausea (54%)
Vomiting (36%) [2]

Respiratory
Cough (26%)
Flu-like syndrome [3]
Rhinitis (6%)
Sinusitis (16%)

Endocrine/Metabolic
Hypocalcemia [10]
Hypophosphatemia [2]
Hypothyroidism (6%)

Genitourinary
Azotemia (prerenal) (4%)
Urinary tract infection (19%)

Renal
Nephrotoxicity [11]

Hematologic
Anemia (43%)
Granulocytopenia (20%)

Ocular
Conjunctivitis [5]
Episcleritis [2]
Orbital inflammation [2]
Scleritis [4]
Uveitis [12]
Vision blurred [2]

Local
Injection-site reactions (18%)

PANDEMIC INFLUENZA VACCINE (H1N1)

Trade names: Celvapan (Baxter), Focetria (Novartis), Pandemrix (GSK), Tamiflu (Roche)
Indications: Pandemic influenza vaccine (H1N1)
Class: Vaccine
Half-life: N/A
Clinically important, potentially hazardous interactions with: none known
Pregnancy category: C
Note: This is the vaccine for swine flu.

Skin
Lymphadenopathy (<10%)

Central Nervous System
Fever [3]
Guillain–Barré syndrome [2]
Headache (>10%)
Seizures [2]

Neuromuscular/Skeletal
Asthenia (fatigue) [2]

Other
Adverse effects [3]

PANITUMUMAB

Trade name: Vectibix (Amgen)
Indications: Metastatic colorectal carcinoma progression
Class: Antineoplastic, Biologic, Epidermal growth factor receptor (EGFR) inhibitor, Monoclonal antibody
Half-life: ~7.5 days
Clinically important, potentially hazardous interactions with: none known
Pregnancy category: C
Important contra-indications noted in the prescribing guidelines for: nursing mothers; pediatric patients
Black Box Warning: DERMATOLOGIC TOXICITY and INFUSION REACTIONS

Skin
Acneform eruption (57%) [17]
Desquamation [3]
Eczema [2]
Erythema (65%) [5]
Exfoliative dermatitis (25%) [2]
Fissures (20%) [4]
Folliculitis [3]
Hand–foot syndrome [3]
Papulopustular eruption [4]
Peripheral edema (12%)
Pruritus (57%) [9]
Rash (22%) [28]
Toxicity (90%) [25]
Xerosis (10%) [12]

Hair
Alopecia [3]
Hair changes (9%) [2]

Nails
Nail changes (9–29%) [2]
Paronychia (25%) [12]

Mucosal
Mucosal inflammation (6%)
Mucositis [4]
Stomatitis (7%) [4]

Central Nervous System
Anorexia [3]
Fever [2]

Neuromuscular/Skeletal
Asthenia (fatigue) (26%) [14]

Gastrointestinal/Hepatic
Abdominal pain (25%) [3]
Constipation (21%) [4]
Diarrhea (21%) [19]
Nausea (23%) [8]
Vomiting (19%) [8]

Respiratory
Cough (14%)
Dyspnea [2]
Pulmonary embolism [3]
Pulmonary fibrosis [3]
Pulmonary toxicity [7]

Endocrine/Metabolic
Dehydration [3]
Hypocalcemia [3]
Hypokalemia [6]
Hypomagnesemia [17]

Hematologic
Anemia [2]
Neutropenia [4]
Thrombocytopenia [3]

Ocular
Conjunctivitis (4%) [2]
Corneal perforation [2]
Eyelashes – hypertrichosis (6%)
Lacrimation (2%)
Ocular toxicity (15%) [2]
Trichomegaly [3]

Local
Infusion-related reactions (3%) [4]
Injection-site reactions (4%)

Other
Adverse effects [4]
Death [2]
Infection [3]

PANOBINOSTAT

Trade name: Farydak (Novartis)
Indications: Multiple myeloma (in combination with bortezomib and dexamethasone)
Class: Histone deacetylase (HDAC) inhibitor
Half-life: 37 hours
Clinically important, potentially hazardous interactions with: antiarrhythmics, QT prolonging agents, sensitive CYP2D6 substrates, strong CYP3A4 inducers

Pregnancy category: N/A (can cause fetal harm)
Important contra-indications noted in the prescribing guidelines for: the elderly; pediatric patients
Black Box Warning: FATAL AND SERIOUS TOXICITIES: SEVERE DIARRHEA AND CARDIAC TOXICITIES

Skin
Edema (<10%)
Erythema (<10%)
Lesions (<10%)
Peripheral edema (29%) [3]
Rash (<10%) [5]

Mucosal
Cheilitis (<10%)
Xerostomia (<10%)

Cardiovascular
Arrhythmias (12%)
Hypertension (<10%)
Hypotension (<10%) [2]
Orthostatic hypotension (<10%)
Palpitation (<10%)
QT prolongation [7]

Central Nervous System
Anorexia [5]
Chills (<10%)
Dysgeusia (taste perversion) (<10%) [3]
Fever (26%) [3]
Headache (<10%) [3]
Insomnia (<10%)
Peripheral neuropathy [6]
Syncope (<10%) [2]
Tremor (<10%)
Vertigo (dizziness) (<10%) [2]

Neuromuscular/Skeletal
Asthenia (fatigue) (60%) [28]
Back pain [2]
Joint disorder (<10%)

Gastrointestinal/Hepatic
Abdominal distension (<10%)
Abdominal pain (<10%) [4]
Colitis (<10%)
Constipation [5]
Diarrhea (68%) [25]
Dyspepsia (<10%) [2]
Flatulence (<10%)
Gastritis (<10%)
Nausea (36%) [16]
Vomiting (26%) [10]

Respiratory
Cough (<10%)
Dyspnea (<10%) [5]
Pneumonia [4]
Respiratory failure (<10%)
Wheezing (<10%)

Endocrine/Metabolic
ALP increased (<10%)
Appetite decreased (28%) [4]
Creatine phosphokinase increased (41%) [4]
Dehydration (<10%) [2]
Hyperbilirubinemia (21%) [3]
Hyperglycemia (<10%)
Hypermagnesemia (27%)
Hyperphosphatemia (29%)
Hyperuricemia (<10%)
Hypoalbuminemia (63%)
Hypocalcemia (67%) [2]
Hypokalemia (52%) [7]
Hypomagnesemia (<10%)
Hyponatremia (49%) [2]
Hypophosphatemia (63%) [4]
Hypothyroidism (<10%)
Weight loss (12%) [3]

Genitourinary
Urinary incontinence (<10%)

Renal
Renal failure (<10%)

Hematologic
Anemia (62%) [13]
Febrile neutropenia [2]
Leukopenia (81%) [5]
Lymphopenia (82%) [6]
Myelosuppression [5]
Neutropenia (75%) [20]
Sepsis [2]
Thrombocytopenia (97%) [32]

Other
Adverse effects [2]
Death (8%)

PANTOPRAZOLE

Trade names: Protium (Nycomed), Protonix (Wyeth)
Indications: Esophagitis associated with gastroesophageal reflux disease (GERD), Zollinger-Ellison syndrome, erosive esophagitis
Class: Proton pump inhibitor (PPI)
Half-life: 1 hour
Clinically important, potentially hazardous interactions with: alcohol, allopurinol, atazanavir, cefditoren, clopidogrel, conivaptan, CYP2C19 inducers and substrates, dabigatran, dasatinib, delavirdine, dexmethylphenidate, digoxin, erlotinib, eucalyptus, fluconazole, indinavir, iron salts, itraconazole, ketoconazole, lapatinib, mesalamine, methotrexate, methylphenidate, mycophenolate, nelfinavir, PEG-interferon, posaconazole, raltegravir, rilpivirine, saquinavir, tipranavir, topotecan, ulipristal, voriconazole, warfarin
Pregnancy category: B
Important contra-indications noted in the prescribing guidelines for: nursing mothers

---

Skin
Anaphylactoid reactions/Anaphylaxis [7]
Edema (<2%)
Facial edema (<4%)
Lupus erythematosus (discoid) [3]
Peripheral edema [2]
Photosensitivity (<2%)
Pruritus (<2%)
Rash (<2%) [2]
Urticaria (<4%) [2]

Mucosal
Xerostomia (<2%)

Central Nervous System
Depression (<2%)
Fever (>4%) [2]
Headache (12%)
Vertigo (dizziness) (3%)

Neuromuscular/Skeletal
Arthralgia (<4%)
Myalgia/Myopathy (<4%)

Gastrointestinal/Hepatic
Abdominal pain (6%)
Constipation (<4%)
Diarrhea (9%)
Flatulence (<4%)
Hepatitis (<2%)
Nausea (7%)
Pancreatitis [2]
Vomiting (4%)

Respiratory
Flu-like syndrome (<10%)
Upper respiratory tract infection (>4%)

Endocrine/Metabolic
Creatine phosphokinase increased (<2%)

Renal
Nephrotoxicity [4]

Hematologic
Leukopenia (<2%)
Thrombocytopenia (<2%) [5]

Ocular
Vision blurred (<2%)

Other
Allergic reactions (<4%)
Infection (<10%)
Kounis syndrome [2]

PAPAVERINE

Indications: Peripheral and cerebral ischemia
Class: Opium alkaloid, Vasodilator, peripheral
Half-life: 0.5–2 hours
Clinically important, potentially hazardous interactions with: levodopa, reboxetine
Pregnancy category: C
Important contra-indications noted in the prescribing guidelines for: nursing mothers; pediatric patients

---

Cardiovascular
Hypotension [2]

Genitourinary
Priapism (11%) [16]

PAROMOMYCIN

Trade name: Humatin (Pfizer)
Indications: Intestinal amebiasis
Class: Antibiotic, aminoglycoside
Half-life: N/A
Clinically important, potentially hazardous interactions with: methotrexate, succinylcholine
Pregnancy category: C

Gastrointestinal/Hepatic
Abdominal pain [2]

Local
Injection-site pain [2]

PAROXETINE HYDRO-CHLORIDE

Trade names: Paxil (GSK), Paxil CR (GSK), Seroxat (GSK)
Indications: Depression, obsessive-compulsive disorder, panic disorder, social and generalized anxiety disorders, post-traumatic stress disorder
Class: Antidepressant, Selective serotonin reuptake inhibitor (SSRI)
Half-life: 21 hours
Clinically important, potentially hazardous interactions with: alcohol, amitriptyline, amphetamines, antiepileptics, aprepitant, aripiprazole, artemether/lumefantrine, asenapine, aspirin, astemizole, atomoxetine, barbiturates, clarithromycin, clozapine, cobicistat/elvitegravir/emtricitabine/tenofovir disoproxil, coumarins, cyproheptadine, darifenacin, darunavir, dexibuprofen, dextroamphetamine, diethylpropion, digitalis, digoxin, duloxetine, entacapone, erythromycin, galantamine, iloperidone, isocarboxazid, linezolid, lithium, MAO inhibitors, mazindol, methadone, methamphetamine, methylene blue, methylphenidate, metoprolol, moclobemide, molindone, NSAIDs, perphenazine, phendimetrazine, phenelzine, phenobarbital, phentermine, phenylpropanolamine, phenytoin, pimozide, primidone, procyclidine, propafenone, propranolol, pseudoephedrine, ranolazine, rasagiline, risperidone, ritonavir, selegiline, sibutramine, St John's wort, sumatriptan, sympathomimetics, tamoxifen, tamsulosin, tetrabenazine, thioridazine, tramadol, tranylcypromine, trazodone, tricyclic antidepressants, troleandomycin, tryptophan, vortioxetine
Pregnancy category: D
Important contra-indications noted in the prescribing guidelines for: nursing mothers; pediatric patients
Note: For menopausal indications see separate entry for paroxetine mesylate.
Black Box Warning: SUICIDALITY AND ANTIDEPRESSANT DRUGS

Skin
Diaphoresis (11%) [10]
Ecchymoses [2]
Exanthems [2]
Hyperhidrosis [2]
Photosensitivity [3]
Pruritus [3]
Rash (2%)
Vasculitis [2]

Mucosal
Xerostomia (18%) [15]

Cardiovascular
Venous thromboembolism [2]

Central Nervous System
Abnormal dreams (3–4%)
Agitation (3–6%)
Akathisia [3]
Anxiety (5%)
Chills (2%) [2]
Delirium [3]
Depression [3]
Dysarthria [2]
Dysgeusia (taste perversion) (2%)
Extrapyramidal symptoms [2]
Headache (17–28%) [11]
Insomnia (11–24%) [4]
Irritability [2]
Mania [2]
Nervousness (4–9%)
Neuroleptic malignant syndrome [4]
Paresthesias (4%)
Parkinsonism [3]
Restless legs syndrome [7]
Serotonin syndrome [19]
Somnolence (drowsiness) (15–24%) [3]
Suicidal ideation [4]
Tic disorder [3]
Tremor (4–11%) [5]
Vertigo (dizziness) (6–14%) [6]
Yawning (2–4%)

Neuromuscular/Skeletal
Asthenia (fatigue) [4]
Myalgia/Myopathy (<10%)

Gastrointestinal/Hepatic
Abdominal pain (4%) [2]
Constipation (5–18%)
Diarrhea (9–12%) [2]
Nausea (26%) [5]

Respiratory
Pharyngitis (4%)
Rhinitis (3%)
Sinusitis (4%)

Endocrine/Metabolic
Galactorrhea [4]
Gynecomastia [2]
Libido decreased (3–15%)
SIADH [18]
Weight gain [7]

Genitourinary
Ejaculatory dysfunction (13–28%)
Erectile dysfunction [2]
Priapism [4]
Sexual dysfunction [7]

Otic
Hallucinations, auditory [3]

Ocular
Glaucoma [2]
Hallucinations, visual [2]
Vision impaired [2]

Other
Adverse effects [2]
Bruxism [4]
Congenital malformations [2]
Death [2]
Infection (5–6%)

PAROXETINE MESYLATE

Trade name: Brisdelle (Noven)
Indications: Vasomotor symptoms associated with the menopause
Class: Selective serotonin reuptake inhibitor (SSRI)
Half-life: N/A
Clinically important, potentially hazardous interactions with: linezolid, MAO inhibitors, methylene blue, pimozide, tamoxifen, thioridazine
Pregnancy category: X
Important contra-indications noted in the prescribing guidelines for: the elderly; nursing mothers; pediatric patients
Note: Brisdelle contains a low dose of paroxetine and is not indicated for psychiatric conditions. Paroxetine mesylate is also available as Pexeva. For psychiatric indications see separate entry for paroxetine hydrochloride.
Black Box Warning: SUICIDAL THOUGHTS AND BEHAVIORS

Central Nervous System
Headache (6%)

Neuromuscular/Skeletal
Asthenia (fatigue) (5%)

Gastrointestinal/Hepatic
Nausea (4%) [2]
Vomiting (4%)

Other
Adverse effects [2]

PATIROMER

Trade name: Veltassa (Relypsa)
Indications: Hyperkalemia
Class: Potassium binder
Half-life: N/A
Clinically important, potentially hazardous interactions with: none known
Pregnancy category: N/A (Not expected to cause fetal risk)
Important contra-indications noted in the prescribing guidelines for: pediatric patients
Black Box Warning: BINDING TO OTHER ORAL MEDICATIONS

Gastrointestinal/Hepatic
Abdominal pain (2%)
Constipation (7%) [9]
Diarrhea (5%) [4]
Flatulence (2%) [3]
Nausea (2%) [2]
Vomiting (<2%) [3]

Endocrine/Metabolic
Hypokalemia (5%) [5]
Hypomagnesemia (5–9%) [5]

PEG-INTERFERON

Trade names: PegIntron (Schering), Sylatron (Schering)
Indications: Chronic hepatitis C, melanoma
Class: Immunomodulator, Interferon
Half-life: ~40 hours
Clinically important, potentially hazardous interactions with: ACE inhibitors, acetaminophen, aldesleukin, bupivacaine, cilostazol, cinacalcet, CYP2C9 substrates, CYP2D6 substrates, delavirdine, duloxetine, estradiol, fesoterodine, fingolimod, fluoxetine, indinavir, melphalan, methadone, methylnaltrexone, pantoprazole, pegloticase, ribavirin, sildenafil, tapentadol, telbivudine, theophylline, theophylline derivatives, tiotropium, trimethoprim, voriconazole, warfarin, zidovudine
Pregnancy category: C (pregnancy category will be X when used in combination with ribavirin)
Important contra-indications noted in the prescribing guidelines for: nursing mothers; pediatric patients
Note: PEG-interferon is commonly administered with ribavirin and many of the reactions listed below are in combination therapy with this drug. Contraindicated in patients with known hypersensitivity reactions, such as urticaria, angioedema, bronchoconstriction, anaphylaxis, Stevens-Johnson syndrome, and toxic epidermal necrolysis to interferon alpha or any other product component; or with autoimmune hepatitis.
Black Box Warning: RISK OF SERIOUS DISORDERS AND RIBAVIRIN-ASSOCIATED EFFECTS
DEPRESSION AND OTHER NEUROPSYCHIATRIC DISORDERS

Skin
Dermatitis (7%)
Diaphoresis (6%)
DRESS syndrome [2]
Eczema [2]
Exanthems [5]
Fixed eruption [2]
Lupus erythematosus [3]
Nummular eczema [2]
Photosensitivity [4]
Pruritus (12%) [9]
Psoriasis [4]
Rash (6%) [23]
Rosacea fulminans [2]
Sarcoidosis [9]
Stevens–Johnson syndrome [2]
Toxic epidermal necrolysis [2]
Toxicity [3]
Vasculitis [2]
Vitiligo [3]
Xerosis (11%)

Hair
Alopecia (22%) [3]
Alopecia areata [2]

Cardiovascular
Flushing (6%)

Central Nervous System
Anorexia (17%)
Cognitive impairment [2]
Depression (16–29%) [9]
Dysgeusia (taste perversion) (<10%) [4]
Fever (37%) [5]
Headache (54%) [13]
Insomnia (19%) [3]
Irritability [2]
Neurotoxicity [2]
Pain (12%)
Parkinsonism [2]
Psychosis [2]
Vertigo (dizziness) (16%)

Neuromuscular/Skeletal
Arthralgia (28%)
Asthenia (fatigue) (56%) [20]
Back pain (9%)
Myalgia/Myopathy (38–42%)

Gastrointestinal/Hepatic
Abdominal pain (15%)
Diarrhea (16%) [3]
Hepatotoxicity [5]
Nausea (24%) [11]
Pancreatitis [4]
Vomiting (24%)

Respiratory
Cough (6%)
Dyspnea (13%)
Flu-like syndrome (46%) [8]
Pneumonitis [2]

Endocrine/Metabolic
ALT increased [2]
AST increased [2]
Diabetes mellitus [2]
Thyroid dysfunction [2]
Weight loss (16%) [3]

Renal
Nephrotoxicity [4]

Hematologic
Anemia (14%) [41]
Hemotoxicity [2]
Leukopenia [5]
Lymphopenia (14%) [2]
Neutropenia (21%) [19]
Sepsis [2]
Thrombocytopenia (5%) [14]

Otic
Hearing loss [2]
Tinnitus [2]

Ocular
Retinopathy [7]
Vision blurred (4%)

Local
Injection-site pain (2%)
Injection-site reactions (22%) [2]

Other
Adverse effects [24]
Death [2]
Infection (3%) [3]

PEGAPTANIB

Trade name: Macugen (Valeant)
Indications: Neovascular (wet) age-related macular degeneration
Class: Vascular endothelial growth factor antagonist
Half-life: 10±4 days
Clinically important, potentially hazardous interactions with: none known
Pregnancy category: B
Important contra-indications noted in the prescribing guidelines for: nursing mothers; pediatric patients
Note: Contraindicated in patients with ocular or periocular infections.

Skin
Dermatitis (<5%)

Cardiovascular
Arterial occlusion (carotid) (<5%)
Chest pain (<5%)
Hypertension (10–40%)
Myocardial ischemia (transient) (<5%)

Central Nervous System
Cerebrovascular accident (<5%)
Headache (6–10%)
Ischemic injury (transient) (<5%)
Vertigo (dizziness) (<10%)

Neuromuscular/Skeletal
Arthralgia (<5%)

Gastrointestinal/Hepatic
Diarrhea (6–10%)
Nausea (6–10%)
Vomiting (<5%)

Respiratory
Bronchitis (6–10%)
Pleural effusion (<5%)

Endocrine/Metabolic
Diabetes mellitus (<5%)

Genitourinary
Urinary retention (<5%)
Urinary tract infection (6–10%)

Otic
Hearing loss (<5%)
Otitis media (<5%)

Ocular
Blepharitis (6–10%)
Cataract (10–40%) [2]
Conjunctival edema (<5%)
Conjunctival hemorrhage (10–40%)
Conjunctivitis (<10%)
Corneal abnormalities (<5%)
Corneal deposits (<5%)
Corneal edema (10–40%)
Endophthalmitis (<5%) [4]
Eyelid irritation (<5%)
Intraocular pressure increased (10–40%)
Meibomianitis (<5%)
Mydriasis (<5%)
Ocular edema (<5%)
Ocular hypertension (10–40%)
Ocular inflammation (<5%) [2]
Ocular pain (10–40%)
Ocular stinging (10–40%)
Ophthalmitis (<5%)
Periorbital hematoma (<5%)

Photopsia (6–10%)
Punctate keratitis (10–40%)
Reduced visual acuity (10–40%)
Retinal detachment (<10%) [5]
Retinal edema (<5%)
Vision blurred (10–40%)
Visual disturbances (10–40%)
Vitreous floaters (10–40%)

PEGASPARGASE

Trade name: Oncaspar (Enzon)
Indications: Acute lymphoblastic leukemia
Class: Antineoplastic
Half-life: 5.7 days
Clinically important, potentially hazardous interactions with: none known
Pregnancy category: C

Skin
Anaphylactoid reactions/Anaphylaxis (<5%) [2]
Angioedema (<5%)
Edema (>5%)
Rash (<5%)
Urticaria (<5%)

Cardiovascular
Hypotension (>5%)
Tachycardia (>5%)

Central Nervous System
Chills (<5%)
Fever (>5%)
Headache (<5%)
Paresthesias (<5%)
Seizures (<5%) [2]

Neuromuscular/Skeletal
Arthralgia (<5%)
Myalgia/Myopathy (<5%)

Gastrointestinal/Hepatic
Abdominal pain (<5%)
Hepatotoxicity [3]
Pancreatitis [2]

Hematologic
Leukopenia [2]
Neutropenia [2]
Thrombocytopenia [2]

Other
Allergic reactions (>5%) [6]

PEGLOTICASE

Trade name: Krystexxa (Savient)
Indications: Chronic gout
Class: Enzyme
Half-life: N/A
Clinically important, potentially hazardous interactions with: PEG-interferon
Pregnancy category: C
Important contra-indications noted in the prescribing guidelines for: nursing mothers; pediatric patients
Note: Contraindicated for patients at higher risk for G6PD deficiency (e.g. those of African and Mediterranean ancestry) who should be screened due to the risk of hemolysis and methemoglobinemia.

Black Box Warning: ANAPHYLAXIS and INFUSION REACTIONS

Skin
Anaphylactoid reactions/Anaphylaxis (5%) [2]
Ecchymoses (11%)

Cardiovascular
Chest pain (6%)

Central Nervous System
Vertigo (dizziness) [3]

Neuromuscular/Skeletal
Arthralgia [3]
Back pain [2]
Gouty tophi (flare) (77%) [6]

Gastrointestinal/Hepatic
Constipation (6%)
Nausea (12%) [3]
Vomiting (5%)

Respiratory
Dyspnea [2]
Nasopharyngitis (7%)

Local
Infusion-related reactions [3]
Infusion-site reactions (26%) [4]

Other
Adverse effects [2]

PEGVISOMANT

Trade name: Somavert (Pfizer)
Indications: Acromegaly
Class: Growth hormone analog
Half-life: 6 days
Clinically important, potentially hazardous interactions with: acarbose, exenatide, hydromorphone, insulin, latex, metformin, opioids, oral hypoglycemics, pioglitazone, saxagliptin, tapentadol
Pregnancy category: B
Important contra-indications noted in the prescribing guidelines for: the elderly; nursing mothers; pediatric patients

---

Skin
Lipohypertrophy (<5%) [2]
Peripheral edema (4–8%)

Cardiovascular
Chest pain (4–8%)
Hypertension (8%)

Central Nervous System
Pain (4–14%)
Paresthesias (7%)
Vertigo (dizziness) (4–8%)

Neuromuscular/Skeletal
Back pain (4–8%)

Gastrointestinal/Hepatic
Diarrhea (4–14%)
Hepatitis [2]
Hepatotoxicity [6]
Nausea (8–14%)

Respiratory
Flu-like syndrome (4–12%)
Sinusitis (4–8%)

Local
Injection-site reactions (8–11%) [4]

Other
Adverse effects [3]
Infection (23%)

PEMBROLIZUMAB

Synonym: lambrolizumab
Trade name: Keytruda (Merck Sharpe & Dohme)
Indications: Unresectable or metastatic melanoma and disease progression following ipilimumab and, if BRAF V600 mutation positive, a BRAF inhibitor
Class: Monoclonal antibody, Programmed death receptor-1 (PD-1) inhibitor
Half-life: 26 days
Clinically important, potentially hazardous interactions with: none known
Pregnancy category: D
Important contra-indications noted in the prescribing guidelines for: nursing mothers; pediatric patients

---

Skin
Bullous pemphigoid [3]
Dermatitis [2]
Lichen planus [2]
Peripheral edema (17%)
Pruritus (30%) [8]
Psoriasis [3]
Rash (29%) [9]
Sarcoidosis [2]
Vitiligo (11%) [6]

Central Nervous System
Chills (14%)
Encephalopathy [2]
Fever (11%) [4]
Headache (16%) [3]
Insomnia (14%)
Peripheral neuropathy [2]
Vertigo (dizziness) (11%)

Neuromuscular/Skeletal
Arthralgia (20%) [4]
Asthenia (fatigue) (47%) [10]
Back pain (12%)
Myalgia/Myopathy (14%) [5]
Myasthenia gravis [3]
Pain in extremities (18%)

Gastrointestinal/Hepatic
Abdominal pain (12%) [2]
Colitis [7]
Constipation (21%)
Diarrhea (20%) [6]
Hepatitis [3]
Hepatotoxicity [4]
Nausea (30%) [4]
Pancreatitis [4]
Vomiting (16%)

Respiratory
Cough (30%) [4]
Dyspnea (18%) [4]
Pneumonitis (3%) [7]
Upper respiratory tract infection (11%)

Endocrine/Metabolic
ALT increased [4]

Appetite decreased (26%) [5]
AST increased (24%) [4]
Diabetes mellitus [3]
Hyperglycemia (40%)
Hyperthyroidism [2]
Hypertriglyceridemia (25%)
Hypoalbuminemia (34%)
Hypocalcemia (24%)
Hyponatremia (35%) [2]
Hypophysitis [5]
Hypothyroidism (8%) [5]
Thyroid dysfunction [3]
Thyroiditis [2]

Renal
Nephrotoxicity [3]
Renal failure [3]

Hematologic
Anemia (14–55%) [3]
Sepsis (<10%)
Thrombocytopenia [2]

Ocular
Uveitis [4]

Other
Adverse effects [10]
Death [2]
Side effects [3]

PEMETREXED

Trade name: Alimta (Lilly)
Indications: Non-squamous non-small cell lung cancer, mesothelioma (in combination with cisplatin)
Class: Antimetabolite, Folic acid antagonist
Half-life: 3.5 hours
Clinically important, potentially hazardous interactions with: clozapine, digoxin, leflunomide, meloxicam, natalizumab, nephrotoxic drugs, NSAIDs, phenytoin, pimecrolimus, probenecid, pyrimethamine, sipuleucel-T, tacrolimus, trastuzumab, vaccines
Pregnancy category: D
Important contra-indications noted in the prescribing guidelines for: nursing mothers; pediatric patients

---

Skin
AGEP [3]
Desquamation (10–14%)
Edema (<5%)
Erythema multiforme (<5%)
Hypersensitivity (<5%)
Peripheral edema [3]
Pruritus (<7%)
Radiation recall dermatitis [5]
Rash (10–14%) [18]
Toxic epidermal necrolysis [4]
Toxicity [2]
Urticaria [2]

Hair
Alopecia (<6%) [3]

Mucosal
Epistaxis (nosebleed) [2]
Mucositis (7%) [6]
Stomatitis (7–15%) [6]

Cardiovascular
Hypertension [6]
Venous thromboembolism [2]

Central Nervous System
Anorexia (19–22%) [8]
Depression (14%)
Dysgeusia (taste perversion) [2]
Fever (<8%) [2]
Headache [4]
Insomnia [2]
Neurotoxicity (<9%)
Peripheral neuropathy [2]

Neuromuscular/Skeletal
Asthenia (fatigue) (25–34%) [31]

Gastrointestinal/Hepatic
Abdominal pain (<5%)
Constipation (<6%) [4]
Diarrhea (5–13%) [11]
Hepatotoxicity [8]
Nausea (19–31%) [14]
Vomiting (9–16%) [9]

Respiratory
Cough [2]
Dysphonia [2]
Dyspnea [4]
Hemoptysis [2]
Pharyngitis (15%)
Pulmonary toxicity [2]

Endocrine/Metabolic
ALT increased (8–10%) [3]
Appetite decreased [5]
AST increased (7–8%) [3]
Creatine phosphokinase increased (<5%) [3]
Hyperglycemia [2]
Hyperkalemia [2]
Hypokalemia [2]
Hypomagnesemia [3]
Hyponatremia [3]

Hematologic
Anemia (15–19%) [20]
Febrile neutropenia (<5%) [9]
Leukocytopenia [2]
Leukopenia (6–12%) [10]
Lymphocytopenia [2]
Neutropenia (6–11%) [21]
Sepsis [2]
Thrombocytopenia (<8%) [14]
Thrombotic complications [2]

Ocular
Conjunctivitis (<5%)
Lacrimation (<5%)

Other
Adverse effects (53%) [13]
Allergic reactions (<5%)
Death [5]
Infection (<5%) [7]

PENICILLAMINE

Trade name: Depen (MedPointe)
Indications: Wilson's disease, rheumatoid arthritis
Class: Antidote, Chelator, Disease-modifying antirheumatic drug (DMARD)
Half-life: 1.7–3.2 hours
Clinically important, potentially hazardous interactions with: aluminum, antacids, ascorbic acid, bone marrow suppressants, chloroquine, clozapine, cytotoxic agents, diclofenac, ferrous sulfate, food, gold & gold compounds, hydroxychloroquine, iron, magnesium, meloxicam, primaquine, probenecid, sodium picosulfate
Pregnancy category: D
Important contra-indications noted in the prescribing guidelines for: nursing mothers; pediatric patients
Note: As an antidote, it is difficult to differentiate side effects due to the drug from those due to the effects of the poison.

Skin
Bullous dermatitis [3]
Bullous pemphigoid [6]
Cicatricial pemphigoid [2]
Cutis laxa [13]
Dermatitis [4]
Dermatomyositis [14]
Edema of lip (<10%)
Ehlers–Danlos syndrome [2]
Elastosis perforans serpiginosa [43]
Epidermolysis bullosa [4]
Epidermolysis bullosa acquisita [2]
Erythema multiforme (<5%)
Exanthems [8]
Fragility [2]
Hypersensitivity [3]
Lichen planus [4]
Lichenoid eruption [7]
Lupus erythematosus [43]
Morphea [2]
Pemphigus [75]
Pemphigus erythematodes (Senear–Usher) [10]
Pemphigus foliaceus [16]
Pemphigus herpetiformis [3]
Pemphigus vulgaris [2]
Peripheral edema (<10%)
Pruritus (44–50%) [2]
Pseudoxanthoma elasticum [16]
Psoriasis [4]
Purpura [5]
Rash (44–50%) [6]
Scleroderma [7]
Toxic epidermal necrolysis [2]
Urticaria (44–50%) [2]
Vasculitis [7]

Hair
Alopecia [3]
Hirsutism [2]

Nails
Nail pigmentation [4]

Mucosal
Aphthous stomatitis [2]
Mucosal lesions (pemphigus-like) [2]
Oral ulceration [5]
Stomatitis [6]

Central Nervous System
Ageusia (taste loss) (12%) [2]
Dysgeusia (taste perversion) (metallic taste) [8]
Hypogeusia (25–33%) [2]

Neuromuscular/Skeletal
Dystonia [4]
Myasthenia gravis [73]
Polymyositis [8]

Respiratory
Pulmonary toxicity [2]

Endocrine/Metabolic
Gynecomastia [5]

Renal
Glomerulonephritis [3]
Nephrotoxicity [5]
Proteinuria [2]

Hematologic
Hemotoxicity [2]

Other
Adverse effects [2]

PENICILLIN G

Trade name: Crystapen (Britannia)
Indications: Anthrax, cellulitis, endocarditis, infections, otitis media, rheumatic fever, respiratory infections, septicemia
Class: Antibiotic, penicillin
Half-life: 4 hours
Clinically important, potentially hazardous interactions with: estrogens, methotrexate, minocycline, phenindione, probenecid, sulfinpyrazone, warfarin
Pregnancy category: B
Important contra-indications noted in the prescribing guidelines for: nursing mothers

---

Skin
Anaphylactoid reactions/Anaphylaxis [5]
Dermatitis [2]
Hypersensitivity [4]
Jarisch–Herxheimer reaction [21]
Nicolau syndrome [2]
Rash [4]
Serum sickness [3]

Central Nervous System
Hoigne's syndrome [16]
Seizures [2]

Gastrointestinal/Hepatic
Hepatotoxicity [2]

Genitourinary
Cystitis [3]

Renal
Nephrotoxicity [2]

Hematologic
Thrombosis [2]

PENICILLIN V

Trade name: V-cillin K (Lilly)
Indications: Cellulitis, endocarditis, erysipelas, oral infections, otitis media, rheumatic fever, scarlet fever, tonsillitis
Class: Antibiotic, penicillin
Half-life: 4 hours
Clinically important, potentially hazardous interactions with: estrogens, methotrexate, minocycline, neomycin, phenindione, probenecid, sulfinpyrazone, warfarin
Pregnancy category: B

Skin
Anaphylactoid reactions/Anaphylaxis [2]
DRESS syndrome [2]
Hypersensitivity [3]
Serum sickness [5]
Urticaria [3]

Central Nervous System
Fever [3]

Neuromuscular/Skeletal
Arthralgia [2]

Gastrointestinal/Hepatic
Diarrhea [2]

PENTAMIDINE

Trade names: NebuPent (Astellas), Pentacarinat (Sanofi-Aventis), Pentam 300 (Astellas)
Indications: *Pneumocystis jiroveci* infection, trypanosomiasis, leishmaniasis
Class: Antiprotozoal
Half-life: 9.1–13.2 hours (intramuscular); 6.5 hours (intravenous)
Clinically important, potentially hazardous interactions with: adefovir, aminoglycosides, amiodarone, amisulpride, amitriptyline, amphotericin B, cisplatin, droperidol, erythromycin, foscarnet, insulin aspart, insulin degludec, insulin detemir, insulin glargine, insulin glulisine, ivabradine, levomepromazine, moxifloxacin, phenothiazines, saquinavir, sparfloxacin, sulpiride, tricyclic antidepressants, trifluoperazine, vancomycin
Pregnancy category: C
Important contra-indications noted in the prescribing guidelines for: nursing mothers; pediatric patients
Note: The rate of adverse side effects is increased in patients with AIDS.

Skin
Exanthems (<15%) [10]
Pruritus [2]
Rash (<47%) [4]
Toxic epidermal necrolysis [3]
Urticaria [3]

Cardiovascular
QT prolongation [8]
Torsades de pointes [4]

Central Nervous System
Dysgeusia (taste perversion) (metallic taste) (2%)
Paresthesias [2]
Vertigo (dizziness) [2]

Neuromuscular/Skeletal
Myalgia/Myopathy (<5%)
Rhabdomyolysis [4]

Gastrointestinal/Hepatic
Pancreatitis [6]

Local
Injection-site irritation [2]
Injection-site pain [2]
Injection-site reactions (>10%)

Other
Adverse effects [3]

PENTOXIFYLLINE

Trade names: Pentoxil (Upsher-Smith), Trental (Sanofi-Aventis)
Indications: Peripheral vascular disease, intermittent claudication
Class: Vasodilator, peripheral, Xanthine alkaloid
Half-life: 0.4–0.8 hours
Clinically important, potentially hazardous interactions with: abciximab, benazepril, captopril, ceftobiprole, cilostazol, ciprofloxacin, citalopram, clevidipine, clopidogrel, diclofenac, enalapril, eptifibatide, fosinopril, insulin degludec, insulin glargine, insulin glulisine, irbesartan, lisinopril, meloxicam, olmesartan, quinapril, ramipril, tinzaparin
Pregnancy category: C

Mucosal
Xerostomia [2]

Cardiovascular
Flushing (2%) [2]

PERAMIVIR *

Trade name: Rapivab (BioCryst)
Indications: Influenza
Class: Antiviral, Neuraminidase inhibitor
Half-life: ~20 hours
Clinically important, potentially hazardous interactions with: live attenuated influenza vaccine
Pregnancy category: C
Important contra-indications noted in the prescribing guidelines for: nursing mothers; pediatric patients

---

Cardiovascular
Hypertension (2%)

Central Nervous System
Behavioral disturbances [2]
Insomnia (3%)

Gastrointestinal/Hepatic
Constipation (4%)
Diarrhea (8%) [6]
Nausea [4]
Vomiting [4]

Endocrine/Metabolic
ALT increased (3%)
AST increased (3%)
Creatine phosphokinase increased (4%)
Hyperglycemia (5%)

Hematologic
Neutropenia (8%) [4]
Thrombocytopenia [2]

PERAMPANEL

Trade name: Fycompa (Eisai)
Indications: Partial-onset seizures, primary generalized tonic-clonic seizures
Class: AMPA glutamate receptor antagonist, Anticonvulsant, Antiepileptic
Half-life: ~105 hours
Clinically important, potentially hazardous interactions with: alcohol, carbamazepine, oral contraceptives, oxcarbazepine, phenobarbital, phenytoin, primidone, rifampin, St John's wort
Pregnancy category: C
Important contra-indications noted in the prescribing guidelines for: the elderly; nursing mothers; pediatric patients
Black Box Warning: SERIOUS PSYCHIATRIC AND BEHAVIORAL REACTIONS

Skin
Peripheral edema (<2%)

Mucosal
Oropharyngeal pain (2%)

Central Nervous System
Aggression (<3%) [9]
Anxiety (2–4%)
Balance disorder (<5%)
Behavioral disturbances [3]
Confusion (<2%)
Depression [2]
Dysarthria (<4%)
Euphoria (<2%)
Gait instability (<4%) [8]
Headache (11–13%) [13]
Hypersomnia (<3%)
Hypoesthesia (<3%)
Incoordination (<2%)
Irritability (4–12%) [13]
Memory loss (<2%)
Mood changes (<2%)
Neurotoxicity [2]
Paresthesias (<2%)
Sedation [2]
Seizures [3]
Somnolence (drowsiness) (9–18%) [24]
Suicidal ideation [2]
Vertigo (dizziness) (16–43%) [30]

Neuromuscular/Skeletal
Arthralgia (<3%)
Asthenia (fatigue) (<12%) [14]
Ataxia (<8%) [5]
Back pain (2–5%)
Bone or joint pain (<2%)
Myalgia/Myopathy (<3%)
Pain in extremities (<3%)

Gastrointestinal/Hepatic
Constipation (2–3%)
Nausea (3–8%) [4]
Vomiting (2–4%)

Respiratory
Cough (<4%)
Upper respiratory tract infection (3–4%)

Endocrine/Metabolic
Hyponatremia (<2%)
Weight gain (4%) [6]

Ocular
Diplopia (<3%)
Vision blurred (<4%)

Other
Adverse effects [3]

PERINDOPRIL

Trade names: Aceon (Solvay), Prestalia (Symplmed)
Indications: Hypertension, coronary disease
Class: Angiotensin-converting enzyme (ACE) inhibitor, Antihypertensive
Half-life: 1.5–3 hours
Clinically important, potentially hazardous interactions with: none known
Pregnancy category: D (category C in first trimester; category D in second and third trimesters)
Important contra-indications noted in the prescribing guidelines for: nursing mothers; pediatric patients
Note: Prestalia is perindopril and amlodipine.
Black Box Warning: FETAL TOXICITY

Skin
Angioedema [6]
Edema (4%)
Peripheral edema [3]
Pruritus (<10%)
Rash (<10%)

Mucosal
Tongue edema [2]

Central Nervous System
Paresthesias (2%)
Vertigo (dizziness) [2]

Neuromuscular/Skeletal
Back pain (6%)

Respiratory
Cough (12%) [16]

Other
Adverse effects [2]

PERPHENAZINE

Trade names: Decentan (Merck), Fentazin (Goldshield), Trilafon (Schering)
Indications: Psychotic disorders, nausea and vomiting
Class: Antiemetic, Antipsychotic, Phenothiazine
Half-life: 9 hours
Clinically important, potentially hazardous interactions with: cobicistat/elvitegravir/emtricitabine/tenofovir disoproxil, paroxetine hydrochloride, sparfloxacin
Pregnancy category: C
Note: Perphenazine is also used in combination with amitriptyline.

Skin
Exanthems [2]
Lupus erythematosus [4]
Rash (<10%)

Neuromuscular/Skeletal
Rhabdomyolysis [2]

Endocrine/Metabolic
Mastodynia (<10%)

Genitourinary
Priapism [2]

PHENOBARBITAL

Synonyms: phenobarbitone; phenylethylmalonylurea
Trade name: Luminal (Sanofi-Aventis)
Indications: Insomnia, seizures
Class: Anticonvulsant, Barbiturate, CYP3A4 inducer
Half-life: 2–6 days
Clinically important, potentially hazardous interactions with: abacavir, abiraterone, afatinib, alcohol, amprenavir, anticoagulants, antihistamines, apremilast, aprepitant, betamethasone, boceprevir, brompheniramine, buclizine, buprenorphine, cabazitaxel, cabozantinib, caffeine, chlorpheniramine, cobicistat/elvitegravir/emtricitabine/tenofovir disoproxil, crizotinib, darunavir, dasatinib, deferasirox, delavirdine, dexamethasone, dicumarol, doxercalciferol, dronedarone, emtricitabine/rilpivirine/tenofovir alafenamide, enzalutamide, estradiol, ethanolamine, ethosuximide, etravirine, fesoterodine, flibanserin, fluconazole, flunisolide, fosamprenavir, gefitinib, hydrocortisone, imatinib, indinavir, influenza vaccine, itraconazole, ixabepilone, lacosamide, lapatinib, ledipasvir & sofosbuvir, lisdexamfetamine, lopinavir, meperidine, methsuximide, methylprednisolone, midazolam, mifepristone, nilotinib, ombitasvir/paritaprevir/ritonavir, oxcarbazepine, oxtriphylline, paroxetine hydrochloride, perampanel, piracetam, pizotifen, prednisolone, prednisone, propranolol, ranolazine, regorafenib, rilpivirine, riociguat, rivaroxaban, roflumilast, romidepsin, rufinamide, simeprevir, sodium oxybate, sofosbuvir, solifenacin, sorafenib, sunitinib, telaprevir, telithromycin, temsirolimus, teniposide, tiagabine, ticagrelor, tipranavir, trabectedin, triamcinolone, ulipristal, vandetanib, vemurafenib, voriconazole, warfarin
Pregnancy category: D
Important contra-indications noted in the prescribing guidelines for: the elderly; nursing mothers
Note: Aromatic antiepileptic drugs, phenytoin, phenobarbital, carbamazepine and primidone, are a frequent cause of severe cutaneous adverse reactions. A strong genetic association between HLA-B*1502 and phenobarbital-induced Stevens-Johnson syndrome and toxic epidermal necrolysis has been shown in Han Chinese patients.

Skin
Anticonvulsant hypersensitivity syndrome [10]
Bullous dermatitis [5]
DRESS syndrome [12]
Erythema multiforme [7]
Erythroderma [2]
Exanthems [13]
Exfoliative dermatitis [6]
Fixed eruption [9]
Hypersensitivity [12]
Lupus erythematosus [2]
Purpura [2]

Rash [4]
Stevens–Johnson syndrome [20]
Toxic epidermal necrolysis [26]

Nails
Nail hypoplasia [2]

Mucosal
Gingival hyperplasia/hypertrophy [3]

Central Nervous System
Behavioral disturbances [3]
Somnolence (drowsiness) [2]
Vertigo (dizziness) [2]

Neuromuscular/Skeletal
Asthenia (fatigue) [2]
Hypoplasia of phalanges [2]

Gastrointestinal/Hepatic
Hepatotoxicity [2]

Local
Injection-site pain (>10%)
Injection-site thrombophlebitis (>10%)

Other
Allergic reactions [2]
Death [2]
Side effects [2]
Teratogenicity [5]

PHENTERMINE

Trade names: Adipex-P (Teva), Ionamin (Celltech), Lomaira (Avanthi), Qsymia (Vivus)
Indications: Obesity
Class: Amphetamine
Half-life: 19–24 hours
Clinically important, potentially hazardous interactions with: fluoxetine, fluvoxamine, MAO inhibitors, paroxetine hydrochloride, phenelzine, sertraline, tranylcypromine
Pregnancy category: X
Important contra-indications noted in the prescribing guidelines for: the elderly; nursing mothers; pediatric patients
Note: Qsymia is phentermine and topiramate.

Mucosal
Xerostomia [6]

Cardiovascular
Cardiotoxicity [3]
Hypertension [11]
Palpitation [3]
Tachycardia [4]
Valvulopathy [17]

Central Nervous System
Anxiety [2]
Cognitive impairment [4]
Depression [3]
Dysgeusia (taste perversion) [4]
Headache [2]
Insomnia [7]
Paresthesias [6]
Vertigo (dizziness) [4]

Gastrointestinal/Hepatic
Constipation [5]

Endocrine/Metabolic
Acidosis [3]

Other
Death [4]
Teratogenicity [2]

PHENTOLAMINE

Trade name: Regitine (Novartis)
Indications: Hypertensive episodes in pheochromocytoma
Class: Adrenergic alpha-receptor antagonist
Half-life: 19 minutes
Clinically important, potentially hazardous interactions with: none known
Pregnancy category: C
Important contra-indications noted in the prescribing guidelines for: nursing mothers

---

Cardiovascular
Flushing (<10%) [2]

Central Nervous System
Headache [2]

Genitourinary
Priapism [4]

PHENYLEPHRINE

Trade names: Rynatan (MedPointe), Tussi-12D (MedPointe)
Indications: Nasal congestion, glaucoma, hypotension
Class: Adrenergic alpha-receptor agonist, Sympathomimetic
Half-life: 2.5 hours
Clinically important, potentially hazardous interactions with: epinephrine, furazolidone, iobenguane, MAO inhibitors, oxprenolol, phenelzine, tranylcypromine
Pregnancy category: C
Important contra-indications noted in the prescribing guidelines for: nursing mothers; pediatric patients

---

Skin
Dermatitis [16]
Hypersensitivity [2]
Stinging (from nasal or ophthalmic preparations) (<10%)

Cardiovascular
Bradycardia [3]
Hypertension [2]

Ocular
Blepharoconjunctivitis [4]
Periorbital dermatitis [3]

Other
Adverse effects [2]

PHENYTOIN

Synonyms: diphenylhydantoin; DPH; phenytoin sodium
Trade name: Dilantin (Pfizer)
Indications: Grand mal seizures
Class: Antiarrhythmic class Ib, Anticonvulsant, Antiepileptic, hydantoin, CYP3A4 inducer
Half-life: 7–42 hours (dose dependent)
Clinically important, potentially hazardous interactions with: abacavir, abiraterone, acitretin, afatinib, amiodarone, amitriptyline, amlodipine, amprenavir, apixaban, apremilast, aprepitant, artemether/lumefantrine, beclomethasone, boceprevir, buprenorphine, cabazitaxel, cabozantinib, caffeine, calcium, capecitabine, caspofungin, cefazolin, chloramphenicol, cimetidine, ciprofloxacin, citalopram, clobazam, clorazepate, cobicistat/elvitegravir/emtricitabine/tenofovir disoproxil, cobimetinib, colesevelam, crizotinib, cyclosporine, cyproterone, dabigatran, daclatasvir, darunavir, dasatinib, deferasirox, delavirdine, dexamethasone, diazoxide, disulfiram, dopamine, doxycycline, dronedarone, efavirenz, emtricitabine/rilpivirine/tenofovir alafenamide, enzalutamide, erlotinib, eslicarbazepine, ethosuximide, etravirine, everolimus, ezogabine, fesoterodine, flibanserin, floxuridine, fluconazole, flunisolide, fluoxetine, fosamprenavir, gefitinib, gold & gold compounds, hydrocortisone, ibrutinib, imatinib, indinavir, influenza vaccine, isoniazid, isotretinoin, isradipine, itraconazole, ixabepilone, lacosamide, lapatinib, ledipasvir & sofosbuvir, leflunomide, levodopa, levomepromazine, levonorgestrel, lisdexamfetamine, lomustine, lopinavir, meperidine, metformin, methsuximide, methylprednisolone, metronidazole, midazolam, mifepristone, mivacurium, nelfinavir, nifedipine, nilotinib, nilutamide, ombitasvir/paritaprevir/ritonavir, omeprazole, ondansetron, osimertinib, oxcarbazepine, oxtriphylline, paroxetine hydrochloride, pemetrexed, perampanel, phenylbutazone, piracetam, ponatinib, posaconazole, prednisolone, prednisone, propranolol, regorafenib, rifapentine, rilpivirine, riociguat, risperidone, ritonavir, rivaroxaban, roflumilast, romidepsin, saquinavir, simeprevir, sofosbuvir, solifenacin, sorafenib, St John's wort, sucralfate, sunitinib, tegafur/gimeracil/oteracil, telaprevir, telithromycin, temsirolimus, teniposide, thalidomide, tiagabine, ticagrelor, ticlopidine, tinidazole, tipranavir, tizanidine, tolvaptan, triamcinolone, trimethoprim, ulipristal, uracil/tegafur, vandetanib, vemurafenib, vigabatrin, voriconazole, vortioxetine, zidovudine, zuclopenthixol
Pregnancy category: D
Note: Aromatic antiepileptic drugs, phenytoin, phenobarbital, carbamazepine and primidone, are a frequent cause of severe cutaneous adverse reactions. A strong genetic association between HLA-B*1502 and phenytoin-induced Stevens-Johnson syndrome and toxic epidermal necrolysis has been shown in Han Chinese patients. Children whose mothers receive phenytoin during pregnancy are born with fetal hydantoin syndrome. The main features of this syndrome are mental and growth retardation, unusual facies,

digital and nail hypoplasia, and coarse scalp hair. Occasionally neonatal acne will be present.

Skin
- Acne keloid [2]
- Acneform eruption [8]
- AGEP [5]
- Angioedema [2]
- Anticonvulsant hypersensitivity syndrome [10]
- Coarse facies [4]
- Dermatomyositis [2]
- DRESS syndrome [28]
- Erythema multiforme [11]
- Erythroderma [8]
- Exanthems (6–71%) [22]
- Exfoliative dermatitis [15]
- Fixed eruption [5]
- Hypersensitivity [46]
- Linear IgA bullous dermatosis [8]
- Lupus erythematosus [19]
- Lymphoma [6]
- Mycosis fungoides [7]
- Pemphigus [2]
- Pigmentation [4]
- Pruritus [5]
- Pseudolymphoma [31]
- Purple glove syndrome [10]
- Purpura [4]
- Pustules [3]
- Rash (<10%) [12]
- Reticular hyperplasia [2]
- Serum sickness [2]
- Stevens–Johnson syndrome (14%) [56]
- Toxic epidermal necrolysis (2%) [63]
- Urticaria [5]
- Vasculitis (2%) [11]

Hair
- Alopecia [3]
- Hirsutism [8]

Nails
- Nail changes [2]
- Nail hypoplasia [3]

Mucosal
- Gingival hyperplasia/hypertrophy (>10%) [56]
- Mucocutaneous eruption [2]

Cardiovascular
- Bradycardia [2]
- Polyarteritis nodosa [2]

Central Nervous System
- Ageusia (taste loss) [2]
- Fetal hydantoin syndrome [8]
- Hallucinations [2]
- Neurotoxicity [2]
- Paresthesias [2]
- Restless legs syndrome [2]

Neuromuscular/Skeletal
- Digital malformations [4]
- Myalgia/Myopathy [2]
- Myasthenia gravis [2]
- Osteoporosis [2]
- Rhabdomyolysis [6]

Gastrointestinal/Hepatic
- Hepatotoxicity [8]

Respiratory
- Cough [2]

Ocular
- Hallucinations, visual [2]

Local
- Injection-site extravasation [2]
- Injection-site necrosis [2]

Other
- Adverse effects [2]
- Death [3]
- Hiccups [2]
- Teratogenicity [3]

PHYSOSTIGMINE

Synonym: eserine
Indications: Miotic in glaucoma treatment, reverses toxic CNS effects caused by anticholinergic drugs
Class: Cholinesterase inhibitor
Half-life: 15–40 minutes
Clinically important, potentially hazardous interactions with: bethanechol, corticosteroids, galantamine, methacholine, succinylcholine
Pregnancy category: C
Important contra-indications noted in the prescribing guidelines for: nursing mothers
Note: Antilirium is a derivative of the Calabar bean, and its active moiety, physostigmine, is also known as eserine. Physostigmine is used to reverse the effect upon the nervous system caused by clinical or toxic dosages of drugs and herbs capable of producing the anticholinergic syndrome. Some of the drugs responsible are: amitriptyline, amoxapine, atropine, benztropine, biperiden, clidinium, cyclobenzaprine, desipramine, doxepin, hyoscyamine, imipramine, lorazepam, maprotiline, nortriptyline, protriptyline, propantheline, scopolamine, trimipramine. Some herbals that can elicit the anticholinergic syndrome are black henbane, deadly nightshade, Devil's apple, Jimson weed, Loco seeds or weeds, Matrimony vine, night blooming jessamine, stinkweed.

Skin
- Diaphoresis (>10%)
- Erythema (<10%)

Mucosal
- Sialorrhea (>10%)

Cardiovascular
- Atrial fibrillation [2]
- Bradycardia [3]

Central Nervous System
- Seizures (<10%) [3]
- Twitching (<10%)

Gastrointestinal/Hepatic
- Nausea [4]
- Vomiting [2]

Ocular
- Epiphora (>10%)
- Ocular burning (<10%)
- Ocular stinging (>10%)

PHYTONADIONE

Synonym: vitamin K_1
Trade names: Mephyton (Valeant), Vitamin K (AbbVie)
Indications: Coagulation disorders
Class: Vitamin
Half-life: 2–4 hours
Clinically important, potentially hazardous interactions with: cholestyramine, orlistat, warfarin
Pregnancy category: C
Important contra-indications noted in the prescribing guidelines for: nursing mothers; pediatric patients

Skin
- Anaphylactoid reactions/Anaphylaxis [4]
- Dermatitis [9]
- Eczema [2]
- Nicolau syndrome [2]
- Scleroderma [12]
- Urticaria [4]

Local
- Injection-site eczematous eruption [10]
- Injection-site erythema [2]
- Injection-site induration [15]

Other
- Allergic reactions [2]

PILOCARPINE

Trade names: Ocusert Pilo (Akorn), Pilopine (Alcon), Salagen (MGI)
Indications: Glaucoma, miosis induction, xerostomia
Class: Miotic, Muscarinic cholinergic agonist
Half-life: N/A
Clinically important, potentially hazardous interactions with: acebutolol, galantamine
Pregnancy category: C
Important contra-indications noted in the prescribing guidelines for: nursing mothers; pediatric patients

Skin
- Burning (<10%)
- Dermatitis [4]
- Diaphoresis [5]
- Edema (4%)
- Hyperhidrosis [2]
- Hypersensitivity (<10%)
- Stinging (<10%)

Central Nervous System
- Dysgeusia (taste perversion) (2%)
- Headache [2]

Ocular
- Cataract [2]

PIMAVANSERIN *

Trade name: Nuplazid (Acadia)
Indications: Hallucinations and delusions associated with Parkinson's disease psychosis
Class: Antipsychotic
Half-life: 57 hours
Clinically important, potentially hazardous interactions with: amiodarone, carbamazepine, chlorpromazine, clarithromycin, disopyramide, drugs known to prolong the QT interval, gatifloxacin, indinavir, itraconazole, ketoconazole, moxifloxacin, phenytoin, procainamide, quinidine, rifampin, sotalol, St John's wort, strong CYP3A4 inhibitors and inducers, thioridazine, ziprasidone
Pregnancy category: N/A (No data available)
Important contra-indications noted in the prescribing guidelines for: the elderly; nursing mothers; pediatric patients
Black Box Warning: INCREASED MORTALITY IN ELDERLY PATIENTS WITH DEMENTIA-RELATED PSYCHOSIS

Skin
Peripheral edema (7%)

Central Nervous System
Confusion (6%)
Gait instability (2%) [2]
Hallucinations (5%)

Gastrointestinal/Hepatic
Constipation (4%)
Nausea (7%)

Cardiovascular
Cardiac arrest [2]

Respiratory
Upper respiratory tract infection (19%)

Local
Application-site burning (8–26%)
Application-site reactions (2%)

Other
Infection (5%) [2]

PIMECROLIMUS

Trade name: Elidel (Valeant)
Indications: Second-line therapy for the short-term and non-continuous chronic treatment of mild to moderate atopic dermatitis
Class: Immunomodulator, Macrolactam
Half-life: N/A
Clinically important, potentially hazardous interactions with: abatacept, alcohol, alefacept, aprepitant, azacitidine, betamethasone, cabazitaxel, calcium channel blockers, cimetidine, conivaptan, CYP3A4 inhibitors, darunavir, delavirdine, denileukin, docetaxel, efavirenz, erythromycin, fingolimod, fluconazole, gefitinib, immunosuppressants, indinavir, itraconazole, ketoconazole, lapatinib, leflunomide, lenalidomide, oxaliplatin, pazopanib, pemetrexed, telithromycin, temsirolimus, triamcinolone, voriconazole
Pregnancy category: C
Important contra-indications noted in the prescribing guidelines for: nursing mothers; pediatric patients
Black Box Warning: LONG-TERM SAFETY OF TOPICAL CALCINEURIN INHIBITORS HAS NOT BEEN ESTABLISHED.

Skin
Burning [4]
Dermatitis [2]
Peripheral edema [3]
Rosacea [5]
Tinea [3]

PIMOZIDE

Trade name: Orap (Teva)
Indications: Tourette's syndrome, schizophrenia
Class: Antipsychotic
Half-life: 50 hours
Clinically important, potentially hazardous interactions with: amitriptyline, amoxapine, amphetamines, amprenavir, aprepitant, arsenic, artemether/lumefantrine, astemizole, atazanavir, azithromycin, azole antifungals, boceprevir, citalopram, clarithromycin, crizotinib, darunavir, dasatinib, degarelix, delavirdine, dirithromycin, dolasetron, droperidol, efavirenz, enzalutamide, erythromycin, fluoxetine, fosamprenavir, grapefruit juice, imatinib, indinavir, itraconazole, ketoconazole, lapatinib, levofloxacin, levomepromazine, lopinavir, lurasidone, methylphenidate, mifepristone, moxifloxacin, nefazodone, nelfinavir, nilotinib, ombitasvir/paritaprevir/ritonavir, paroxetine hydrochloride, pazopanib, pemoline, phenothiazines, posaconazole, protease inhibitors, quinidine, quinine, ritonavir, saquinavir, sertraline, sotalol, sparfloxacin, sulpiride, telaprevir, telavancin, telithromycin, thioridazine, tipranavir, tricyclic antidepressants, trifluoperazine, troleandomycin, vandetanib, voriconazole, vorinostat, zileuton, ziprasidone
Pregnancy category: C
Important contra-indications noted in the prescribing guidelines for: nursing mothers; pediatric patients

---

Skin
Facial edema (<10%)
Rash (8%)

Mucosal
Sialorrhea (14%)
Xerostomia (>10%) [3]

Cardiovascular
QT prolongation [4]

Neuromuscular/Skeletal
Myalgia/Myopathy (3%)

Endocrine/Metabolic
Gynecomastia (>10%)

PIOGLITAZONE

Trade name: Actos (Takeda)
Indications: Type II diabetes
Class: Antidiabetic, CYP3A4 inducer, Thiazolidinedione
Half-life: 3–7 hours
Clinically important, potentially hazardous interactions with: alcohol, conivaptan, corticosteroids, CYP2C8 inhibitors and inducers, dapagliflozin, deferasirox, gemfibrozil, insulin, pegvisomant, pregabalin, rifampin, saxagliptin, somatropin, teriflunomide, trimethoprim
Pregnancy category: C
Important contra-indications noted in the prescribing guidelines for: nursing mothers; pediatric patients
Note: Contraindicated in patients with established NYHA Class III or IV heart failure.
Black Box Warning: CONGESTIVE HEART FAILURE

Skin
Edema (4–11%) [27]
Peripheral edema [12]

Cardiovascular
Cardiac failure (<10%) [13]
Cardiomyopathy [3]
Cardiotoxicity [2]
Myocardial infarction [3]

Central Nervous System
Headache (9%) [4]
Stroke [2]

Neuromuscular/Skeletal
Asthenia (fatigue) (4%)
Bone loss [4]
Fractures [8]
Myalgia/Myopathy (5%)

Gastrointestinal/Hepatic
Diarrhea [4]
Hepatotoxicity [8]
Nausea [3]
Vomiting [2]

Respiratory
Nasopharyngitis [3]
Pharyngitis (5%)
Sinusitis (6%)
Upper respiratory tract infection (13%)

Endocrine/Metabolic
Hypoglycemia [10]
Weight gain [17]

Genitourinary
Bladder cancer [7]

Hematologic
Anemia (<2%) [2]
Pancytopenia [2]

Ocular
Macular edema [2]

Other
Adverse effects [4]
Death [3]
Tooth disorder (5%)

PIPERACILLIN/ TAZOBACTAM

Trade name: Zosyn (Wyeth)
Indications: Moderate to severe infections
Class: Antibacterial
Half-life: 0.7-1.2 hours
Clinically important, potentially hazardous interactions with: heparin, methotrexate
Pregnancy category: B
Important contra-indications noted in the prescribing guidelines for: nursing mothers

---

Skin
AGEP [2]
DRESS syndrome [3]
Rash [5]

Central Nervous System
Fever [3]
Neurotoxicity [2]

Gastrointestinal/Hepatic
Diarrhea [4]
Hepatotoxicity [3]
Nausea [2]
Vomiting [2]

Endocrine/Metabolic
Hypokalemia [2]

Renal
Nephrotoxicity [3]

Hematologic
Hemolytic anemia [3]
Hemotoxicity [2]
Thrombocytopenia [4]

Other
Adverse effects [3]

PIRFENIDONE

Trade name: Esbriet (Intermune)
Indications: Idiopathic pulmonary fibrosis
Class: Immunosuppressant, Pyridone
Half-life: 3 hours
Clinically important, potentially hazardous interactions with: ciprofloxacin, fluvoxamine
Pregnancy category: C
Important contra-indications noted in the prescribing guidelines for: nursing mothers; pediatric patients

---

Skin
Photosensitivity (9%) [20]
Phototoxicity [2]
Pruritus (8%) [3]
Rash (30%) [13]

Cardiovascular
Chest pain (5%) [3]

Central Nervous System
Anorexia (13%) [10]
Dysgeusia (taste perversion) (6%)
Headache (22%) [3]
Insomnia (10%)
Sedation [2]
Vertigo (dizziness) (18%) [6]

Neuromuscular/Skeletal
Arthralgia (10%)
Asthenia (fatigue) (6–26%) [7]

Gastrointestinal/Hepatic
Abdominal pain (24%) [7]
Diarrhea (26%) [10]
Dyspepsia (19%) [9]
Gastroesophageal reflux (11%) [5]
Hepatotoxicity [4]
Nausea (36%) [17]
Vomiting (13%) [6]

Respiratory
Cough [2]
Dyspnea [2]
Nasopharyngitis [2]
Sinusitis (11%)
Upper respiratory tract infection (27%) [2]

Endocrine/Metabolic
ALT increased [5]
Appetite decreased (8%) [3]
AST increased [5]
Weight loss (10%) [3]

Other
Adverse effects [9]

PIROXICAM

Trade name: Feldene (Pfizer)
Indications: Arthritis
Class: Non-steroidal anti-inflammatory (NSAID)
Half-life: 50 hours
Clinically important, potentially hazardous interactions with: ACE inhibitors, aspirin, furosemide, lithium, methotrexate, ritonavir, warfarin
Pregnancy category: C
Important contra-indications noted in the prescribing guidelines for: the elderly; nursing mothers
Note: NSAIDs may cause an increased risk of serious cardiovascular and gastrointestinal adverse events, which can be fatal. This risk may increase with duration of use.
Elderly patients are at greater risk for serious gastrointestinal events.
Black Box Warning: CARDIOVASCULAR AND GASTROINTESTINAL RISKS

Skin
AGEP [2]
Angioedema [3]
Dermatitis [5]
Erythema multiforme [12]
Erythroderma [2]
Exanthems (>5%) [8]
Fixed eruption [15]
Lichenoid eruption [5]
Linear IgA bullous dermatosis [3]
Pemphigus [3]
Photosensitivity [40]
Pruritus (<10%) [6]
Purpura [2]
Rash (>10%)
Stevens–Johnson syndrome [2]
Toxic epidermal necrolysis [12]
Urticaria [7]
Vasculitis [3]
Vesiculation [2]

Hair
Alopecia [3]

Mucosal
Aphthous stomatitis [4]

Central Nervous System
Anorexia (<10%)
Vertigo (dizziness) (<10%)

Gastrointestinal/Hepatic
Abdominal pain (<10%)
Constipation (<10%)
Diarrhea (<10%)
Dyspepsia (<10%)
Flatulence (<10%)
Gastrointestinal ulceration (<10%)
Nausea (<10%)
Vomiting (<10%)

Renal
Renal function abnormal (<10%)

Otic
Hearing loss [2]
Tinnitus [2]

Other
Adverse effects [2]
Side effects (47%)

PITAVASTATIN

Trade name: Livalo (Kowa)
Indications: Primary hyperlipidemia, mixed dyslipidemia
Class: Statin
Half-life: 12 hours
Clinically important, potentially hazardous interactions with: alcohol, cyclosporine, erythromycin, gemfibrozil, lopinavir, niacin, rifampin, ritonavir
Pregnancy category: X
Important contra-indications noted in the prescribing guidelines for: nursing mothers; pediatric patients
Note: Contraindicated in patients with active liver disease.

Skin
Hypersensitivity (<2%)
Rash (<2%)
Urticaria (<2%)

Central Nervous System
Headache (<2%)

Neuromuscular/Skeletal
Arthralgia (<2%)
Back pain (2–4%)
Myalgia/Myopathy (2–3%) [5]
Pain in extremities (<2%)

Gastrointestinal/Hepatic
Constipation (2–4%)
Diarrhea (2–3%)

Respiratory
Influenza (<2%)
Nasopharyngitis (<2%) [2]

Endocrine/Metabolic
ALT increased [2]
AST increased [2]
Creatine phosphokinase increased [2]

Other
Adverse effects [3]

PNEUMOCOCCAL VACCINE

Trade names: PCV (Lederle), PncOMP (Merck), Pneumovax II (Sanofi-Aventis), Pnu-Immune (Lederle), PPV (Lederle), Prevnar (Wyeth)
Indications: Prevention of bacteremia, meningitis, pneumonia, respiratory tract infections, otitis media, sinusitis
Class: Vaccine
Half-life: N/A
Clinically important, potentially hazardous interactions with: none known
Pregnancy category: C

Skin
Anaphylactoid reactions/Anaphylaxis [2]
Rash [2]
Serum sickness [2]
Urticaria [5]

Central Nervous System
Fever [20]
Headache [3]
Irritability [3]
Seizures [4]
Sleep disturbances [2]

Neuromuscular/Skeletal
Arthralgia [2]
Asthenia (fatigue) [6]
Myalgia/Myopathy [3]

Respiratory
Respiratory tract infection [2]

Endocrine/Metabolic
Appetite decreased [2]

Local
Injection-site edema [8]
Injection-site erythema [10]
Injection-site induration [3]
Injection-site pain [10]
Injection-site reactions [9]

POLIDOCANOL

Trade names: Asclera (Chemische Fabrik Kreussler), Varithena (BTG)
Indications: Uncomplicated spider veins and uncomplicated reticular veins in the lower extremity
Class: Sclerosant, local
Half-life: 1.5 hours
Clinically important, potentially hazardous interactions with: none known
Pregnancy category: C
Important contra-indications noted in the prescribing guidelines for: nursing mothers; pediatric patients
Note: Severe allergic reactions have been reported following polidocanol use, including anaphylactic reactions, some of them fatal. Severe reactions are more frequent with use of larger volumes (>3 mL).
Contraindicated in patients with acute thromboembolic diseases.

Skin
Anaphylactoid reactions/Anaphylaxis [4]
Pigmentation [2]
Urticaria [2]

Cardiovascular
Cardiac arrest [2]
Phlebitis [2]

Central Nervous System
Migraine [2]

Neuromuscular/Skeletal
Leg pain [2]

Hematologic
Thrombosis [2]

Local
Injection-site hematoma (42%)
Injection-site irritation (41%)
Injection-site pain (24%)
Injection-site pigmentation (38%)
Injection-site pruritus (19%)
Injection-site reactions [3]
Injection-site thrombosis (6%)

POMALIDOMIDE

Trade name: Pomalyst (Celgene)
Indications: Multiple myeloma in patients who have received at least two prior therapies including lenalidomide and bortezomib
Class: Immunomodulator, Thalidomide analog
Half-life: 7.5–9.5 hours
Clinically important, potentially hazardous interactions with: ketoconazole, P-glycoprotein, rifampin
Pregnancy category: X
Important contra-indications noted in the prescribing guidelines for: nursing mothers; pediatric patients
Black Box Warning: EMBRYO-FETAL TOXICITY and VENOUS AND ARTERIAL THROMBOEMBOLISM

Skin
Edema [2]
Hyperhidrosis (6%)
Peripheral edema (23%)
Pruritus (15%)
Rash (22%) [2]
Xerosis (9%)

Mucosal
Epistaxis (nosebleed) (15%)

Cardiovascular
Chest pain (22%)
Venous thromboembolism [8]

Central Nervous System
Anxiety (11%)
Chills (9%)
Confusion (10%)
Fever (19%) [3]
Headache (13%)
Insomnia (7%)
Neurotoxicity (18%) [3]
Pain (6%)
Peripheral neuropathy (10%) [2]
Tremor (9%) [2]
Vertigo (dizziness) (20%)

Neuromuscular/Skeletal
Arthralgia (16%)
Asthenia (fatigue) (12–55%) [9]
Back pain (32%) [3]
Bone or joint pain (11–12%) [2]
Muscle spasm (19%)
Myalgia/Myopathy [2]
Pain in extremities (5%)

Gastrointestinal/Hepatic
Constipation (36%) [2]
Diarrhea (34%) [2]
Nausea (36%)
Vomiting (14%)

Respiratory
Cough (14%)
Dyspnea (34%) [5]
Pneumonia (23%) [6]
Upper respiratory tract infection (32%)

Endocrine/Metabolic
Appetite decreased (22%)
Dehydration [2]
Hypercalcemia (21%)
Hyperglycemia (12%)
Hypocalcemia (6%)
Hypokalemia (10%)
Hyponatremia (10%)
Serum creatinine increased (15%)
Weight loss (14%)

Genitourinary
Urinary tract infection (8%)

Renal
Renal failure (15%)

Hematologic
Anemia (38%) [12]
Febrile neutropenia [2]
Leukopenia (11%) [3]
Lymphopenia (4%) [2]
Myelosuppression [3]
Neutropenia (52%) [18]
Sepsis [2]
Thrombocytopenia (25%) [12]

Other
Death [3]
Infection [5]

POSACONAZOLE

Trade name: Noxafil (Schering)
Indications: *Aspergillus* and *Candida* infection prophylaxis in immunocompromised patients
Class: Antibiotic, triazole, Antifungal, azole
Half-life: 35 hours
Clinically important, potentially hazardous interactions with: alprazolam, atazanavir, atorvastatin, boceprevir, cabozantinib, calcium channel blockers, cimetidine, cyclosporine, digoxin, dihydroergotamine, diltiazem, dronedarone, efavirenz, ergotamine, esomeprazole, everolimus, felodipine, flibanserin, fosamprenavir, HMG-CoA reductase inhibitors, lapatinib, lomitapide, lovastatin, metoclopramide, midazolam, mifepristone, nicardipine, nifedipine, omeprazole, pantoprazole, phenytoin, pimozide, ponatinib, quinidine, regorafenib, rifabutin, rilpivirine, ritonavir, rivaroxaban, ruxolitinib, simeprevir, simvastatin, sirolimus, tacrolimus,

telaprevir, temsirolimus, triazolam, venetoclax, verapamil, vinblastine, vincristine
Pregnancy category: C
Important contra-indications noted in the prescribing guidelines for: nursing mothers; pediatric patients

---

Skin
- Edema (9%)
- Herpes (14%)
- Herpes simplex (3–15%)
- Hyperhidrosis (2–10%)
- Jaundice (<5%)
- Peripheral edema (15%)
- Petechiae (11%)
- Pruritus (11%)
- Rash (3–19%) [2]
- Thrombocytopenic purpura (<5%)

Mucosal
- Epistaxis (nosebleed) (14%)
- Mucositis (17%)
- Oral candidiasis (<12%)

Cardiovascular
- Hypertension (18%)
- Hypotension (14%)
- QT prolongation [3]
- Tachycardia (12%)
- Torsades de pointes (<5%)

Central Nervous System
- Anorexia (2–19%)
- Anxiety (9%)
- Dysgeusia (taste perversion) (~2%)
- Fever (6–45%)
- Headache (8–28%) [4]
- Insomnia (<17%)
- Neurotoxicity [2]
- Paresthesias (<5%)
- Rigors (<20%)
- Tremor (~2%)
- Vertigo (dizziness) (11%) [3]

Neuromuscular/Skeletal
- Arthralgia (11%)
- Asthenia (fatigue) (3–17%)
- Back pain (10%)
- Bone or joint pain (16%)
- Myalgia/Myopathy (16%)

Gastrointestinal/Hepatic
- Abdominal pain (5–27%) [3]
- Constipation (21%)
- Diarrhea (10–42%) [4]
- Dyspepsia (10%)
- Hepatitis (<5%)
- Hepatomegaly (<5%)
- Hepatotoxicity (<5%) [3]
- Nausea (9–38%) [9]
- Vomiting (7–29%) [4]

Respiratory
- Cough (3–25%)
- Dyspnea (<20%)
- Pharyngitis (12%)
- Pneumonia (3–10%)
- Pulmonary embolism (<5%)
- Upper respiratory tract infection (7%)

Endocrine/Metabolic
- Adrenal insufficiency (<5%)
- ALP increased (3–13%)
- ALT increased (3–11%) [2]
- AST increased (6–17%) [2]
- Dehydration (<11%)
- Hyperglycemia (11%)
- Hypocalcemia (9%)
- Hypokalemia (30%)
- Hypomagnesemia (18%)
- Weight loss (<14%)

Genitourinary
- Vaginal bleeding (10%)

Renal
- Renal failure (<5%)

Hematologic
- Anemia (2–25%)
- Febrile neutropenia (20%)
- Hemolytic uremic syndrome (<5%)
- Neutropenia (4–23%)
- Thrombocytopenia (29%)

Ocular
- Vision blurred (~2%)

Other
- Adverse effects [11]
- Allergic reactions (<5%)
- Infection (18%)

POTASSIUM IODIDE

Synonyms: KI; Lugol's solution
Trade name: SSKI (Upsher-Smith)
Indications: Hyperthyroidism, erythema nodosum, sporotrichosis
Class: Antihyperthyroid, Antimycobacterial
Half-life: N/A
Clinically important, potentially hazardous interactions with: ACE inhibitors, potassium-sparing diuretics, spironolactone, triamterene
Pregnancy category: D
Important contra-indications noted in the prescribing guidelines for: nursing mothers

---

Skin
- Acneform eruption (<10%) [3]
- Angioedema (<10%)
- Bullous pemphigoid [2]
- Dermatitis herpetiformis [2]
- Iododerma [17]
- Psoriasis [2]
- Urticaria (<10%)
- Vasculitis [3]

Central Nervous System
- Dysgeusia (taste perversion) (<10%) [2]

Gastrointestinal/Hepatic
- Gastrointestinal disorder [2]

Endocrine/Metabolic
- Hypothyroidism [2]

PRALIDOXIME

Trade name: Protopam (Baxter)
Indications: Muscle weakness and respiratory depression caused by organophosphate drugs which have anticholinesterase activity, antidote to overdose of anticholinesterase drugs
Class: Antidote
Half-life: 2.4–5.3 hours
Clinically important, potentially hazardous interactions with: succinylcholine
Pregnancy category: C
Important contra-indications noted in the prescribing guidelines for: the elderly; nursing mothers
Note: Pralidoxime is not effective in the treatment of poisoning due to phosphorus, inorganic phosphates, or organophosphates not having anticholinesterase activity. Pralidoxime is not indicated as an antidote for intoxication by pesticides of the carbamate class since it may increase the toxicity of carbaryl. In therapy it has been difficult to differentiate side effects due to the drug from those due to the effects of the poison.

PRAMIPEXOLE

Trade name: Mirapex (Boehringer Ingelheim)
Indications: Parkinsonism, restless legs syndrome
Class: Dopamine receptor agonist
Half-life: ~8 hours
Clinically important, potentially hazardous interactions with: levomepromazine, risperidone, zuclopenthixol
Pregnancy category: C
Important contra-indications noted in the prescribing guidelines for: nursing mothers; pediatric patients

---

Skin
- Edema (5%)
- Peripheral edema (5%) [3]

Mucosal
- Xerostomia (7%) [3]

Cardiovascular
- Chest pain (3%)
- Hypotension (~53%) [2]
- Orthostatic hypotension [2]

Central Nervous System
- Abnormal dreams (11%)
- Akathisia (2–3%)
- Amnesia (4–6%)
- Anorexia (<5%)
- Compulsions [6]
- Confusion [2]
- Depression (2%)
- Dyskinesia (17–47%) [2]
- Hallucinations (5–17%) [4]
- Headache (4–7%) [3]
- Hyperesthesia (3%)
- Impulse control disorder [10]
- Insomnia (4–27%)
- Restless legs syndrome [2]
- Somnolence (drowsiness) (9–36%) [7]
- Tremor (4%)
- Twitching (2%)
- Vertigo (dizziness) (2–26%) [5]

Neuromuscular/Skeletal
- Antecollis [2]
- Arthralgia (4%)
- Asthenia (fatigue) (<14%) [2]

Gastrointestinal/Hepatic
- Constipation [4]
- Nausea [7]
- Vomiting (4%) [3]

Respiratory
Cough (3%)
Dyspnea (4%)
Rhinitis (3%)

Genitourinary
Urinary frequency (6%)
Urinary tract infection (4%)

Other
Adverse effects (2%) [5]

PRASUGREL

Trade name: Effient (Lilly)
Indications: Acute coronary syndrome in patients who are to be managed with percutaneous coronary intervention
Class: Antiplatelet, thienopyridine
Half-life: 2–15 hours
Clinically important, potentially hazardous interactions with: clopidogrel, conivaptan, coumarins, darunavir, delavirdine, diclofenac, indinavir, meloxicam, NSAIDs, phenindione, telithromycin, voriconazole, warfarin
Pregnancy category: B
Important contra-indications noted in the prescribing guidelines for: the elderly; nursing mothers; pediatric patients
Note: Contraindicated in patients with active pathological bleeding, prior transient ischemic attack or stroke.
Black Box Warning: BLEEDING RISK

Skin
Hypersensitivity [2]
Peripheral edema (3%)
Rash (3%) [4]

Mucosal
Epistaxis (nosebleed) (6%)

Cardiovascular
Atrial fibrillation (3%)
Bradycardia (3%)
Chest pain (3%)
Hypertension (8%)
Hypotension (4%)

Central Nervous System
Fever (3%)
Headache (6%)
Vertigo (dizziness) (4%)

Neuromuscular/Skeletal
Asthenia (fatigue) (4%)
Back pain (5%)
Pain in extremities (3%)

Gastrointestinal/Hepatic
Diarrhea (3%)
Gastrointestinal bleeding (2%)
Nausea (5%)

Respiratory
Cough (4%)
Dyspnea (5%)
Respiratory distress [2]

Endocrine/Metabolic
Hypercholesterolemia (7%)
Hyperlipidemia (7%)

Hematologic
Anemia (2%)
Bleeding (<14%) [23]
Hemorrhage [2]
Leukopenia (3%)

Other
Malignant neoplasms (2%)

PRAVASTATIN

Trade names: Lipostat (Bristol-Myers Squibb), Pravachol (Bristol-Myers Squibb)
Indications: Hypercholesterolemia
Class: HMG-CoA reductase inhibitor, Statin
Half-life: ~2–3 hours
Clinically important, potentially hazardous interactions with: azithromycin, ciprofibrate, clarithromycin, colchicine, cyclosporine, darunavir, efavirenz, erythromycin, gemfibrozil, imatinib, red rice yeast, telithromycin
Pregnancy category: X
Important contra-indications noted in the prescribing guidelines for: nursing mothers

Skin
Dermatomyositis [2]
Edema (3%)
Lichenoid eruption [2]
Pruritus [2]
Rash (5–7%) [7]

Cardiovascular
Angina (5%)
Chest pain (3–10%)

Central Nervous System
Anxiety (5%)
Fever (2%)
Headache (6%)
Nervousness (5%)
Paresthesias (3%)
Sleep disturbances (3%)
Vertigo (dizziness) (4–7%)

Neuromuscular/Skeletal
Asthenia (fatigue) (3–8%)
Bone or joint pain (25%)
Cramps (5%)
Myalgia/Myopathy (2–3%) [9]
Rhabdomyolysis [24]

Gastrointestinal/Hepatic
Abdominal distension (2%)
Diarrhea (7%)
Dyspepsia (3%)
Flatulence (3%)
Nausea (7%)
Pancreatitis [4]
Vomiting (7%)

Respiratory
Bronchitis (3%)
Cough (3–8%)
Influenza (9%)
Pharyngitis (2%)
Pulmonary toxicity (4%)
Rhinitis (4%)
Upper respiratory tract infection (6–21%)

Endocrine/Metabolic
ALT increased (3%)
Creatine phosphokinase increased (4%) [3]
GGT increased (2%)
Weight gain (4%)
Weight loss (3%)

Genitourinary
Urinary tract infection (3%)

Renal
Renal failure [2]

Ocular
Diplopia (3%)
Vision blurred (3%)

Other
Adverse effects [2]
Infection (3%)

PRAZIQUANTEL

Trade name: Biltricide (Bayer)
Indications: Helmintic infections
Class: Anthelmintic
Half-life: 0.8–1.5 hours
Clinically important, potentially hazardous interactions with: dexamethasone, efavirenz, oxcarbazepine, rifampin, rifapentine
Pregnancy category: B
Important contra-indications noted in the prescribing guidelines for: nursing mothers

Skin
Diaphoresis (<10%)
Edema [2]
Pruritus [3]
Rash [2]
Urticaria [5]

Central Nervous System
Fever [2]
Headache [7]
Seizures [2]
Somnolence (drowsiness) [2]
Vertigo (dizziness) [7]

Neuromuscular/Skeletal
Asthenia (fatigue) [3]

Gastrointestinal/Hepatic
Abdominal pain [8]
Diarrhea [4]
Nausea [5]
Vomiting [5]

Other
Adverse effects [2]
Allergic reactions [2]

PREDNISOLONE

Trade names: Blephamide (Allergan), Delta-Cortef (Pharmacia), Hydeltrasol (Merck), Inflamase (Novartis), Pediapred (UCB), Prelone (Teva)
Indications: Arthralgias, asthma, dermatoses, inflammatory ocular conditions
Class: Corticosteroid, systemic
Half-life: 2–4 hours
Clinically important, potentially hazardous interactions with: aluminum, aminophylline, carbamazepine, carbimazole, cyclosporine, daclizumab, diuretics, etoposide, etretinate, grapefruit juice, indomethacin, isoniazid, itraconazole, ketoconazole, live vaccines,

methotrexate, naproxen, oral contraceptives, pancuronium, phenobarbital, phenytoin, rifampin, troleandomycin
Pregnancy category: C

Skin
Acneform eruption [4]
AGEP [2]
Candidiasis [2]
Dermatitis [3]
Edema [6]
Erythema [2]
Erythema multiforme [2]
Exanthems [3]
Kaposi's sarcoma [3]
Pruritus [2]
Stevens–Johnson syndrome [2]
Toxicity [2]

Hair
Alopecia [2]

Cardiovascular
Atrial fibrillation [2]
Cardiotoxicity [4]
Flushing [2]
Hypertension [12]
Tachycardia [2]

Central Nervous System
Behavioral disturbances [2]
Depression [4]

Neuromuscular/Skeletal
Arthralgia [4]
Asthenia (fatigue) [4]
Back pain [4]
Bone or joint pain [4]
Myalgia/Myopathy [2]
Osteonecrosis [4]
Osteoporosis [32]

Gastrointestinal/Hepatic
Constipation [3]
Diarrhea [2]
Hepatotoxicity [6]
Nausea [2]
Pancreatitis [2]

Respiratory
Upper respiratory tract infection [2]

Endocrine/Metabolic
Cushing's syndrome [2]
Diabetes mellitus [4]
Hyperglycemia [3]
Hypokalemia [6]

Hematologic
Anemia [3]
Febrile neutropenia [3]
Neutropenia [4]
Thrombocytopenia [2]

Ocular
Cataract [5]
Chorioretinopathy [2]
Glaucoma [2]
Intraocular pressure increased [4]

Other
Adverse effects [10]
Allergic reactions [2]
Death [2]
Infection [17]
Side effects [4]

PREDNISONE

Trade names: Deltasone (Pharmacia), Meticorten (Schering)
Indications: Arthralgias, asthma, dermatoses, inflammatory ocular conditions
Class: Corticosteroid, systemic
Half-life: N/A
Clinically important, potentially hazardous interactions with: aluminum, aminophylline, aspirin, chlorambucil, cimetidine, clarithromycin, cyclophosphamide, cyclosporine, dicumarol, diuretics, docetaxel, estrogens, grapefruit juice, indomethacin, influenza vaccine, itraconazole, ketoconazole, lansoprazole, live vaccines, methotrexate, montelukast, omeprazole, oral contraceptives, pancuronium, phenobarbital, phenytoin, ranitidine, rifampin, timolol, tolbutamide, vitamin A, yellow fever vaccine
Pregnancy category: B
Important contra-indications noted in the prescribing guidelines for: the elderly; nursing mothers

---

Skin
Dermatitis [4]
Ecchymoses [2]
Erythema [3]
Kaposi's sarcoma [7]
Squamous cell carcinoma [2]
Thinning [2]
Toxicity [2]

Hair
Alopecia [2]

Mucosal
Stomatitis [2]

Cardiovascular
Cardiotoxicity [2]
Hypertension [7]

Central Nervous System
Headache [3]
Leukoencephalopathy [3]
Peripheral neuropathy [4]

Neuromuscular/Skeletal
Arthralgia [2]
Asthenia (fatigue) [7]
Fractures [3]
Myalgia/Myopathy [2]
Osteonecrosis [3]
Osteoporosis [23]

Gastrointestinal/Hepatic
Constipation [2]
Diarrhea [4]
Nausea [4]
Vomiting [2]

Endocrine/Metabolic
Hyperglycemia [3]

Hematologic
Anemia [4]
Febrile neutropenia [2]
Leukopenia [2]
Lymphopenia [2]
Neutropenia [12]
Thrombocytopenia [8]

Ocular
Cataract [3]

Other
Adverse effects [9]
Death [2]
Infection [11]
Side effects [3]

PREGABALIN

Trade name: Lyrica (Pfizer)
Indications: Neuropathy, post-herpetic neuralgia, partial epilepsy, fibromyalgia
Class: Anticonvulsant, GABA analog
Half-life: 6 hours
Clinically important, potentially hazardous interactions with: lacosamide, pioglitazone
Pregnancy category: C
Important contra-indications noted in the prescribing guidelines for: nursing mothers; pediatric patients

---

Skin
Edema (2%) [8]
Peripheral edema (9%) [12]

Mucosal
Xerostomia (5%) [11]

Cardiovascular
Cardiac failure [3]
Chest pain (2%)

Central Nervous System
Anorgasmia [2]
Confusion [2]
Depression [2]
Gait instability [4]
Headache (7%) [7]
Impaired concentration [2]
Insomnia [3]
Memory loss [2]
Neurotoxicity [2]
Pain (5%)
Sedation [5]
Somnolence (drowsiness) [42]
Suicidal ideation [4]
Tremor [2]
Vertigo (dizziness) (4%) [54]

Neuromuscular/Skeletal
Asthenia (fatigue) (5%) [8]
Ataxia [8]
Back pain (2%)
Muscle spasm [2]
Myoclonus [4]
Rhabdomyolysis [3]

Gastrointestinal/Hepatic
Constipation [5]
Diarrhea [2]
Nausea [8]
Vomiting [2]

Endocrine/Metabolic
Appetite increased [2]
Weight gain [20]

Genitourinary
Erectile dysfunction [3]

Ocular
Diplopia (9%) [2]
Ocular edema [2]
Vision blurred (6%) [7]

Other
- Adverse effects [5]
- Infection (7%)
- Side effects [2]

PRILOCAINE

Trade name: Citanest (AstraZeneca)
Indications: Local anesthetic
Class: Membrane integrity antagonist, Potassium channel antagonist, Sodium channel antagonist
Half-life: 2 hours
Clinically important, potentially hazardous interactions with: adenosine, amide-type anesthetics, antimalarials, co-trimoxazole, dronedarone, nitric compounds, sulfonamides
Pregnancy category: B
Important contra-indications noted in the prescribing guidelines for: nursing mothers; pediatric patients

---

Skin
- Angioedema [3]
- Contact dermatitis [3]
- Hypersensitivity [2]
- Petechiae [3]
- Purpura [3]

Central Nervous System
- Coma [4]
- Paresthesias [3]
- Seizures [2]

Hematologic
- Methemoglobinemia [11]

Other
- Adverse effects [2]

PROBENECID

Indications: Gouty arthritis
Class: Uricosuric
Half-life: 6–12 hours (dose-dependent)
Clinically important, potentially hazardous interactions with: acemetacin, acetaminophen, amphotericin B, ampicillin/sulbactam, benzodiazepines, captopril, cefazolin, cefditoren, cefixime, ceftaroline fosamil, ceftriaxone, ciprofloxacin, deferiprone, doripenem, ertapenem, flucloxacillin, furosemide, gemifloxacin, glibenclamide, ketoprofen, ketorolac, levodopa, levofloxacin, meloxicam, methotrexate, moxifloxacin, norfloxacin, NSAIDs, ofloxacin, pemetrexed, penicillamine, penicillin G, penicillin V, salicylates, sulfamethoxazole, sulfonamides, torsemide, zidovudine
Pregnancy category: C
Important contra-indications noted in the prescribing guidelines for: nursing mothers; pediatric patients

---

Skin
- Pruritus (<10%)
- Rash (<10%)
- Urticaria (<5%)

Mucosal
- Gingivitis (<10%)

Cardiovascular
- Flushing (<10%)

Renal
- Nephrotoxicity [3]

Hematologic
- Thrombocytopenia [2]

PROCAINAMIDE

Trade names: Procan (Pfizer), Procanbid (Pfizer)
Indications: Ventricular arrhythmias
Class: Antiarrhythmic, Antiarrhythmic class Ia
Half-life: 2.5–4.5 hours
Clinically important, potentially hazardous interactions with: abarelix, amiodarone, amisulpride, arsenic, artemether/lumefantrine, asenapine, astemizole, ciprofloxacin, enoxacin, ethoxzolamide, gatifloxacin, glycopyrrolate, glycopyrronium, imidapril, lomefloxacin, lurasidone, metformin, mivacurium, moxifloxacin, nilotinib, norfloxacin, ofloxacin, quinine, quinolones, rocuronium, sotalol, sparfloxacin, tetrabenazine, trimethoprim, trospium, vandetanib, zofenopril
Pregnancy category: C
Important contra-indications noted in the prescribing guidelines for: nursing mothers; pediatric patients

---

Skin
- Dermatitis (6%)
- Exanthems (<8%) [5]
- Hypersensitivity [2]
- Lupus erythematosus (>10%) [175]
- Purpura [3]
- Urticaria (<5%)
- Vasculitis [5]

Mucosal
- Oral mucosal eruption (2%)

Cardiovascular
- Hypotension [2]
- QT prolongation [4]
- Torsades de pointes [3]

Central Nervous System
- Dysgeusia (taste perversion) (3–4%)
- Psychosis [2]

Neuromuscular/Skeletal
- Myalgia/Myopathy [2]
- Myasthenia gravis [3]

Gastrointestinal/Hepatic
- Hepatotoxicity [3]
- Nausea [3]

Respiratory
- Pulmonary toxicity [2]

Hematologic
- Agranulocytosis [4]
- Neutropenia [3]
- Pancytopenia [2]
- Pure red cell aplasia [3]

PROCHLORPERAZINE

Trade name: Compazine (GSK)
Indications: Psychotic disorders, control of severe nausea and vomiting
Class: Antiemetic, Antipsychotic, Muscarinic antagonist, Phenothiazine
Half-life: 23 hours
Clinically important, potentially hazardous interactions with: antihistamines, arsenic, chlorpheniramine, dofetilide, pericyazine, piperazine, quinine, quinolones, sparfloxacin
Pregnancy category: C
Important contra-indications noted in the prescribing guidelines for: the elderly; nursing mothers; pediatric patients

---

Skin
- Anaphylactoid reactions/Anaphylaxis (<10%)
- Fixed eruption [3]
- Photosensitivity (<10%) [3]
- Pruritus (<10%)
- Rash (<10%)
- Toxic epidermal necrolysis [2]

Mucosal
- Xerostomia (>10%)

Central Nervous System
- Akathisia [14]
- Extrapyramidal symptoms [3]
- Neuroleptic malignant syndrome [3]
- Parkinsonism [4]

Neuromuscular/Skeletal
- Dystonia [6]

Endocrine/Metabolic
- Gynecomastia (<10%)

PROGESTINS

Trade names: Aygestin (Barr), Megace (Bristol-Myers Squibb), Micronor (Ortho), Ovrette (Wyeth), Provera (Pfizer)
Indications: Prevention of pregnancy
Class: Progestogen
Half-life: N/A
Clinically important, potentially hazardous interactions with: acitretin, aprepitant, dofetilide, rosuvastatin, voriconazole

---

Skin
- Acneform eruption [3]
- Dermatitis [4]
- Diaphoresis (31%)
- Erythema multiforme [2]
- Urticaria [2]

Cardiovascular
- Flushing (12%)

Endocrine/Metabolic
- Amenorrhea [2]

PROMETHAZINE

Trade name: Phenergan (Wyeth)
Indications: Allergic rhinitis, urticaria
Class: Histamine H1 receptor antagonist
Half-life: 10–14 hours
Clinically important, potentially hazardous interactions with: antihistamines, arsenic, chlorpheniramine, dofetilide, nalbuphine, piperazine, quinolones, sparfloxacin, zaleplon
Pregnancy category: C
Important contra-indications noted in the prescribing guidelines for: the elderly; nursing mothers; pediatric patients
Note: Not for intra-arterial or subcutaneous injection and contraindicated in comatose states.
Black Box Warning: RESPIRATORY DEPRESSION and SEVERE TISSUE INJURY, INCLUDING GANGRENE

Skin
Dermatitis [3]
Erythema multiforme [2]
Lupus erythematosus [2]
Photosensitivity [12]
Purpura [2]
Toxic epidermal necrolysis [2]
Urticaria [3]

Mucosal
Xerostomia (<10%) [2]

Cardiovascular
QT prolongation [2]

Central Nervous System
Neuroleptic malignant syndrome [2]
Somnolence (drowsiness) [3]

PROPAFENONE

Trade name: Rythmol (Reliant)
Indications: Ventricular arrhythmias
Class: Antiarrhythmic, Antiarrhythmic class Ic
Half-life: 10–32 hours
Clinically important, potentially hazardous interactions with: amitriptyline, boceprevir, carvedilol, clozapine, cobicistat/elvitegravir/emtricitabine/tenofovir disoproxil, delavirdine, digoxin, efavirenz, fosamprenavir, grapefruit juice, mirabegron, neostigmine, paroxetine hydrochloride, propranolol, pyridostigmine, rifapentine, ritonavir, telaprevir, tipranavir
Pregnancy category: C
Important contra-indications noted in the prescribing guidelines for: nursing mothers; pediatric patients

---

Skin
Lupus erythematosus [3]
Psoriasis [2]
Rash (<3%)

Mucosal
Oral lesions (>5%)
Xerostomia (2%)

Cardiovascular
Bradycardia [2]
Brugada syndrome [7]
Cardiotoxicity [3]
Congestive heart failure [2]
Hypotension [2]

Central Nervous System
Dysgeusia (taste perversion) (3–23%)
Seizures [3]
Syncope [2]

Gastrointestinal/Hepatic
Hepatotoxicity [8]

Local
Injection-site pain (28–90%) [4]

PROPOFOL

Trade name: Diprivan (AstraZeneca)
Indications: Induction and maintenance of anesthesia
Class: Anesthetic, general
Half-life: initial: 40 minutes; terminal: 3 days
Clinically important, potentially hazardous interactions with: zinc
Pregnancy category: B
Important contra-indications noted in the prescribing guidelines for: nursing mothers; pediatric patients

---

Skin
Anaphylactoid reactions/Anaphylaxis (<10%) [8]
Angioedema [2]
Exanthems (6%) [2]
Rash (5%)
Urticaria [2]

Hair
Hair pigmentation [2]

Cardiovascular
Bradycardia [14]
Brugada syndrome [2]
Cardiac failure [2]
Hypotension [17]
Tachycardia [2]

Central Nervous System
Amnesia [10]
Hallucinations [3]
Seizures [8]
Twitching (<10%)

Neuromuscular/Skeletal
Ataxia [2]
Rhabdomyolysis [9]

Gastrointestinal/Hepatic
Nausea [2]
Pancreatitis [6]
Vomiting [3]

Respiratory
Apnea [3]
Cough [2]
Hypoxia [7]
Respiratory depression [2]

Endocrine/Metabolic
Acidosis [2]

Renal
Green urine [7]

Local
Infusion-related reactions [3]
Injection-site pain (>10%) [34]

Other
Adverse effects [2]
Death [7]
Hiccups [3]

PROPRANOLOL

Trade names: Hemangeol (Pierre Fabre), Inderal (Wyeth)
Indications: Hypertension, angina pectoris, atrial fibrillation, myocardial infarction, migraine, tremor, infantile hemangioma
Class: Antiarrhythmic, Antiarrhythmic class II, Beta adrenergic blocker, Beta blocker
Half-life: 2–6 hours
Clinically important, potentially hazardous interactions with: alcohol, aluminum hydroxide, aminophylline, amiodarone, barbiturates, bupivacaine, chlorpromazine, cholestyramine, cimetidine, ciprofloxacin, clonidine, colestipol, delavirdine, diazepam, dronedarone, epinephrine, ethanol, fluconazole, fluoxetine, fluvoxamine, haloperidol, imipramine, insulin, insulin detemir, insulin glargine, insulin glulisine, isoniazid, levothyroxine, lidocaine, neostigmine, nicardipine, nifedipine, nilutamide, nisoldipine, oxtriphylline, paroxetine hydrochloride, phenobarbital, phenytoin, propafenone, pyridostigmine, quinidine, rifampin, ritonavir, rizatriptan, sodium iodide I-131, teniposide, terbutaline, tolbutamide, verapamil, warfarin, zileuton, zolmitriptan
Pregnancy category: C
Important contra-indications noted in the prescribing guidelines for: nursing mothers; pediatric patients
Note: Cutaneous side effects of beta-receptor blockers are clinically polymorphous. They apparently appear after several months of continuous therapy.

Skin
Acneform eruption [2]
Angioedema [2]
Cold extremities [6]
Dermatitis [2]
Eczema [2]
Exanthems [4]
Lichenoid eruption [3]
Lupus erythematosus [2]
Necrosis [3]
Pemphigus [2]
Psoriasis [20]
Rash (<10%) [2]
Raynaud's phenomenon [3]
Stevens–Johnson syndrome [2]
Urticaria [3]

Hair
Alopecia [6]

Nails
Nail thickening [2]

Cardiovascular
Bradycardia [19]
Cardiac arrest [2]
Flushing [2]
Hypertension [2]
Hypotension [18]

Central Nervous System
Agitation [2]

Amnesia [2]
Confusion [2]
Delirium [3]
Hallucinations [5]
Headache [2]
Insomnia [2]
Nightmares [2]
Psychosis [3]
Sleep disturbances [9]
Somnolence (drowsiness) [4]
Vertigo (dizziness) [3]

Neuromuscular/Skeletal
Asthenia (fatigue) [4]
Myalgia/Myopathy [3]

Gastrointestinal/Hepatic
Constipation [2]
Diarrhea [6]
Gastroesophageal reflux [2]
Nausea [2]

Respiratory
Bronchospasm [3]
Wheezing [3]

Endocrine/Metabolic
Hyperkalemia [4]
Hypoglycemia [15]
Weight gain [2]

Genitourinary
Peyronie's disease [6]

Ocular
Hallucinations, visual [4]

Other
Adverse effects [10]
Death [3]
Tooth decay [2]

PROTAMINE SULFATE

Indications: Heparin overdose
Class: Heparin antagonist
Half-life: 2 hours
Clinically important, potentially hazardous interactions with: none known
Pregnancy category: C

Skin
Anaphylactoid reactions/Anaphylaxis [42]
Angioedema [3]
Hypersensitivity [10]
Rash [2]
Urticaria [5]

Cardiovascular
Hypertension [2]
Hypotension [6]

Other
Adverse effects [2]
Allergic reactions [13]
Death [13]

PROTHROMBIN COMPLEX CONCENTRATE (HUMAN)

Synonym: PCC
Trade name: Kcentra (CSL Behring)
Indications: Urgent reversal of acquired coagulation factor deficiency induced by vitamin K antagonist therapy in adult patients with acute major bleeding
Class: Coagulant
Half-life: 4–60 hours
Clinically important, potentially hazardous interactions with: none known
Pregnancy category: C
Important contra-indications noted in the prescribing guidelines for: nursing mothers; pediatric patients
Black Box Warning: ARTERIAL AND VENOUS THROMBOEMBOLIC COMPLICATIONS

Skin
Hematoma (3%)

Cardiovascular
Hypertension (3%)
Hypotension (5%)
Orthostatic hypotension (4%)
Tachycardia (3%)

Central Nervous System
Headache (8%)
Intracranial hemorrhage (3%)
Neurotoxicity (3%)

Neuromuscular/Skeletal
Arthralgia (4%)

Gastrointestinal/Hepatic
Constipation (2%)
Nausea (4%)
Vomiting (4%)

Respiratory
Dyspnea (2%)
Hypoxia (2%)
Respiratory distress (2%)

Endocrine/Metabolic
Hypokalemia (2%)

Hematologic
Prothrombin time increased (3%)

PSEUDOEPHEDRINE

Trade names: Allegra-D (Sanofi-Aventis), Benadryl (Pfizer), Bromfed (Muro), Entex (Andrx), Robitussin-CF (Wyeth), Sudafed (Pfizer), Trinalin (Schering)
Indications: Nasal congestion
Class: Adrenergic alpha-receptor agonist
Half-life: 9–16 hours
Clinically important, potentially hazardous interactions with: bromocriptine, fluoxetine, fluvoxamine, furazolidone, iobenguane, MAO inhibitors, paroxetine hydrochloride, phenelzine, rasagiline, sertraline, tranylcypromine
Pregnancy category: C

Skin
AGEP [2]
Baboon syndrome (SDRIFE) [2]
Dermatitis [3]
Diaphoresis (<10%)
Erythroderma [2]
Exanthems [4]
Fixed eruption [13]

Cardiovascular
Myocardial infarction [2]
Palpitation [2]

Central Nervous System
Somnolence (drowsiness) [2]

Ocular
Hallucinations, visual [2]

PSORALENS

Trade names: Oxsoralen (Valeant), Trisoralen (Valeant)
Indications: Psoriasis, eczema, vitiligo, cutaneous T-cell lymphoma
Class: Psoralen
Half-life: 2 hours
Clinically important, potentially hazardous interactions with: none known
Pregnancy category: C

Skin
Anaphylactoid reactions/Anaphylaxis [2]
Basal cell carcinoma [3]
Bullous pemphigoid (with UVA) [12]
Burning (<10%) [3]
Dermatitis [11]
Eczema [2]
Edema (<10%)
Ephelides (<10%) [5]
Erythema [2]
Herpes simplex [2]
Herpes zoster [2]
Hypomelanosis (<10%)
Lupus erythematosus [5]
Melanoma [3]
Photosensitivity [14]
Phototoxicity [14]
Pigmentation [9]
Porokeratosis (actinic) [3]
Pruritus (>10%) [4]
Rash (<10%)
Squamous cell carcinoma [4]
Tumors (for the most part malignant) [18]
Vesiculation [2]
Vitiligo [2]

Hair
Hypertrichosis [4]

Nails
Nail pigmentation [4]
Photo-onycholysis [3]

Mucosal
Cheilitis (<10%)

Central Nervous System
Pain [3]

PYRIDOSTIGMINE

Trade names: Mestinon (Valeant), Regonol (Novartis)
Indications: Myasthenia gravis
Class: Acetylcholinesterase inhibitor
Half-life: ~2 hours
Clinically important, potentially hazardous interactions with: aminoglycosides, bacitracin, clindamycin, colistin, edrophonium, polymyxin B, propafenone, propranolol, quinidine, tetracyclines
Pregnancy category: B
Important contra-indications noted in the prescribing guidelines for: nursing mothers; pediatric patients

---

Central Nervous System
Neurotoxicity [3]
Parkinsonism [2]

Gastrointestinal/Hepatic
Abdominal pain [5]
Diarrhea [2]
Nausea [3]

Other
Adverse effects [2]
Side effects [2]

PYRIMETHAMINE

Trade names: Daraprim (GSK), Fansidar (Roche)
Indications: Malaria
Class: Antimalarial, Antiprotozoal
Half-life: 80–95 hours
Clinically important, potentially hazardous interactions with: dapsone, pemetrexed, trimethoprim, zidovudine
Pregnancy category: C
Important contra-indications noted in the prescribing guidelines for: the elderly; nursing mothers
Note: Fansidar is pyrimethamine and sulfadoxine. Sulfadoxine is a sulfonamide and can be absorbed systemically. Sulfonamides can produce severe, possibly fatal, reactions such as toxic epidermal necrolysis and Stevens-Johnson syndrome.

Skin
Angioedema [2]
Bullous dermatitis [2]
DRESS syndrome [2]
Erythema multiforme [4]
Exanthems [3]
Exfoliative dermatitis [2]
Fixed eruption [3]
Hypersensitivity (>10%)
Lichenoid eruption [2]
Photosensitivity (>10%) [3]
Pigmentation [5]
Pruritus [2]
Stevens–Johnson syndrome (<10%) [25]
Toxic epidermal necrolysis [15]

Central Nervous System
Vertigo (dizziness) [2]

Neuromuscular/Skeletal
Asthenia (fatigue) [2]

Gastrointestinal/Hepatic
Diarrhea [2]
Nausea [2]
Vomiting [2]

Other
Adverse effects [2]
Death [4]

QUETIAPINE

Trade name: Seroquel (AstraZeneca)
Indications: Schizophrenia, bipolar I disorder
Class: Antipsychotic, Mood stabilizer
Half-life: ~6 hours
Clinically important, potentially hazardous interactions with: alcohol, amoxapine, antihypertensive agents, arsenic, atazanavir, azithromycin, CNS acting drugs, darunavir, dolasetron, dopamine, drugs known to cause electrolyte imbalance or increase QT interval, erythromycin, fluconazole, hepatic enzyme inducers, itraconazole, ketoconazole, levodopa, methadone, P4503A inhibitors, pazopanib, telavancin, tipranavir, tricyclic antidepressants, voriconazole
Pregnancy category: C
Important contra-indications noted in the prescribing guidelines for: the elderly; nursing mothers; pediatric patients
Black Box Warning: INCREASED MORTALITY IN ELDERLY PATIENTS WITH DEMENTIA-RELATED PSYCHOSIS
SUICIDALITY AND ANTIDEPRESSANT DRUGS

Skin
Diaphoresis (<10%)
Hyperhidrosis (2%)
Peripheral edema [5]
Rash (4%)

Mucosal
Sialorrhea [2]
Xerostomia (9%) [19]

Cardiovascular
Bradycardia [2]
Hypertension (41%)
Hypotension [5]
Postural hypotension [2]
QT prolongation [7]
Tachycardia (6%) [2]

Central Nervous System
Abnormal dreams (2–3%)
Agitation (20%)
Akathisia (8%) [4]
Anxiety (2–4%)
Compulsions [3]
Delirium [2]
Depression (3%) [2]
Extrapyramidal symptoms [3]
Headache (21%) [6]
Hypoesthesia (2%)
Hypomania [3]
Impulse control disorder [2]
Insomnia (9%)
Mania [2]
Neuroleptic malignant syndrome [15]
Pain (7%)
Paresthesias (3%)
Parkinsonism (4%) [2]
Psychosis [2]
Restless legs syndrome [7]
Sedation [12]
Seizures [5]
Serotonin syndrome [2]
Sleep related disorder [2]
Somnambulism [2]
Somnolence (drowsiness) (18%) [20]
Suicidal ideation [2]
Tardive dyskinesia (5%) [2]
Tic disorder [2]
Vertigo (dizziness) (11%) [10]

Neuromuscular/Skeletal
Asthenia (fatigue) (5%) [5]
Ataxia (2%)
Dystonia [2]
Pisa syndrome [2]
Rhabdomyolysis [4]

Gastrointestinal/Hepatic
Abdominal pain (4–7%)
Colitis [3]
Constipation (8%) [3]
Dyspepsia (5%)
Hepatotoxicity [2]
Nausea (7%)
Pancreatitis [3]
Vomiting (6%)

Endocrine/Metabolic
ALT increased (5%)
Appetite increased [2]
Hyperglycemia [3]
Hypertriglyceridemia [3]
Libido decreased (2%)
Metabolic syndrome [2]
SIADH [2]
Weight gain (5%) [19]

Genitourinary
Priapism [14]
Sexual dysfunction [2]
Urinary retention [2]

Hematologic
Leukopenia [2]
Neutropenia [2]
Thrombocytopenia [3]

Ocular
Amblyopia (2–3%)
Vision blurred (<4%)

Other
Adverse effects [11]
Death [7]
Toothache (2–3%)

QUINACRINE

Synonym: mepacrine
Trade name: Atabrine (Winthrop)
Indications: Various infections caused by susceptible helminths
Class: Antibiotic, Antimalarial
Half-life: 4–10 hours
Clinically important, potentially hazardous interactions with: none known
Pregnancy category: N/A

Skin
Exanthems [3]
Exfoliative dermatitis (8%) [3]
Fixed eruption [3]
Lichenoid eruption (12%) [6]
Ochronosis [2]
Pigmentation [9]
Squamous cell carcinoma [2]

Hair
Alopecia (80%) [2]

Nails
Nail pigmentation (ala nasi) (blue-gray) [2]

Mucosal
Oral pigmentation [4]

Gastrointestinal/Hepatic
Nausea [2]
Vomiting [2]

QUINAPRIL

Trade names: Accupril (Pfizer), Accupro (Pfizer), Accuretic (Pfizer)
Indications: Hypertension, heart failure
Class: Angiotensin-converting enzyme (ACE) inhibitor, Antihypertensive, Vasodilator
Half-life: 2 hours
Clinically important, potentially hazardous interactions with: alcohol, aldesleukin, allopurinol, alpha blockers, alprostadil, amifostine, amiloride, angiotensin II receptor antagonists, antacids, antidiabetics, antihypertensives, antipsychotics, anxiolytics and hypnotics, aprotinin, azathioprine, baclofen, beta blockers, calcium channel blockers, chlortetracycline, ciprofloxacin, clonidine, corticosteroids, cyclosporine, demeclocycline, diazoxide, diuretics, doxycycline, eplerenone, estrogens, everolimus, gemifloxacin, general anesthetics, gold & gold compounds, heparins, hydralazine, insulin, levodopa, lithium, lymecycline, MAO inhibitors, metformin, methyldopa, methylphenidate, minocycline, minoxidil, moxifloxacin, moxisylyte, moxonidine, nitrates, nitroprusside, NSAIDs, ofloxacin, oxytetracycline, pentoxifylline, phosphodiesterase 5 inhibitors, potassium salts, prostacyclin analogues, quinine, quinolones, rituximab, salicylates, sirolimus, spironolactone, sulfonylureas, temsirolimus, tetracycline, tetracyclines, tigecycline, tizanidine, tolvaptan, triamterene, trimethoprim
Pregnancy category: D (category C in first trimester; category D in second and third trimesters)
Important contra-indications noted in the prescribing guidelines for: nursing mothers; pediatric patients
Note: Contraindicated in patients with a history of angioedema related to previous treatment with an ACE inhibitor.
Black Box Warning: FETAL TOXICITY

Skin
Angioedema [9]
Diaphoresis [3]
Edema [4]
Peripheral edema [3]
Photosensitivity [2]
Pruritus [7]
Rash [5]

Central Nervous System
Dysgeusia (taste perversion) [3]

Neuromuscular/Skeletal
Myalgia/Myopathy (2%)

Respiratory
Cough [9]

Other
Adverse effects [2]

QUINIDINE

Indications: Tachycardia, atrial fibrillation
Class: Antiarrhythmic, Antiarrhythmic class Ia, Antimalarial, Antiprotozoal
Half-life: 6–8 hours
Clinically important, potentially hazardous interactions with: abarelix, afatinib, amiloride, amiodarone, amisulpride, amitriptyline, amprenavir, anisindione, anticoagulants, aripiprazole, arsenic, artemether/lumefantrine, asenapine, astemizole, atazanavir, boceprevir, celiprolol, ciprofloxacin, clevidipine, clozapine, cobicistat/elvitegravir/emtricitabine/tenofovir disoproxil, crizotinib, dabigatran, darunavir, dasatinib, degarelix, delavirdine, dicumarol, digoxin, duloxetine, enoxacin, enzalutamide, ethoxzolamide, fosamprenavir, gatifloxacin, glycopyrrolate, glycopyrronium, indinavir, itraconazole, ketoconazole, lomefloxacin, lopinavir, lurasidone, metformin, mifepristone, mivacurium, moxifloxacin, nelfinavir, nilotinib, norfloxacin, ofloxacin, osimertinib, oxprenolol, pimozide, pipecuronium, posaconazole, pristinamycin, propranolol, pyridostigmine, quinine, quinolones, ranolazine, rifapentine, ritonavir, rocuronium, sertindole, sotalol, sparfloxacin, sulpiride, telaprevir, telithromycin, tetrabenazine, tipranavir, tramadol, vecuronium, venetoclax, verapamil, voriconazole, vortioxetine, warfarin, zuclopenthixol
Pregnancy category: C
Important contra-indications noted in the prescribing guidelines for: nursing mothers; pediatric patients

---

Skin
Acneform eruption [2]
AGEP [2]
Dermatitis [4]
Exanthems [6]
Exfoliative dermatitis [5]
Fixed eruption [2]
Lichen planus [7]
Lichenoid eruption [6]
Livedo reticularis [6]
Lupus erythematosus [35]
Photosensitivity [21]
Pigmentation [3]
Pruritus [3]
Psoriasis [5]
Purpura [13]
Rash (<10%)
Toxic epidermal necrolysis [2]
Vasculitis [5]

Mucosal
Oral mucosal eruption [2]

Cardiovascular
Congestive heart failure [2]
Flushing [2]
QT prolongation [8]
Torsades de pointes [13]

Central Nervous System
Dysgeusia (taste perversion) (>10%)
Headache (<10%)
Syncope [2]
Tremor (2%)

Gastrointestinal/Hepatic
Diarrhea (>10%) [5]

Genitourinary
Urinary tract infection [2]

Hematologic
Thrombocytopenia [2]

QUININE

Trade name: Qualaquin (URL Pharma)
Indications: Malaria
Class: Antimalarial, Antiprotozoal
Half-life: 8–14 hours
Clinically important, potentially hazardous interactions with: amantadine, amiodarone, amitriptyline, amoxapine, anisindione, anticoagulants, arsenic, artemether/lumefantrine, astemizole, atazanavir, atorvastatin, cimetidine, cisapride, citalopram, class Ia or III antiarrhythmics, clevidipine, CYP3A4 and CYP2D6 substrates, CYP3A4 inducers or inhibitors, darunavir, dasatinib, degarelix, dicumarol, digoxin, disopyramide, dofetilide, dolasetron, droperidol, enalapril, flecainide, fosamprenavir, halofantrine, haloperidol, histamine, indinavir, lapatinib, levofloxacin, mefloquine, metformin, moxifloxacin, nelfinavir, neuromuscular blocking agents, olmesartan, oral typhoid vaccine, pazopanib, pimozide, procainamide, prochlorperazine, quinapril, quinidine, ramipril, rifampin, ritonavir, saquinavir, sotalol, succinylcholine, telavancin, telithromycin, terfenadine, tipranavir, voriconazole, vorinostat, warfarin, ziprasidone
Pregnancy category: C
Important contra-indications noted in the prescribing guidelines for: nursing mothers; pediatric patients
Note: Qualaquin (quinine sulfate) is not idicated for the prevention or treatment of nocturnal leg cramps.
Contraindicated in patients with prolongation of QT interval, G6PD deficiency, myasthenia gravis, or optic neuritis.

Skin
Acneform eruption [2]
Acral necrosis [2]
Dermatitis [6]
Erythema multiforme [2]
Exanthems (<5%) [3]
Exfoliative dermatitis [2]
Fixed eruption [12]
Lichen planus [3]
Lichenoid eruption [3]
Livedo reticularis (photosensitive) [3]
Photosensitivity [19]
Pigmentation [6]
Purpura [13]
Raynaud's phenomenon [2]
Stevens–Johnson syndrome [2]
Thrombocytopenic purpura [8]
Toxic epidermal necrolysis [3]
Urticaria [2]
Vasculitis [5]

Cardiovascular
Cardiotoxicity [2]

Neuromuscular/Skeletal
Leg cramps [2]
Rhabdomyolysis [2]

Endocrine/Metabolic
Hypoglycemia [3]

Hematologic
Hemolytic anemia [2]
Hemolytic uremic syndrome [16]
Thrombocytopenia [11]

Otic
Hearing loss [4]
Ototoxicity [2]
Tinnitus [9]

Ocular
Amblyopia [8]

Other
Adverse effects [3]
Death [2]

RABEPRAZOLE

Trade name: Aciphex (Eisai) (Janssen)
Indications: Gastroesophageal reflux disease (GERD), duodenal ulcers, Zollinger-Ellison syndrome
Class: Proton pump inhibitor (PPI)
Half-life: 1–2 hours
Clinically important, potentially hazardous interactions with: atazanavir, clopidogrel, cyclosporine, digoxin, ketoconazole, rilpivirine, simvastatin, warfarin
Pregnancy category: B
Important contra-indications noted in the prescribing guidelines for: nursing mothers

---

Skin
Pruritus [2]
Rash [2]

Central Nervous System
Dysgeusia (taste perversion) [2]
Headache (2–5%) [3]
Pain (3%)
Vertigo (dizziness) [4]

Neuromuscular/Skeletal
Asthenia (fatigue) [2]

Gastrointestinal/Hepatic
Abdominal pain [5]
Constipation (2%)
Diarrhea (3%) [7]
Dyspepsia [3]
Flatulence [2]
Gastrointestinal bleeding [2]
Nausea [4]
Vomiting [4]

Respiratory
Cough [2]

Endocrine/Metabolic
Hypomagnesemia [2]

Renal
Nephrotoxicity [2]

Other
Adverse effects [4]

RADIUM-223 DICHLORIDE

Synonym: Ra-223 dichloride
Trade name: Xofigo (Bayer)
Indications: Castration-resistant prostate cancer
Class: Radiopharmaceutical, alpha-emitting
Half-life: 11.4 days
Clinically important, potentially hazardous interactions with: none known
Pregnancy category: X
Important contra-indications noted in the prescribing guidelines for: nursing mothers; pediatric patients

---

Skin
Peripheral edema (13%) [3]

Neuromuscular/Skeletal
Bone or joint pain [2]

Gastrointestinal/Hepatic
Diarrhea (25%) [6]
Nausea (36%) [5]
Vomiting (19%) [4]

Endocrine/Metabolic
Dehydration (3%)

Renal
Renal failure (3%)
Renal function abnormal (<3%)

Hematologic
Anemia (93%) [5]
Leukopenia (35%) [3]
Lymphocytopenia (72%) [2]
Myelosuppression [2]
Neutropenia (18%) [5]
Pancytopenia (2%)
Thrombocytopenia (31%) [5]

Other
Adverse effects [2]

RALOXIFENE

Trade name: Evista (Lilly)
Indications: Osteoporosis, reduction in risk of invasive breast cancer in postmenopausal women with osteoporosis or at high risk for invasive breast cancer
Class: Selective estrogen receptor modulator (SERM)
Half-life: 27.7 hours
Clinically important, potentially hazardous interactions with: cholestyramine, levothyroxine
Pregnancy category: X
Important contra-indications noted in the prescribing guidelines for: nursing mothers; pediatric patients
Black Box Warning: INCREASED RISK OF VENOUS THROMBOEMBOLISM AND DEATH FROM STROKE

Skin
Diaphoresis (3%)
Hot flashes (8–29%) [14]
Peripheral edema (3–5%) [4]
Rash (6%)

Cardiovascular
Chest pain (3%)
Venous thromboembolism [5]

Central Nervous System
Insomnia (6%)
Stroke [4]

Neuromuscular/Skeletal
Arthralgia (11–16%)
Leg cramps (6–12%) [5]
Myalgia/Myopathy (8%)

Gastrointestinal/Hepatic
Abdominal pain (7%)
Vomiting (5%)

Respiratory
Bronchitis (10%)
Flu-like syndrome (~2%)
Pharyngitis (8%)
Pneumonia (3%)
Sinusitis (10%)

Endocrine/Metabolic
Mastodynia (4%) [2]
Weight gain (9%)

Genitourinary
Vaginal bleeding (6%)
Vaginitis (4%)

Hematologic
Thrombosis [2]

Other
Adverse effects [2]
Infection (11%)

RALTEGRAVIR

Trade name: Isentress (Merck)
Indications: HIV-1 infection
Class: Antiretroviral, Integrase strand transfer inhibitor
Half-life: 9 hours
Clinically important, potentially hazardous interactions with: atazanavir, efavirenz, histamine H_2 antagonists, omeprazole, pantoprazole, proton pump inhibitors, rifampin, St John's wort, strong UGT inducers, tipranavir
Pregnancy category: C
Important contra-indications noted in the prescribing guidelines for: nursing mothers; pediatric patients

---

Skin
DRESS syndrome [2]
Herpes zoster (<2%)
Hypersensitivity (<2%) [6]
Pruritus (4%)
Rash [8]

Central Nervous System
Depression (<2%) [2]
Headache (2%) [8]
Insomnia (4%) [4]
Neurotoxicity [2]
Vertigo (dizziness) (<2%)

Neuromuscular/Skeletal
Asthenia (fatigue) (<2%) [4]
Myalgia/Myopathy [3]
Rhabdomyolysis [8]

Gastrointestinal/Hepatic
Abdominal pain (<2%) [2]
Diarrhea [7]
Dyspepsia (<2%)
Gastritis (<2%)
Hepatitis [2]
Hepatotoxicity (<2%) [3]
Nausea (<2%) [7]
Vomiting (<2%)

Endocrine/Metabolic
ALT increased [3]
Creatine phosphokinase increased [3]

Renal
Nephrolithiasis (<2%)
Renal failure (<2%)

Other
Adverse effects [6]

RAMELTEON

Trade name: Rozerem (Takeda)
Indications: Insomnia
Class: Hypnotic, Melatonin receptor agonist
Half-life: 1–2.6 hours
Clinically important, potentially hazardous interactions with: alcohol, antifungals, CNS depressants, conivaptan, CYP1A2 inhibitors, donepezil, doxepin, droperidol, fluconazole, fluvoxamine, food, ketoconazole, levomepromazine, rifampin, rifapentine, St John's wort, voriconazole, zolpidem
Pregnancy category: C
Important contra-indications noted in the prescribing guidelines for: nursing mothers; pediatric patients

---

Central Nervous System
Depression (2%)
Dysgeusia (taste perversion) (2%)
Headache (7%) [8]
Insomnia (exacerbation) (3%)
Somnolence (drowsiness) (3%) [9]
Vertigo (dizziness) (4%) [6]

Neuromuscular/Skeletal
Arthralgia (2%)
Asthenia (fatigue) (3%) [4]
Myalgia/Myopathy (2%)

Gastrointestinal/Hepatic
Nausea (3%) [3]

Respiratory
Upper respiratory tract infection (3%)

Genitourinary
Urinary tract infection [2]

Other
Adverse effects [7]

RAMIPRIL

Trade names: Altace (Monarch), Tritace (Sanofi-Aventis)
Indications: Hypertension
Class: Angiotensin-converting enzyme (ACE) inhibitor, Antihypertensive, Vasodilator
Half-life: 2–17 hours
Clinically important, potentially hazardous interactions with: alcohol, aldesleukin, allopurinol, alpha blockers, alprostadil, amifostine, amiloride, angiotensin II receptor antagonists, antacids, antihypertensives, antipsychotics, azathioprine, baclofen, beta blockers, calcium channel blockers, clonidine, corticosteroids, cyclosporine, diazoxide, diuretics, eplerenone, estrogens, everolimus, general anesthetics, gold & gold compounds, heparins, hydralazine, hypotensives, insulin, levodopa, lithium, MAO inhibitors, metformin, methyldopa, minoxidil, moxisylyte, moxonidine, nitrates, nitroprusside, NSAIDs, pentoxifylline, phosphodiasterase 5 inhibitors, potassium salts, prostacyclin analogues, quinine, rituximab, sirolimus, spironolactone, sulfonylureas, telmisartan, temsirolimus, tizanidine, tolvaptan, triamterene, trimethoprim
Pregnancy category: D (category C in first trimester; category D in second and third trimesters)
Important contra-indications noted in the prescribing guidelines for: nursing mothers; pediatric patients
Note: Contraindicated in patients with a history of angioedema related to previous treatment with an ACE inhibitor, or a history of hereditary or idiopathic angioedema.
Black Box Warning: FETAL TOXICITY

Skin
Angioedema [11]
Diaphoresis [2]
Lichen planus pemphigoides [3]
Photosensitivity [2]
Pruritus [3]
Rash [4]

Hair
Alopecia (<10%)

Cardiovascular
Angina (3%)
Flushing [2]
Hypotension (11%) [3]
Postural hypotension (2%)

Central Nervous System
Headache (5%) [2]
Syncope (2%)
Vertigo (dizziness) (2–4%) [4]

Neuromuscular/Skeletal
Asthenia (fatigue) (2%)

Gastrointestinal/Hepatic
Hepatotoxicity [2]
Nausea (2%)
Pancreatitis [2]
Vomiting (2%)

Respiratory
Cough (8–12%) [22]

Endocrine/Metabolic
Hyperkalemia [2]

Other
Adverse effects [4]

RAMUCIRUMAB

Trade name: Cyramza (Lilly)
Indications: Gastric cancer
Class: Monoclonal antibody, Vascular endothelial growth factor antagonist
Half-life: N/A
Clinically important, potentially hazardous interactions with: none known
Pregnancy category: C
Important contra-indications noted in the prescribing guidelines for: nursing mothers; pediatric patients
Black Box Warning: HEMORRHAGE, GASTROINSTINAL PERFORATION, AND IMPAIRED WOUND HEALING

Skin
Peripheral edema [2]
Rash (4%)

Mucosal
Epistaxis (nosebleed) (5%) [2]
Stomatitis [3]

Cardiovascular
Hypertension (16%) [18]
Thromboembolism (2%) [2]
Venous thromboembolism [2]

Central Nervous System
Headache (9%) [2]

Neuromuscular/Skeletal
Asthenia (fatigue) [11]

Gastrointestinal/Hepatic
Ascites [2]
Constipation [3]
Diarrhea (14%) [5]
Gastric obstruction (2%)
Gastrointestinal perforation [3]
Hepatotoxicity [2]
Nausea [4]
Vomiting [4]

Respiratory
Dyspnea [3]

Endocrine/Metabolic
Appetite decreased [2]
Hyponatremia (6%)

Renal
Proteinuria [8]

Hematologic
Anemia [5]
Bleeding [4]
Febrile neutropenia [7]
Hemorrhage [3]
Leukopenia [4]
Neutropenia (5%) [10]
Thrombocytopenia [5]

Local
Infusion-related reactions [3]

Other
Death [3]

RANIBIZUMAB

Trade name: Lucentis (Genentech)
Indications: Neovascular (wet) age-related macular degeneration, macular edema (following retinal vein occlusion)
Class: Monoclonal antibody, Vascular endothelial growth factor antagonist
Half-life: 9 days
Clinically important, potentially hazardous interactions with: none known
Pregnancy category: C
Important contra-indications noted in the prescribing guidelines for: nursing mothers; pediatric patients
Note: Contraindicated in patients with ocular or periocular infections.

Cardiovascular
Atrial fibrillation (<5%)
Hypertension [4]
Myocardial infarction [2]
Thromboembolism [3]

Central Nervous System
Anxiety (<4%)
Headache (3–12%)
Insomnia (<5%)

Stroke [3]

Neuromuscular/Skeletal
Arthralgia (2–11%)
Pain in extremities (<5%)

Gastrointestinal/Hepatic
Gastroenteritis (<4%)
Nausea (<9%)

Respiratory
Bronchitis (<12%)
COPD (<7%)
Cough (2–9%)
Dyspnea (<5%)
Influenza (3–7%)
Nasopharyngitis (5–16%) [2]
Sinusitis (3–8%)
Upper respiratory tract infection (2–9%)

Endocrine/Metabolic
Hypercholesterolemia (<5%)

Genitourinary
Urinary tract infection (<9%)

Hematologic
Anemia (<8%)

Ocular
Blepharitis (<13%)
Cataract (2–17%) [4]
Conjunctival hemorrhage (48–74%) [4]
Conjunctival hyperemia (<8%)
Endophthalmitis [9]
Hallucinations, visual [2]
Intraocular inflammation (<18%) [5]
Intraocular pressure increased (7–24%) [7]
Iridocyclitis [2]
Lacrimation (increased) (2–14%)
Maculopathy (6–11%)
Ocular adverse effects [3]
Ocular hemorrhage [4]
Ocular hyperemia (5–11%)
Ocular pain (17–35%) [3]
Ocular pruritus (<12%)
Ocular stinging (7–15%)
Posterior capsule opacification (<8%)
Retinal atrophy [2]
Retinal detachment [2]
Retinal vein occlusion [2]
Vision blurred (5–18%)
Visual disturbances (5–18%)
Vitreous detachment (4–21%)
Vitreous floaters (7–27%) [2]
Xerophthalmia (3–12%)

Local
Injection-site bleeding (<6%)

Other
Adverse effects [4]
Systemic reactions [2]

RANITIDINE

Trade name: Zantac (Concordia)
Indications: Duodenal ulcer
Class: Histamine H2 receptor antagonist
Half-life: 2.5 hours
Clinically important, potentially hazardous interactions with: alfentanil, delavirdine, fentanyl, gefitinib, metformin, prednisone, rilpivirine, risperidone
Pregnancy category: B
Important contra-indications noted in the prescribing guidelines for: nursing mothers

---

Skin
AGEP [2]
Anaphylactoid reactions/Anaphylaxis [18]
Dermatitis [6]
Eczema [2]
Exanthems [5]
Hypersensitivity [2]
Photosensitivity [2]
Pseudolymphoma [2]
Purpura [2]
Rash (<10%)
Toxic epidermal necrolysis [2]
Urticaria [4]

Central Nervous System
Confusion [2]

Endocrine/Metabolic
Gynecomastia [3]
Porphyria [3]

Other
Adverse effects [2]

RANOLAZINE

Trade name: Ranexa (CV Therapeutics)
Indications: Angina
Class: Anti-ischemic, Fatty acid oxidation inhibitor
Half-life: 7 hours
Clinically important, potentially hazardous interactions with: aprepitant, atazanavir, clarithromycin, conivaptan, cyclosporine, CYP3A inducers, CYP3A inhibitors, darunavir, delavirdine, diltiazem, dofetilide, efavirenz, erythromycin, grapefruit juice, indinavir, itraconazole, ketoconazole, lopinavir, nelfinavir, ombitasvir/paritaprevir/ritonavir, oxcarbazepine, paroxetine hydrochloride, phenobarbital, quinidine, rifampin, rifapentine, ritonavir, simvastatin, sotalol, telithromycin, thioridazine, tipranavir, venetoclax, verapamil, voriconazole, ziprasidone
Pregnancy category: C
Important contra-indications noted in the prescribing guidelines for: nursing mothers
Note: Ranolazine is contraindicated in patients with existing QT prolongation, and in patients with liver disease.

Mucosal
Xerostomia (<2%)

Cardiovascular
Palpitation (<2%)
QT prolongation [7]
Torsades de pointes [2]

Central Nervous System
Headache (3%) [4]
Vertigo (dizziness) [10]

Neuromuscular/Skeletal
Asthenia (fatigue) [3]

Gastrointestinal/Hepatic
Abdominal pain (<2%)
Constipation [8]
Nausea [9]
Vomiting [2]

Otic
Tinnitus (<2%)

RASAGILINE

Trade name: Azilect (Teva)
Indications: Parkinsonism
Class: Monoamine oxidase B inhibitor
Half-life: 0.6–2.0 hours
Clinically important, potentially hazardous interactions with: aminophylline, amitriptyline, ciprofloxacin, citalopram, dextromethorphan, entacapone, fluoxetine, fluvoxamine, MAO inhibitors, meperidine, paroxetine hydrochloride, pethidine, pseudoephedrine, SSRIs
Pregnancy category: C
Important contra-indications noted in the prescribing guidelines for: nursing mothers; pediatric patients

---

Skin
Ecchymoses (2%)

Mucosal
Xerostomia (3%)

Cardiovascular
Hypotension (5%)

Central Nervous System
Depression (5%) [2]
Dyskinesia (>10%)
Fever (3%)
Gait instability (5%)
Headache (14%) [2]
Paresthesias (2%)
Somnolence (drowsiness) [2]
Vertigo (dizziness) (2%) [3]

Neuromuscular/Skeletal
Arthralgia (7%) [2]
Asthenia (fatigue) (2%)
Dystonia (2%)
Neck pain (2%)

Gastrointestinal/Hepatic
Dyspepsia (7%)
Gastroenteritis (3%)

Respiratory
Flu-like syndrome (5%)
Rhinitis (3%)

Ocular
Conjunctivitis (3%)

REBOXETINE

Trade name: Edronax (Pfizer)
Indications: Clinical depression, panic disorder
Class: Antidepressant, Noradrenaline reuptake inhibitor
Half-life: 13 hours
Clinically important, potentially hazardous interactions with: azithromycin, bosentan, itraconazole, ketoconazole, MAO inhibitors, papaverine, voriconazole

Pregnancy category: N/A (not recommended in pregnancy)
Important contra-indications noted in the prescribing guidelines for: the elderly; nursing mothers; pediatric patients

---

Skin
Diaphoresis [8]
Mucosal
Xerostomia [12]
Central Nervous System
Headache [5]
Insomnia [9]
Somnolence (drowsiness) [2]
Genitourinary
Ejaculatory dysfunction [2]

RESLIZUMAB *

Trade name: Cinqair (Teva)
Indications: Adjunctive treatment for severe eosinophilic asthma
Class: Interleukin-5 antagonist, Monoclonal antibody
Half-life: 24 days
Clinically important, potentially hazardous interactions with: none known
Pregnancy category: N/A (Insufficient evidence to inform drug-associated risk)
Important contra-indications noted in the prescribing guidelines for: nursing mothers; pediatric patients
Black Box Warning: ANAPHYLAXIS

Mucosal
Oropharyngeal pain (3%)
Central Nervous System
Headache [3]
Respiratory
Asthma (exacerbation) [3]
Nasopharyngitis [4]
Upper respiratory tract infection [3]
Endocrine/Metabolic
Creatine phosphokinase increased (14%)

RIBAVIRIN

Trade names: Copegus (Roche), Rebetol (Schering-Plough), Rebetron (Schering), Virazole (Valeant)
Indications: Respiratory syncytial viral infections
Class: Antiviral, nucleoside analog
Half-life: 24 hours
Clinically important, potentially hazardous interactions with: abacavir, azathioprine, didanosine, emtricitabine, interferon alfa, PEG-interferon, stavudine, zidovudine
Pregnancy category: X
Important contra-indications noted in the prescribing guidelines for: nursing mothers
Note: [INH] = Inhalation; [O] = Oral. Rebetron is ribavirin and interferon.
Black Box Warning: RISK OF SERIOUS DISORDERS AND RIBAVIRIN-ASSOCIATED EFFECTS

Skin
Dermatitis [O] (16%)
DRESS syndrome [2]
Eczema [O] (4–5%) [3]
Exanthems [5]
Lichenoid eruption [2]
Nummular eczema [2]
Peripheral edema [2]
Photosensitivity [6]
Pruritus [O] (13–29%) [24]
Psoriasis [2]
Rash [O] (5–28%) [36]
Sarcoidosis [16]
Stevens-Johnson syndrome [2]
Toxic epidermal necrolysis [2]
Toxicity [2]
Vasculitis [2]
Vitiligo [2]
Xerosis [O] (10–24%) [2]
Hair
Alopecia [O] (27–36%) [4]
Alopecia areata [2]
Cardiovascular
Flushing [O] (4%)
Central Nervous System
Depression [O] (20–36%) [10]
Dysgeusia (taste perversion) [O] (4–9%) [4]
Fever [O] (32–55%) [6]
Headache [INH] (Insomnia [O] (25–41%) [23]
Irritability [9]
Neurotoxicity [2]
Pain [O] (10%)
Rigors [O] (25–48%)
Suicidal ideation [O] (2%) [2]
Vertigo (dizziness) [O] (14–26%) [4]
Neuromuscular/Skeletal
Arthralgia [INH] (22–34%) [7]
Asthenia (fatigue) [50]
Muscle spasm [3]
Myalgia/Myopathy [INH] (40–64%)
Gastrointestinal/Hepatic
Diarrhea [15]
Hepatotoxicity [5]
Nausea [INH] (<10%) [33]
Pancreatitis [4]
Vomiting [O] (9–25%)
Respiratory
Cough [O] (7–23%) [8]
Dyspnea [O] (13–26%) [5]
Flu-like syndrome [O] (13–18%) [7]
Nasopharyngitis [3]
Pneumonitis [2]
Rhinitis [O] (8%)
Upper respiratory tract infection [3]
Endocrine/Metabolic
ALT increased [5]
AST increased [5]
Diabetes mellitus [2]
Hyperuricemia [O] (33–38%)
Thyroid dysfunction [2]
Weight loss [O] (10–29%) [2]
Genitourinary
Erectile dysfunction [2]
Renal
Nephrotoxicity [5]
Hematologic
Anemia [INH] (<10%) [65]
Hemoglobin decreased [2]
Hemotoxicity [2]
Leukopenia [O] (6–45%) [2]
Lymphopenia [O] (12–14%) [2]
Neutropenia [O] (8–42%) [18]
Thrombocytopenia [INH] (<15%) [10]
Otic
Hearing loss [2]
Tinnitus [2]
Ocular
Retinopathy [6]
Local
Injection-site reactions [2]
Other
Adverse effects [21]
Death [3]
Infection [INH] [3]
Vogt-Koyanagi-Harada syndrome [6]

RIFABUTIN

Trade name: Mycobutin (Pfizer)
Indications: Disseminated *Mycobacterium avium* infection
Class: Antibiotic, rifamycin, CYP3A4 inducer
Half-life: 45 hours
Clinically important, potentially hazardous interactions with: abiraterone, amiodarone, amprenavir, anisindione, anticoagulants, atazanavir, atovaquone, atovaquone/proguanil, azithromycin, bedaquiline, boceprevir, cabazitaxel, cabozantinib, cobicistat/elvitegravir/emtricitabine/tenofovir disoproxil, corticosteroids, crizotinib, cyclosporine, dapsone, darunavir, delavirdine, dicumarol, efavirenz, enzalutamide, etravirine, flibanserin, fosamprenavir, indinavir, itraconazole, ixabepilone, lapatinib, ledipasvir & sofosbuvir, levonorgestrel, lopinavir, midazolam, mifepristone, nelfinavir, oral contraceptives, posaconazole, rilpivirine, ritonavir, romidepsin, simeprevir, sofosbuvir, solifenacin, sorafenib, sunitinib, tacrolimus, temsirolimus, thalidomide, tipranavir, tolvaptan, vandetanib, vemurafenib, voriconazole
Pregnancy category: B
Important contra-indications noted in the prescribing guidelines for: the elderly; nursing mothers; pediatric patients

---

Skin
Lupus erythematosus [2]
Pigmentation [2]
Rash (11%) [2]
Central Nervous System
Anorexia (2%)
Dysgeusia (taste perversion) (3%)
Fever (2%)
Headache (3%)
Neuromuscular/Skeletal
Arthralgia [6]
Myalgia/Myopathy (2%)

Gastrointestinal/Hepatic
Abdominal pain (4%)
Diarrhea (3%)
Dyspepsia (3%)
Eructation (belching) (3%)
Flatulence (2%)
Hepatotoxicity [2]
Nausea (6%)

Ocular
Intraocular inflammation [2]
Ocular toxicity [2]
Uveitis [31]
Visual disturbances [2]

RIFAMPIN

Synonym: rifampicin
Trade names: Rifadin (Sanofi-Aventis), Rimactane (Novartis)
Indications: Tuberculosis
Class: Antibiotic, rifamycin, CYP1A2 inducer, CYP3A4 inducer
Half-life: 3–5 hours
Clinically important, potentially hazardous interactions with: abacavir, abiraterone, afatinib, amiodarone, amprenavir, anisindione, antacids, anticoagulants, apixaban, apremilast, aprepitant, artemether/lumefantrine, atazanavir, atorvastatin, atovaquone, atovaquone/proguanil, beclomethasone, bedaquiline, betamethasone, bisoprolol, boceprevir, bosentan, brentuximab vedotin, buprenorphine, cabazitaxel, cabozantinib, canagliflozin, caspofungin, clobazam, clozapine, cobimetinib, corticosteroids, cortisone, crizotinib, cyclosporine, cyproterone, dabigatran, daclatasvir, dapsone, darunavir, dasatinib, deferasirox, delavirdine, dexamethasone, diclofenac, dicumarol, digoxin, doxycycline, dronedarone, efavirenz, emtricitabine/rilpivirine/tenofovir alafenamide, enzalutamide, estradiol, eszopiclone, etoricoxib, etravirine, everolimus, fesoterodine, flibanserin, fludrocortisone, flunisolide, fosamprenavir, gadoxetate, gefitinib, gestrinone, halothane, hydrocortisone, imatinib, indinavir, isoniazid, itraconazole, ixabepilone, ketoconazole, lapatinib, ledipasvir & sofosbuvir, leflunomide, lesinurad, levodopa, levonorgestrel, linagliptin, linezolid, lopinavir, lorcainide, losartan, lurasidone, macitentan, maraviroc, methylprednisolone, midazolam, mifepristone, nelfinavir, nevirapine, nifedipine, nilotinib, ombitasvir/paritaprevir/ritonavir, ondansetron, oral contraceptives, osimertinib, ospemifene, oxtriphylline, paclitaxel, pazopanib, perampanel, phenylbutazone, pioglitazone, pitavastatin, ponatinib, praziquantel, prednisolone, prednisone, propranolol, propyphenazone, protease inhibitors, pyrazinamide, quinine, raltegravir, ramelteon, ranolazine, regorafenib, rilpivirine, riociguat, ritonavir, rivaroxaban, roflumilast, romidepsin, rosiglitazone, saquinavir, simeprevir, simvastatin, sofosbuvir, solifenacin, sorafenib, sunitinib, tacrolimus, tadalafil, tasimelteon, telaprevir, telithromycin, temsirolimus, terbinafine, thalidomide, ticagrelor, tipranavir, tofacitinib, tolvaptan, trabectedin, treprostinil, triamcinolone, triazolam, trimethoprim, troleandomycin, ulipristal, vandetanib, vemurafenib, voriconazole, vortioxetine, warfarin, zaleplon, zidovudine, zolpidem
Pregnancy category: C

Skin
Acneform eruption [3]
AGEP [2]
Anaphylactoid reactions/Anaphylaxis [6]
Dermatitis [3]
Diaphoresis (<10%)
DRESS syndrome [5]
Erythema multiforme [4]
Exanthems (<5%) [6]
Fixed eruption [6]
Hypersensitivity [5]
Linear IgA bullous dermatosis [3]
Pemphigus [9]
Pruritus (<62%) [9]
Purpura [6]
Rash (<5%) [4]
Red man syndrome [7]
Stevens–Johnson syndrome [5]
Thrombocytopenic purpura [2]
Toxic epidermal necrolysis [6]
Urticaria [8]
Vasculitis [5]

Cardiovascular
Flushing (7%) [8]

Central Nervous System
Fever [2]
Seizures [3]
Vertigo (dizziness) [2]

Neuromuscular/Skeletal
Asthenia (fatigue) [3]

Gastrointestinal/Hepatic
Abdominal pain [3]
Diarrhea [2]
Hepatitis [3]
Hepatotoxicity [17]
Nausea [4]
Vomiting [2]

Respiratory
Pneumonitis [2]

Endocrine/Metabolic
Amenorrhea [2]
Porphyria [2]

Renal
Nephrotoxicity [9]

Hematologic
Agranulocytosis [2]
Anemia [3]
Thrombocytopenia [11]

Other
Adverse effects [11]
Death [7]
Side effects (5%)

RIFAXIMIN

Trade names: Xifaxan (Salix), Xifaxanta (Norgine)
Indications: Diarrhea in travelers (caused by non-invasive strains of *E. coli*), reduction in risk of overt hepatic encephalopathy recurrence (in adults)
Class: Antibiotic, rifamycin
Half-life: 2–5 hours
Clinically important, potentially hazardous interactions with: BCG vaccine
Pregnancy category: C
Important contra-indications noted in the prescribing guidelines for: nursing mothers; pediatric patients
Note: Safety and effectiveness in pediatric patients with travelers' diarrhea <12 years of age have not been established.

Skin
Cellulitis (2–5%)
Clammy skin (<2%)
Diaphoresis (<2%)
Edema (2–5%)
Hot flashes (<2%)
Hyperhidrosis (<2%)
Peripheral edema (15%) [2]
Pruritus (9%)
Rash (<5%)
Sunburn (<2%)

Mucosal
Epistaxis (nosebleed) (2–5%)
Gingival lesions (<2%)
Rhinorrhea (<2%)
Xerostomia (2–5%)

Cardiovascular
Chest pain (<5%) [2]
Hypotension (2–5%)

Central Nervous System
Abnormal dreams (<2%)
Ageusia (taste loss) (<2%)
Amnesia (2–5%)
Anorexia (<5%)
Confusion (2–5%)
Depression (7%)
Dysgeusia (taste perversion) (<2%)
Fever (3–6%)
Headache (10%) [8]
Hypoesthesia (2–5%)
Impaired concentration (2–5%)
Insomnia (<7%)
Migraine (<2%)
Pain (<5%)
Syncope (<2%)
Tremor (2–5%)
Vertigo (dizziness) (<13%) [3]

Neuromuscular/Skeletal
Arthralgia (<6%)
Asthenia (fatigue) (<12%) [3]
Back pain (6%)
Muscle spasm (<9%)
Myalgia/Myopathy (<5%)
Neck pain (<2%)
Pain in extremities (2–5%)

Gastrointestinal/Hepatic
Abdominal distension (<8%)
Abdominal pain (2–9%) [10]

Ascites (11%)
Black stools (<2%)
Constipation (4–6%)
Diarrhea (<2%) [5]
Fecal urgency (6%)
Flatulence (11%) [2]
Hernia (<2%)
Nausea (5–14%) [7]
Tenesmus (7%)
Vomiting (2%) [3]

Respiratory
Cough (7%)
Dyspnea (<6%)
Flu-like syndrome (2–5%)
Nasopharyngitis (<7%) [4]
Pharyngitis (<2%)
Pharyngolaryngeal pain (<2%)
Pneumonia (2–5%)
Rhinitis (<5%)
Sinusitis [2]
Upper respiratory tract infection (2–5%) [6]

Endocrine/Metabolic
AST increased (<2%)
Dehydration (<5%)
Hyperglycemia (2–5%)
Hyperkalemia (2–5%)
Hypoglycemia (2–5%)
Hyponatremia (2–5%)
Weight gain (2–5%)

Genitourinary
Dysuria (<2%)
Hematuria (<2%)
Polyuria (<2%)
Urinary frequency (<2%)

Renal
Proteinuria (<2%)

Hematologic
Anemia (8%)
Lymphocytosis (<2%)
Monocytosis (<2%)
Neutropenia (<2%)

Otic
Ear pain (<2%)
Tinnitus (<2%)

Other
Breast cancer [2]

RIOCIGUAT

Trade name: Adempas (Bayer)
Indications: Pulmonary hypertension
Class: Soluble guanylate cyclase (sGC) stimulator
Half-life: 7–12 hours
Clinically important, potentially hazardous interactions with: antacids, carbamazepine, dipyridamole, nitrates or nitric oxide donors, phenobarbital, phenytoin, rifampin, sildenafil, St John's wort, tadalafil, theophylline, vardenafil
Pregnancy category: X
Important contra-indications noted in the prescribing guidelines for: nursing mothers; pediatric patients
Black Box Warning: EMBRYO-FETAL TOXICITY

Skin
Peripheral edema [2]

Cardiovascular
Hypotension (10%) [6]

Central Nervous System
Headache (27%) [3]
Syncope [2]
Vertigo (dizziness) (20%)

Gastrointestinal/Hepatic
Constipation (5%)
Diarrhea (12%)
Dyspepsia (21%) [2]
Gastroesophageal reflux (5%)
Nausea (14%)
Vomiting (10%)

Hematologic
Anemia (7%)
Bleeding (2%) [2]

Other
Adverse effects [4]

RISEDRONATE

Trade names: Actonel (Procter & Gamble), Atelvia (Warner Chilcott)
Indications: Paget's disease of bone, osteoporosis
Class: Bisphosphonate
Half-life: terminal: 220 hours
Clinically important, potentially hazardous interactions with: antacids, calcium supplements, iron preparations, laxatives, magnesium-based supplements
Pregnancy category: C
Important contra-indications noted in the prescribing guidelines for: nursing mothers; pediatric patients

---

Skin
Ecchymoses (4%)
Peripheral edema (8%)
Pruritus (3%)
Rash (8%)

Cardiovascular
Chest pain (5%)
Hypertension (11%)

Central Nervous System
Depression (7%)
Fever [2]
Headache (10%) [3]
Insomnia (5%)
Pain (14%)
Paresthesias (2%)
Vertigo (dizziness) (7%)

Neuromuscular/Skeletal
Arthralgia (10–24%) [6]
Asthenia (fatigue) (5%)
Back pain (28%) [4]
Bone or joint pain (7%) [5]
Fractures (9%) [9]
Myalgia/Myopathy (7%) [3]
Neck pain (5%) [3]
Osteonecrosis [5]
Tendinopathy/Tendon rupture (3%)

Gastrointestinal/Hepatic
Abdominal pain (12%) [3]
Constipation (13%) [3]
Diarrhea (11%) [4]
Dyspepsia (11%) [2]
Esophagitis [2]
Gastrointestinal disorder [3]
Hepatotoxicity [6]
Nausea (11%) [2]

Respiratory
Bronchitis (10%)
Cough (6%)
Flu-like syndrome (11%) [2]
Influenza [3]
Nasopharyngitis [3]
Pharyngitis (6%)
Rhinitis (6%)
Sinusitis (9%)

Genitourinary
Urinary tract infection (11%)

Ocular
Cataract (7%)
Ocular adverse effects [3]
Scleritis [2]

Other
Adverse effects [5]
Allergic reactions (4%)
Infection (31%) [2]
Tooth disorder (2%)

RISPERIDONE

Trade names: Risperdal (Ortho-McNeil) (Janssen), Risperdal Consta (Ortho-McNeil) (Janssen)
Indications: Schizophrenia, bipolar mania, irritability associated with autistic disorder
Class: Antipsychotic, Mood stabilizer
Half-life: 3–30 hours
Clinically important, potentially hazardous interactions with: ACE inhibitors, alcohol, alpha blockers, amantadine, angiotensin II receptor antagonists, anxiolytics and hypnotics, apomorphine, artemether/lumefantrine, barbiturates, bromocriptine, cabergoline, calcium channel blockers, carbamazepine, cimetidine, citalopram, clozapine, cobicistat/elvitegravir/emtricitabine/tenofovir disoproxil, ethosuximide, fluoxetine, general anesthetics, histamine, levodopa, memantine, methyldopa, metoclopramide, opioid analgesics, oxcarbazepine, paliperidone, paroxetine hydrochloride, pergolide, phenytoin, pramipexole, primidone, ranitidine, ritonavir, ropinirole, rotigotine, sodium oxybate, sympathomimetics, tetrabenazine, tramadol, tricyclics, valproic acid
Pregnancy category: C
Important contra-indications noted in the prescribing guidelines for: nursing mothers; pediatric patients
Note: Safety and effectiveness have not been established for pediatric patients with schizophrenia <13 years of age, for bipolar mania <10 years of age, and for autistic disorder <5 years of age. [C] = in children.
Black Box Warning: INCREASED MORTALITY IN ELDERLY PATIENTS WITH DEMENTIA-RELATED PSYCHOSIS

Skin
Angioedema [6]

Edema [3]
Peripheral edema (16%) [4]
Photosensitivity (<10%) [2]
Rash [C] (11%) (2–4%)
Seborrhea (2%)
Urticaria [2]
Xerosis (2%)

Hair
Alopecia [2]

Mucosal
Sialopenia (5%)
Sialorrhea [C] (22%) (<3%) [10]
Xerostomia [C] (13%) (4%) [6]

Cardiovascular
Bradycardia [2]
Cardiotoxicity [2]
Hypotension [2]
QT prolongation [4]
Tachycardia [C] (7%) (<5%)
Venous thromboembolism [5]
Ventricular arrhythmia [2]

Central Nervous System
Agitation [2]
Akathisia [C] (16%) (5–9%) [15]
Anorexia [C] (8%) (2%)
Anxiety [C] (16%) (2–16%) [4]
Catatonia [2]
Compulsions [3]
Depression (14%) [6]
Extrapyramidal symptoms [14]
Fever [C] (20%) (<2%)
Headache [7]
Insomnia [7]
Neuroleptic malignant syndrome [24]
Neurotoxicity [2]
Parkinsonism [C] (2–16%) (12–20%) [5]
Psychosis [3]
Rabbit syndrome [3]
Restless legs syndrome [2]
Sedation [2]
Seizures [2]
Serotonin syndrome [3]
Somnolence (drowsiness) [C] (12–67%) (5–14%) [14]
Suicidal ideation [2]
Tardive dyskinesia [3]
Tremor [C] (10–12%) (6%) [4]
Vertigo (dizziness) [C] (7–16%) (4–10%) [5]

Neuromuscular/Skeletal
Arthralgia (2–3%)
Asthenia (fatigue) [C] (18–42%) (<3%) [3]
Back pain (2–3%)
Dystonia [C] (9–18%) (5–11%) [3]
Pisa syndrome [2]
Rhabdomyolysis [7]

Gastrointestinal/Hepatic
Abdominal pain [C] (15–18%) (3–4%)
Constipation [C] (21%) (8–9%) [3]
Diarrhea [C] (7%) (73%)
Dyspepsia [C] (5–16%) (4–10%)
Dysphagia [2]
Nausea [C] (8–16%) (4–9%) [4]
Pancreatitis [2]
Vomiting [C] (10–25%)

Respiratory
Cough [C] (34%) (3%)
Dyspnea [C] (2–5%) (2%)
Pneumonia [2]
Pulmonary embolism [3]
Rhinitis [C] (13–36%) (7–11%)
Upper respiratory tract infection [C] (34%) (2–3%)

Endocrine/Metabolic
Amenorrhea [5]
Appetite increased [C] (49%) [3]
Galactorrhea (<10%) [12]
Gynecomastia (<10%) [6]
Hyperprolactinemia [17]
Metabolic syndrome [5]
Weight gain [C] (5%) [29]

Genitourinary
Priapism (<10%) [27]
Sexual dysfunction [2]
Urinary incontinence [C] (5–22%) (2%)
Urinary tract infection (3%)

Renal
Enuresis [3]

Ocular
Abnormal vision [C] (4–7%) (<3%)

Local
Injection-site pain [2]

Other
Adverse effects [8]
Death [2]
Tooth disorder (<3%)

RITODRINE

Indications: Preterm labor
Class: Beta-2 adrenergic agonist, Tocolytic
Half-life: 1.3–12 hours
Clinically important, potentially hazardous interactions with: glycopyrrolate
Pregnancy category: B

Skin
Anaphylactoid reactions/Anaphylaxis (<3%)
Diaphoresis (<14%)
Erythema (10–15%) [2]
Pustules [2]
Rash (<3%)
Toxic epidermal necrolysis [2]
Vasculitis [2]

Cardiovascular
Chest pain [2]
Myocardial ischemia [2]
Pulmonary edema [3]

Central Nervous System
Chills (3–10%)
Tremor (>10%)

Neuromuscular/Skeletal
Rhabdomyolysis [3]

Gastrointestinal/Hepatic
Hepatotoxicity [3]

Endocrine/Metabolic
Hypokalemia [2]

Ocular
Glaucoma [2]

Other
Adverse effects [2]

RITONAVIR

Trade names: Kaletra (AbbVie), Norvir (AbbVie)
Indications: HIV infection
Class: Antiretroviral, CYP3A4 inhibitor, HIV-1 protease inhibitor
Half-life: 3–5 hours
Clinically important, potentially hazardous interactions with: abiraterone, afatinib, alfentanil, alfuzosin, alprazolam, amiodarone, amitriptyline, amprenavir, aprepitant, astemizole, atazanavir, atorvastatin, atovaquone, atovaquone/proguanil, avanafil, azithromycin, bepridil, boceprevir, bosentan, buprenorphine, bupropion, buspirone, cabazitaxel, cabozantinib, carbamazepine, chlordiazepoxide, ciclesonide, citalopram, clozapine, cobicistat/elvitegravir/emtricitabine/tenofovir disoproxil, colchicine, conivaptan, crizotinib, cyclosporine, cyproterone, darifenacin, dasatinib, deferasirox, delavirdine, diazepam, diclofenac, dihydroergotamine, docetaxel, dronedarone, dutasteride, efavirenz, eletriptan, ergot alkaloids, ergotamine, erlotinib, estazolam, estradiol, eszopiclone, etravirine, everolimus, ezetimibe, fentanyl, fesoterodine, flecainide, flibanserin, flurazepam, fluticasone propionate, halazepam, indacaterol, itraconazole, ivabradine, ixabepilone, ketoconazole, lapatinib, ledipasvir & sofosbuvir, levomepromazine, levothyroxine, lomitapide, macitentan, maraviroc, meloxicam, meperidine, meptazinol, methylergonovine, methysergide, midazolam, mifepristone, nelfinavir, nifedipine, nilotinib, oral contraceptives, osimertinib, paclitaxel, paroxetine hydrochloride, pazopanib, phenytoin, pimozide, piroxicam, pitavastatin, ponatinib, posaconazole, propafenone, propoxyphene, propranolol, quazepam, quinidine, quinine, ranolazine, rifabutin, rifampin, rifapentine, rilpivirine, rimonabant, risperidone, rivaroxaban, romidepsin, rosuvastatin, ruxolitinib, saquinavir, sildenafil, silodosin, simeprevir, simvastatin, sofosbuvir, solifenacin, St John's wort, sunitinib, tadalafil, telaprevir, telithromycin, temsirolimus, tenofovir disoproxil, ticagrelor, tolvaptan, trabectedin, triazolam, ulipristal, vardenafil, vemurafenib, venetoclax, voriconazole, zolpidem, zuclopenthixol
Pregnancy category: B
Important contra-indications noted in the prescribing guidelines for: nursing mothers
Note: Protease inhibitors cause dyslipidemia which includes elevated triglycerides and cholesterol and redistribution of body fat centrally to produce the so-called 'protease paunch', breast enlargement, facial atrophy, and 'buffalo hump'. Kaletra is ritonavir and lopinavir. See also separate entry for ombitasvir/paritaprevir/ritonavir.
Black Box Warning: DRUG-DRUG INTERACTIONS LEADING TO POTENTIALLY SERIOUS AND/OR LIFE THREATENING REACTIONS

Skin
Acneform eruption (4%)
Bullous dermatitis (<2%)
Dermatitis (<2%)
Diaphoresis (<10%)
Ecchymoses (<2%)

Eczema (<2%)
Edema (6%)
Exanthems (<2%) [2]
Facial edema (8%)
Folliculitis (<2%)
Hypersensitivity (8%)
Jaundice [3]
Lipodystrophy [4]
Peripheral edema (6%)
Photosensitivity (<2%)
Pruritus (12%)
Psoriasis (<2%)
Rash (27%) [12]
Seborrhea (<2%)
Toxicity [2]
Urticaria (8%)
Xanthomas [2]
Xerosis (<2%)

Hair

Alopecia [2]

Mucosal

Cheilitis (<2%)
Gingivitis (<2%)
Oral candidiasis (<2%)
Oral ulceration (<2%)
Oropharyngeal pain (16%)
Xerostomia (<2%)

Cardiovascular

Cardiotoxicity [2]
Flushing (13%)
Hypertension (3%)
Hypotension (2%)
Orthostatic hypotension (2%)

Central Nervous System

Ageusia (taste loss) (<2%)
Confusion (3%)
Dysgeusia (taste perversion) (16%)
Headache [7]
Hyperesthesia (<2%)
Impaired concentration (3%)
Insomnia [2]
Neurotoxicity [2]
Paresthesias (51%)
Parosmia (<2%)
Peripheral neuropathy (10%)
Syncope (3%)
Vertigo (dizziness) (16%) [2]

Neuromuscular/Skeletal

Arthralgia (19%)
Asthenia (fatigue) (46%) [3]
Back pain (19%)
Myalgia/Myopathy (4–9%)
Rhabdomyolysis [2]

Gastrointestinal/Hepatic

Abdominal pain (26%) [2]
Diarrhea (68%) [14]
Dyspepsia (12%)
Flatulence (8%)
Gastrointestinal bleeding (2%)
Gastrointestinal disorder [4]
Hepatotoxicity (9%) [5]
Nausea (57%) [11]
Vomiting (32%) [7]

Respiratory

Cough (22%)
Nasopharyngitis [2]
Upper respiratory tract infection [2]

Endocrine/Metabolic

ALT increased [3]
Cushing's syndrome [7]
Gynecomastia [2]
Hyperbilirubinemia [5]
Hypercholesterolemia (3%) [2]
Hyperlipidemia [2]
Hypertriglyceridemia (9%) [2]

Genitourinary

Urinary frequency (4%)

Renal

Fanconi syndrome [4]
Nephrolithiasis [3]
Nephrotoxicity [2]
Renal failure [2]

Ocular

Vision blurred (6%)

Other

Adverse effects [9]
Allergic reactions (<2%)

RITUXIMAB

Trade names: MabThera (Roche), Rituxan (Genentech)
Indications: Non-Hodgkin's lymphoma, chronic lymphocytic leukemia, rhematoid arthritis (in combination with methotrexate), granulomatosis with polyangiitis and mycroscopic polyangiitis (in combination with glucocorticoids)
Class: Biologic, CD20-directed cytolytic monoclonal antibody, Disease-modifying antirheumatic drug (DMARD), Immunosuppressant, Monoclonal antibody
Half-life: 60 hours (after first infusion)
Clinically important, potentially hazardous interactions with: benazepril, captopril, certolizumab, cisplatin, clevidipine, enalapril, fosinopril, irbesartan, lisinopril, olmesartan, quinapril, ramipril
Pregnancy category: C
Important contra-indications noted in the prescribing guidelines for: nursing mothers; pediatric patients
Black Box Warning: FATAL INFUSION REACTIONS, SEVERE MUCOCUTANEOUS REACTIONS, HEPATITIS B VIRUS REACTIVATION and PROGRESSIVE MULTIFOCAL LEUKOENCEPHALOPATHY

Skin

Anaphylactoid reactions/Anaphylaxis [7]
Angioedema (11%) [4]
Dermatitis [2]
Diaphoresis (15%) [2]
Herpes simplex [2]
Herpes zoster [6]
Hypersensitivity [5]
Kaposi's sarcoma [3]
Paraneoplastic pemphigus [2]
Peripheral edema (8%)
Pruritus (14%) [8]
Psoriasis [3]
Rash (15%) [12]
Serum sickness [22]
Stevens–Johnson syndrome [5]
Toxic epidermal necrolysis [3]
Toxicity [2]
Urticaria (8%) [5]
Vasculitis [3]

Mucosal

Mucocutaneous reactions [2]
Stomatitis [2]

Cardiovascular

Cardiotoxicity [5]
Flushing (5%)
Hypertension (6%) [2]
Hypotension (10%) [9]
Myocardial infarction [2]

Central Nervous System

Anxiety (5%)
Chills (33%) [15]
Encephalitis [3]
Fever (53%) [22]
Headache (19%) [4]
Leukoencephalopathy [25]
Neurotoxicity [3]
Pain (12%)
Peripheral neuropathy [5]
Rigors [4]
Vertigo (dizziness) (10%)

Neuromuscular/Skeletal

Arthralgia (10%) [2]
Asthenia (fatigue) (26%) [14]
Back pain (10%)
Myalgia/Myopathy (10%)

Gastrointestinal/Hepatic

Abdominal pain (14%)
Colitis [4]
Constipation [2]
Diarrhea (10%) [7]
Hepatitis [2]
Hepatotoxicity [6]
Nausea (23%) [9]
Pancreatitis [2]
Vomiting (10%) [6]

Respiratory

Acute respiratory distress syndrome [3]
Bronchospasm (8%) [6]
Cough (increased) (13%) [6]
Dyspnea (7%) [7]
Flu-like syndrome [3]
Nasopharyngitis [2]
Pneumonia [17]
Pneumonitis [2]
Pulmonary toxicity [13]
Rhinitis (12%) [2]
Sinusitis (6%) [4]
Upper respiratory tract infection [6]

Endocrine/Metabolic

ALT increased [2]
Hyperglycemia (9%)
Hyponatremia [2]

Genitourinary

Urinary tract infection [7]

Renal

Nephrotoxicity [3]

Hematologic

Anemia (8%) [9]
Cytopenia [3]
Febrile neutropenia [12]
Hemotoxicity [2]
Hypogammaglobulinemia [4]
Leukopenia (14%) [10]
Lymphocytopenia [2]

Lymphopenia (48%) [7]
Myelosuppression [5]
Myelotoxicity [2]
Neutropenia (14%) [37]
Sepsis [3]
Thrombocytopenia (12%) [26]
Thrombosis [2]

Local

Application-site reactions [4]
Infusion-related reactions [18]
Infusion-site reactions [11]
Injection-site pain [2]
Injection-site reactions [4]

Other

Adverse effects [26]
Allergic reactions [2]
Death [22]
Infection (31%) [40]

RIVAROXABAN

Trade name: Xarelto (Janssen)
Indications: Prevention of venous thromboembolism in patients undergoing knee or hip replacement surgery, treatment of deep vein thrombosis and pulmonary embolism
Class: Anticoagulant, Direct factor Xa inhibitor
Half-life: 5–9 hours
Clinically important, potentially hazardous interactions with: anticoagulants, aspirin, atazanavir, atorvastatin, carbamazepine, clarithromycin, clopidogrel, combined P-glycoprotein and strong CYP3A4 inhibitors and inducers, conivaptan, dabigatran, darunavir, delavirdine, diclofenac, efavirenz, enoxaparin, erythromycin, fosamprenavir, HIV protease inhibitors, indinavir, itraconazole, ketoconazole, ketorolac, lapatinib, lopinavir, nelfinavir, phenobarbital, phenytoin, posaconazole, rifampin, ritonavir, saquinavir, St John's wort, telithromycin, tipranavir, voriconazole
Pregnancy category: C
Important contra-indications noted in the prescribing guidelines for: nursing mothers; pediatric patients
Note: Contraindicated in patients with active pathological bleeding.
Black Box Warning: PREMATURE DISCONTINUATION OF XARELTO INCREASES THE RISK OF THROMBOTIC EVENTS
SPINAL/EPIDURAL HEMATOMA

Skin

Hematoma [2]
Pruritus (2%)
Rash [2]

Mucosal

Epistaxis (nosebleed) [6]
Gingival bleeding [2]

Gastrointestinal/Hepatic

Abdominal pain [2]
Hepatotoxicity [4]

Genitourinary

Hematuria [5]

Hematologic

Anemia (3%)
Bleeding [13]
Hemorrhage [5]

Other

Adverse effects [3]

RIVASTIGMINE

Trade name: Exelon (Novartis)
Indications: Alzheimer's disease and dementia
Class: Acetylcholinesterase inhibitor, Cholinesterase inhibitor
Half-life: 1–2 hours
Clinically important, potentially hazardous interactions with: galantamine
Pregnancy category: B
Important contra-indications noted in the prescribing guidelines for: nursing mothers; pediatric patients

---

Skin

Dermatitis [2]
Diaphoresis (10%)
Exanthems [2]
Hyperhidrosis (4%)
Peripheral edema (>2%)
Rash (>2%) [2]

Cardiovascular

Bradycardia [5]
Chest pain (>2%)
Hypertension (3%)
QT prolongation [2]
Thrombophlebitis (<2%)

Central Nervous System

Aggression (3%)
Agitation (>2%)
Anorexia (6–17%) [2]
Anxiety (4–5%)
Confusion (8%)
Delusions of parasitosis (>2%)
Depression (6%)
Hallucinations (4%)
Headache (4–17%)
Insomnia (3–9%)
Nervousness (>2%)
Pain (>2%)
Parkinsonism (2%)
Restlessness [2]
Somnolence (drowsiness) (3–5%)
Syncope (3%) [3]
Tremor (4–10%) [3]
Vertigo (dizziness) (6–21%) [4]

Neuromuscular/Skeletal

Arthralgia (>2%)
Asthenia (fatigue) (2–9%)
Back pain (>2%)
Dystonia [2]
Fractures (>2%)
Myalgia/Myopathy (20%)

Gastrointestinal/Hepatic

Abdominal pain (4–13%)
Constipation (5%) [2]
Diarrhea (7–19%) [4]
Dyspepsia (9%)
Eructation (belching) (2%)
Flatulence (4%)
Nausea (29–47%) [11]
Vomiting (17–31%) [11]

Respiratory

Bronchitis (>2%)
Cough (>2%)
Flu-like syndrome (3%)
Pharyngitis (>2%)
Rhinitis (4%)

Endocrine/Metabolic

Dehydration (2%)
Weight loss (3%) [2]

Genitourinary

Urinary incontinence (>2%)
Urinary tract infection (7%)

Local

Application-site pruritus [2]
Application-site reactions [3]

Other

Adverse effects [5]
Death [2]
Infection (>2%)

RIZATRIPTAN

Trade name: Maxalt (Merck)
Indications: Migraine
Class: 5-HT1 agonist, Serotonin receptor agonist, Triptan
Half-life: 2–3 hours
Clinically important, potentially hazardous interactions with: dihydroergotamine, ergot-containing drugs, isocarboxazid, MAO inhibitors, methysergide, naratriptan, phenelzine, propranolol, sibutramine, SSRIs, St John's wort, sumatriptan, tranylcypromine, zolmitriptan
Pregnancy category: C
Important contra-indications noted in the prescribing guidelines for: nursing mothers
Note: Safety and effectiveness in pediatric patients <6 years of age have not been established.

Mucosal

Xerostomia (3%)

Cardiovascular

Chest pain (<3%) [2]

Central Nervous System

Headache (<2%)
Neurotoxicity [2]
Pain (3%)
Paresthesias (3–4%)
Somnolence (drowsiness) (4–6%)
Vertigo (dizziness) (4–9%) [10]

Neuromuscular/Skeletal

Asthenia (fatigue) (4–7%) [9]
Jaw pain (<2%)
Neck pain (<2%)

Gastrointestinal/Hepatic

Nausea (4–6%)

Other

Adverse effects [4]

ROFLUMILAST

Trade names: Daliresp (Takeda), Daxas (Takeda)
Indications: To reduce the risk of COPD exacerbations in patients with severe COPD associated with chronic bronchitis and a history of exacerbations
Class: Anti-inflammatory, Phosphodiesterase inhibitor, Phosphodiesterase type 4 (PDE4) inhibitor
Half-life: 17 hours
Clinically important, potentially hazardous interactions with: aminophylline, carbamazepine, cimetidine, denileukin, efavirenz, enoxacin, erythromycin, fingolimod, fluvoxamine, ketoconazole, oral contraceptives, pazopanib, phenobarbital, phenytoin, rifampin
Pregnancy category: C
Important contra-indications noted in the prescribing guidelines for: nursing mothers; pediatric patients
Note: Contraindicated in patients with moderate to severe liver impairment (Child-Pugh B or C class).

Cardiovascular
Cardiotoxicity [2]
Hypertension [3]

Central Nervous System
Anorexia [2]
Anxiety (<2%) [2]
Depression (<2%)
Headache (4%) [21]
Insomnia (2%) [6]
Neurotoxicity [3]
Suicidal ideation [2]
Tremor (<2%)
Vertigo (dizziness) [3]

Neuromuscular/Skeletal
Back pain (3%) [4]
Muscle spasm (<2%)

Gastrointestinal/Hepatic
Abdominal pain (<2%) [2]
Diarrhea (10%) [25]
Dyspepsia (<2%)
Gastritis (<2%)
Nausea (5%) [24]
Vomiting (<2%) [2]

Respiratory
Bronchitis [3]
COPD [3]
Dyspnea [3]
Influenza (3%) [3]
Nasopharyngitis [4]
Pneumonia [3]
Rhinitis (<2%)
Sinusitis (<2%)
Upper respiratory tract infection [4]

Endocrine/Metabolic
Appetite decreased (2%) [4]
Weight loss (8%) [24]

Genitourinary
Urinary tract infection (<2%)

Other
Adverse effects [6]

ROLAPITANT

Synonym: SCH 619734
Trade name: Varubi (Tesaro)
Indications: Delayed nausea and vomiting from chemotherapy, in combination with dexamethasone and a 5HT3-receptor antagonist
Class: Antiemetic, Neurokinin 1 receptor antagonist
Half-life: ~7 days
Clinically important, potentially hazardous interactions with: thioridazine
Pregnancy category: N/A (No data available)
Important contra-indications noted in the prescribing guidelines for: nursing mothers; pediatric patients

---

Mucosal
Stomatitis (4%)

Central Nervous System
Headache [5]
Vertigo (dizziness) (6%)

Neuromuscular/Skeletal
Asthenia (fatigue) [4]

Gastrointestinal/Hepatic
Abdominal pain (3%)
Constipation [5]
Dyspepsia (4%) [3]

Endocrine/Metabolic
Appetite decreased (9%)

Genitourinary
Urinary tract infection (4%)

Hematologic
Anemia (3%)
Neutropenia (7–9%) [2]

Other
Hiccups (5%) [3]

ROMIDEPSIN

Trade name: Istodax (Celgene)
Indications: Cutaneous T-cell lymphoma (CTCL)
Class: Histone deacetylase (HDAC) inhibitor
Half-life: 3 hours
Clinically important, potentially hazardous interactions with: atazanavir, carbamazepine, clarithromycin, conivaptan, coumadin derivatives, CYP3A4 inhibitors and inducers, darunavir, delavirdine, dexamethasone, efavirenz, indinavir, itraconazole, ketoconazole, nefazodone, nelfinavir, oxcarbazepine, phenobarbital, phenytoin, rifabutin, rifampin, rifapentine, ritonavir, saquinavir, St John's wort, telithromycin, voriconazole, warfarin
Pregnancy category: D
Important contra-indications noted in the prescribing guidelines for: nursing mothers; pediatric patients

---

Skin
Dermatitis (4–27%)
Edema (>2%)
Exfoliative dermatitis (4–27%)
Peripheral edema (6–10%)
Pruritus (7–31%)

Mucosal
Stomatitis (6–10%)

Cardiovascular
Hypotension (7–23%)
Supraventricular arrhythmias (>2%)
Tachycardia (10%)
Ventricular arrhythmia (>2%)

Central Nervous System
Anorexia (23–54%) [5]
Chills (11–17%)
Dysgeusia (taste perversion) (15–40%)
Fever (20–47%)
Headache (15–34%)

Neuromuscular/Skeletal
Asthenia (fatigue) (53–77%) [10]

Gastrointestinal/Hepatic
Abdominal pain (13–14%)
Constipation (12–40%)
Diarrhea (20–36%)
Nausea (56–86%) [9]
Vomiting (34–52%) [5]

Respiratory
Cough (18–21%)
Dyspnea (13–21%)

Endocrine/Metabolic
ALT increased (3–22%)
AST increased (3–28%)
Hyperglycemia (2–51%)
Hypermagnesemia (27%)
Hyperuricemia (33%)
Hypoalbuminemia (3–48%)
Hypocalcemia (4–52%)
Hypokalemia (6–20%)
Hypomagnesemia (22–28%)
Hyponatremia (<20%)
Hypophosphatemia (27%)
Weight loss (10–15%)

Hematologic
Anemia (19–72%) [3]
Leukopenia (4–55%)
Lymphopenia (4–57%)
Neutropenia (11–66%) [4]
Sepsis (>2%)
Thrombocytopenia (17–72%) [7]

Other
Adverse effects [2]
Infection (46–54%) [2]

ROPINIROLE

Trade name: Requip (GSK)
Indications: Parkinsonism
Class: Dopamine receptor agonist
Half-life: ~6 hours
Clinically important, potentially hazardous interactions with: ciprofloxacin, estradiol, levomepromazine, norfloxacin, risperidone, warfarin, zuclopenthixol
Pregnancy category: C
Important contra-indications noted in the prescribing guidelines for: nursing mothers; pediatric patients

---

Skin
Diaphoresis (3–6%)
Herpes simplex (5%)

Hyperhidrosis (3%)
Peripheral edema (2–7%) [2]
Rash [2]

Mucosal
Xerostomia (5%)

Cardiovascular
Cardiotoxicity [2]
Chest pain (4%)
Flushing (3%)
Hypotension [2]
Orthostatic hypotension [4]

Central Nervous System
Amnesia (3%)
Dyskinesia [8]
Hallucinations (<5%) [7]
Headache (6%) [5]
Hyperesthesia (4%)
Impulse control disorder [3]
Insomnia [2]
Pain (3–8%)
Paresthesias (5%)
Psychosis [5]
Sleep related disorder [2]
Somnolence (drowsiness) (11–40%) [12]
Syncope (<12%) [3]
Tremor (6%)
Vertigo (dizziness) (6–40%) [16]
Yawning (3%)

Neuromuscular/Skeletal
Arthralgia (4%)
Asthenia (fatigue) (8–11%) [4]
Back pain [2]
Myalgia/Myopathy (3%)

Gastrointestinal/Hepatic
Abdominal pain (3–7%) [2]
Constipation [2]
Diarrhea (5%)
Dyspepsia (4–10%) [3]
Nausea (40–60%) [17]
Vomiting (11%) [3]

Respiratory
Cough (3%)
Dyspnea (3%)
Flu-like syndrome (3%)
Pharyngitis (6–9%)
Rhinitis (4%)
Sinusitis (4%)

Genitourinary
Impotence (3%)
Urinary tract infection (5%)

Ocular
Abnormal vision (6%)
Xerophthalmia (2%)

Other
Adverse effects [5]
Infection (viral) (11%)

ROSIGLITAZONE

Trade names: Avandamet (GSK), Avandaryl (GSK), Avandia (GSK)
Indications: Type II diabetes
Class: Antidiabetic, Thiazolidinedione
Half-life: 3–4 hours
Clinically important, potentially hazardous interactions with: CYP2C8 inhibitors and inducers, gemfibrozil, grapefruit juice, paclitaxel, rifampin, teriflunomide
Pregnancy category: C
Important contra-indications noted in the prescribing guidelines for: nursing mothers
Note: Thiazolidinediones, including rosiglitazone, cause or exacerbate congestive heart failure in some patients.
Contraindicated in patients with established NYHA Class III or IV heart failure. Avandaryl is rosiglitazone and glimepiride; Avandamet is rosiglitazone and metformin.
Black Box Warning: CONGESTIVE HEART FAILURE

Skin
Edema (5%) [12]
Peripheral edema [11]

Cardiovascular
Cardiac failure [13]
Congestive heart failure [2]
Myocardial infarction [9]
Myocardial ischemia [3]

Central Nervous System
Headache (6%)
Stroke [2]

Neuromuscular/Skeletal
Arthralgia (5%)
Back pain (4%)
Fractures [5]

Gastrointestinal/Hepatic
Hepatotoxicity [9]
Nausea [2]

Respiratory
Dyspnea [2]
Nasopharyngitis (6%)
Respiratory tract infection (10%)

Endocrine/Metabolic
Weight gain [4]

Genitourinary
Bladder disorder [2]

Hematologic
Anemia [2]

Ocular
Macular edema [8]
Proptosis [2]

Other
Adverse effects [3]
Death [6]

ROSUVASTATIN

Trade name: Crestor (AstraZeneca)
Indications: Hypercholesterolemia, mixed dyslipidemia
Class: HMG-CoA reductase inhibitor, Statin
Half-life: ~19 hours
Clinically important, potentially hazardous interactions with: alcohol, amiodarone, antacids, atazanavir, ciprofibrate, colchicine, conivaptan, coumarins, cyclosporine, daptomycin, darunavir, dronedarone, eltrombopag, erythromycin, ethinylestradiol, fenofibrate, fibrates, fosamprenavir, fusidic acid, gemfibrozil, indinavir, ledipasvir & sofosbuvir, lopinavir, nelfinavir, niacin, niacinamide, phenindione, progestins, protease inhibitors, ritonavir, saquinavir, tipranavir, trabectedin, vitamin K antagonists, warfarin
Pregnancy category: X
Important contra-indications noted in the prescribing guidelines for: nursing mothers

---

Skin
Peripheral edema (>2%)
Rash (>2%)

Central Nervous System
Depression (>2%)
Headache (6%)
Pain (>2%)
Paresthesias (>2%)
Vertigo (dizziness) (4%) [3]

Neuromuscular/Skeletal
Arthralgia (>2%)
Asthenia (fatigue) (3%) [2]
Back pain (3%)
Myalgia/Myopathy (3%) [18]
Rhabdomyolysis [16]

Gastrointestinal/Hepatic
Abdominal pain (>2%)
Constipation (2%)
Hepatotoxicity [5]
Nausea (3%)

Respiratory
Cough (>2%)
Flu-like syndrome (2%)
Rhinitis (2%)
Sinusitis (2%)

Endocrine/Metabolic
Creatine phosphokinase increased [2]
Diabetes mellitus [3]

Renal
Nephrotoxicity [4]
Renal failure [3]

Other
Adverse effects [6]

ROTAVIRUS VACCINE

Trade names: Rotarix (GSK), RotaTeq (Merck)
Indications: Prevention of rotavirus gastroenteritis
Half-life: N/A
Clinically important, potentially hazardous interactions with: none known

Pregnancy category: C

Central Nervous System
Fever [3]

Gastrointestinal/Hepatic
Intussusception [2]

ROTIGOTINE

Trade name: Neupro (Schwarz)
Indications: Parkinsonism, restless legs syndrome
Class: Dopamine receptor agonist
Half-life: 5–7 hours
Clinically important, potentially hazardous interactions with: antipsychotics, levomepromazine, memantine, methyldopa, metoclopramide, risperidone, zuclopenthixol
Pregnancy category: C
Important contra-indications noted in the prescribing guidelines for: nursing mothers; pediatric patients
Note: Neupro contains sodium metabisulfite which is capable of causing anaphylactoid reactions in patients with sulfite allergy.

Skin
Diaphoresis (4%)
Erythema (2%)
Peripheral edema (7%) [3]
Rash (2%) [3]

Mucosal
Xerostomia (3%) [3]

Cardiovascular
Chest pain (>2%)
Hypertension (3%)
Hypotension [2]

Central Nervous System
Abnormal dreams (3%)
Anorexia (3%)
Anxiety (>2%)
Depression (>2%)
Dyskinesia [4]
Gait instability [2]
Hallucinations (2%) [3]
Headache (14%) [8]
Impulse control disorder [4]
Insomnia (10%) [3]
Somnolence (drowsiness) (25%) [16]
Tremor (>2%) [2]
Vertigo (dizziness) (3–18%) [7]

Neuromuscular/Skeletal
Arthralgia (4%)
Asthenia (fatigue) (8%) [10]
Back pain (6%)
Myalgia/Myopathy (2%)

Gastrointestinal/Hepatic
Abdominal pain (>2%)
Constipation (5%)
Diarrhea (>2%)
Dyspepsia (4%)
Gastrointestinal disorder [2]
Nausea (38%) [23]
Vomiting (13%) [6]

Respiratory
Cough (>2%)
Flu-like syndrome (>2%)
Rhinitis (>2%)
Sinusitis (3%)
Upper respiratory tract infection (>2%)

Genitourinary
Urinary frequency (>2%)
Urinary tract infection (3%)

Ocular
Abnormal vision (3%)
Hallucinations, visual (2%) [2]
Visual disturbances (3%)

Local
Application-site erythema [4]
Application-site pruritus [4]
Application-site reactions (37%) [31]

Other
Adverse effects [5]

SACCHARIN

Indications: Sugar substitute
Class: Sweetening agent
Half-life: N/A
Clinically important, potentially hazardous interactions with: none known
Pregnancy category: N/A
Note: Saccharin is a sulfonamide and can be absorbed systemically. Sulfonamides can produce severe, possibly fatal, reactions such as toxic epidermal necrolysis and Stevens-Johnson syndrome.

Skin
Dermatitis [3]
Exanthems [2]
Photosensitivity [3]
Pruritus [3]
Urticaria [5]

SACUBITRIL/ VALSARTAN

Synonym: LCZ696
Trade name: Entresto (Novartis)
Indications: To reduce risk of cardiovascular death and hospitalization for heart failure in chronic heart failure
Class: Angiotensin receptor neprilysin inhibitor (ARNI)
Half-life: <12 hours
Clinically important, potentially hazardous interactions with: ACE inhibitors, aliskiren, lithium, NSAIDs, potassium-sparing diuretics
Pregnancy category: N/A (Can cause fetal harm)
Important contra-indications noted in the prescribing guidelines for: nursing mothers; pediatric patients
Note: Contraindicated in patients with a history of angioedema related to previous therapy with angiotensin-converting enzyme inhibitor or angiotensin II receptor blocker. See also separate profile for valsartan.
Black Box Warning: FETAL TOXICITY

Skin
Angioedema (<2%)
Peripheral edema [2]

Cardiovascular
Hypotension (18%) [3]
Orthostatic hypotension (2%)

Central Nervous System
Gait instability (2%)
Vertigo (dizziness) (6%) [2]

Neuromuscular/Skeletal
Arthralgia [2]

Gastrointestinal/Hepatic
Constipation [2]

Respiratory
Cough (9%) [3]
Nasopharyngitis [2]

Endocrine/Metabolic
Creatine phosphokinase increased (16%)
Hyperkalemia (12%) [3]

Renal
Nephrotoxicity [2]
Renal failure (5%)

Other
Adverse effects [2]

SALSALATE

Trade name: Mono-Gesic (Schwarz)
Indications: Arthritis
Class: Non-steroidal anti-inflammatory (NSAID), Salicylate
Half-life: 7–8 hours
Clinically important, potentially hazardous interactions with: dichlorphenamide, methotrexate
Pregnancy category: C
Important contra-indications noted in the prescribing guidelines for: nursing mothers; pediatric patients
Note: NSAIDs may cause an increased risk of serious cardiovascular and gastrointestinal adverse events, which can be fatal. This risk may increase with duration of use.

Skin
Anaphylactoid reactions/Anaphylaxis (<10%)
Rash (<10%)

SAQUINAVIR

Trade name: Invirase (Roche)
Indications: Advanced HIV infection
Class: Antiretroviral, CYP3A4 inhibitor, HIV-1 protease inhibitor
Half-life: 12 hours
Clinically important, potentially hazardous interactions with: abiraterone, afatinib, alprazolam, amitriptyline, amprenavir, astemizole, atazanavir, atorvastatin, avanafil, cabazitaxel, cabozantinib, clindamycin, clozapine, crizotinib, darifenacin, darunavir, dasatinib, delavirdine, dihydroergotamine, dronedarone, efavirenz, eplerenone, ergot derivatives, everolimus, fentanyl, fesoterodine, flibanserin, fluticasone propionate, itraconazole, ixabepilone, ketoconazole, lapatinib, levomepromazine, lomitapide, lopinavir, maraviroc, methysergide, midazolam, mifepristone, nelfinavir, omeprazole, paclitaxel, pantoprazole, pazopanib, pentamidine, phenytoin, pimozide, ponatinib, quinine, rifampin, rilpivirine, ritonavir, rivaroxaban, romidepsin, rosuvastatin, ruxolitinib, sildenafil, simeprevir, simvastatin, solifenacin, St John's wort, sunitinib, tadalafil, telithromycin, temsirolimus, ticagrelor, tipranavir, tolvaptan, vardenafil, vemurafenib, voriconazole
Pregnancy category: B
Important contra-indications noted in the prescribing guidelines for: nursing mothers
Note: Protease inhibitors cause dyslipidemia which includes elevated triglycerides and cholesterol and redistribution of body fat centrally to produce the so-called 'protease paunch', breast enlargement, facial atrophy, and 'buffalo hump'.

Skin
Acneform eruption (<2%)
Candidiasis (<2%)
Dermatitis (<2%)
Diaphoresis (<2%)
Eczema (<2%)
Erythema (<2%)
Exanthems (<2%)
Folliculitis (<2%)
Herpes simplex (<2%)
Herpes zoster (<2%)
Photosensitivity (<2%)
Pigmentation (<2%)
Seborrheic dermatitis (<2%)
Ulcerations (<2%)
Urticaria (<2%)
Verrucae (<2%)
Xerosis (<2%)

Hair
Hair changes (<2%)

Mucosal
Cheilitis (<2%)
Gingivitis (<2%)
Glossitis (<2%)
Oral ulceration (2%)
Stomatitis (<2%)
Xerostomia (<2%)

Cardiovascular
QT prolongation [3]

Central Nervous System
Dysesthesia (<2%)
Dysgeusia (taste perversion) (<2%)
Hyperesthesia (<2%)
Paresthesias (3%)

Gastrointestinal/Hepatic
Hepatotoxicity [2]

Endocrine/Metabolic
Gynecomastia [2]

SAXAGLIPTIN

Trade name: Onglyza (Bristol-Myers Squibb)
Indications: Type II diabetes mellitus
Class: Antidiabetic, Dipeptidyl peptidase-4 (DPP-4) inhibitor
Half-life: 2.5–3.1 hours
Clinically important, potentially hazardous interactions with: ACE inhibitors, alcohol, aprepitant, beta blockers, bexarotene, colchicine, conivaptan, corticosteroids, CYP3A4 inducers, darunavir, dasatinib, delavirdine, diazoxide, diuretics, efavirenz, estradiol, estrogens, hypoglycemic agents, indinavir, ketoconazole, lapatinib, MAO inhibitors, oxcarbazepine, P-glycoprotein inhibitors and inducers, pegvisomant, pioglitazone, rifapentine, somatropin, strong CYP3A4/5 inhibitors, telithromycin, terbinafine, testosterone, voriconazole
Pregnancy category: B
Important contra-indications noted in the prescribing guidelines for: nursing mothers; pediatric patients

---

Skin
Hypersensitivity (<2%)
Peripheral edema (2–3%)

Cardiovascular
Cardiac disorder [2]
Cardiac failure [2]

Central Nervous System
Headache (7%) [7]

Gastrointestinal/Hepatic
Abdominal pain (2%)
Diarrhea [4]
Gastroenteritis (2%)
Vomiting (2%)

Respiratory
Nasopharyngitis [4]
Sinusitis (3%) [2]
Upper respiratory tract infection (8%) [7]

Endocrine/Metabolic
Hypoglycemia [9]

Genitourinary
Urinary tract infection (7%) [7]

Other
Adverse effects [7]
Infection [2]

SEBELIPASE ALFA *

Trade name: Kanuma (Alexion)
Indications: Lysosomal acid lipase deficiency
Class: Enzyme replacement
Half-life: 5–7 minutes
Clinically important, potentially hazardous interactions with: none known
Pregnancy category: N/A (No available data)
Important contra-indications noted in the prescribing guidelines for: nursing mothers

---

Skin
Hypersensitivity (20%)
Urticaria (33%)

Mucosal
Oropharyngeal pain (17%)

Cardiovascular
Chest pain (<8%)
Tachycardia (<30%)

Central Nervous System
Anxiety (<8%)
Fever (25–56%)
Headache (28%)

Neuromuscular/Skeletal
Asthenia (fatigue) (8%)
Hypotonia (<30%)

Gastrointestinal/Hepatic
Constipation (8%)
Diarrhea (67%)
Nausea (8%)
Vomiting (67%)

Respiratory
Cough (33%)
Nasopharyngitis (11–33%)
Rhinitis (56%)

Hematologic
Anemia (44%)

Other
Sneezing (<30%)

SECUKINUMAB

Trade name: Cosentyx (Novartis)
Indications: Plaque psoriasis, psoriatic arthritis, ankylosing spondylitis
Class: Interleukin 17A (IL-17A) antagonist, Monoclonal antibody
Half-life: 22–31 days
Clinically important, potentially hazardous interactions with: live vaccines
Pregnancy category: B
Important contra-indications noted in the prescribing guidelines for: nursing mothers; pediatric patients
Note: Use with caution in patients with inflammatory bowel disease.

Skin
Candidiasis [3]
Neoplasms [2]
Pruritus [2]

Cardiovascular
Hypertension [2]

Central Nervous System
Headache [10]

Neuromuscular/Skeletal
Arthralgia [2]

Gastrointestinal/Hepatic
Diarrhea (3–4%) [3]

Respiratory
Nasopharyngitis (11–12%) [16]
Upper respiratory tract infection (3%) [9]

Hematologic
Neutropenia [4]

Local
Injection-site reactions [2]

Other
Adverse effects [4]
Infection (29%) [12]

SELEGILINE

Synonyms: deprenyl; L-deprenyl
Trade names: Eldepryl (Somerset), Emsam (Mylan Specialty), Zelapar (Valeant)
Indications: Parkinsonism
Class: Antidepressant, Monoamine oxidase B inhibitor
Half-life: 9 minutes
Clinically important, potentially hazardous interactions with: amitriptyline, carbidopa, citalopram, doxepin, ephedra, ephedrine, escitalopram, fluoxetine, fluvoxamine, levodopa, meperidine, methadone, moclobemide, naratriptan, nefazodone, oral contraceptives, oxcarbazepine, paroxetine hydrochloride, propoxyphene, sertraline, tramadol, venlafaxine
Pregnancy category: C
Important contra-indications noted in the prescribing guidelines for: nursing mothers; pediatric patients
Black Box Warning: SUICIDALITY IN CHILDREN AND ADOLESCENTS

Mucosal
Xerostomia (>10%) [2]

Cardiovascular
Hypertension [2]

Central Nervous System
Hallucinations [2]
Headache [2]
Serotonin syndrome [2]

Gastrointestinal/Hepatic
Nausea [2]

Local
Application-site reactions [5]

Other
Bruxism (<10%)

SELEXIPAG *

Trade name: Uptravi (Actelion)
Indications: Pulmonary arterial hypertension
Class: Prostacyclin receptor agonist
Half-life: <3 hours
Clinically important, potentially hazardous interactions with: gemfibrozil, strong CYP2C8 inhibitors
Pregnancy category: N/A (No data available)
Important contra-indications noted in the prescribing guidelines for: nursing mothers

---

Skin
Rash (11%)

Cardiovascular
Flushing (12%)

Central Nervous System
Headache (65%) [5]

Neuromuscular/Skeletal
Arthralgia (11%)
Jaw pain (26%) [3]
Myalgia/Myopathy (16%)
Pain in extremities (17%)

Gastrointestinal/Hepatic
Diarrhea (42%)
Nausea (33%) [3]
Vomiting (18%)

Endocrine/Metabolic
Appetite decreased (6%)

Hematologic
Anemia (8%)

SERTRALINE

Trade name: Zoloft (Pfizer)
Indications: Depression, panic disorders, obsessive compulsive disorders
Class: Antidepressant, Selective serotonin reuptake inhibitor (SSRI)
Half-life: 24–26 hours
Clinically important, potentially hazardous interactions with: amphetamines, astemizole, clarithromycin, clozapine, darunavir, dextroamphetamine, diethylpropion, droperidol, efavirenz, erythromycin, isocarboxazid, linezolid, MAO inhibitors, mazindol, methamphetamine, metoclopramide, phendimetrazine, phenelzine, phentermine, phenylpropanolamine, pimozide, pseudoephedrine, selegiline, sibutramine, St John's wort, sumatriptan, sympathomimetics, tranylcypromine, trazodone, troleandomycin, zolmitriptan
Pregnancy category: C

Skin
Angioedema [3]
Diaphoresis (8%) [6]
Rash (<10%)
Stevens–Johnson syndrome [2]

Hair
Alopecia [3]

Mucosal
Xerostomia (16%) [7]

Cardiovascular
Chest pain (<10%)
Flushing (2%)
Palpitation (<10%)
QT prolongation [2]

Central Nervous System
Akathisia [6]
Anxiety (<10%)
Coma [2]
Headache (>10%)
Hypoesthesia (5%)
Insomnia (>10%)
Mania [3]
Pain (<10%)
Paresthesias (<10%)
Restless legs syndrome [3]
Seizures [2]
Serotonin syndrome [10]
Somnolence (drowsiness) (>10%)
Tremor (<10%) [3]
Vertigo (dizziness) (>10%) [3]
Yawning (<10%)

Neuromuscular/Skeletal
Asthenia (fatigue) (>10%)
Back pain (<10%)

Gastrointestinal/Hepatic
Constipation (<10%)
Diarrhea (>10%) [3]
Hepatotoxicity [4]
Nausea (10%)
Vomiting (>10%)

Respiratory
Rhinitis (<10%)

Endocrine/Metabolic
Galactorrhea [2]
Gynecomastia [2]
Hyponatremia [3]
Libido decreased (>10%)
SIADH [14]
Weight gain (<10%)

Genitourinary
Impotence (<10%)
Priapism [5]
Sexual dysfunction (10%) [4]

Otic
Tinnitus (<10%)

Ocular
Abnormal vision (<10%)
Hallucinations, visual [3]

Other
Adverse effects [4]
Allergic reactions [2]
Bruxism [2]
Death [5]

SILDENAFIL

Trade names: Revatio (Pfizer), Viagra (Pfizer)
Indications: Erectile dysfunction, hypertension
Class: Phosphodiesterase type 5 (PDE5) inhibitor
Half-life: 4 hours
Clinically important, potentially hazardous interactions with: alfuzosin, alpha blockers, amlodipine, amprenavir, amyl nitrite, antifungals, antihypertensives, atazanavir, boceprevir, bosentan, cimetidine, clarithromycin, cobicistat/elvitegravir/emtricitabine/tenofovir disoproxil, conivaptan, CYP3A4 inhibitors and inducers, darunavir, dasatinib, deferasirox, delavirdine, disopyramide, erythromycin, etravirine, fosamprenavir, grapefruit juice, high-fat foods, HMG-CoA reductase inhibitors, indinavir, isosorbide, isosorbide dinitrate, isosorbide mononitrate, itraconazole, ketoconazole, lopinavir, macrolide antibiotics, nelfinavir, nicorandil, nitrates, nitroglycerin, ombitasvir/paritaprevir/ritonavir, other phosphodiesterase 5 inhibitors, paclitaxel, PEG-interferon, riociguat, ritonavir, sapropterin, saquinavir, St John's wort, telaprevir, telithromycin, tipranavir
Pregnancy category: B
Important contra-indications noted in the prescribing guidelines for: nursing mothers; pediatric patients

---

Skin
Dermatitis (<2%)
Diaphoresis (<2%)
Edema (<2%)
Erythema (6%)
Exfoliative dermatitis (<2%)
Facial edema (<2%)
Genital edema (<2%)
Herpes simplex (<2%)
Lichenoid eruption [2]
Peripheral edema (<2%)
Photosensitivity (<2%)
Pruritus (<2%)
Rash (2%)
Ulcerations (<2%)
Urticaria (<2%)

Mucosal
Epistaxis (nosebleed) (9–13%) [2]
Gingivitis (<2%)
Glossitis (<2%)
Nasal congestion [7]
Rectal hemorrhage (<2%)
Stomatitis (<2%)
Xerostomia (<2%)

Cardiovascular
Angina (<2%)
Atrial fibrillation [2]
Atrioventricular block (<2%)
Cardiac arrest (<2%) [2]
Cardiac failure (<2%)
Cardiomyopathy (<2%)
Chest pain (<2%) [2]
Congestive heart failure [2]
Flushing (10–25%) [31]
Hypotension (<2%) [4]
Myocardial infarction [4]
Myocardial ischemia (<2%)
Palpitation (<2%)
Postural hypotension (<2%)
Tachycardia (<2%)
Vasodilation [3]
Ventricular arrhythmia [2]

Central Nervous System
Abnormal dreams (<2%)
Amnesia [3]
Anorgasmia (<2%)
Chills (<2%)
Depression (<2%)
Fever (6%)
Headache (16–46%) [37]
Hyperesthesia (<2%)
Insomnia (7%)
Migraine (<2%)
Neurotoxicity (<2%)
Pain (<2%)
Paresthesias (3%)
Seizures [3]
Somnolence (drowsiness) (<2%)
Stroke [2]
Subarachnoid hemorrhage [2]
Syncope (<2%)
Tremor (<2%)
Vertigo (dizziness) (2%) [6]

Neuromuscular/Skeletal
Arthralgia (<2%)
Asthenia (fatigue) (<2%) [2]
Ataxia (<2%)
Back pain [3]
Bone or joint pain (<2%)
Gouty tophi (<2%)
Hypertonia (<2%)
Myalgia/Myopathy (7%) [4]
Tendinopathy/Tendon rupture (<2%)

Gastrointestinal/Hepatic
Abdominal pain (<2%) [3]
Colitis (<2%)
Diarrhea (3–9%) [3]
Dyspepsia (7–17%) [13]
Dysphagia (<2%)
Esophagitis (<2%)
Gastritis (<2%)
Gastroenteritis (<2%)
Nausea [3]
Vomiting (<2%)

Respiratory
Asthma (<2%)
Bronchitis (<2%)

Cough (<2%)
Dyspnea (7%) [4]
Hemoptysis [2]
Hypoxia [3]
Laryngitis (<2%)
Pharyngitis (<2%)
Pneumonia [2]
Respiratory failure [3]
Rhinitis (4%) [6]
Sinusitis (<2%)
Stridor [2]
Upper respiratory tract infection [2]

Endocrine/Metabolic
Gynecomastia (<2%)
Hyperglycemia (<2%)
Hypernatremia (<2%)
Hyperuricemia (<2%)

Genitourinary
Cystitis (<2%)
Ejaculatory dysfunction (<2%)
Nocturia (<2%)
Priapism [6]
Urinary frequency (<2%)
Urinary incontinence (<2%)
Urinary tract infection (3%)

Hematologic
Anemia (<2%)
Leukopenia (<2%)

Otic
Ear pain (<2%)
Hearing loss (<2%) [4]
Tinnitus (<2%) [2]

Ocular
Abnormal vision [3]
Cataract (<2%)
Conjunctivitis (<2%)
Dyschromatopsia (blue-green vision) (3–11%) [5]
Mydriasis (<2%)
Ocular hemorrhage (<2%)
Ocular pain (<2%)
Ocular pigmentation (<2%)
Optic neuropathy [18]
Photophobia (<2%)
Retinal vein occlusion [2]
Vision blurred [4]
Visual disturbances [3]
Xerophthalmia (<2%)

Other
Adverse effects [5]
Allergic reactions (<2%)
Death [3]
Dipsia (thirst) (<2%)

SILODOSIN

Trade names: Rapaflo (Watson), Urief (Kissei)
Indications: Benign prostatic hyperplasia
Class: Adrenergic alpha-receptor antagonist
Half-life: 4.7–6 hours
Clinically important, potentially hazardous interactions with: alpha blockers, antihypertensives, atorvastatin, clarithromycin, conivaptan, cyclosporine, darunavir, delavirdine, diltiazem, erythromycin, indinavir, itraconazole, ketoconazole, lapatinib, ritonavir, stong CYP3A4 inhibitors, telithromycin, vasodilators, verapamil, voriconazole
Pregnancy category: B (not indicated for use in women)
Important contra-indications noted in the prescribing guidelines for: pediatric patients
Note: Contraindicated in patients with severe hepatic or renal impairment.

Mucosal
Nasal congestion (2%) [3]
Rhinorrhea (<2%)

Cardiovascular
Orthostatic hypotension (3%) [9]
Postural hypotension [2]

Central Nervous System
Headache (2%) [3]
Insomnia (<2%)
Vertigo (dizziness) (3%) [8]

Neuromuscular/Skeletal
Asthenia (fatigue) (<2%)

Gastrointestinal/Hepatic
Abdominal pain (<2%)
Diarrhea (3%) [2]

Respiratory
Nasopharyngitis (2%)
Sinusitis (<2%)

Genitourinary
Ejaculatory dysfunction (25%) [28]
Retrograde ejaculation (28%) [4]

Other
Adverse effects [2]
Dipsia (thirst) (7%) [2]

SIMEPREVIR

Trade name: Olysio (Janssen)
Indications: Hepatitis C
Class: Antiviral, Hepatitis C virus NS3/4A protease inhibitor
Half-life: 10–13 hours
Clinically important, potentially hazardous interactions with: atazanavir, carbamazepine, cisapride, clarithromycin, cobicistat/elvitegravir/emtricitabine/tenofovir disoproxil, darunavir, delavirdine, dexamethasone, efavirenz, erythromycin, etravirine, fluconazole, fosamprenavir, indinavir, itraconazole, ketoconazole, ledipasvir & sofosbuvir, lopinavir, milk thistle, nelfinavir, nevirapine, oxcarbazepine, phenobarbital, phenytoin, posaconazole, rifabutin, rifampin, rifapentine, ritonavir, saquinavir, St John's wort, telithromycin, tipranavir, voriconazole
Pregnancy category: X (simeprevir is pregnancy category C but must not be used in monotherapy)
Important contra-indications noted in the prescribing guidelines for: nursing mothers; pediatric patients
Note: Must be used in combination with PEG-interferon and ribavirin (see separate entries).

Skin
Photosensitivity (28%) [5]
Pruritus (22%) [7]
Rash (28%) [10]

Central Nervous System
Fever [2]
Headache [12]
Insomnia [3]

Neuromuscular/Skeletal
Asthenia (fatigue) [9]
Myalgia/Myopathy (16%)

Gastrointestinal/Hepatic
Nausea (22%) [8]
Vomiting [2]

Respiratory
Dyspnea (12%)
Flu-like syndrome [2]

Endocrine/Metabolic
Hyperbilirubinemia [8]

Hematologic
Anemia [10]
Neutropenia [3]

Other
Adverse effects [6]

SIMVASTATIN

Trade names: Inegy (MSD), Simcor (AbbVie), Vytorin (MSD), Zocor (Merck)
Indications: Hypercholesterolemia
Class: HMG-CoA reductase inhibitor, Statin
Half-life: 1.9 hours
Clinically important, potentially hazardous interactions with: alitretinoin, amiodarone, amlodipine, amprenavir, atazanavir, azithromycin, boceprevir, bosentan, carbamazepine, ciprofibrate, clarithromycin, clopidogrel, colchicine, conivaptan, coumarins, cyclosporine, danazol, darunavir, dasatinib, delavirdine, diltiazem, dronedarone, efavirenz, erythromycin, fosamprenavir, fusidic acid, gemfibrozil, grapefruit juice, HIV protease inhibitors, imatinib, imidazoles, indinavir, itraconazole, ketoconazole, lomitapide, lopinavir, miconazole, mifepristone, nefazodone, nelfinavir, ombitasvir/paritaprevir/ritonavir, paclitaxel, pazopanib, posaconazole, rabeprazole, ranolazine, red rice yeast, rifampin, ritonavir, roxithromycin, saquinavir, selenium, St John's wort, tacrolimus, telaprevir, telithromycin, ticagrelor, tipranavir, triazoles, verapamil, voriconazole, warfarin
Pregnancy category: X
Important contra-indications noted in the prescribing guidelines for: nursing mothers; pediatric patients
Note: Simcor is simvastatin and niacin; Vytorin is simvastatin and ezetimibe.

Skin
Dermatomyositis [5]
Eczema (5%) [4]
Edema (3%)
Eosinophilic fasciitis [2]
Erythema multiforme [2]
Lichen planus pemphigoides [2]
Lupus erythematosus [5]
Peripheral edema [2]
Photosensitivity [7]
Pruritus [3]

Purpura [3]
Rash (<10%) [3]
Vasculitis [2]

Cardiovascular
Atrial fibrillation (6%)

Central Nervous System
Cognitive impairment [3]
Headache (3–7%)
Memory loss [2]
Vertigo (dizziness) (5%)

Neuromuscular/Skeletal
Asthenia (fatigue) (9%) [3]
Compartment syndrome [2]
Myalgia/Myopathy (<10%) [35]
Rhabdomyolysis [87]
Tendinopathy/Tendon rupture [3]

Gastrointestinal/Hepatic
Abdominal pain (7%)
Constipation (2–7%)
Diarrhea [4]
Gastritis (5%)
Hepatitis [4]
Hepatotoxicity [6]
Nausea (5%)
Pancreatitis [7]

Respiratory
Bronchitis (7%)
Upper respiratory tract infection (9%)

Endocrine/Metabolic
Diabetes mellitus [4]

Renal
Nephrotoxicity [2]
Renal failure [9]

Hematologic
Leukopenia [2]

Other
Adverse effects [8]
Death [5]

SIROLIMUS

Synonym: rapamycin
Trade name: Rapamune (Wyeth)
Indications: Prophylaxis of organ rejection in renal transplants, lymphangioleiomyomatosis
Class: Immunosuppressant, Macrolactam, Non-calcineurin inhibitor
Half-life: 62 hours
Clinically important, potentially hazardous interactions with: atazanavir, benazepril, boceprevir, captopril, cobicistat/elvitegravir/emtricitabine/tenofovir disoproxil, crizotinib, cyclosporine, darunavir, dasatinib, delavirdine, dronedarone, efavirenz, enalapril, enzalutamide, fosinopril, Hemophilus B vaccine, indinavir, itraconazole, lisinopril, lopinavir, micafungin, mifepristone, posaconazole, quinapril, ramipril, St John's wort, tacrolimus, telaprevir, telithromycin, tipranavir, voriconazole, zotarolimus
Pregnancy category: C
Important contra-indications noted in the prescribing guidelines for: the elderly; nursing mothers; pediatric patients
Black Box Warning: IMMUNOSUPPRESSION, USE IS NOT RECOMMENDED IN LIVER OR LUNG TRANSPLANT PATIENTS

Skin
Abscess (3–20%)
Acneform eruption (20–31%) [9]
Angioedema [5]
Cellulitis (3–20%)
Dermatitis [3]
Diaphoresis (3–20%)
Ecchymoses (3–20%)
Edema (16–24%) [6]
Facial edema (3–20%) [2]
Folliculitis [3]
Fungal dermatitis (3–20%)
Hypertrophy (3–20%)
Lymphedema [2]
Peripheral edema (54–64%) [3]
Pruritus (3–20%)
Purpura (3–20%)
Rash (10–20%) [5]
Toxicity [2]
Ulcerations (3–20%)
Vasculitis [2]

Hair
Hirsutism (3–20%)

Nails
Onychopathy [2]

Mucosal
Aphthous stomatitis (9%) [8]
Gingival hyperplasia/hypertrophy (3–20%)
Gingivitis (3–20%)
Mucositis [2]
Oral candidiasis (3–20%)
Oral ulceration (3–20%) [8]
Stomatitis (3–20%) [5]

Cardiovascular
Thrombophlebitis (3–20%)

Central Nervous System
Chills (3–20%)
Depression (3–20%)
Fever [2]
Hyperesthesia (3–20%)
Paresthesias (3–20%)
Tremor (21–31%)

Neuromuscular/Skeletal
Arthralgia (25–31%) [3]
Asthenia (fatigue) [3]
Myalgia/Myopathy [2]

Gastrointestinal/Hepatic
Diarrhea [3]
Hepatitis [2]
Hepatotoxicity [3]

Respiratory
Cough [2]
Flu-like syndrome (3–20%)
Pneumonitis [7]
Pulmonary toxicity [3]
Upper respiratory tract infection (20–26%) [2]

Endocrine/Metabolic
Hypercholesterolemia [2]
Hyperlipidemia [2]
Hypertriglyceridemia [2]

Renal
Nephrotoxicity [2]
Proteinuria [5]

Hematologic
Anemia [3]
Dyslipidemia [4]
Hemolytic uremic syndrome [2]
Leukopenia [2]
Neutropenia [2]
Thrombosis [2]

Otic
Tinnitus (3–20%)

Ocular
Eyelid edema (40%) [2]

Local
Application-site pruritus [2]

Other
Adverse effects [5]
Death [3]
Infection [5]

SITAGLIPTIN

Trade names: Janumet (Merck Sharpe & Dohme), Januvia (Merck Sharpe & Dohme)
Indications: Type II diabetes mellitus
Class: Antidiabetic, Dipeptidyl peptidase-4 (DPP-4) inhibitor
Half-life: 12 hours
Clinically important, potentially hazardous interactions with: alcohol, anabolic steroids, beta blockers, corticosteroids, diazoxide, digoxin, estrogens, loop diuretics, MAO inhibitors, progestogens, testosterone, thiazides
Pregnancy category: B
Important contra-indications noted in the prescribing guidelines for: the elderly; nursing mothers; pediatric patients
Note: Janumet is sitagliptin and metformin.

Skin
Angioedema [3]
Bullous pemphigoid [2]
Edema [3]

Central Nervous System
Headache [5]

Neuromuscular/Skeletal
Arthralgia [2]
Rhabdomyolysis [4]

Gastrointestinal/Hepatic
Abdominal pain (2%)
Constipation [2]
Diarrhea [9]
Hepatotoxicity [2]
Nausea [9]
Pancreatitis [9]
Vomiting [6]

Respiratory
Nasopharyngitis [5]
Upper respiratory tract infection [2]

Endocrine/Metabolic
Creatine phosphokinase increased [2]
Hypoglycemia [10]

Weight gain [3]
Weight loss [2]

Renal
Renal failure [2]

Other
Adverse effects [7]
Cancer [2]

SMALLPOX VACCINE

Trade name: Dryvax (Wyeth)
Indications: Prevention of smallpox (variola)
Class: Vaccine
Half-life: ~5 years
Clinically important, potentially hazardous interactions with: corticosteroids
Pregnancy category: C

Skin
Basal cell carcinoma [4]
Bullous dermatitis [2]
Carcinoma [2]
Dermatitis [2]
Eczema vaccinatum [13]
Erythema multiforme [8]
Exanthems [7]
Folliculitis [2]
Herpes simplex [2]
Herpes zoster [2]
Melanoma [2]
Photosensitivity [2]
Purpura [11]
Rash [2]
Scar [2]
Stevens–Johnson syndrome [3]
Toxic epidermal necrolysis [5]
Tumors [3]
Urticaria [5]
Vaccinia [25]
Vaccinia gangrenosum [3]
Vaccinia necrosum [6]

Central Nervous System
Headache [2]

Other
Allergic reactions [2]
Death [8]

SOFOSBUVIR

Trade name: Sovaldi (Gilead)
Indications: Hepatitis C
Class: Hepatitis C virus nucleotide analog NS5B polymerase inhibitor
Half-life: <27 hours
Clinically important, potentially hazardous interactions with: carbamazepine, oxcarbazepine, phenobarbital, phenytoin, rifabutin, rifampin, rifapentine, ritonavir, St John's wort, tipranavir
Pregnancy category: X (Sofosbuvir is pregnancy category B in monotherapy)
Important contra-indications noted in the prescribing guidelines for: nursing mothers; pediatric patients
Note: Used in combination with daclatasvir, ledipasvir, ribavirin, velpatasvir or with PEG-interferon and ribavirin (see separate entries).

Skin
Pruritus (11–27%) [10]
Rash (8–18%) [9]

Cardiovascular
Bradyarrhythmia [2]

Central Nervous System
Chills (2–18%) [2]
Fever (4–18%) [2]
Headache (24–44%) [44]
Insomnia (15–29%) [17]
Irritability (10–16%) [5]
Vertigo (dizziness) [2]

Neuromuscular/Skeletal
Arthralgia [2]
Asthenia (fatigue) (30–59%) [42]
Back pain [2]
Myalgia/Myopathy (6–16%) [2]

Gastrointestinal/Hepatic
Diarrhea (9–17%) [5]
Nausea (13–34%) [34]

Respiratory
Cough [3]
Flu-like syndrome (3–18%) [2]
Nasopharyngitis [2]
Upper respiratory tract infection [4]

Endocrine/Metabolic
Appetite decreased (6–18%)

Hematologic
Anemia (6–21%) [26]
Lymphopenia [2]
Neutropenia (<17%) [4]

Other
Adverse effects [6]

SOFOSBUVIR & VELPATASVIR *

Trade name: Epclusa (Gilead)
Indications: Hepatitis C
Class: Hepatitis C virus NS5A inhibitor (velpatasvir), Hepatitis C virus nucleotide analog NS5B polymerase inhibitor (sofosbuvir)
Half-life: <27 hours (sofosbuvir); 15 hours (velpatasvir)
Clinically important, potentially hazardous interactions with: amiodarone, carbamazepine, efavirenz, omeprazole, oxcarbazepine, phenobarbital, phenytoin, rifabutin, rifampin, rifapentine, St John's wort, topotecan
Pregnancy category: N/A (Insufficient evidence to inform drug-associated risk; contraindicated in pregnancy when given with ribavirin)
Important contra-indications noted in the prescribing guidelines for: nursing mothers; pediatric patients
Note: See also separate entry for sofosbuvir.

Skin
Rash (2%)

Central Nervous System
Headache (22%) [7]
Insomnia (5%) [3]

Neuromuscular/Skeletal
Asthenia (fatigue) (5–15%) [7]

Gastrointestinal/Hepatic
Hepatotoxicity (2–6%)
Nausea (9%) [6]

Endocrine/Metabolic
Creatine phosphokinase increased (<2%)

Hematologic
Anemia [2]

SOLIFENACIN

Trade name: Vesicare (Astellas)
Indications: Overactive bladder
Class: Antimuscarinic, Muscarinic antagonist
Half-life: 45–68 hours
Clinically important, potentially hazardous interactions with: atazanavir, carbamazepine, clarithromycin, indinavir, itraconazole, ketoconazole, nefazodone, nelfinavir, phenobarbital, phenytoin, rifabutin, rifampin, rifapentine, ritonavir, saquinavir, St John's wort, troleandomycin, voriconazole
Pregnancy category: C
Important contra-indications noted in the prescribing guidelines for: nursing mothers; pediatric patients

Mucosal
Xerostomia (11–27%) [19]

Cardiovascular
QT prolongation [2]

Central Nervous System
Vertigo (dizziness) (2%) [2]

Neuromuscular/Skeletal
Asthenia (fatigue) (<2%)

Gastrointestinal/Hepatic
Abdominal pain (2%)
Constipation [10]

Ocular
Vision blurred (4–5%) [5]
Xerophthalmia (2%)

Other
Adverse effects [4]

SONIDEGIB

Trade name: Odomzo (Novartis)
Indications: Basal cell carcinoma
Class: Hedgehog (Hh) signaling pathway inhibitor
Half-life: 28 days
Clinically important, potentially hazardous interactions with: atazanavir, carbamazepine, diltiazem, efavirenz, fluconazole, itraconazole, ketoconazole, modafinil, nefazodone, phenobarbital, phenytoin, posaconazole, rifabutin, rifampin, saquinavir, St John's wort, telithromycin, voriconazole
Pregnancy category: N/A (Can cause fetal harm)
Important contra-indications noted in the prescribing guidelines for: nursing mothers; pediatric patients
Note: Patients should not donate blood or blood products while receiving sonidegib and for at least

20 months after the last dose.
Black Box Warning: EMBRYO-FETAL TOXICITY

Skin
Pruritus (10%)

Hair
Alopecia (53%) [5]

Central Nervous System
Anorexia [2]
Dysgeusia (taste perversion) (46%) [5]
Headache (15%)
Pain (14%)
Vertigo (dizziness) [2]

Neuromuscular/Skeletal
Asthenia (fatigue) (41%) [4]
Bone or joint pain (32%)
Muscle spasm (54%) [5]
Myalgia/Myopathy (19%) [5]

Gastrointestinal/Hepatic
Abdominal pain (18%)
Diarrhea (32%)
Hepatotoxicity [2]
Nausea (39%) [3]
Vomiting (11%) [3]

Endocrine/Metabolic
ALT increased (19%)
Appetite decreased (30%)
AST increased (19%)
Creatine phosphokinase increased (61%) [6]
Hyperbilirubinemia [2]
Hyperglycemia (51%)
Weight loss (30%) [3]

Hematologic
Anemia (32%)
Lymphopenia (28%)

SORAFENIB

Trade name: Nexavar (Bayer)
Indications: Advanced renal cell carcinoma
Class: Antineoplastic, Epidermal growth factor receptor (EGFR) inhibitor, Tyrosine kinase inhibitor
Half-life: 25–48 hours
Clinically important, potentially hazardous interactions with: bevacizumab, carbamazepine, clozapine, conivaptan, coumarins, CYP3A4 inducers, darunavir, delavirdine, dexamethasone, digoxin, docetaxel, doxorubicin, efavirenz, indinavir, irinotecan, neomycin, oxcarbazepine, phenobarbital, phenytoin, rifabutin, rifampin, rifapentine, St John's wort, telithromycin, voriconazole, warfarin
Pregnancy category: D
Important contra-indications noted in the prescribing guidelines for: nursing mothers; pediatric patients
Note: In combination with carboplatin and paclitaxel, Nexavar is contraindicated in patients with squamous cell lung cancer.

Skin
Acneform eruption (<10%) [5]
Actinic keratoses [3]
AGEP [2]
Desquamation (19–40%) [9]
Edema [3]
Erythema (>10%) [4]
Erythema multiforme [10]
Exanthems [3]
Exfoliative dermatitis (<10%)
Facial erythema [3]
Folliculitis [3]
Hand–foot syndrome (21–30%) [97]
Hyperkeratosis [4]
Hypersensitivity [2]
Keratoacanthoma [3]
Nevi [2]
Palmar–plantar toxicity [2]
Pigmentation [2]
Pruritus (14–19%) [10]
Psoriasis [2]
Radiation recall dermatitis [3]
Rash (19–40%) [47]
Recall reaction [2]
Squamous cell carcinoma [7]
Toxicity [14]
Xerosis (10–11%) [6]

Hair
Alopecia (14–27%) [24]

Nails
Splinter hemorrhage [3]

Mucosal
Epistaxis (nosebleed) [2]
Glossodynia (<10%)
Mucositis (<10%) [12]
Stomatitis (<10%) [11]
Xerostomia (<10%)

Cardiovascular
Cardiac failure [2]
Cardiotoxicity (3%) [2]
Congestive heart failure (<10%)
Flushing (<10%)
Hypertension (9–17%) [46]
Myocardial infarction (<10%)

Central Nervous System
Anorexia (16–29%) [15]
Depression (<10%)
Encephalopathy [2]
Fever (<10%) [6]
Headache (10%) [5]
Neurotoxicity (2–40%) [4]
Pain (>10%) [4]

Neuromuscular/Skeletal
Arthralgia (<10%)
Asthenia (fatigue) (37–46%) [51]
Back pain [3]
Bone or joint pain (>10%) [3]
Myalgia/Myopathy (<10%)

Gastrointestinal/Hepatic
Abdominal pain (11–31%) [9]
Ascites [2]
Constipation (14–15%) [4]
Diarrhea (43–55%) [59]
Dyspepsia (<10%)
Dysphagia (<10%)
Gastrointestinal bleeding [5]
Hepatotoxicity (11%) [24]
Nausea (23–24%) [12]
Pancreatitis [6]
Pneumatosis intestinalis [2]
Vomiting (15–16%) [8]

Respiratory
Cough (13%) [2]
Dysphonia [5]
Dyspnea (14%) [4]
Flu-like syndrome (<10%)
Hoarseness (<10%)
Pulmonary toxicity [2]

Endocrine/Metabolic
ALT increased [7]
Appetite decreased (<10%) [5]
AST increased [6]
Creatine phosphokinase increased [2]
Hyperbilirubinemia [2]
Hypoalbuminemia (56%)
Hypocalcemia [2]
Hypokalemia [2]
Hyponatremia [2]
Hypophosphatemia (35–45%) [6]
Hypothyroidism [7]
Thyroid dysfunction [4]
Weight loss (10–30%) [12]

Genitourinary
Erectile dysfunction (<10%)

Renal
Proteinuria [3]
Renal failure (<10%) [2]

Hematologic
Anemia (44%) [8]
Hemorrhage (15–18%) [4]
Hemotoxicity [2]
Leukopenia (>10%) [3]
Lymphopenia (23–47%) [5]
Myelosuppression [2]
Neutropenia (<10%) [7]
Thrombocytopenia (12–46%) [12]
Thrombosis [2]

Other
Adverse effects [15]
Death [9]
Infection [2]
Side effects (71%) [4]

SOTALOL

Trade name: Betapace (Bayer)
Indications: Ventricular arrhythmias
Class: Antiarrhythmic, Antiarrhythmic class II, Antiarrhythmic class III, Beta adrenergic blocker, Beta blocker
Half-life: 7–18 hours
Clinically important, potentially hazardous interactions with: abarelix, amiodarone, amisulpride, amitriptyline, arsenic, artemether/lumefantrine, asenapine, astemizole, atomoxetine, bepridil, ciprofloxacin, class I and class III antiarrhythmics, clonidine, degarelix, disopyramide, dronedarone, droperidol, enoxacin, gatifloxacin, guanethidine, haloperidol, insulin, isoprenaline, ivabradine, levomepromazine, lomefloxacin, loop diuretics, mizolastine, moxifloxacin, nilotinib, norfloxacin, ofloxacin, oral macrolides, phenothiazines, pimozide, procainamide, quinidine, quinine, quinolones, ranolazine, reserpine, salbutamol, sertindole, sparfloxacin, sulpiride, terbutaline, tetrabenazine, thiazides and related diruetics, tolterodine, tricyclic antidepressants, trifluoperazine, vandetanib, zuclopenthixol

Pregnancy category: B
Important contra-indications noted in the prescribing guidelines for: nursing mothers; pediatric patients
Note: Contraindicated in patients with bronchial asthma, sinus bradycardia, second and third degree AV block, unless a functioning pacemaker is present, congenital or acquired long QT syndromes, cardiogenic shock, or uncontrolled congestive heart failure.

Skin
Edema (5%)
Pruritus (<10%)
Psoriasis [3]
Rash (3%)
Scleroderma [3]

Cardiovascular
Arrhythmias [2]
Bradycardia [9]
Cardiac failure [2]
Cardiogenic shock [2]
Cardiotoxicity [2]
Hypotension [3]
QT prolongation [18]
Torsades de pointes [24]

Central Nervous System
Depression [2]
Paresthesias (3%)

Neuromuscular/Skeletal
Asthenia (fatigue) (6%) [2]

Other
Adverse effects [2]

SPIRONOLACTONE

Trade names: Aldactazide (Pfizer), Aldactone (Pfizer)
Indications: Hyperaldosteronism, hirsutism, hypertension, edema for patients with congestive heart failure, cirrhosis of the liver or nephrotic syndrome
Class: Aldosterone antagonist, Diuretic
Half-life: 78–84 minutes
Clinically important, potentially hazardous interactions with: ACE inhibitors, alcohol, amiloride, barbiturates, benazepril, captopril, cyclosporine, enalapril, fosinopril, lisinopril, mitotane, moexipril, narcotics, NSAIDs, potassium chloride, potassium iodide, quinapril, ramipril, trandolapril, triamterene, zofenopril
Pregnancy category: C
Important contra-indications noted in the prescribing guidelines for: nursing mothers; pediatric patients
Note: Aldactazide is spironolactone and hydrochlorothiazide. Hydrochlorothiazide is a sulfonamide and can be absorbed systemically. Sulfonamides can produce severe, possibly fatal, reactions such as toxic epidermal necrolysis and Stevens-Johnson syndrome.
Black Box Warning: Spironolactone has been shown to be a tumorigen in chronic toxicity studies in rats

---

Skin
Bullous pemphigoid [2]
Dermatitis [6]
Eczema [2]
Exanthems (<5%) [6]
Lichenoid eruption [2]
Melasma [2]
Pigmentation [3]
Pruritus [3]
Rash (<10%) [2]
Urticaria [2]
Xerosis (40%) [2]

Hair
Alopecia [2]

Endocrine/Metabolic
Amenorrhea [2]
Gynecomastia [29]
Hyperkalemia [8]

STANOZOLOL

Trade name: Winstrol (Ovation)
Indications: Hereditary angioedema
Class: Anabolic steroid
Half-life: N/A
Clinically important, potentially hazardous interactions with: anticoagulants, warfarin
Pregnancy category: X
Important contra-indications noted in the prescribing guidelines for: nursing mothers

---

Skin
Acneform eruption (>10%) [2]
Pigmentation (<10%)

Hair
Hirsutism (in women) [3]

Cardiovascular
Hypertension [2]
Myocardial infarction [2]
Myocardial ischemia [2]

Central Nervous System
Chills (<10%)

Gastrointestinal/Hepatic
Hepatotoxicity [2]

Endocrine/Metabolic
Gynecomastia (>10%)

Genitourinary
Priapism (>10%)

Renal
Nephrotoxicity [2]

Other
Death [2]

STAVUDINE

Synonym: D4T
Trade name: Zerit (Bristol-Myers Squibb)
Indications: HIV infection
Class: Antiretroviral, Nucleoside analog reverse transcriptase inhibitor
Half-life: 1.44 hours
Clinically important, potentially hazardous interactions with: doxorubicin, ribavirin, zidovudine
Pregnancy category: C
Important contra-indications noted in the prescribing guidelines for: nursing mothers
Black Box Warning: LACTIC ACIDOSIS and HEPATOMEGALY with STEATOSIS; PANCREATITIS

Skin
Diaphoresis (19%)
Lipoatrophy [7]
Lipodystrophy [8]
Rash (40%)
Toxic epidermal necrolysis [2]
Toxicity [2]

Central Nervous System
Chills (50%)
Neurotoxicity [4]
Peripheral neuropathy (52%) [11]

Neuromuscular/Skeletal
Myalgia/Myopathy (32%) [2]

Gastrointestinal/Hepatic
Diarrhea (50%)
Hepatotoxicity [2]
Nausea (39%)
Pancreatitis [6]
Vomiting (39%)

Endocrine/Metabolic
Acidosis [11]
Diabetes mellitus [2]
Fat distribution abnormality [4]
Gynecomastia [4]

Renal
Fanconi syndrome [2]

Other
Adverse effects [3]
Allergic reactions (9%)

STREPTOKINASE

Trade names: Kabikinase (Pfizer), Streptase (AstraZeneca)
Indications: Pulmonary embolism, acute myocardial infarction
Class: Fibrinolytic
Half-life: 83 minutes
Clinically important, potentially hazardous interactions with: bivalirudin, lepirudin
Pregnancy category: C

Skin
Anaphylactoid reactions/Anaphylaxis [2]
Angioedema (>10%) [2]
Diaphoresis (<10%)
Exanthems (<5%) [2]
Pruritus (<10%)
Rash (<10%)
Serum sickness [7]
Urticaria (<5%)
Vasculitis [7]

Neuromuscular/Skeletal
Rhabdomyolysis [2]

Ocular
Periorbital edema (>10%)

Other
Allergic reactions (4%) [4]

STREPTOMYCIN

Trade name: Streptomycin (Pfizer)
Indications: Tuberculosis
Class: Antibiotic, aminoglycoside
Half-life: 2–5 hours
Clinically important, potentially hazardous interactions with: aldesleukin, aminoglycosides, atracurium, bacitracin, bumetanide, doxacurium, ethacrynic acid, furosemide, methoxyflurane, neostigmine, non-depolarizing muscle relaxants, pancuronium, polypeptide antibiotics, rocuronium, succinylcholine, teicoplanin, torsemide, vecuronium
Pregnancy category: D
Important contra-indications noted in the prescribing guidelines for: nursing mothers
Note: Aminoglycosides may cause neurotoxicity and/or nephrotoxicity.

Skin
Anaphylactoid reactions/Anaphylaxis [3]
Dermatitis [2]
DRESS syndrome [2]
Erythema multiforme [4]
Exanthems (>5%) [8]
Exfoliative dermatitis [11]
Lupus erythematosus [5]
Nicolau syndrome [2]
Photosensitivity [2]
Pruritus [2]
Purpura [3]
Stevens–Johnson syndrome [3]
Toxic epidermal necrolysis [9]
Urticaria [3]

Mucosal
Cheilitis (2%)
Glossitis (2%)
Oral mucosal eruption [2]
Stomatitis [2]

Renal
Nephrotoxicity [2]

Otic
Ototoxicity [6]

Ocular
Optic neuropathy [2]

Other
Adverse effects [2]
Allergic reactions [2]

STREPTOZOCIN

Trade name: Zanosar (Gensia)
Indications: Carcinoma of the pancreas, carcinoid tumor, Hodgkin's disease
Class: Alkylating agent, Antineoplastic
Half-life: 35 minutes
Clinically important, potentially hazardous interactions with: aldesleukin
Pregnancy category: D
Important contra-indications noted in the prescribing guidelines for: nursing mothers

---

Neuromuscular/Skeletal
Asthenia (fatigue) [2]

Gastrointestinal/Hepatic
Abdominal pain [2]
Nausea [2]
Vomiting [2]

Renal
Nephrotoxicity [2]

Hematologic
Neutropenia [2]

Local
Injection-site pain (<10%)

SUCCIMER

Synonym: DMSA
Trade name: Chemet (Sanofi-Aventis)
Indications: Heavy metal poisoning
Class: Chelator
Half-life: 2 days
Clinically important, potentially hazardous interactions with: other chelating agents
Pregnancy category: C
Important contra-indications noted in the prescribing guidelines for: nursing mothers; pediatric patients

---

Skin
Candidiasis (16%)
Exanthems (11%)
Pruritus (11%)
Rash (<11%) [2]

Mucosal
Mucocutaneous eruption (11%)

Central Nervous System
Chills (16%)
Dysgeusia (taste perversion) (metallic) (21%)
Fever (16%)
Headache (16%)
Pain (3%)
Paresthesias (13%)

Neuromuscular/Skeletal
Back pain (16%)

Gastrointestinal/Hepatic
Abdominal pain (16%)

Respiratory
Flu-like syndrome (16%)

SUCCINYLCHOLINE

Synonym: suxamethonium
Trade name: Anectine (Sabex)
Indications: Skeletal muscle relaxation during general anesthesia
Class: Cholinesterase inhibitor, Depolarizing muscle relaxant
Half-life: N/A
Clinically important, potentially hazardous interactions with: amikacin, aminoglycosides, donepezil, galantamine, gentamicin, hydromorphone, kanamycin, levomepromazine, neomycin, neostigmine, paromomycin, physostigmine, pipecuronium, pralidoxime, quinine, streptomycin, tapentadol, thalidomide, tobramycin, vancomycin, vecuronium
Pregnancy category: C
Important contra-indications noted in the prescribing guidelines for: the elderly; nursing mothers
Black Box Warning: RISK OF CARDIAC ARREST FROM HYPERKALEMIC RHABDOMYOLYSIS

Skin
Anaphylactoid reactions/Anaphylaxis [12]

Mucosal
Sialorrhea (<10%)

Cardiovascular
Bradycardia [2]

Central Nervous System
Malignant hyperthermia [7]
Paralysis [3]
Twitching [4]

Neuromuscular/Skeletal
Myalgia/Myopathy [11]
Rhabdomyolysis [26]

Endocrine/Metabolic
Hyperkalemia [8]

Other
Death [3]

SUCRALFATE

Trade name: Carafate (Aptalis)
Indications: Duodenal ulcer
Class: Chelator
Half-life: N/A
Clinically important, potentially hazardous interactions with: anagrelide, chlortetracycline, ciprofloxacin, clorazepate, demeclocycline, doxycycline, gemifloxacin, ketoconazole, lansoprazole, levofloxacin, lomefloxacin, lymecycline, minocycline, moxifloxacin, norfloxacin, ofloxacin, oxtriphylline, oxytetracycline, paricalcitol, phenytoin, sparfloxacin, tetracycline, tigecycline, voriconazole
Pregnancy category: B
Important contra-indications noted in the prescribing guidelines for: the elderly; nursing mothers; pediatric patients
Note: Sucralfate use can lead to symptoms of aluminum toxicity.

Mucosal
Xerostomia [2]

Gastrointestinal/Hepatic
Constipation (2%)

SUCRALOSE

Trade name: Splenda (McNeil)
Indications: Weight reduction
Class: Sweetening agent
Half-life: 2–5 hours
Clinically important, potentially hazardous interactions with: none known
Pregnancy category: N/A

Central Nervous System
Migraine [3]

SUGAMMADEX *

Trade name: Bridion (Organon)
Indications: Reversal of neuromuscular blockade induced by rocuronium bromide and vecuronium bromide in adults undergoing surgery
Class: Cyclodextrin, Selective relaxant binding agent
Half-life: ~2 hours
Clinically important, potentially hazardous interactions with: toremifene
Pregnancy category: N/A (No data available)
Important contra-indications noted in the prescribing guidelines for: the elderly; nursing mothers; pediatric patients

---

Skin
Anaphylactoid reactions/Anaphylaxis [8]
Erythema (<2%)
Hypersensitivity [7]
Pruritus (2–3%)

Mucosal
Oropharyngeal pain (3–5%)
Xerostomia (<2%) [2]

Cardiovascular
Bradycardia (<5%)
QT prolongation (<6%) [2]
Tachycardia (2–5%)

Central Nervous System
Anxiety (<3%)
Chills (3–7%)
Depression (<2%)
Dysgeusia (taste perversion) [3]
Fever (5–9%)
Headache (5–10%) [2]
Hypoesthesia (<3%)
Insomnia (2–5%)
Pain (36–52%)
Restlessness (<2%)
Somnolence (drowsiness) [2]
Vertigo (dizziness) (3–6%)

Neuromuscular/Skeletal
Bone or joint pain (<2%)
Myalgia/Myopathy (<2%)
Pain in extremities (<6%)

Gastrointestinal/Hepatic
Abdominal pain (4–6%)
Diarrhea [2]
Flatulence (<3%)
Nausea (23–26%) [2]
Vomiting (11–15%)

Respiratory
Bronchospasm [2]
Cough (<8%)

Endocrine/Metabolic
Creatine phosphokinase increased (<2%)
Hypocalcemia (<2%)

Hematologic
Anemia (<2%)

Local
Injection-site pain (4–6%)

Other
Allergic reactions [2]

SULFADOXINE

Trade name: Fansidar (Roche)
Indications: Malaria
Class: Antibiotic, sulfonamide, Antimalarial
Half-life: 5–8 days
Clinically important, potentially hazardous interactions with: none known
Pregnancy category: C
Important contra-indications noted in the prescribing guidelines for: the elderly; nursing mothers; pediatric patients
Note: Sulfadoxine is a sulfonamide and can be absorbed systemically. Sulfonamides can produce severe, possibly fatal, reactions such as toxic epidermal necrolysis and Stevens-Johnson syndrome.
Fansidar is sulfadoxine and pyrimethamine (this combination is almost always prescribed).

Skin
Erythema multiforme [3]
Exfoliative dermatitis [3]
Fixed eruption [2]
Hypersensitivity (>10%)
Photosensitivity (>10%) [2]
Pruritus [2]
Stevens–Johnson syndrome (<10%) [24]
Toxic epidermal necrolysis [17]

Mucosal
Glossitis (>10%)

Central Nervous System
Tremor (>10%)
Vertigo (dizziness) [2]

Neuromuscular/Skeletal
Asthenia (fatigue) [2]

Gastrointestinal/Hepatic
Diarrhea [2]

Other
Death [7]

SULFA-METHOXAZOLE

Trade names: Bactrim (Women First), Septra (Monarch)
Indications: Various infections caused by susceptible organisms
Class: Antibiotic, sulfonamide, Folic acid antagonist
Half-life: 7–12 hours
Clinically important, potentially hazardous interactions with: anticoagulants, azathioprine, cyclosporine, methotrexate, pralatrexate, probenecid, warfarin
Pregnancy category: C
Note: Sulfamethoxazole is a sulfonamide and can be absorbed systemically. Sulfonamides can produce severe, possibly fatal, reactions such as toxic epidermal necrolysis and Stevens-Johnson syndrome.
Sulfamethoxazole is commonly used in conjunction with trimethoprim (see separate entry for co-trimoxazole).

Skin
AGEP [3]
Anaphylactoid reactions/Anaphylaxis [4]
Angioedema (<5%)
Dermatitis [4]
DRESS syndrome [4]
Erythema multiforme [15]
Erythema nodosum [2]
Exanthems (<5%) [30]
Exfoliative dermatitis [3]
Fixed eruption [29]
Hypersensitivity [6]
Linear IgA bullous dermatosis [3]
Lupus erythematosus [3]
Photosensitivity (>10%) [3]
Pruritus (10%) [7]
Purpura [3]
Pustules [6]
Radiation recall dermatitis [3]
Rash (>10%) [3]
Stevens–Johnson syndrome (<10%) [22]
Sweet's syndrome [3]
Toxic epidermal necrolysis (<10%) [32]
Urticaria [9]
Vasculitis [6]

Mucosal
Oral mucosal eruption [2]
Oral ulceration [2]

Neuromuscular/Skeletal
Rhabdomyolysis [4]

Renal
Nephrotoxicity [2]

Hematologic
Thrombocytopenia [2]

Other
Allergic reactions [2]
Side effects (2%) [2]

SULFASALAZINE

Synonyms: salicylazosulfapyridine; salazopyrin
Trade name: Azulfidine (Pfizer)
Indications: Inflammatory bowel disease, ulcerative colitis, rheumatoid arthritis
Class: Aminosalicylate, Disease-modifying antirheumatic drug (DMARD), Sulfonamide
Half-life: 5–10 hours
Clinically important, potentially hazardous interactions with: cholestyramine, methotrexate
Pregnancy category: B
Important contra-indications noted in the prescribing guidelines for: nursing mothers; pediatric patients
Note: Sulfasalazine is a sulfonamide and can be absorbed systemically. Sulfonamides can produce severe, possibly fatal, reactions such as toxic epidermal necrolysis and Stevens-Johnson syndrome.
Safety and effectiveness in pediatric patients <2 years of age have not been established.
Contraindicated in patients with intestinal or urinary obstruction, or with porphyria.

Skin
AGEP [3]
Anaphylactoid reactions/Anaphylaxis [4]

Angioedema [2]
Bullous pemphigoid [3]
Cyanosis (<10%)
Dermatitis [2]
DRESS syndrome [31]
Erythema multiforme [8]
Erythema nodosum [2]
Exanthems (2–23%) [23]
Exfoliative dermatitis [5]
Fixed eruption [7]
Hypersensitivity (<5%) [16]
Lichen planus [3]
Lupus erythematosus [34]
Photosensitivity (10%) [4]
Pigmentation [3]
Pruritus (10%) [7]
Pseudolymphoma [2]
Pustules [2]
Rash (>10%) [19]
Raynaud's phenomenon [3]
Serum sickness [3]
Stevens–Johnson syndrome [9]
Toxic epidermal necrolysis (<10%) [13]
Urticaria (<5%) [10]
Vasculitis [4]

Hair
Alopecia [6]

Mucosal
Mucocutaneous reactions (6%) [2]
Oral mucosal eruption [4]
Oral ulceration [3]
Stomatitis (<10%)

Cardiovascular
Flushing [2]

Central Nervous System
Anorexia (10%)
Aseptic meningitis [3]
Fever [4]
Headache (10%) [7]
Vertigo (dizziness) (<10%)

Neuromuscular/Skeletal
Arthralgia [2]
Asthenia (fatigue) [5]

Gastrointestinal/Hepatic
Abdominal pain (<10%)
Dyspepsia (10%) [3]
Hepatotoxicity [13]
Nausea (10%) [7]
Pancreatitis [6]
Vomiting (10%) [2]

Respiratory
Pulmonary toxicity [3]
Upper respiratory tract infection [3]

Renal
Nephrotoxicity [4]
Renal failure [2]

Hematologic
Agranulocytosis [5]
Anemia (<10%)
Leukopenia (<10%) [4]
Neutropenia [2]
Thrombocytopenia (<10%)

Ocular
Conjunctival pigmentation [2]

Other
Adverse effects [9]
Death [3]
Side effects (5%)

SULINDAC

Trade name: Clinoril (Merck)
Indications: Arthritis
Class: Non-steroidal anti-inflammatory (NSAID)
Half-life: 7.8–16.4 hours
Clinically important, potentially hazardous interactions with: methotrexate, warfarin
Pregnancy category: C (category C in first and second trimesters; category D in third trimester)
Important contra-indications noted in the prescribing guidelines for: nursing mothers; pediatric patients
Note: NSAIDs may cause an increased risk of serious cardiovascular and gastrointestinal adverse events, which can be fatal. This risk may increase with duration of use.

Skin
Anaphylactoid reactions/Anaphylaxis [4]
Erythema multiforme [8]
Exanthems (<5%) [9]
Fixed eruption [5]
Photosensitivity [2]
Pruritus (<10%) [5]
Purpura [2]
Rash (>10%)
Stevens–Johnson syndrome [5]
Toxic epidermal necrolysis [13]
Urticaria [4]

Mucosal
Oral mucosal eruption (3%) [2]
Stomatitis [2]
Xerostomia [2]

Gastrointestinal/Hepatic
Hepatotoxicity [4]
Pancreatitis [3]

SUMATRIPTAN

Trade names: Alsuma (King), Imigran (GSK), Imitrex (GSK), Onzetra Xsail (Avanir), Sumavel DosePro (Endo), Zecuity (Teva)
Indications: Migraine attacks, cluster headaches
Class: 5-HT1 agonist, Serotonin receptor agonist, Triptan
Half-life: 2.5 hours
Clinically important, potentially hazardous interactions with: citalopram, dihydroergotamine, ergot-containing drugs, escitalopram, fluoxetine, fluvoxamine, isocarboxazid, MAO inhibitors, methysergide, naratriptan, nefazodone, paroxetine hydrochloride, phenelzine, rizatriptan, sertraline, sibutramine, SNRIs, SSRIs, St John's wort, tranylcypromine, venlafaxine, zolmitriptan
Pregnancy category: C
Important contra-indications noted in the prescribing guidelines for: the elderly; nursing mothers; pediatric patients
Note: Contraindicated in patients with Wolff-Parkinson-White syndrome, peripheral vascular disease, ischemic bowel disease, uncontrolled hypertension, severe hepatic impairment or a history of coronary artery disease, coronary vasospasm, stroke, transient ischemic attack, or hemiplegic or basilar migraine; or with recent (within 24 hours) use of another 5-HT1 agonist (e.g. another triptan) or an ergotamine-containing medication, or current or recent (past 2 weeks) use of a monoamine oxidase-A inhibitor.

Skin
Burning (<10%)
Diaphoresis (2%)
Hot flashes (>10%)

Mucosal
Nasal discomfort [2]
Xerostomia [2]

Cardiovascular
Chest pain (<2%) [6]
Flushing (7%) [3]
Hypertension [2]
Myocardial infarction [5]

Central Nervous System
Dysgeusia (taste perversion) [9]
Headache [2]
Neurotoxicity [3]
Pain (<2%) [2]
Paresthesias (3–5%) [10]
Somnolence (drowsiness) [3]
Stroke [2]
Vertigo (dizziness) (<2%) [10]
Warm feeling (2–3%)

Neuromuscular/Skeletal
Asthenia (fatigue) (2–3%) [5]
Jaw pain (<3%)
Myalgia/Myopathy (2%) [2]
Neck pain (<3%)

Gastrointestinal/Hepatic
Colitis [2]
Nausea [12]

Respiratory
Nasopharyngitis [2]
Upper respiratory tract infection [2]

Local
Application-site erythema [2]
Injection-site reactions (10–58%) [2]

Other
Adverse effects [10]

SUNITINIB

Trade name: Sutent (Pfizer)
Indications: Gastrointestinal stromal tumor, advanced renal cell carcinoma, advanced pancreatic neuroendocrine tumor
Class: Antineoplastic, Epidermal growth factor receptor (EGFR) inhibitor, Tyrosine kinase inhibitor
Half-life: 40–60 hours
Clinically important, potentially hazardous interactions with: atazanavir, bevacizumab, carbamazepine, clarithromycin, clozapine, dexamethasone, digoxin, efavirenz, grapefruit juice, indinavir, itraconazole, ketoconazole, nefazodone, nelfinavir, phenobarbital, phenytoin, rifabutin, rifampin, rifapentine, ritonavir, saquinavir, St John's wort, telithromycin, temsirolimus, voriconazole

Pregnancy category: D
Important contra-indications noted in the prescribing guidelines for: nursing mothers; pediatric patients
Note: [G] = treated for gastrointestinal tumor; [R] = treated for renal cell carcinoma; [P] treated for pancreatic neuroendocrine tumor.
Black Box Warning: HEPATOTOXICITY

Skin
Acral erythema [2]
Edema [6]
Erythema [5]
Facial edema [2]
Hand–foot syndrome (12–14%) [61]
Lesions [2]
Nevi [2]
Peripheral edema [R] (17%)
Pigmentation [12]
Pruritus [R] [3]
Pyoderma gangrenosum [4]
Rash (14–38%) [14]
Thrombocytopenic purpura [4]
Toxicity [20]
Xerosis (17%) [3]

Hair
Alopecia (5–12%) [3]
Hair pigmentation [G] [7]

Nails
Subungual hemorrhage [3]

Mucosal
Epistaxis (nosebleed) [2]
Glossodynia [R] [P] (15%)
Mucosal inflammation [4]
Mucositis (29–53%) [16]
Stomatitis [15]
Xerostomia [R] [P] [2]

Cardiovascular
Aortic dissection [2]
Cardiac failure [2]
Cardiomyopathy [2]
Cardiotoxicity [7]
Congestive heart failure [2]
Hypertension [46]
QT prolongation [2]
Ventricular arrhythmia [2]

Central Nervous System
Anorexia [8]
Dysgeusia (taste perversion) (21–43%) [6]
Fever [R] (15–18%) [2]
Headache (13–25%) [4]
Leukoencephalopathy [3]
Neurotoxicity [R] (10%)
Pain [R] (18%)
Vertigo (dizziness) [R] (16%)

Neuromuscular/Skeletal
Arthralgia [R] (12–28%)
Asthenia (fatigue) (22%) [63]
Back pain [R] (11–17%)
Myalgia/Myopathy [G] (14–17%)
Osteonecrosis [3]

Gastrointestinal/Hepatic
Abdominal pain (20–33%) [2]
Constipation [3]
Diarrhea [34]
Dyspepsia [R] [P] [3]
Gastrointestinal bleeding [3]
Gastrointestinal disorder [2]
Hepatotoxicity [8]
Nausea [15]
Pneumatosis intestinalis [2]
Vomiting [14]

Respiratory
Cough [R] (8–17%) [2]
Dyspnea [5]
Pulmonary toxicity [3]
Radiation recall pneumonitis [2]

Endocrine/Metabolic
ALT increased [3]
Appetite decreased [2]
AST increased [2]
Hypothyroidism [R] [24]
Serum creatinine increased [2]
Thyroid dysfunction [7]

Renal
Nephrotoxicity [4]
Proteinuria [3]

Hematologic
Anemia [17]
Bleeding [5]
Bone marrow suppression [2]
Cytopenia [2]
Hemorrhage [2]
Hemotoxicity [3]
Hyperlipasemia [2]
Leukopenia [15]
Lymphocytopenia [2]
Lymphopenia [8]
Myelosuppression [2]
Neutropenia [39]
Thrombocytopenia [33]

Ocular
Epiphora [R] (6%)
Periorbital edema [R] (7%)

Other
Adverse effects [17]
Death [6]
Side effects [3]

SUVOREXANT

Trade name: Belsomra (Merck Sharpe & Dohme)
Indications: Insomnia
Class: Orexin receptor antagonist
Half-life: 10–22 hours
Clinically important, potentially hazardous interactions with: none known
Pregnancy category: C
Important contra-indications noted in the prescribing guidelines for: nursing mothers; pediatric patients
Note: Contraindicated in patients with narcolepsy.

Mucosal
Xerostomia (2%)

Central Nervous System
Abnormal dreams (2%)
Headache (7%) [2]
Sedation [2]
Somnolence (drowsiness) (7%) [6]
Vertigo (dizziness) (3%)

Gastrointestinal/Hepatic
Diarrhea (2%)

Respiratory
Cough (2%)
Upper respiratory tract infection (2%)

TACROLIMUS

Trade names: Envarsus XR (Veloxis), Prograf (Astellas), Protopic (Astellas)
Indications: Prophylaxis of organ rejection, atopic dermatitis (topical)
Class: Calcineurin inhibitor, Immunosuppressant, Macrolactam
Half-life: ~8.7 hours
Clinically important, potentially hazardous interactions with: abatacept, afatinib, alefacept, amiodarone, amprenavir, atazanavir, azacitidine, beta blockers, betamethasone, boceprevir, bosentan, cabazitaxel, caspofungin, cinacalcet, cobicistat/elvitegravir/emtricitabine/tenofovir disoproxil, crizotinib, cyclosporine, CYP3A4 inhibitors and inducers, dabigatran, dairy products, danazol, darunavir, dasatinib, delavirdine, denileukin, dexlansoprazole, diclofenac, docetaxel, dronedarone, efavirenz, enzalutamide, erythromycin, etoricoxib, fingolimod, gefitinib, grapefruit juice, Hemophilus B vaccine, HMG-CoA reductase inhibitors, ibuprofen, immunosuppressants, indinavir, irbesartan, itraconazole, ketoconazole, leflunomide, lenalidomide, lopinavir, lovastatin, meloxicam, mifepristone, mycophenolate, nelfinavir, nifedipine, olmesartan, omeprazole, oxaliplatin, pazopanib, pemetrexed, posaconazole, potassium, potassium-sparing diuretics, pralatrexate, rifabutin, rifampin, rifapentine, sevelamer, simvastatin, sirolimus, St John's wort, telaprevir, telithromycin, temsirolimus, tinidazole, tipranavir, tofacitinib, triamcinolone, vaccines, voriconazole
Pregnancy category: C
Important contra-indications noted in the prescribing guidelines for: the elderly; nursing mothers; pediatric patients
Black Box Warning: MALIGNANCIES AND SERIOUS INFECTIONS

Skin
Anaphylactoid reactions/Anaphylaxis [3]
Burning (46%) [13]
Dermatitis [2]
Diaphoresis (>3%)
Ecchymoses (>3%)
Edema (>10%)
Erythema (12%) [2]
Exanthems (4%) [2]
Folliculitis (10%) [2]
Graft-versus-host reaction [2]
Herpes simplex (13%) [4]
Kaposi's sarcoma [2]
Kaposi's varicelliform eruption [2]
Lymphoma [2]
Peripheral edema (26%)
Photosensitivity (>3%)
Pigmentation [2]
Pruritus (25–36%) [11]
Pustules (6%)
Rash (24%)
Rosacea [5]
Thrombocytopenic purpura [2]
Toxicity [2]

Hair
Alopecia (>3%) [6]
Hypertrichosis [2]

Mucosal
Gingival hyperplasia/hypertrophy [6]
Oral candidiasis (>3%)
Oral pigmentation [2]
Oral ulceration [2]

Cardiovascular
Cardiomyopathy [3]
Flushing [4]
Hypertension (49%) [8]
QT prolongation [2]

Central Nervous System
Encephalopathy [10]
Fever (>10%)
Headache [9]
Leukoencephalopathy [14]
Neurotoxicity [9]
Paresthesias (40%) [4]
Parkinsonism [2]
Seizures (<10%) [4]
Tremor (>10%) [8]
Vertigo (dizziness) [3]

Neuromuscular/Skeletal
Arthralgia (>10%) [2]
Asthenia (fatigue) (>10%) [3]
Back pain (>10%)
Myalgia/Myopathy (>3%)

Gastrointestinal/Hepatic
Abdominal pain [3]
Constipation (>10%)
Diarrhea (>10%) [5]
Dyspepsia (>10%)
Dysphagia (>3%)
Hepatotoxicity [9]
Nausea (>10%) [2]
Pancreatitis [3]
Vomiting (>10%)

Respiratory
Cough (>10%)
Dyspnea (>10%)
Pulmonary toxicity [2]

Endocrine/Metabolic
Creatine phosphokinase increased (>10%) [3]
Diabetes mellitus [5]
Diabetic ketoacidosis [5]
Gynecomastia [3]
Hyperglycemia [8]
Hyperkalemia [2]
Hyperlipidemia [2]
Hypomagnesemia (>10%) [2]
Hypophosphatemia (>10%)
SIADH [2]

Renal
Nephrotoxicity [42]
Renal failure [2]
Renal function abnormal [2]

Hematologic
Anemia (>10%)
Angiopathy [4]
Dyslipidemia [3]
Hemolytic anemia [2]
Hemolytic uremic syndrome [17]
Leukopenia (>10%) [4]
Neutropenia [3]
Thrombotic complications [5]

Otic
Tinnitus [2]

Ocular
Diplopia [2]
Ocular burning [3]
Optic neuropathy [2]
Vision blurred [2]
Vision loss [3]

Local
Application-site burning [5]
Application-site erythema [2]
Application-site infection [2]
Application-site irritation [2]
Application-site pruritus [6]

Other
Adverse effects [11]
Cancer [2]
Infection (>10%) [14]

TADALAFIL

Trade names: Adcirca (Lilly), Cialis (Lilly)
Indications: Erectile dysfunction, pulmonary arterial hypertension
Class: Phosphodiesterase type 5 (PDE5) inhibitor
Half-life: 15–18 hours
Clinically important, potentially hazardous interactions with: alcohol, alfuzosin, alpha blockers, amlodipine, amyl nitrite, angiotensin II receptor blockers, antifungals, antihypertensives, atazanavir, bendroflumethiazide, boceprevir, bosentan, clarithromycin, cobicistat/elvitegravir/emtricitabine/tenofovir disoproxil, conivaptan, CYP3A4 inhibitors or inducers, darunavir, dasatinib, delavirdine, disopyramide, doxazosin, efavirenz, enalapril, erythromycin, etravirine, fosamprenavir, grapefruit juice, indinavir, itraconazole, ketoconazole, lopinavir, macrolide antibiotics, metoprolol, nelfinavir, nicorandil, nitrates, nitroglycerin, oxcarbazepine, phosphodiesterase 5 inhibitors, rifampin, rifapentine, riociguat, ritonavir, sapropterin, saquinavir, St John's wort, tamsulosin, telaprevir, telithromycin, voriconazole
Pregnancy category: B (Cialis is not indicated for use in women)
Important contra-indications noted in the prescribing guidelines for: pediatric patients

---

Skin
Diaphoresis (<2%)
Facial edema (<2%)
Peripheral edema [2]
Pruritus (<2%)
Rash (<2%)

Mucosal
Epistaxis (nosebleed) (<2%)
Nasal congestion [4]
Rectal hemorrhage (<2%)
Xerostomia (<2%)

Cardiovascular
Angina (<2%)
Chest pain (<2%)
Flushing (2–3%) [15]
Hypotension (<2%)
Myocardial infarction (<2%)
Palpitation (<2%)
Postural hypotension (<2%)
Tachycardia (<2%)

Central Nervous System
Amnesia [3]
Headache (4–15%) [33]
Hyperesthesia (<2%)
Hypoesthesia (<2%)
Insomnia (<2%)
Pain (<3%)
Paresthesias (<2%)
Somnolence (drowsiness) (<2%)
Syncope (<2%)
Vertigo (dizziness) (<2%) [6]

Neuromuscular/Skeletal
Arthralgia (<2%)
Asthenia (fatigue) (<2%)
Back pain (2–6%) [19]
Myalgia/Myopathy (<4%) [12]
Neck pain (<2%)

Gastrointestinal/Hepatic
Dyspepsia [7]
Dysphagia (<2%)
Esophagitis (<2%)
Gastritis (<2%)
Gastroesophageal reflux (<2%)
Loose stools (<2%)
Nausea (<2%) [2]
Vomiting (<2%)

Respiratory
Dyspnea (<2%)
Pharyngitis (<2%)

Endocrine/Metabolic
GGT increased (<2%)

Genitourinary
Erection (<2%)
Priapism (spontaneous) (<2%) [2]

Otic
Hearing loss (<2%) [4]
Tinnitus (<2%)

Ocular
Chorioretinopathy [2]
Conjunctival hyperemia (<2%)
Conjunctivitis (<2%)
Dyschromatopsia (<2%)
Eyelid edema (<2%)
Eyelid pain (<2%)
Lacrimation (<2%)
Optic neuropathy [7]
Vision blurred (<2%)

Other
Adverse effects [3]

TAFLUPROST

Trade names: Saflutan (Merck Sharpe & Dohme), Zioptan (Merck Sharpe & Dohme)
Indications: Reduction of elevated intraocular pressure in open angle glaucoma or ocular hypertension
Class: Antiglaucoma, Prostaglandin analog
Half-life: 0.5 hours
Clinically important, potentially hazardous interactions with: none known
Pregnancy category: C
Important contra-indications noted in the prescribing guidelines for: nursing mothers; pediatric patients

Central Nervous System
Headache (6%)

Respiratory
Cough (3%)

Genitourinary
Urinary tract infection (2%)

Ocular
Cataract (3%)
Conjunctival hyperemia (4–20%) [6]
Conjunctivitis (5%)
Deepening of upper lid sulcus [4]
Eyelashes – hypertrichosis (2%)
Eyelashes – pigmentation (2%) [2]
Eyelid erythema (<10%)
Eyelid pigmentation [3]
Keratoconjunctivitis (<10%)
Lacrimation (<10%)
Ocular burning [3]
Ocular hyperemia [2]
Ocular itching [5]
Ocular pain (3%)
Ocular pigmentation (<10%)
Ocular pruritus (5%) [2]
Ocular stinging (7%) [4]
Photophobia (<10%)
Vision blurred (2%)
Visual disturbances (<10%)
Xerophthalmia (3%)

Other
Adverse effects [5]

TALIMOGENE LAHERPAREPVEC *

Synonym: T-VEC
Trade name: Imlygic (Amgen)
Indications: Unresectable cutaneous, subcutaneous, and nodal lesions in patients with melanoma recurrent after initial surgery
Class: Oncolytic virus immunotherapy
Half-life: N/A
Clinically important, potentially hazardous interactions with: none known
Pregnancy category: N/A (Contraception advised to prevent pregnancy during treatment)
Important contra-indications noted in the prescribing guidelines for: nursing mothers; pediatric patients

Skin
Cellulitis (<5%) [3]
Herpes (oral) (<5%)
Vitiligo (<5%)

Mucosal
Oropharyngeal pain (6%)

Central Nervous System
Chills (49%) [2]
Fever (43%) [2]
Headache (19%)
Vertigo (dizziness) (10%)

Neuromuscular/Skeletal
Arthralgia (17%)
Asthenia (fatigue) (50%) [2]
Myalgia/Myopathy (18%)
Pain in extremities (16%)

Gastrointestinal/Hepatic
Abdominal pain (9%)
Constipation (12%)
Diarrhea (19%)
Nausea (36%)
Vomiting (21%)

Respiratory
Flu-like syndrome (31%)

Endocrine/Metabolic
Weight loss (6%)

Renal
Glomerulonephritis (<5%)

Local
Injection-site pain (28%)

TAMOXIFEN

Trade name: Nolvadex (AstraZeneca)
Indications: Advanced breast cancer
Class: Selective estrogen receptor modulator (SERM)
Half-life: 5–7 days
Clinically important, potentially hazardous interactions with: anastrozole, bexarotene, cinacalcet, delavirdine, droperidol, duloxetine, gadobenate, paroxetine hydrochloride, rifapentine, terbinafine, tipranavir
Pregnancy category: D
Important contra-indications noted in the prescribing guidelines for: nursing mothers; pediatric patients

Skin
Carcinosarcoma [2]
Diaphoresis [4]
Edema (2–6%) [3]
Exanthems (3%) [3]
Hot flashes [17]
Lupus erythematosus [2]
Pruritus ani et vulvae [2]
Radiation recall dermatitis [5]
Rash (<10%) [2]
Sarcoma [9]
Toxicity [3]
Tumors [3]
Vasculitis [5]
Xerosis (7%)

Hair
Alopecia [7]
Hirsutism [2]

Mucosal
Stomatitis [2]
Xerostomia (7%) [2]

Cardiovascular
Flushing (>10%) [9]
Myocardial ischemia [2]
QT prolongation [3]
Thromboembolism [6]
Thrombophlebitis [3]
Venous thromboembolism [6]

Central Nervous System
Depression [5]
Headache [3]
Insomnia [4]
Mood changes [3]
Parkinsonism [2]

Stroke [4]
Vertigo (dizziness) [3]

Neuromuscular/Skeletal
Asthenia (fatigue) [5]
Bone or joint pain [3]
Fractures [2]
Leg cramps [2]
Myalgia/Myopathy [3]

Gastrointestinal/Hepatic
Hepatic steatosis [2]
Hepatotoxicity [10]
Nausea [4]
Pancreatitis [4]
Vomiting [3]

Respiratory
Pulmonary embolism [7]

Endocrine/Metabolic
ALP increased [2]
Amenorrhea [8]
Galactorrhea (<10%)
Hypercholesterolemia [2]
Hypertriglyceridemia [7]
Libido decreased [4]
Weight gain [4]

Genitourinary
Dyspareunia [4]
Endometrial cancer [5]
Ovarian hyperstimulation syndrome [2]
Sexual dysfunction [2]
Vaginal bleeding [4]
Vaginal discharge [5]
Vaginal dryness [5]

Hematologic
Hemolytic uremic syndrome [2]
Thrombosis [9]

Ocular
Cataract [9]
Keratopathy [3]
Macular edema [2]
Maculopathy [5]
Ocular adverse effects [5]
Ocular toxicity [5]
Retinopathy [5]
Vision impaired [3]

TAMSULOSIN

Trade names: Flomax (Boehringer Ingelheim), Jalyn (GSK)
Indications: Benign prostatic hypertrophy
Class: Adrenergic alpha-receptor antagonist
Half-life: 9–13 hours
Clinically important, potentially hazardous interactions with: alpha adrenergic blockers, cimetidine, conivaptan, darunavir, delavirdine, erythromycin, indinavir, ketoconazole, paroxetine hydrochloride, phosphodiesterase 5 inhibitors, tadalafil, telithromycin, terbinafine, vardenafil, voriconazole, warfarin
Pregnancy category: B (not indicated for use in women; Jalyn is pregnancy category X)
Important contra-indications noted in the prescribing guidelines for: nursing mothers; pediatric patients
Note: Jalyn is tamsulosin and dutasteride.

Mucosal
Xerostomia [4]

Cardiovascular
Chest pain (4%)
Hypotension (6–19%) [3]
Postural hypotension [3]

Central Nervous System
Headache (19–21%) [6]
Insomnia (<2%)
Somnolence (drowsiness) (3–4%)
Vertigo (dizziness) (15–17%) [16]

Neuromuscular/Skeletal
Asthenia (fatigue) (8–9%) [2]
Back pain (7–8%)

Gastrointestinal/Hepatic
Constipation [2]
Diarrhea (4–6%)
Nausea (3–4%)

Respiratory
Cough (3–5%)
Pharyngitis (5–6%)
Rhinitis (13–18%) [2]
Sinusitis (2–4%)

Endocrine/Metabolic
Libido decreased (<2%)

Genitourinary
Ejaculatory dysfunction (8–18%) [9]
Erectile dysfunction [2]
Priapism [4]
Urinary retention [3]

Ocular
Floppy iris syndrome [34]
Vision blurred (<2%)

Other
Adverse effects [3]
Infection (9–11%)
Tooth disorder (<2%)

TAPENTADOL

Trade names: Nucynta (Janssen), Nucynta ER (Janssen), Palexia (Grunenthal)
Indications: Immediate release formulation: moderate to severe acute pain, extended release formulation: moderate to severe chronic pain and neuropathic pain associated with diabetic peripheral neuropathy when a continuous analgesic is needed for an extended period of time
Class: Analgesic, opioid
Half-life: 5 hours
Clinically important, potentially hazardous interactions with: alcohol, alvimopan, amphetamines, anesthetics, anitemetics, anticholinergics, buprenorphine, butorphanol, CNS depressants, desmopressin, droperidol, hypnotics, linezolid, MAO inhibitors, mirtazapine, nalbuphine, PEG-interferon, pegvisomant, pentazocine, phenothiazines, sedatives, sibutramine, SNRIs, SSRIs, St John's wort, succinylcholine, thiazide diuretics, tramadol, tranquilizers, trazodone, tricyclic antidepressants, triptans
Pregnancy category: C
Important contra-indications noted in the prescribing guidelines for: the elderly; nursing mothers; pediatric patients
Note: Contraindicated in patients with impaired pulmonary function or paralytic ileus. Should not be used in patients currently using or within 14 days of using a monoamine oxidase inhibitor.
Black Box Warning: For extended release oral tablets: ABUSE POTENTIAL, LIFE-THREATENING RESPIRATORY DEPRESSION, ACCIDENTAL EXPOSURE, and INTERACTION WITH ALCOHOL

Mucosal
Xerostomia [4]

Central Nervous System
Headache [4]
Neurotoxicity [2]
Somnolence (drowsiness) [8]
Vertigo (dizziness) (4%) [9]

Neuromuscular/Skeletal
Asthenia (fatigue) [3]

Gastrointestinal/Hepatic
Constipation [15]
Diarrhea [2]
Gastrointestinal disorder [2]
Nausea (4%) [21]
Vomiting (3%) [14]

Other
Adverse effects [4]

TARTRAZINE

Class: Food additive
Half-life: N/A
Clinically important, potentially hazardous interactions with: none known
Note: Tartrazine intolerance has been estimated to affect between 0.01% and 0.1% of the population. Adverse reactions are most common in people who are sensitive to aspirin.
Banned in Austria and Norway.

Skin
Anaphylactoid reactions/Anaphylaxis [8]
Angioedema [11]
Atopic dermatitis [2]
Hypersensitivity [9]
Pruritus [2]
Purpura [5]
Urticaria (often related to aspirin intolerance) [33]
Vasculitis [3]

Other
Adverse effects [3]
Allergic reactions [9]

TASIMELTEON

Trade name: Hetlioz (Vanda)
Indications: Non-24-hour sleep-wake disorder
Class: Melatonin receptor agonist
Half-life: 2–3 hours
Clinically important, potentially hazardous interactions with: fluvoxamine, ketoconazole, rifampin
Pregnancy category: C
Important contra-indications noted in the prescribing guidelines for: the elderly; nursing mothers; pediatric patients

---

Central Nervous System
Abnormal dreams (10%) [3]
Headache (17%) [3]
Nightmares (10%) [3]

Respiratory
Upper respiratory tract infection (7%) [2]

Endocrine/Metabolic
ALT increased (10%) [2]

Genitourinary
Urinary tract infection (7%) [3]

TAVABOROLE

Indications: Onychomycosis
Class: Antifungal, oxaborole
Half-life: N/A
Clinically important, potentially hazardous interactions with: none known
Pregnancy category: C
Important contra-indications noted in the prescribing guidelines for: nursing mothers; pediatric patients

---

Nails
Onychocryptosis (3%)

Local
Application-site erythema (2%) [2]
Application-site exfoliation (3%)

TAZAROTENE

Trade names: Avage (Allergan), Fabior (GSK), Tazorac (Allergan), Zorac (Allergan)
Indications: Acne vulgaris, mild to moderate plaque psoriasis involving up to 10% body surface area
Half-life: 18 hours
Clinically important, potentially hazardous interactions with: none known
Pregnancy category: X
Important contra-indications noted in the prescribing guidelines for: the elderly; nursing mothers; pediatric patients

---

Skin
Burning (10–20%) [5]
Contact dermatitis (5–10%)
Desquamation (5–10%)
Erythema (10–20%) [5]
Pruritus (10–25%) [11]
Psoriasis (5–10%)
Rash (5–10%)
Scaling [2]
Stinging (<3%) [2]
Xerosis (<3%) [5]

Other
Adverse effects [2]
Side effects [2]

TEDIZOLID

Trade name: Sivextro (Cubist)
Indications: Acute bacterial skin and skin structure infections caused by susceptible bacteria
Class: Antibiotic, oxazolidinone
Half-life: 12 hours
Clinically important, potentially hazardous interactions with: none known
Pregnancy category: C
Important contra-indications noted in the prescribing guidelines for: nursing mothers; pediatric patients

---

Skin
Dermatitis (<2%)
Hypersensitivity (<2%)
Pruritus (<2%)
Urticaria (<2%)

Cardiovascular
Flushing (<2%)
Hypertension (<2%)
Palpitation (<2%)
Tachycardia (<2%)

Central Nervous System
Headache (6%) [2]
Hypoesthesia (<2%)
Insomnia (<2%)
Vertigo (dizziness) (2%) [2]

Gastrointestinal/Hepatic
Diarrhea (4%) [3]
Nausea (8%) [4]
Vomiting (3%) [3]

Hematologic
Anemia (<2%)

Ocular
Asthenopia (<2%)
Vision blurred (<2%)
Vision impaired (<2%)
Vitreous floaters (<2%)

Local
Infusion-related reactions (<2%)

Other
Adverse effects [2]
Infection (<2%)

TEDUGLUTIDE

Trade name: Gattex (Hospira)
Indications: Treatment of short bowel syndrome in adult patients dependent on parenteral support
Class: Glucagon-like peptide-2 (GLP-2) analog
Half-life: 1–2 hours
Clinically important, potentially hazardous interactions with: none known
Pregnancy category: B
Important contra-indications noted in the prescribing guidelines for: nursing mothers; pediatric patients

---

Skin
Edema [4]
Hypersensitivity (<10%)

Central Nervous System
Headache (16%) [6]
Sleep disturbances (<10%)

Gastrointestinal/Hepatic
Abdominal distension (14%) [4]
Abdominal pain (30%) [8]
Constipation [3]
Flatulence (<10%)
Gastrointestinal disorder [2]
Hepatotoxicity [3]
Nausea (18%) [7]
Vomiting (<10%) [2]

Respiratory
Cough (<10%)
Nasopharyngitis [2]
Upper respiratory tract infection (12%)

Local
Injection-site erythema [2]
Injection-site reactions (22%)

Other
Adverse effects [9]

TEGAFUR/GIMERACIL/OTERACIL

Synonyms: TS-1; S-1
Trade name: Teysuno (Taiho Pharma)
Indications: Gastric, colorectal, head and neck cancers, non-small cell lung cancer, inoperable or recurrent breast cancer, pancreatic cancer
Class: Antineoplastic
Half-life: N/A
Clinically important, potentially hazardous interactions with: capecitabine, flucytosine, fluorouracil, other fluoropyrimidine-group antineoplastics, phenytoin, uracil/tegafur, warfarin
Pregnancy category: N/A (Contraindicated in pregnancy)
Important contra-indications noted in the prescribing guidelines for: the elderly; nursing mothers; pediatric patients
Note: Contraindicated in patients with severe bone marrow depression, hepatic or renal impairment.
Not available in the USA.

Skin
Dermatitis (<5%)
Desquamation (<5%)
Edema (<5%) [3]
Erythema (<5%)
Hand-foot syndrome (<5%) [8]
Herpes simplex (<5%)
Jaundice (<5%)
Pigmentation (21%) [8]
Pruritus (<5%)
Rash (12%) [4]
Raynaud's phenomenon (<5%)

Ulcerations (<5%)
Xerosis (<5%) [2]

Hair
Alopecia (<5%) [3]

Nails
Nail disorder (<5%)
Paronychia (<5%) [2]

Mucosal
Mucositis [7]
Stomatitis (17%) [8]

Cardiovascular
Flushing (<5%)
Hypertension (<5%)
Hypotension (<5%)

Central Nervous System
Anorexia (34%) [21]
Fever (<5%) [2]
Headache (<5%)
Paresthesias (<5%)
Peripheral neuropathy [3]
Vertigo (dizziness) (<5%)
Warm feeling (<5%)

Neuromuscular/Skeletal
Arthralgia (<5%)
Asthenia (fatigue) (22%) [11]
Myalgia/Myopathy (<5%)

Gastrointestinal/Hepatic
Diarrhea (19%) [29]
Hepatotoxicity [6]
Nausea (23%) [16]
Vomiting (8%) [10]

Respiratory
Pharyngitis (<5%)
Pneumonitis [4]
Rhinitis (<5%)

Endocrine/Metabolic
ALT increased (12%) [4]
Appetite decreased [4]
AST increased (12%) [2]
Hyponatremia [3]
Weight loss (<5%)

Genitourinary
Glycosuria (<5%)
Hematuria (<5%)

Renal
Nephrotoxicity [2]
Proteinuria (<5%)

Hematologic
Anemia [22]
Bleeding (<5%)
Bone marrow suppression [2]
Febrile neutropenia [9]
Hemotoxicity [5]
Leukocytopenia [2]
Leukopenia (87%) [23]
Myelosuppression [6]
Neutropenia (44%) [39]
Thrombocytopenia (11%) [14]

Ocular
Conjunctivitis (<5%)
Keratitis (<5%)
Lacrimation (<5%)
Ocular adverse effects [2]
Ocular pain (<5%)
Reduced visual acuity (<5%)

Other
Adverse effects [19]

TEICOPLANIN

Trade name: Targocid (Sanofi-Aventis)
Indications: Staphylococcal infections
Class: Antibiotic, glycopeptide
Half-life: 150 hours
Clinically important, potentially hazardous interactions with: amikacin, cephaloridine, colistin, gentamicin, kanamycin, neomycin, streptomycin, tobramycin, vancomycin
Pregnancy category: N/A (Not recommended in pregnancy)
Important contra-indications noted in the prescribing guidelines for: nursing mothers

---

Skin
DRESS syndrome [2]
Erythema (<10%)
Exanthems [2]
Hypersensitivity [3]
Pruritus (<10%)
Rash (<10%) [4]
Red man syndrome [3]
Urticaria [2]

Central Nervous System
Fever (<10%)

Gastrointestinal/Hepatic
Hepatotoxicity (2%) [2]

Renal
Nephrotoxicity [2]

Hematologic
Neutropenia [2]

Otic
Ototoxicity [2]

TELAPREVIR

Trade name: Incivek (Vertex)
Indications: Hepatitis C (must only be used in combination with PEG-interferon alfa and ribavirin)
Class: Antiviral, CYP3A4 inhibitor, Hepatitis C virus NS3/4A protease inhibitor
Half-life: 4–11 hours
Clinically important, potentially hazardous interactions with: alfuzosin, alprazolam, amiodarone, amlodipine, atazanavir, atorvastatin, bepridil, bosentan, budesonide, carbamazepine, cisapride, dabigatran, darunavir, desipramine, dexamethasone, digoxin, dihydroergotamine, diltiazem, efavirenz, ergotamine, escitalopram, estradiol, felodipine, flecainide, flibanserin, fluticasone propionate, fosamprenavir, itraconazole, ketoconazole, lidocaine, lomitapide, lovastatin, methylergonovine, methylprednisolone, midazolam, mifepristone, nicardipine, nisoldipine, phenobarbital, phenytoin, pimozide, ponatinib, posaconazole, propafenone, quinidine, rifampin, ritonavir, ruxolitinib, salmeterol, sildenafil, simvastatin, sirolimus, St John's wort, tacrolimus, tadalafil, telithromycin, tenofovir disoproxil, trazodone, triazolam, vardenafil, venetoclax, verapamil, voriconazole, warfarin, zolpidem
Pregnancy category: X
Important contra-indications noted in the prescribing guidelines for: the elderly; nursing mothers; pediatric patients
Note: Must be used in combination with PEG-interferon alfa and ribavirin (see separate entries).
Black Box Warning: SERIOUS SKIN REACTIONS

Skin
Dermatitis [2]
DRESS syndrome [6]
Exanthems [6]
Pruritus (including anal pruritus) (53%) [14]
Rash (56%) [37]
Stevens–Johnson syndrome [3]
Toxic epidermal necrolysis [2]
Toxicity [2]

Central Nervous System
Dysgeusia (taste perversion) (10%)

Neuromuscular/Skeletal
Asthenia (fatigue) (56%) [4]

Gastrointestinal/Hepatic
Anorectal discomfort (11%)
Diarrhea (26%) [2]
Hemorrhoids (12%)
Hepatotoxicity [5]
Nausea (39%) [4]
Vomiting (13%)

Renal
Nephrotoxicity [3]

Hematologic
Anemia [35]
Neutropenia [5]
Thrombocytopenia [6]

Other
Adverse effects [19]
Infection [4]

TELBIVUDINE

Trade names: Sebvio (Novartis), Tyzeka (Novartis)
Indications: Hepatitis B (chronic)
Class: Nucleoside analog reverse transcriptase inhibitor
Half-life: ~15 hours
Clinically important, potentially hazardous interactions with: interferon alfa, PEG-interferon
Pregnancy category: B
Important contra-indications noted in the prescribing guidelines for: the elderly; nursing mothers; pediatric patients

---

Skin
Pruritus (2%)
Rash (4%)

Cardiovascular
Arrhythmias [2]

Central Nervous System
Fever (4%)
Headache (11%)

Insomnia (3%)
Neurotoxicity [2]
Vertigo (dizziness) (4%)

Neuromuscular/Skeletal
Arthralgia (4%)
Asthenia (fatigue) (>5%) [2]
Back pain (4%)
Myalgia/Myopathy (3%) [8]

Gastrointestinal/Hepatic
Abdominal distension (3%)
Abdominal pain (12%)
Diarrhea [2]
Dyspepsia (3%)
Hepatitis (exacerbation) (2%)

Respiratory
Cough (7%)
Flu-like syndrome (7%)
Pharyngolaryngeal pain (5%)
Upper respiratory tract infection (>5%)

Endocrine/Metabolic
ALT increased (3%)
Creatine phosphokinase increased [4]

Hematologic
Neutropenia (2%)

TELMISARTAN

Trade name: Micardis (Boehringer Ingelheim)
Indications: Hypertension
Class: Angiotensin II receptor antagonist (blocker), Antihypertensive
Half-life: 24 hours
Clinically important, potentially hazardous interactions with: ramipril
Pregnancy category: D (category C in first trimester; category D in second and third trimesters)
Important contra-indications noted in the prescribing guidelines for: nursing mothers; pediatric patients
Black Box Warning: FETAL TOXICITY

Skin
Angioedema [2]
Peripheral edema [2]

Cardiovascular
Hypotension [2]

Central Nervous System
Headache [4]
Vertigo (dizziness) [5]

Neuromuscular/Skeletal
Asthenia (fatigue) [4]

Respiratory
Cough [9]

Endocrine/Metabolic
Hyperkalemia [2]

TEMAZEPAM

Trade name: Restoril (Mallinckrodt)
Indications: Insomnia, anxiety
Class: Benzodiazepine
Half-life: 8–15 hours
Clinically important, potentially hazardous interactions with: amprenavir, chlorpheniramine, clarithromycin, efavirenz, esomeprazole, imatinib, mianserin, nelfinavir
Pregnancy category: X
Important contra-indications noted in the prescribing guidelines for: the elderly; nursing mothers; pediatric patients

---

Skin
Dermatitis (<10%)
Diaphoresis (>10%)
Rash (>10%)

Mucosal
Sialopenia (>10%)
Sialorrhea (<10%)
Xerostomia (2%)

Other
Adverse effects [2]

TEMOZOLOMIDE

Trade name: Temodar (MSD)
Indications: Anaplastic astrocytoma, newly diagnosed glioblastoma multiforme concomitantly with radiotherapy and then as maintenance treatment
Class: Alkylating agent, Antineoplastic
Half-life: 1.8 hours
Clinically important, potentially hazardous interactions with: clozapine, digoxin, valproic acid
Pregnancy category: D
Important contra-indications noted in the prescribing guidelines for: the elderly; nursing mothers; pediatric patients

---

Skin
Peripheral edema (11%)
Pruritus (8%)
Rash (8%) [6]
Toxicity [2]

Hair
Alopecia [3]

Cardiovascular
Thromboembolism [2]

Central Nervous System
Anorexia [3]
Fever [2]
Headache [3]
Paresthesias (9%)

Neuromuscular/Skeletal
Asthenia (fatigue) [12]
Myalgia/Myopathy (5%)

Gastrointestinal/Hepatic
Constipation [2]
Diarrhea [6]
Hepatotoxicity [5]
Nausea [8]
Vomiting [3]

Endocrine/Metabolic
Mastodynia (6%)

Hematologic
Anemia [3]
Febrile neutropenia [2]
Hemotoxicity [5]
Leukopenia [5]
Lymphocytopenia [4]
Lymphopenia [2]
Myelosuppression [2]
Neutropenia [10]
Thrombocytopenia [11]

Other
Death [6]
Infection [5]

TEMSIROLIMUS

Trade name: Torisel (Wyeth)
Indications: Renal cell carcinoma, other cancers
Class: Analog of sirolimus, Antineoplastic, mTOR inhibitor
Half-life: 17 hours
Clinically important, potentially hazardous interactions with: ACE inhibitors, atazanavir, BCG vaccine, benazepril, captopril, carbamazepine, clarithromycin, clozapine, conivaptan, cyclosporine, darunavir, dasatinib, denosumab, dexamethasone, digoxin, enalapril, fluconazole, fosinopril, grapefruit juice, hypoglycemic agents, indinavir, itraconazole, ketoconazole, leflunomide, lisinopril, live and inactive vaccines, macolide antibiotics, natalizumab, nefazodone, nelfinavir, P-glycoprotein inhibitors, phenobarbital, phenytoin, pimecrolimus, posaconazole, protease inhibitors, quinapril, ramipril, rifabutin, rifampin, rifapentine, ritonavir, saquinavir, St John's wort, sunitinib, tacrolimus, telithromycin, tipranavir, trastuzumab, voriconazole
Pregnancy category: D
Important contra-indications noted in the prescribing guidelines for: the elderly; nursing mothers; pediatric patients
Note: Contraindicated in patients with bilirubin >1.5xULN.

Skin
Acneform eruption (10%) [3]
Edema [2]
Exanthems [3]
Hypersensitivity (9%) [3]
Pruritus (19%) [3]
Rash (47%) [14]
Toxicity [3]
Xerosis (11%)

Nails
Nail disorder (14%)
Paronychia [2]

Mucosal
Mucositis (30%) [12]
Stomatitis [15]

Cardiovascular
Chest pain (16%)
Hypertension (7%) [3]

Central Nervous System
Anorexia (30%) [3]

Chills (8%)
Depression (4%)
Dysgeusia (taste perversion) (20%) [2]
Fever (24%)
Headache (15%)
Insomnia (12%)
Neurotoxicity [2]
Pain (28%)

Neuromuscular/Skeletal
Arthralgia (18%)
Asthenia (fatigue) (30%) [19]
Back pain (20%)
Myalgia/Myopathy (8%)

Gastrointestinal/Hepatic
Abdominal pain (21%)
Diarrhea [5]
Nausea [5]
Vomiting [2]

Respiratory
Cough (26%) [3]
Dyspnea [7]
Pharyngitis (12%)
Pneumonia [2]
Pneumonitis (36%) [11]
Rhinitis (10%)
Upper respiratory tract infection (7%)

Endocrine/Metabolic
ALT increased [4]
AST increased [2]
Dehydration [2]
Hypercholesterolemia [4]
Hyperglycemia [14]
Hyperlipidemia [2]
Hypertriglyceridemia [5]
Hypokalemia [3]
Hypophosphatemia [4]
Serum creatinine increased [2]

Genitourinary
Urinary tract infection (15%)

Hematologic
Anemia [9]
Febrile neutropenia [2]
Hemorrhage [2]
Immunosupression [2]
Leukopenia [4]
Lymphopenia [4]
Neutropenia [5]
Thrombocytopenia [16]

Ocular
Conjunctivitis (7%)

Other
Adverse effects [9]
Death [2]
Infection (20%) [5]

TENOFOVIR ALAFENAMIDE *

Trade names: Descovy (Gilead), Vemlidy (Gilead)
Indications: Hepatitis B
Class: Antiviral, Hepatitis B virus necleoside analog reverse transcriptase inhibitor
Half-life: < 1 hour
Clinically important, potentially hazardous interactions with: carbamazepine, oxcarbazepine, phenobarbital, phenytoin, rifabutin, rifampin, rifapentine, St John's wort
Pregnancy category: N/A (No data available)
Important contra-indications noted in the prescribing guidelines for: nursing mothers; pediatric patients
Note: Descovy is tenofovir alafenamide and emtricitabine. See also separate profile for tenofovir alafenamide in combination with cobicistat, elvitegravir and emtricitabine.
Black Box Warning: LACTIC ACIDOSIS/ SEVERE HEPATOMEGALY WITH STEATOSIS and POST TREATMENT SEVERE ACUTE EXACERBATION OF HEPATITIS B

Central Nervous System
Headache (9%)

Neuromuscular/Skeletal
Asthenia (fatigue) (6%)
Back pain (5%)

Gastrointestinal/Hepatic
Abdominal pain (7%)
Nausea (5%)

Respiratory
Cough (6%)

Endocrine/Metabolic
ALT increased (8%)
AST increased (3%)
Creatine phosphokinase increased (3%)
Hyperamylasemia (3%)
Hypercholesterolemia (4%)

Genitourinary
Glycosuria (5%)

Other
Adverse effects [2]

TENOFOVIR DISOPROXIL

Trade names: Atripla (Gilead), Complera (Gilead), Truvada (Gilead), Viread (Gilead)
Indications: HIV infection in combination with at least two other antiretroviral agents
Class: Antiretroviral, Nucleoside analog reverse transcriptase inhibitor
Half-life: 12–18 hours
Clinically important, potentially hazardous interactions with: acyclovir, adefovir, atazanavir, cidofovir, cobicistat/elvitegravir/emtricitabine/ tenofovir disoproxil, darunavir, didanosine, ganciclovir, high-fat foods, indinavir, ledipasvir & sofosbuvir, lopinavir, protease inhibitors, ritonavir, telaprevir, tipranavir, trospium, valacyclovir, valganciclovir
Pregnancy category: B
Important contra-indications noted in the prescribing guidelines for: nursing mothers; pediatric patients
Note: Atripla is tenofovir disoproxil, efavirenz and emtricitabine; Complera is tenofovir disoproxil, emtricitabine and rilpivirine; Truvada is tenofovir disoproxil and emtricitabine. See also separate profile for tenofovir disoproxil in combination with cobicistat, elvitegravir and emtricitabine.
Black Box Warning: LACTIC ACIDOSIS/ SEVERE HEPATOMEGALY WITH STEATOSIS and POST TREATMENT EXACERBATION OF HEPATITIS

Skin
Diaphoresis (3%)
Lichenoid eruption [2]
Rash (5–18%) [4]
Stevens–Johnson syndrome [2]

Cardiovascular
Chest pain (3%)

Central Nervous System
Abnormal dreams [3]
Anorexia (3%)
Anxiety (6%) [2]
Depression (4–11%)
Fever (2–8%)
Headache (5–14%) [6]
Insomnia (3–5%) [2]
Neurotoxicity (3%) [6]
Pain (7–13%)
Peripheral neuropathy (<3%)
Somnolence (drowsiness) [2]
Vertigo (dizziness) (<3%) [4]

Neuromuscular/Skeletal
Arthralgia (5%)
Asthenia (fatigue) (6–7%) [5]
Back pain (3–9%)
Bone or joint pain [4]
Fractures [2]
Myalgia/Myopathy (3%) [2]
Osteomalacia [5]

Gastrointestinal/Hepatic
Abdominal pain (4–7%) [2]
Diarrhea (11%) [5]
Dyspepsia (3–4%)
Flatulence (3%)
Hepatic failure [2]
Hepatotoxicity [3]
Nausea (8%) [7]
Pancreatitis [5]
Vomiting (4–5%) [4]

Respiratory
Pneumonia (2–5%)

Endocrine/Metabolic
Acidosis [3]
Creatine phosphokinase increased [2]
Hypokalemia [2]
Hypophosphatemia [3]
Weight loss (2%)

Renal
Fanconi syndrome [23]
Nephrotoxicity [40]
Proteinuria [4]
Renal failure [10]
Renal tubular necrosis [2]

Other
Adverse effects [10]

TERAZOSIN

Trade name: Hytrin (AbbVie)
Indications: Hypertension, benign prostatic hypertrophy
Class: Adrenergic alpha-receptor antagonist
Half-life: 12 hours
Clinically important, potentially hazardous interactions with: vardenafil
Pregnancy category: C

Skin
Edema (<10%)
Lichenoid eruption [2]
Peripheral edema (6%)

Mucosal
Xerostomia (<10%)

Cardiovascular
Postural hypotension [2]

Central Nervous System
Paresthesias (3%)
Vertigo (dizziness) [3]

Genitourinary
Priapism [2]

Ocular
Floppy iris syndrome [2]

TERBINAFINE

Trade name: Lamisil (Novartis)
Indications: Fungal infections of the skin and nails
Class: Antifungal
Half-life: ~36 hours
Clinically important, potentially hazardous interactions with: amitriptyline, amphotericin B, atomoxetine, caffeine, carbamazepine, cimetidine, codeine, conivaptan, cyclosporine, CYP2D6 substrates, desipramine, estrogens, fesoterodine, fluconazole, nebivolol, progestogens, rifampin, rifapentine, saxagliptin, tamoxifen, tamsulosin, tetrabenazine, thioridazine, tramadol, tricyclic antidepressants
Pregnancy category: B
Important contra-indications noted in the prescribing guidelines for: nursing mothers; pediatric patients

---

Skin
AGEP [24]
Baboon syndrome (SDRIFE) [2]
Dermatitis (<10%)
Eczema [2]
Erythema multiforme [9]
Erythroderma [2]
Exanthems [5]
Fixed eruption [3]
Hypersensitivity [3]
Lichenoid eruption [2]
Lupus erythematosus [29]
Pityriasis rosea [2]
Pruritus (3%) [5]
Psoriasis [14]
Pustules [3]
Rash (6%) [3]
Stevens–Johnson syndrome [2]
Toxic epidermal necrolysis [3]
Urticaria [7]

Hair
Alopecia (<10%)

Nails
Onychocryptosis [2]

Central Nervous System
Ageusia (taste loss) [17]
Dysgeusia (taste perversion) (3%) [7]
Headache (13%)

Gastrointestinal/Hepatic
Abdominal pain (2%)
Diarrhea (6%)
Dyspepsia (4%)
Flatulence (2%)
Hepatotoxicity [10]
Nausea (3%)

Other
Adverse effects [3]
Allergic reactions (<10%)
Side effects (3%)

TERBUTALINE

Trade names: Brethine (aaiPharma), Bricanyl (AstraZeneca)
Indications: Bronchospasm
Class: Beta-2 adrenergic agonist, Bronchodilator, Tocolytic
Half-life: 11–16 hours
Clinically important, potentially hazardous interactions with: alpha blockers, atomoxetine, beta blockers, betahistine, cannabinoids, epinephrine, insulin aspart, insulin degludec, insulin detemir, insulin glargine, insulin glulisine, iobenguane, loop diuretics, MAO inhibitors, propranolol, sotalol, sympathomimetics, tricyclic antidepressants, yohimbine
Pregnancy category: C
Important contra-indications noted in the prescribing guidelines for: nursing mothers; pediatric patients
Black Box Warning: PROLONGED TOCOLYSIS

Skin
Diaphoresis (<10%)

Mucosal
Xerostomia (<10%)

Cardiovascular
Arrhythmias [2]

Central Nervous System
Dysgeusia (taste perversion) (<10%)
Tremor [2]

Gastrointestinal/Hepatic
Nausea [2]

Other
Side effects [2]

TERIFLUNOMIDE

Trade name: Aubagio (Sanofi-Aventis)
Indications: Relapsing forms of multiple sclerosis
Class: Pyrimidine synthesis inhibitor
Half-life: N/A
Clinically important, potentially hazardous interactions with: alosetron, caffeine, duloxetine, ethinylestradiol, leflunomide, live vaccines, oral contraceptives, paclitaxel, pioglitazone, repaglinide, rosiglitazone, theophylline, tizanidine, warfarin
Pregnancy category: X
Important contra-indications noted in the prescribing guidelines for: the elderly; nursing mothers; pediatric patients
Black Box Warning: HEPATOTOXICITY and RISK OF TERATOGENICITY

Skin
Acneform eruption (<3%)
Burning (2–3%)
Herpes (oral) (2–4%)
Pruritus (3–4%)

Hair
Alopecia (10–13%) [13]

Cardiovascular
Hypertension (4%) [3]
Palpitation (2–3%)

Central Nervous System
Anxiety (3–4%)
Carpal tunnel syndrome (<3%)
Headache (19–22%) [3]
Paresthesias (9–10%) [3]
Peripheral neuropathy (<2%) [2]

Neuromuscular/Skeletal
Asthenia (fatigue) [2]
Back pain (<3%) [2]
Bone or joint pain (4–5%)
Myalgia/Myopathy (3–4%)

Gastrointestinal/Hepatic
Abdominal distension (<2%)
Abdominal pain (5–6%)
Diarrhea (15–18%) [10]
Gastroenteritis (2–4%)
Hepatotoxicity [4]
Nausea (9–14%) [8]

Respiratory
Bronchitis (5–8%)
Influenza (9–12%) [2]
Nasopharyngitis [2]
Sinusitis (4–6%)
Upper respiratory tract infection (9%)

Endocrine/Metabolic
ALT increased (12–14%) [10]
AST increased (2–3%)
GGT increased (3–5%)
Hypophosphatemia (mild) (18%)
Weight loss (2–3%)

Genitourinary
Cystitis (2–4%)

Renal
Renal failure [2]

Hematologic
Immunosupression (10–15%)
Leukopenia (<2%) [2]

Lymphopenia [2]
Neutropenia (2–4%) [3]

Ocular
Conjunctivitis (<3%)
Vision blurred (3%)

Other
Adverse effects [4]
Allergic reactions (2–3%)
Infection [5]
Side effects [2]
Toothache (4%)

TERIPARATIDE

Trade name: Forteo (Lilly)
Indications: Osteoporosis in postmenopausal women and men at increased risk of fractures
Class: Parathyroid hormone analog
Half-life: 1 hour
Clinically important, potentially hazardous interactions with: alcohol, digoxin
Pregnancy category: C
Important contra-indications noted in the prescribing guidelines for: nursing mothers; pediatric patients
Black Box Warning: POTENTIAL RISK OF OSTEOSARCOMA

Skin
Diaphoresis (2%)
Herpes zoster (3%)
Rash (5%)

Cardiovascular
Angina (3%)
Hypertension (7%)

Central Nervous System
Anxiety (4%)
Depression (4%)
Dysgeusia (taste perversion) (<2%)
Headache (8%) [8]
Insomnia (4–5%)
Pain (21%)
Paresthesias (<2%)
Syncope (3%)
Vertigo (dizziness) (4–8%) [7]

Neuromuscular/Skeletal
Arthralgia (10%) [3]
Asthenia (fatigue) (9%)
Bone tumor [2]
Leg cramps (3%) [4]
Myalgia/Myopathy [2]
Neck pain (3%)
Pain in extremities [3]

Gastrointestinal/Hepatic
Constipation (5%)
Diarrhea (5%)
Dyspepsia (5%)
Gastritis (2–7%)
Nausea (9–14%) [8]
Vomiting (3%)

Respiratory
Cough (6%)
Dyspnea (4–6%)
Pharyngitis (6%)
Pneumonia (4–6%)
Rhinitis (10%)

Endocrine/Metabolic
Hypercalcemia [4]

Local
Injection-site pain (<2%)

Other
Adverse effects [4]
Tooth disorder (2%)

TERLIPRESSIN

Trade names: Glypressin (IS Pharma), Terlipressin (Ferring) (Bissendorf Peptide)
Indications: Esophageal variceal hemorrhage
Class: Vasopressin agonist
Half-life: 50–70 minutes
Clinically important, potentially hazardous interactions with: none known
Pregnancy category: N/A
Note: Contraindicated in pregnancy.

Skin
Gangrene [2]
Necrosis [12]

Cardiovascular
Myocardial infarction [3]
QT prolongation [2]
Torsades de pointes [2]

Central Nervous System
Seizures [3]

Neuromuscular/Skeletal
Rhabdomyolysis [3]

Endocrine/Metabolic
Hyponatremia [8]

TESTOSTERONE

Trade names: Androderm (Actavis), AndroGel (AbbVie), Delatestryl (Endo), Fortesta (Endo), Natesto (Endo), Testim (Auxilium)
Indications: Androgen replacement, hypogonadism, postpartum breast pain
Class: Androgen
Half-life: 10–100 minutes
Clinically important, potentially hazardous interactions with: acarbose, anisindione, anticoagulants, cyclosporine, dicumarol, metformin, saxagliptin, sitagliptin, warfarin
Pregnancy category: X
Important contra-indications noted in the prescribing guidelines for: nursing mothers; pediatric patients
Note: Contraindicated in men with carcinoma of the breast or known or suspected carcinoma of the prostate; and in pregnant or breastfeeding women.
Black Box Warning: SECONDARY EXPOSURE TO TESTOSTERONE

Skin
Acneform eruption (>10%) [19]
Carcinoma [2]
Dermatitis (4%) [2]
Edema (<10%)
Rash (2%)

Hair
Alopecia [3]
Hirsutism (<10%) [12]

Cardiovascular
Cardiotoxicity [2]
Flushing (<10%)
Myocardial infarction [3]

Endocrine/Metabolic
Gynecomastia [2]
Mastodynia (>10%)

Genitourinary
Priapism (>10%) [10]

Hematologic
Thrombosis [2]

Local
Application-site bullae (12%)
Application-site burning (3%)
Application-site erythema (7%)
Application-site induration (3%)
Application-site pruritus (37%)
Application-site vesicles (6%)

Other
Adverse effects [3]

THALLIUM

Indications: For diagnostic use in myocardial perfusion imaging
Class: Radioactive element
Half-life: 73.1 hours
Clinically important, potentially hazardous interactions with: none known
Pregnancy category: C

Hair
Alopecia [11]

Nails
Leukonychia (Mees' lines) [2]

Cardiovascular
Tachycardia [3]

Central Nervous System
Encephalopathy [5]
Peripheral neuropathy [5]

Gastrointestinal/Hepatic
Abdominal pain [5]

Other
Death [2]

THIABENDAZOLE

Synonym: tiabendazole
Indications: Various infections caused by susceptible helminths
Class: Anthelmintic, Antibiotic, imidazole
Half-life: 1.2 hours
Clinically important, potentially hazardous interactions with: none known
Pregnancy category: C

Skin
Dermatitis [3]
Erythema multiforme [3]
Exanthems (>5%) [4]

Fixed eruption [2]
Rash (<10%)
Sjögren's syndrome [3]
Stevens–Johnson syndrome (<10%)
Toxic epidermal necrolysis [2]
Urticaria (<5%)

Central Nervous System
Vertigo (dizziness) [3]

Gastrointestinal/Hepatic
Abdominal pain [2]
Nausea [2]

TIAGABINE

Trade name: Gabitril (Cephalon)
Indications: Partial seizures
Class: Anticonvulsant, Mood stabilizer
Half-life: 7–9 hours
Clinically important, potentially hazardous interactions with: alcohol, antipsychotics, carbamazepine, chloroquine, conivaptan, CYP3A4 inhibitors and inducers, dasatinib, deferasirox, droperidol, hydroxychloroquine, ketorolac, levomepromazine, MAO inhibitors, mefloquine, orlistat, phenobarbital, phenytoin, SSRIs, St John's wort, tricyclic antidepressants
Pregnancy category: C
Important contra-indications noted in the prescribing guidelines for: the elderly; nursing mothers; pediatric patients

---

Skin
Ecchymoses (<6%)
Pruritus (2%)
Rash (5%) [2]

Cardiovascular
Vasodilation (2%)

Central Nervous System
Confusion (5%)
Depression (<7%) [4]
Emotional lability (3%)
Gait instability (3–5%)
Headache [8]
Hostility (2–5%)
Impaired concentration (6–14%) [2]
Insomnia (5–6%)
Nervousness (10–14%) [10]
Pain (2–7%)
Paresthesias (4%)
Seizures [4]
Somnolence (drowsiness) (18–21%) [9]
Speech disorder (4%)
Status epilepticus (non-convulsive) [17]
Syncope [2]
Tremor (9–21%) [7]
Vertigo (dizziness) (27–31%) [22]

Neuromuscular/Skeletal
Asthenia (fatigue) (18–23%) [16]
Ataxia (5–9%)
Dystonia [5]
Myalgia/Myopathy (2–5%)

Gastrointestinal/Hepatic
Abdominal pain (5–7%)
Diarrhea (2–10%)
Nausea (11%) [7]
Vomiting (7%)

Respiratory
Cough (4%)
Flu-like syndrome (6–9%)
Pharyngitis (7–8%)

Endocrine/Metabolic
Appetite increased (2%)

Genitourinary
Urinary tract infection (<5%)

Ocular
Amblyopia (4–9%)
Nystagmus (2%)

Other
Adverse effects [6]
Infection (10–19%) [3]

TICAGRELOR

Trade name: Brilinta (AstraZeneca)
Indications: Thrombotic cardiovascular events
Class: Antiplatelet, Antiplatelet, cyclopentyl triazolo-pyrimidine (CPTP)
Half-life: 7 hours
Clinically important, potentially hazardous interactions with: atazanavir, carbamazepine, clarithromycin, dexamethasone, digoxin, efavirenz, indinavir, itraconazole, ketoconazole, lovastatin, nefazodone, nelfinavir, phenobarbital, phenytoin, rifampin, ritonavir, saquinavir, simvastatin, telithromycin, venetoclax, voriconazole
Pregnancy category: C
Important contra-indications noted in the prescribing guidelines for: nursing mothers; pediatric patients
Note: Maintenance doses of aspirin above 100 mg reduce the effectiveness of ticagrelor and should be avoided. Contraindicated in patients with a history of intracranial hemorrhage, or active pathological bleeding, and in patients with severe hepatic impairment.
Black Box Warning: BLEEDING RISK

Cardiovascular
Atrial fibrillation (4%)
Chest pain (3–4%)
Hypertension (4%)
Hypotension (3%)
Ventricular arrhythmia [6]

Central Nervous System
Headache (7%)
Vertigo (dizziness) (5%)

Neuromuscular/Skeletal
Asthenia (fatigue) (3%)
Back pain (4%)
Rhabdomyolysis [2]

Gastrointestinal/Hepatic
Diarrhea (4%)
Nausea (4%)

Respiratory
Cough (5%)
Dyspnea (14%) [15]
Pneumonitis [2]

Hematologic
Bleeding (12%) [8]

Other
Adverse effects [2]

TINZAPARIN

Trade name: Innohep (Leo Pharma)
Indications: Acute symptomatic deep vein thrombosis
Class: Anticoagulant, Heparin, low molecular weight
Half-life: 3–4 hours
Clinically important, potentially hazardous interactions with: aliskiren, angiotensin II recepton antagonists, aspirin, butabarbital, clopidogrel, collagenase, dasatinib, dextran, diclofenac, dipyridamole, drotrecogin alfa, glyceryl trinitrate, ibritumomab, iloprost, ketorolac, NSAIDs, oral anticoagulants, pentosan, pentoxifylline, platelet inhibitors, prostacyclin analogues, salicylates, sulfinpyrazone, throbolytics, ticlopidine, tositumomab & iodine[131]
Pregnancy category: B
Important contra-indications noted in the prescribing guidelines for: the elderly; nursing mothers; pediatric patients
Black Box Warning: SPINAL / EPIDURAL HEMATOMAS

Skin
Bullous dermatitis (<10%)
Pruritus (<10%)

Mucosal
Epistaxis (nosebleed) (2%)

Cardiovascular
Chest pain (2%)

Central Nervous System
Fever (2%)
Headache (2%)
Pain (2%)

Neuromuscular/Skeletal
Back pain (2%)

Respiratory
Pulmonary embolism (2%)

Endocrine/Metabolic
ALT increased (13%)
AST increased (9%)

Genitourinary
Urinary tract infection (4%)

Hematologic
Bleeding [4]
Hemorrhage (2%)

Local
Injection-site hematoma (16%)

TIOTROPIUM

Trade names: Spiriva (Boehringer Ingelheim), Stiolto Respimat (Boehringer Ingelheim)
Indications: Bronchospasm (associated with COPD)
Class: Anticholinergic, Muscarinic antagonist
Half-life: 5–6 days
Clinically important, potentially hazardous interactions with: acetylcholinesterase inhibitors, anticholinergics, antihistamines, botulinum toxin (A & B), cannabinoids, conivaptan, disopyramide, domperidone, haloperidol, ketoconazole, levodopa, MAO

inhibitors, memantine, metoclopramide, nefopam, parasympathomimetics, PEG-interferon, phenothiazines, potassium chloride, pramlintide, secretin, sublingual nitrates, tricyclic antidepressants
Pregnancy category: C
Important contra-indications noted in the prescribing guidelines for: nursing mothers; pediatric patients
Note: Stiolto Respimat is tiotropium and olodaterol.

Skin
Candidiasis (4%)
Edema (5%)
Herpes zoster (<3%)
Rash (4%)

Mucosal
Epistaxis (nosebleed) (4%)
Oral candidiasis [2]
Stomatitis (<3%)
Xerostomia (10–16%) [22]

Cardiovascular
Angina (<3%)
Cardiotoxicity [2]
Chest pain (7%)
Hypertension [2]

Central Nervous System
Depression (<3%)
Headache [6]
Paresthesias (<3%)
Vertigo (dizziness) [2]

Neuromuscular/Skeletal
Arthralgia (>3%)
Back pain [4]
Bone or joint pain (<3%)
Leg pain (<3%)
Myalgia/Myopathy (4%)

Gastrointestinal/Hepatic
Abdominal pain (5%)
Constipation (4%) [2]
Diarrhea [3]
Dyspepsia (6%)
Gastroesophageal reflux (<3%)
Vomiting (4%)

Respiratory
Asthma [4]
Bronchitis [4]
COPD (exacerbation) [4]
Cough (>3%) [8]
Dysphonia (<3%)
Dyspnea [4]
Flu-like syndrome (>3%)
Influenza [3]
Laryngitis (<3%)
Nasopharyngitis [11]
Pharyngitis (9%)
Pneumonia [3]
Rhinitis (6%) [3]
Sinusitis (11%)
Upper respiratory tract infection (41%) [4]

Endocrine/Metabolic
Hypercholesterolemia (<3%)
Hyperglycemia (<3%)

Genitourinary
Urinary tract infection (7%)

Ocular
Cataract (<3%)

Other
Adverse effects [12]
Allergic reactions (<3%)
Death [7]
Infection (4%)

TIPRANAVIR

Trade name: Aptivus (Boehringer Ingelheim)
Indications: Antiretroviral treatment of HIV-1
Class: HIV-1 protease inhibitor, Sulfonamide
Half-life: 4.8–6.0 hours
Clinically important, potentially hazardous interactions with: abacavir, alcohol, alfuzosin, alprazolam, amiodarone, antacids, antifungals, apixaban, artemether/lumefantrine, atazanavir, atomoxetine, atorvastatin, bepridil, bosentan, buprenorphine, calcium channel blockers, carbamazepine, cisapride, clarithromycin, codeine, conivaptan, corticosteroids, cyclosporine, CYP2D6 substrates, CYP3A4 inducers, dabigatran, darifenacin, deferasirox, delavirdine, didanosine, digoxin, dihydroergotamine, disulfiram, efavirenz, enfuvirtide, eplerenone, ergotamine, esomeprazole, estradiol, estrogens, etravirine, fesoterodine, flecainide, fluconazole, fosamprenavir, fusidic acid, garlic, HMG-CoA reductase inhibitors, lopinavir, lovastatin, meperidine, methadone, metoprolol, metronidazole, midazolam, nebivolol, nefazodone, omeprazole, P-glycoprotein substrates, pantoprazole, phenobarbital, phenytoin, pimozide, propafenone, protease inhibitors, proton pump inhibitors, quetiapine, quinidine, quinine, raltegravir, ranolazine, rifabutin, rifampin, rilpivirine, rivaroxaban, rosuvastatin, salmeterol, saquinavir, sildenafil, simeprevir, simvastatin, sirolimus, sofosbuvir, St John's wort, tacrolimus, tamoxifen, telithromycin, temsirolimus, tenofovir disoproxil, tetrabenazine, theophylline, thioridazine, tramadol, trazodone, triazolam, tricyclic antidepressants, valproic acid, vardenafil, vitamin E, zidovudine
Pregnancy category: C
Important contra-indications noted in the prescribing guidelines for: the elderly; nursing mothers; pediatric patients
Note: Tipranavir is a sulfonamide and can be absorbed systemically. Sulfonamides can produce severe, possibly fatal, reactions such as toxic epidermal necrolysis and Stevens-Johnson syndrome.
Tipranavir is co-administered with ritonavir. Contraindicated in patients with moderate or severe (Child-Pugh Class B or C) hepatic impairment.
Black Box Warning: HEPATOTOXICITY and INTRACRANIAL HEMORRHAGE

Skin
Exanthems (<2%)
Herpes simplex (<2%)
Herpes zoster (<2%)
Hypersensitivity (<2%)
Lipoatrophy (<2%)
Lipodystrophy (<2%)
Lipohypertrophy (<2%)
Pruritus (<2%)
Rash (3%) [2]

Central Nervous System
Anorexia (<2%)
Depression (2%)
Fever (14%)
Headache (5%)
Insomnia (2%)
Intracranial hemorrhage (<2%) [3]
Neurotoxicity (<2%)
Peripheral neuropathy (2%)
Sleep related disorder (<2%)
Somnolence (drowsiness) (<2%)
Vertigo (dizziness) (<2%)

Neuromuscular/Skeletal
Asthenia (fatigue) (2%)
Cramps (<2%)
Myalgia/Myopathy (2%)

Gastrointestinal/Hepatic
Abdominal distension (<2%)
Abdominal pain (6%)
Dyspepsia (<2%)
Flatulence (<2%)
Gastroesophageal reflux (<2%)
Hepatic failure (<2%)
Hepatitis (<2%)
Hepatotoxicity [4]
Nausea (9%)
Pancreatitis (<2%)
Vomiting (6%)

Respiratory
Dyspnea (2%)
Flu-like syndrome (<2%)

Endocrine/Metabolic
ALT increased (2%) [2]
Appetite decreased (<2%)
Dehydration (2%)
Diabetes mellitus (<2%)
GGT increased (2%)
Hyperamylasemia (<2%)
Hypercholesterolemia (<2%)
Hyperglycemia (<2%)
Hyperlipidemia (3%)
Hypertriglyceridemia (4%) [2]
Weight loss (3%)

Hematologic
Anemia (3%)
Neutropenia (2%)
Thrombocytopenia (<2%)

Other
Adverse effects [3]

TIZANIDINE

Trade name: Zanaflex (Acorda)
Indications: Muscle spasticity, multiple sclerosis
Class: Adrenergic alpha2-receptor agonist
Half-life: 2.5 hours
Clinically important, potentially hazardous interactions with: acebutolol, alfuzosin, benazepril, captopril, cilazapril, ciprofloxacin, enalapril, fluvoxamine, fosinopril, irbesartan, lisinopril, norfloxacin, obeticholic acid, olmesartan, phenytoin, quinapril, ramipril, rofecoxib, teriflunomide, trandolapril

Pregnancy category: C
Important contra-indications noted in the prescribing guidelines for: the elderly; pediatric patients

---

Skin
Pallor [2]
Pruritus (<10%)
Rash (<10%)

Mucosal
Xerostomia (49–88%) [14]

Cardiovascular
Bradycardia (<10%) [5]
Hypotension (16–33%) [3]

Central Nervous System
Dyskinesia (3%)
Nervousness (3%)
Somnolence (drowsiness) (48–92%) [4]
Speech disorder (3%)
Tremor (<10%)
Vertigo (dizziness) (41–45%) [3]

Neuromuscular/Skeletal
Asthenia (fatigue) (41–78%) [5]

Gastrointestinal/Hepatic
Constipation (4%)
Hepatotoxicity (6%) [4]
Vomiting (3%)

Respiratory
Flu-like syndrome (3%)
Pharyngitis (3%)
Rhinitis (3%)

Genitourinary
Urinary frequency (3%)
Urinary tract infection (10%)

Ocular
Amblyopia (3%)

Other
Infection (6%)

TOBRAMYCIN

Trade names: TOBI (Chiron), TobraDex (Alcon)
Indications: Various serious infections caused by susceptible organisms, superficial ocular infections
Class: Antibiotic, aminoglycoside
Half-life: 2–3 hours
Clinically important, potentially hazardous interactions with: adefovir, aldesleukin, aminoglycosides, atracurium, bumetanide, daptomycin, doxacurium, ethacrynic acid, furosemide, neuromuscular blockers, pancuronium, polypeptide antibiotics, rocuronium, succinylcholine, teicoplanin, torsemide, vecuronium
Pregnancy category: D (category D for injection and inhalation; category B for ophthalmic use)
Important contra-indications noted in the prescribing guidelines for: the elderly; nursing mothers; pediatric patients
Note: Aminoglycosides may cause neurotoxicity and/or nephrotoxicity.
TobraDex is tobramycin and dexamethasone.

Skin
Exanthems [4]
Hypersensitivity [3]
Rash [2]

Central Nervous System
Dysgeusia (taste perversion) [2]
Fever [2]

Respiratory
Cough [3]

Renal
Nephrotoxicity [6]

Ocular
Conjunctivitis [2]
Eyelid dermatitis [2]
Intraocular pressure increased [2]

TOCILIZUMAB

Trade name: Actemra (Roche)
Indications: Rheumatoid arthritis, juvenile idiopathic arthritis, Castleman's disease
Class: Anti-interleukin-6 receptor monoclonal antibody, Disease-modifying antirheumatic drug (DMARD), Monoclonal antibody
Half-life: 8–14 days
Clinically important, potentially hazardous interactions with: efavirenz, fesoterodine, fingolimod, infliximab, lurasidone, paricalcitol, pazopanib, typhoid vaccine, yellow fever vaccine
Pregnancy category: C
Important contra-indications noted in the prescribing guidelines for: nursing mothers; pediatric patients
Black Box Warning: RISK OF SERIOUS INFECTIONS

Skin
Anaphylactoid reactions/Anaphylaxis [4]
Cellulitis [7]
Herpes zoster [7]
Hypersensitivity [4]
Malignancies [2]
Peripheral edema (<2%)
Psoriasis [2]
Rash (2%) [6]

Mucosal
Mucosal ulceration [2]
Oral ulceration (2%)
Stomatitis (<2%)

Cardiovascular
Cardiotoxicity [3]
Hypertension (6%) [3]

Central Nervous System
Headache (7%) [6]
Neurotoxicity [2]
Vertigo (dizziness) (3%)

Neuromuscular/Skeletal
Arthralgia [4]
Fractures [2]

Gastrointestinal/Hepatic
Abdominal pain (2%)
Gastroenteritis [4]
Gastrointestinal bleeding [2]
Gastrointestinal perforation [7]
Gastrointestinal ulceration (<2%)
Hepatotoxicity [12]
Nausea [3]

Respiratory
Bronchitis (3%) [5]
Cough (<2%)
Dyspnea (<2%)
Influenza [3]
Nasopharyngitis (7%) [6]
Pharyngitis [2]
Pneumonia [8]
Pneumothorax [2]
Pulmonary toxicity [4]
Upper respiratory tract infection (7%) [9]

Endocrine/Metabolic
ALT increased (6%) [7]
Hypercholesterolemia [2]
Hyperlipidemia [5]
Hypertriglyceridemia [2]
Hypothyroidism (<2%)
Weight gain (<2%)

Genitourinary
Urinary tract infection [2]

Renal
Nephrolithiasis (<2%)
Pyelonephritis [3]

Hematologic
Hemotoxicity [2]
Leukopenia (<2%) [4]
Lymphopenia [2]
Neutropenia [15]
Sepsis [2]

Ocular
Conjunctivitis (<2%)

Local
Infusion-related reactions [3]
Infusion-site reactions [2]

Other
Adverse effects [10]
Death [4]
Infection [35]

TOFACITINIB

Trade name: Xeljanz (Pfizer)
Indications: Rheumatoid arthritis
Class: Janus kinase (JAK) inhibitor
Half-life: ~3 hours
Clinically important, potentially hazardous interactions with: azathioprine, biologic disease-modifying antirheumatics, cyclosporine, CYP3A4 inhibitors, fluconazole, ketoconazole, live vaccines, potent immunosuppressives, rifampin, strong CYP inducers, strong CYP2C19 inhibitors, tacrolimus
Pregnancy category: C
Important contra-indications noted in the prescribing guidelines for: the elderly; nursing mothers; pediatric patients
Black Box Warning: SERIOUS INFECTIONS AND MALIGNANCY

Skin
Erythema (<2%)
Herpes zoster [4]
Peripheral edema (<2%)
Pruritus (<2%)
Rash (<2%) [2]

Mucosal
Nasal congestion (<2%)

Cardiovascular
Hypertension (2%)

Central Nervous System
Fever (<2%)
Headache (3–4%) [10]
Insomnia (<2%)
Paresthesias (<2%)

Neuromuscular/Skeletal
Arthralgia (<2%)
Bone or joint pain (<2%)
Tendinitis (<2%)

Gastrointestinal/Hepatic
Abdominal pain (<2%) [2]
Diarrhea (3–4%) [7]
Dyspepsia (<2%) [2]
Gastritis (<2%)
Nausea (<2%) [2]
Vomiting (<2%)

Respiratory
Bronchitis [3]
Cough (<2%)
Dyspnea (<2%)
Influenza [2]
Nasopharyngitis (3–4%) [8]
Tuberculosis [3]
Upper respiratory tract infection (4–5%) [7]

Endocrine/Metabolic
ALT increased [2]
AST increased [2]
Creatine phosphokinase increased [2]
Dehydration (<2%)

Genitourinary
Urinary tract infection (2%) [5]

Hematologic
Anemia (<2%)
Neutropenia [3]

Other
Adverse effects [8]
Infection (20–22%) [11]

TOLTERODINE

Trade name: Detrol (Pharmacia & Upjohn)
Indications: Urinary incontinence
Class: Muscarinic antagonist
Half-life: 2–4 hours
Clinically important, potentially hazardous interactions with: itraconazole, ketoconazole, lopinavir, nelfinavir, sotalol, voriconazole, warfarin
Pregnancy category: C
Important contra-indications noted in the prescribing guidelines for: nursing mothers; pediatric patients

---

Skin
Erythema (2%)
Rash (2%)

Mucosal
Xerostomia (35%) [38]

Cardiovascular
Chest pain (2%)

Central Nervous System
Headache (7%) [4]
Somnolence (drowsiness) (3%)
Vertigo (dizziness) (5%) [4]

Neuromuscular/Skeletal
Arthralgia (2%)
Asthenia (fatigue) (4%)

Gastrointestinal/Hepatic
Abdominal pain (5%) [2]
Constipation (7%) [13]
Diarrhea (4%)
Dyspepsia (4%)

Respiratory
Flu-like syndrome (3%)
Upper respiratory tract infection (6%)

Genitourinary
Dysuria (2%)

Ocular
Vision blurred [3]
Xerophthalmia (3%) [2]

Other
Adverse effects [6]

TOPIRAMATE

Trade names: Qsymia (Vivus), Qudexy (Upsher-Smith), Topamax (Janssen), Trokendi XR (Supernus)
Indications: Partial onset seizures, migraine
Class: Anticonvulsant, Mood stabilizer
Half-life: 21 hours
Clinically important, potentially hazardous interactions with: eslicarbazepine, levonorgestrel, metformin, rufinamide, ulipristal, valproic acid
Pregnancy category: D
Important contra-indications noted in the prescribing guidelines for: nursing mothers; pediatric patients
Note: Qsymia is topiramate and phentermine.

Skin
Anhidrosis [2]
Bromhidrosis (2%)
Diaphoresis (2%)
Edema (2%)
Fixed eruption [2]
Hot flashes (<10%)
Hypohidrosis [2]
Palmar erythema [2]
Pruritus (2%) [3]
Rash (4%) [3]

Hair
Alopecia [2]

Mucosal
Gingivitis (2%)
Xerostomia (3%) [5]

Cardiovascular
Flushing (>5%)
Tachycardia [3]

Central Nervous System
Anorexia (>5%) [4]
Anxiety [2]
Cognitive impairment (>5%) [15]
Confusion (>5%)
Depression [10]
Dysgeusia (taste perversion) (>5%) [9]
Encephalopathy [3]
Fever (>5%)
Hyperthermia [3]
Impaired concentration [3]
Insomnia [7]
Nervousness (>5%)
Neurotoxicity [5]
Palinopsia [3]
Paresthesias (>5%) [31]
Psychosis [3]
Seizures [3]
Somnambulism [2]
Somnolence (drowsiness) (>5%) [3]
Suicidal ideation [2]
Tremor (>10%)
Vertigo (dizziness) (>5%) [11]

Neuromuscular/Skeletal
Asthenia (fatigue) (>5%) [8]

Gastrointestinal/Hepatic
Constipation [5]
Diarrhea [3]
Nausea [5]

Respiratory
Flu-like syndrome (<2%)

Endocrine/Metabolic
Acidosis [4]
Appetite decreased [2]
Gynecomastia (8%)
Hyperammonemia [2]
Mastodynia (3–9%)
Weight gain [2]
Weight loss (>5%) [14]

Genitourinary
Erectile dysfunction [2]

Renal
Nephrolithiasis [5]

Ocular
Glaucoma [15]
Myopia [9]
Uveitis [5]
Vision loss [2]

Other
Adverse effects [10]
Death [2]
Infection (>5%)
Side effects [3]
Teratogenicity [8]

TOPOTECAN

Trade name: Hycamtin (GSK)
Indications: Metastatic ovarian carcinoma
Class: Antineoplastic, Topoisomerase I inhibitor
Half-life: 3–6 hours
Clinically important, potentially hazardous interactions with: atorvastatin, darunavir, gefitinib, lapatinib, oxaliplatin, pantoprazole
Pregnancy category: D
Important contra-indications noted in the prescribing guidelines for: nursing mothers; pediatric patients
Black Box Warning: BONE MARROW SUPPRESSION

Hair
Alopecia (59%) [7]

Mucosal
Mucositis [2]
Stomatitis (24%) [4]

Central Nervous System
Fever [2]
Paresthesias (9%)

Neuromuscular/Skeletal
Asthenia (fatigue) [9]

Gastrointestinal/Hepatic
Abdominal pain [2]
Diarrhea [5]
Hepatotoxicity [3]
Nausea [3]
Vomiting [4]

Respiratory
Dyspnea [3]

Renal
Nephrotoxicity [2]

Hematologic
Anemia [11]
Febrile neutropenia [5]
Granulocytopenia [2]
Myelosuppression [2]
Neutropenia [16]
Thrombocytopenia [15]

Other
Adverse effects [2]
Death [5]
Infection [2]

TOREMIFENE

Trade name: Fareston (ProStrakan)
Indications: Metastatic breast cancer
Class: Selective estrogen receptor modulator (SERM)
Half-life: ~5 days
Clinically important, potentially hazardous interactions with: amoxapine, arsenic, dolasetron, efavirenz, pazopanib, sugammadex, telavancin
Pregnancy category: D
Important contra-indications noted in the prescribing guidelines for: nursing mothers; pediatric patients
Black Box Warning: QT PROLONGATION

Skin
Diaphoresis (20%) [6]
Edema (5%) [2]
Hot flashes (35%) [4]

Cardiovascular
Flushing [3]
Thromboembolism [3]
Venous thromboembolism [2]

Central Nervous System
Headache [2]
Vertigo (dizziness) [2]

Gastrointestinal/Hepatic
Hepatotoxicity [3]
Nausea [2]
Vomiting [2]

Endocrine/Metabolic
ALP increased [2]
Galactorrhea (<10%)

Genitourinary
Priapism (<10%)
Vaginal bleeding [2]
Vaginal discharge [2]

Ocular
Cataract [3]

TORSEMIDE

Trade names: Demadex (Roche), Torem (Roche)
Indications: Essential hypertension, edema due to congestive heart failure, hepatic, pulmonary or renal edema
Class: Diuretic, loop
Half-life: 2–4 hours
Clinically important, potentially hazardous interactions with: ACE inhibitors, amikacin, aminoglycosides, aminophylline, anti-diabetics, antihypertensives, cephalosporins, cisplatin, gentamicin, indomethacin, kanamycin, neomycin, probenecid, salicylates, streptomycin, tobramycin
Pregnancy category: B
Important contra-indications noted in the prescribing guidelines for: nursing mothers; pediatric patients
Note: Torsemide is a sulfonamide and can be absorbed systemically. Sulfonamides can produce severe, possibly fatal, reactions such as toxic epidermal necrolysis and Stevens-Johnson syndrome.

Skin
Photosensitivity (<10%)
Urticaria (<10%)
Vasculitis [2]

Central Nervous System
Headache (7%)
Vertigo (dizziness) (3%)

Neuromuscular/Skeletal
Arthralgia (2%)
Asthenia (fatigue) (2%)
Myalgia/Myopathy (2%)

Gastrointestinal/Hepatic
Constipation (2%)
Diarrhea (2%)
Dyspepsia (2%)
Nausea (2%)

Respiratory
Cough (2%)
Pharyngolaryngeal pain (2%)
Rhinitis (3%)

Endocrine/Metabolic
Pseudoporphyria [2]

TRAMADOL

Trade names: Rybix ODT (Victory Pharma), Ultracet (Ortho-McNeil), Ultram (Ortho-McNeil)
Indications: Pain
Class: Opiate agonist
Half-life: 6–7 hours
Clinically important, potentially hazardous interactions with: alcohol, amitriptyline, carbamazepine, cinacalcet, citalopram, delavirdine, desflurane, desvenlafaxine, duloxetine, erythromycin, fluoxetine, fluvoxamine, ketoconazole, levomepromazine, linezolid, lorcaserin, MAO inhibitors, nefazodone, ondansetron, paroxetine hydrochloride, phenelzine, quinidine, risperidone, tapentadol, terbinafine, tianeptine, tipranavir, tranylcypromine, venlafaxine, vilazodone, zuclopenthixol
Pregnancy category: C
Important contra-indications noted in the prescribing guidelines for: the elderly; nursing mothers; pediatric patients

---

Skin
Anaphylactoid reactions/Anaphylaxis [2]
Angioedema [2]
Contact dermatitis [2]
Diaphoresis (9%) [3]
Hypersensitivity [2]
Peripheral edema [2]
Pruritus (<10%) [4]
Rash (<5%) [2]
Urticaria (<18%)

Mucosal
Xerostomia (10%) [4]

Cardiovascular
Flushing [2]
Vasodilation (<5%)

Central Nervous System
Anorexia (<5%)
Anxiety (<5%)
Catatonia [2]
Confusion (<5%)
Euphoria (<5%)
Fever [2]
Headache [7]
Insomnia [3]
Nervousness (<5%)
Restless legs syndrome [5]
Seizures [16]
Serotonin syndrome [16]
Sleep related disorder (<5%)
Somnolence (drowsiness) [7]
Tremor (5–10%)
Vertigo (dizziness) [18]

Neuromuscular/Skeletal
Asthenia (fatigue) (<5%) [3]
Hypertonia (<5%)

Gastrointestinal/Hepatic
Abdominal pain (<5%) [3]
Constipation [7]
Diarrhea [2]
Flatulence (<5%)
Nausea [21]
Vomiting [19]

Respiratory
Apnea [2]
Respiratory depression [2]

Endocrine/Metabolic
Adrenal insufficiency [2]
Hypoglycemia [6]
Hyponatremia [3]

Genitourinary
Urinary frequency (<5%)
Urinary retention (<5%)

Otic
Hallucinations, auditory [2]

Ocular
Hallucinations, visual [3]
Mydriasis [2]
Visual disturbances (<5%)

Other
Adverse effects [6]
Death [2]

TRAMETINIB

Trade name: Mekinist (Novartis)
Indications: Melanoma (unresectable or metastatic) in patients with BRAF V600E or V600K mutations
Class: MEK inhibitor
Half-life: 4–5 days
Clinically important, potentially hazardous interactions with: none known
Pregnancy category: D
Important contra-indications noted in the prescribing guidelines for: nursing mothers; pediatric patients

---

Skin
Acneform eruption (19%) [6]
Actinic keratoses [2]
Cellulitis (<10%)
Dermatitis (19%) [2]
Edema (32%)
Folliculitis (<10%)
Lymphedema (32%)
Panniculitis [3]
Papulopustular eruption [2]
Peripheral edema (32%) [5]
Pruritus (10%) [2]
Pustules (<10%)
Rash (57%) [12]
Squamous cell carcinoma [2]
Toxicity (87%) [5]
Xerosis (11%)

Hair
Alopecia [2]

Nails
Paronychia (10%)

Mucosal
Aphthous stomatitis (15%)
Epistaxis (nosebleed) (13%)
Gingival bleeding (13%)
Mucosal inflammation (15%)
Oral ulceration (15%)
Rectal hemorrhage (13%)
Stomatitis (15%) [2]
Xerostomia (<10%)

Cardiovascular
Bradycardia (<10%)
Cardiomyopathy (7%)
Cardiotoxicity [4]
Hypertension (15%) [3]

Central Nervous System
Dysgeusia (taste perversion) (<10%)
Fever [3]
Vertigo (dizziness) (<10%)

Neuromuscular/Skeletal
Arthralgia [2]
Asthenia (fatigue) [8]
Rhabdomyolysis (<10%)

Gastrointestinal/Hepatic
Abdominal pain (13%)
Black stools (13%)
Diarrhea (43%) [11]
Nausea [6]
Vomiting [3]

Respiratory
Pneumonitis (2%)

Endocrine/Metabolic
ALP increased (24%)
ALT increased (39%)
AST increased (60%)
Hypoalbuminemia (42%)

Genitourinary
Hematuria (13%)
Vaginal bleeding (13%)

Hematologic
Anemia (38%) [2]
Hemorrhage (13%)
Neutropenia [2]
Thrombocytopenia [2]

Ocular
Conjunctival hemorrhage (13%)
Retinopathy [2]
Vision blurred (<10%)
Xerophthalmia (<10%)

Other
Adverse effects [2]

TRANDOLAPRIL

Trade names: Mavik (AbbVie), Tarka (AbbVie)
Indications: Hypertension
Class: Angiotensin-converting enzyme (ACE) inhibitor, Antihypertensive, Vasodilator
Half-life: 6 hours
Clinically important, potentially hazardous interactions with: alcohol, aldesleukin, aliskiren, allopurinol, alpha blockers, amiloride, angiotensin II receptor antagonists, antacids, antidiabetics, antipsychotics, anxiolytics and hypnotics, baclofen, beta blockers, calcium channel blockers, clonidine, corticosteroids, cyclosporine, diazoxide, diuretics, estrogens, general anesthetics, gold & gold compounds, heparins, hydralazine, insulin, levodopa, lithium, MAO inhibitors, metformin, methyldopa, minoxidil, moxisylyte, moxonidine, nitrates, nitroprusside, NSAIDs, potassium salts, spironolactone, sulfonylureas, tizanidine, triamterene, trimethoprim
Pregnancy category: D (category C in first trimester; category D in second and third trimesters)
Important contra-indications noted in the prescribing guidelines for: nursing mothers; pediatric patients
Note: Contraindicated in patients with hereditary/idiopathic angioedema and in patients with a history of angioedema related to previous treatment with an ACE inhibitor. Tarka is trandolapril and verapamil.
Black Box Warning: FETAL TOXICITY

Skin
Angioedema [3]
Edema (>3%)

Mucosal
Xerostomia (>3%)

Cardiovascular
Bradycardia (5%)
Cardiogenic shock (4%)
Hypotension (11%)

Central Nervous System
Hyperesthesia (>3%)
Stroke (3%)
Syncope (6%)
Vertigo (dizziness) (23%)

Neuromuscular/Skeletal
Asthenia (fatigue) (3%)
Myalgia/Myopathy (5%)

Gastrointestinal/Hepatic
Dyspepsia (6%)
Gastritis (4%)

Respiratory
Cough (35%) [5]

Endocrine/Metabolic
Creatine phosphokinase increased (5%)
Hyperkalemia (5%)
Hypocalcemia (5%)

TRANEXAMIC ACID

Trade name: Cyklokapron (Pharmacia)
Indications: Fibrinolysis
Class: Antifibrinolytic
Half-life: 2 hours
Clinically important, potentially hazardous interactions with: none known
Pregnancy category: B

Skin
Fixed eruption [2]

Central Nervous System
Headache [2]
Seizures [11]

Renal
Nephrotoxicity [2]

Other
Adverse effects [2]

TRASTUZUMAB

Trade name: Herceptin (Genentech)
Indications: Metastatic breast cancer
Class: Antineoplastic, Monoclonal antibody
Half-life: 2–16 days (dose dependent)
Clinically important, potentially hazardous interactions with: abatacept, abciximab, alefacept, antineoplastics, azacitidine, betamethasone, cabazitaxel, denileukin, docetaxel, doxorubicin, fingolimod, gefitinib, immunosuppressants, leflunomide, lenalidomide, oxaliplatin, paclitaxel, pazopanib, pemetrexed, temsirolimus

Pregnancy category: D
Important contra-indications noted in the prescribing guidelines for: nursing mothers; pediatric patients
Black Box Warning: CARDIOMYOPATHY, INFUSION REACTIONS, EMBRYO-FETAL TOXICITY, and PULMONARY TOXICITY

Skin
- Acneform eruption (2%) [4]
- Edema (8%)
- Hand–foot syndrome [9]
- Herpes simplex (2%)
- Hypersensitivity [2]
- Peripheral edema (5–10%)
- Photosensitivity [2]
- Pruritus (2%)
- Radiation recall dermatitis [2]
- Rash (4–18%) [9]
- Toxicity [3]

Hair
- Alopecia [6]

Nails
- Nail disorder (2%)

Mucosal
- Epistaxis (nosebleed) (2%)
- Mucositis [3]
- Stomatitis [3]

Cardiovascular
- Arrhythmias (3%)
- Cardiac disorder [3]
- Cardiac failure [4]
- Cardiomyopathy [2]
- Cardiotoxicity [22]
- Congestive heart failure (2–7%) [5]
- Hypertension (4%) [3]
- Myocardial toxicity [3]
- Palpitation (3%)
- Tachycardia (5%)

Central Nervous System
- Anorexia (14%)
- Chills (5–32%) [8]
- Depression (6%)
- Fever (6–36%) [6]
- Headache (10–26%) [2]
- Insomnia (14%)
- Neurotoxicity [3]
- Pain (47%) [2]
- Paresthesias (2–9%)
- Peripheral neuropathy [4]
- Vertigo (dizziness) (4–13%)

Neuromuscular/Skeletal
- Arthralgia (6–8%) [4]
- Asthenia (fatigue) (5–47%) [17]
- Back pain (5–22%)
- Bone or joint pain (3–7%)
- Muscle spasm (3%)
- Myalgia/Myopathy (4%) [3]

Gastrointestinal/Hepatic
- Abdominal pain (2–22%)
- Constipation (2%)
- Diarrhea (7–25%) [22]
- Dyspepsia (2%)
- Hepatotoxicity [8]
- Nausea (6–33%) [6]
- Vomiting (4–23%) [4]

Respiratory
- Cough (5–26%)
- Dyspnea (3–22%)
- Flu-like syndrome (10%) [3]
- Influenza (4%)
- Nasopharyngitis (8%)
- Pharyngitis (12%)
- Pharyngolaryngeal pain (2%)
- Pulmonary toxicity [2]
- Rhinitis (2–14%)
- Sinusitis (2–9%)
- Upper respiratory tract infection (3%)

Endocrine/Metabolic
- ALT increased [5]
- Appetite decreased [2]
- AST increased [3]
- Hyperbilirubinemia [2]
- Hyperglycemia [3]

Genitourinary
- Urinary tract infection (3–5%)

Hematologic
- Anemia (4%) [6]
- Febrile neutropenia [15]
- Leukopenia (3%) [9]
- Neutropenia [19]
- Thrombocytopenia [6]

Local
- Infusion-related reactions [4]
- Injection-site reactions (21–40%) [6]

Other
- Adverse effects [3]
- Allergic reactions (3%)
- Death [4]
- Infection (20%) [2]

TRAVOPROST

Trade names: Izba (Alcon), Travatan (Alcon), Travatan Z (Alcon)
Indications: Reduction of elevated intraocular pressure in open-angle glaucoma or ocular hypertension
Class: Prostaglandin analog
Half-life: N/A
Clinically important, potentially hazardous interactions with: none known
Pregnancy category: C
Important contra-indications noted in the prescribing guidelines for: nursing mothers; pediatric patients

---

Cardiovascular
- Angina (<5%)
- Bradycardia (<5%)
- Chest pain (<5%)
- Hypertension (<5%)
- Hypotension (<5%)

Central Nervous System
- Anxiety (<5%)
- Depression (<5%)
- Dysgeusia (taste perversion) [3]
- Headache (<5%)
- Pain (<5%)

Neuromuscular/Skeletal
- Arthralgia (<5%)
- Back pain (<5%)

Gastrointestinal/Hepatic
- Dyspepsia (<5%)
- Gastrointestinal disorder (<5%)
- Nausea [2]

Respiratory
- Bronchitis (<5%)
- Flu-like syndrome (<5%)
- Sinusitis (<5%)

Endocrine/Metabolic
- Hypercholesterolemia (<5%)

Genitourinary
- Prostatitis (<5%)
- Urinary incontinence (<5%)
- Urinary tract infection (<5%)

Ocular
- Abnormal vision (<4%)
- Blepharitis (<4%)
- Cataract (<4%)
- Conjunctival hyperemia [10]
- Conjunctivitis (<4%)
- Corneal staining (<4%)
- Deepening of upper lid sulcus [6]
- Eyelashes – hypertrichosis [2]
- Eyelid crusting (<4%)
- Foreign body sensation (5–10%)
- Iris pigmentation (<4%) [2]
- Keratitis (<4%)
- Lacrimation (<4%)
- Ocular adverse effects [4]
- Ocular hemorrhage (35–50%)
- Ocular hyperemia [5]
- Ocular inflammation (<4%)
- Ocular pain (5–10%)
- Ocular pigmentation (<5%) [4]
- Ocular pruritus (5–10%) [4]
- Ocular stinging (5–10%)
- Photophobia (<4%)
- Reduced visual acuity (5–10%)
- Subconjunctival hemorrhage (<4%)
- Uveitis [5]
- Xerophthalmia (<4%)

Other
- Allergic reactions (<5%)
- Infection (<5%)

TRAZODONE

Trade names: Desyrel (Bristol-Myers Squibb), Oleptro (Angelini)
Indications: Depression
Class: Antidepressant, tricyclic, Serotonin reuptake inhibitor
Half-life: 3–6 hours
Clinically important, potentially hazardous interactions with: amiodarone, amprenavir, atazanavir, boceprevir, citalopram, cobicistat/elvitegravir/emtricitabine/tenofovir disoproxil, darunavir, delavirdine, fluoxetine, fluvoxamine, ginkgo biloba, indinavir, linezolid, lopinavir, MAO inhibitors, nefazodone, paroxetine hydrochloride, sertraline, tapentadol, telaprevir, tipranavir, venlafaxine
Pregnancy category: C
Important contra-indications noted in the prescribing guidelines for: nursing mothers; pediatric patients
Black Box Warning: SUICIDALITY IN CHILDREN AND ADOLESCENTS

Skin
Edema (<10%)
Exanthems [6]
Photosensitivity [2]
Psoriasis (exacerbation) [2]
Urticaria [3]

Hair
Alopecia [2]

Mucosal
Xerostomia (>10%) [6]

Cardiovascular
Arrhythmias [2]
QT prolongation [2]

Central Nervous System
Dysgeusia (taste perversion) (>10%)
Headache [3]
Sedation (>5%)
Serotonin syndrome [7]
Somnolence (drowsiness) (>5%) [3]
Tremor (<10%)
Vertigo (dizziness) (>5%) [4]

Neuromuscular/Skeletal
Myalgia/Myopathy (<10%)

Gastrointestinal/Hepatic
Constipation (>5%)
Nausea [2]

Genitourinary
Priapism (12%) [23]
Sexual dysfunction [2]

Ocular
Vision blurred (>5%)

TRETINOIN

Synonyms: all-trans-retinoic acid; ATRA
Trade names: Aknemycin Plus (EM Industries), Renova (Ortho), Retin-A Micro (Ortho), Solage (Galderma), Vesanoid (Roche)
Indications: Acne vulgaris, skin aging, facial roughness, fine wrinkles, hyperpigmentation [T], acute promyelocytic leukemia [O]
Class: Antineoplastic, Retinoid
Half-life: 0.5–2 hours
Clinically important, potentially hazardous interactions with: aldesleukin, bexarotene
Pregnancy category: D (category B (topical), category C (oral), category D in third trimester)
Important contra-indications noted in the prescribing guidelines for: nursing mothers; pediatric patients
Note: Oral retinoids can cause birth defects, and women should avoid tretinoin when pregnant or trying to conceive. Avoid prolonged exposure to sunlight.
[T] = Topical; [O] = Oral.

Skin
Bullous dermatitis [2]
Burning [O][T] (10–40%) [20]
Cellulitis [O] (<10%)
Crusting [2]
Dermatitis [7]
Desquamation (14%)
Diaphoresis (20%)
Differentiation syndrome [O] (25%) [19]
Edema (29%) [8]
Erythema [O][T] (<49%) [19]
Erythema nodosum [4]
Exfoliative dermatitis [O] (8%) [3]
Facial edema [O] (<10%)
Flaking [O] (23%)
Hyperkeratosis [O] (78%)
Hypomelanosis (5%) [2]
Pallor [O] (<10%)
Palmar–plantar desquamation [O] (<10%)
Peeling [4]
Photosensitivity [O][T] (10%) [3]
Pigmentation (5%) [3]
Pruritus [O][T] (5–40%) [14]
Rash [O][T] (54%) [3]
Scaling (10–40%) [16]
Stinging (<26%) [8]
Sweet's syndrome [21]
Ulcerations (scrotal) [9]
Vasculitis [2]
Xerosis [O] (49–100%) [19]

Hair
Alopecia areata [O] (14%)

Nails
Pyogenic granuloma [3]

Mucosal
Cheilitis [O] (10%)
Xerostomia [O] (10%)

Cardiovascular
Phlebitis (11%)

Central Nervous System
Depression [O] (14%)
Fever [O] [6]
Headache [2]
Intracranial pressure increased [2]
Pain [O] (37%)
Paresthesias [O] (17%)
Pseudotumor cerebri [O] [11]
Shivering [O] (63%)
Tremor [O] (<10%)

Neuromuscular/Skeletal
Arthralgia [O] (10%) [3]
Bone or joint pain [O] (77%) [3]
Myalgia/Myopathy (14%) [3]

Gastrointestinal/Hepatic
Hepatotoxicity [3]
Pancreatitis [2]

Hematologic
Hemorrhage [2]

Ocular
Diplopia [2]
Ocular pigmentation [O] (<10%)
Ocular pruritus [O] (10%)
Xerophthalmia [O] (<10%) [2]

Local
Injection-site reactions (17%)

Other
Death [O] [2]
Infection [O] (58%)

TRIAMTERENE

Trade names: Dyazide (GSK), Dyrenium (Concordia)
Indications: Edema
Class: Diuretic, potassium-sparing
Half-life: 1–2 hours
Clinically important, potentially hazardous interactions with: ACE inhibitors, acemetacin, benazepril, captopril, cyclosporine, enalapril, fosinopril, indomethacin, lisinopril, metformin, moexipril, potassium iodide, potassium salts, quinapril, ramipril, spironolactone, trandolapril, zofenopril
Pregnancy category: C
Important contra-indications noted in the prescribing guidelines for: nursing mothers; pediatric patients
Note: Dyazide and Maxzide are triamterene and hydrochlorothiazide. Hydrochlorothiazide is a sulfonamide and can be absorbed systemically. Sulfonamides can produce severe, possibly fatal, reactions such as toxic epidermal necrolysis and Stevens-Johnson syndrome.

Skin
Edema (<10%)
Lupus erythematosus (with hydrochlorothiazide) [2]
Photosensitivity [2]
Rash (<10%)

TRIFLURIDINE & TIPIRACIL

Trade name: Lonsurf (Monarch)
Indications: Metastatic colorectal cancer in patients who have been previously treated with fluoropyrimidine-, oxaliplatin-and irinotecan-based chemotherapy, an anti-VEGF biological therapy, and if RAS wild-type, an anti-EGFR therapy
Class: Antineoplastic, Thymidine phosphorylase inhibitor, Thymidine-based nucleoside analogue
Half-life: 2 hours
Clinically important, potentially hazardous interactions with: none known
Pregnancy category: N/A (Can cause fetal harm)
Important contra-indications noted in the prescribing guidelines for: nursing mothers; pediatric patients

---

Hair
Alopecia (7%)

Mucosal
Stomatitis (8%)

Central Nervous System
Dysgeusia (taste perversion) (7%)
Fever (19%)

Neuromuscular/Skeletal
Asthenia (fatigue) (52%) [3]

Gastrointestinal/Hepatic
Abdominal pain (21%) [2]
Diarrhea (32%) [2]
Nausea (48%) [2]

Vomiting (28%)

Respiratory
Nasopharyngitis (4%)
Pulmonary embolism (2%)

Endocrine/Metabolic
Appetite decreased (39%)

Genitourinary
Urinary tract infection (4%)

Hematologic
Anemia (77%) [6]
Febrile neutropenia [3]
Granulocytopenia [3]
Leukopenia [7]
Neutropenia (67%) [8]
Thrombocytopenia (42%) [3]

Other
Infection (27%)

TRIMETHOPRIM

Trade names: Bactrim (Women First), Septra (Monarch)
Indications: Various urinary tract infections caused by susceptible organisms, acute otitis media in children, acute and chronic bronchitis
Class: Antibiotic
Half-life: 8–10 hours
Clinically important, potentially hazardous interactions with: ACE inhibitors, amantadine, angiotensin II receptor antagonists, antidiabetics, azathioprine, benazepril, captopril, carvedilol, cilazapril, conivaptan, coumarins, cyclosporine, CYP2C8 substrates, CYP2C9 inhibitors, CYP3A4 inducers, dapsone, deferasirox, digoxin, dofetilide, enalapril, eplerenone, fosinopril, irbesartan, lamivudine, leucovorin, levoleucovorin, lisinopril, memantine, mercaptopurine, metformin, methotrexate, olmesartan, oral typhoid vaccine, PEG-interferon, phenytoin, pioglitazone, pralatrexate, procainamide, pyrimethamine, quinapril, ramipril, repaglinide, rifampin, sulfonylureas, trandolapril
Pregnancy category: C
Important contra-indications noted in the prescribing guidelines for: nursing mothers
Note: Although trimethoprim has been known to elicit occasional adverse reactions by itself, it is most commonly used in conjunction with sulfamethoxazole (co-trimoxazole - see separate entry).

Skin
DRESS syndrome [2]
Fixed eruption [6]
Pruritus (<10%)
Rash (3–7%)
Stevens–Johnson syndrome [5]
Toxic epidermal necrolysis [3]

Central Nervous System
Aseptic meningitis [3]

Neuromuscular/Skeletal
Rhabdomyolysis [3]

Gastrointestinal/Hepatic
Hepatotoxicity [2]

Endocrine/Metabolic
Hyperkalemia [3]
Hyponatremia [2]

Hematologic
Anemia [2]
Thrombocytopenia [2]

TRIMIPRAMINE

Trade name: Surmontil (Odyssey)
Indications: Major depression
Class: Antidepressant, tricyclic
Half-life: 20–26 hours
Clinically important, potentially hazardous interactions with: amprenavir, arbutamine, bupropion, clonidine, epinephrine, formoterol, guanethidine, isocarboxazid, linezolid, MAO inhibitors, phenelzine, quinolones, sparfloxacin, tranylcypromine, venlafaxine
Pregnancy category: C
Important contra-indications noted in the prescribing guidelines for: pediatric patients
Black Box Warning: SUICIDALITY AND ANTIDEPRESSANT DRUGS

Skin
Diaphoresis (<10%)

Mucosal
Xerostomia (>10%) [2]

Cardiovascular
QT prolongation [2]

Central Nervous System
Dysgeusia (taste perversion) (>10%)
Parkinsonism (<10%)
Seizures [4]

TYPHOID VACCINE

Trade names: Typherix (GSK), Typhim Vi (Sanofi Pasteur), Vivotif (Berna Biotech)
Indications: Immunization against typhoid fever
Class: Vaccine
Half-life: N/A
Clinically important, potentially hazardous interactions with: alcohol, antibiotics, antimalarials, atovaquone/proguanil, azathioprine, belimumab, cefixime, ceftaroline fosamil, ceftobiprole, chloroquine, ciprofloxacin, corticosteroids, daptomycin, fingolimod, gemifloxacin, hydroxychloroquine, immunosuppressants, interferon gamma, leflunomide, mefloquine, mercaptopurine, sulfonamides, telavancin, tigecycline, tinidazole, tocilizumab, ustekinumab
Pregnancy category: C
Important contra-indications noted in the prescribing guidelines for: nursing mothers; pediatric patients
Note: Vivotif is a live oral vaccine.

Central Nervous System
Fever (<3%) [5]
Headache (5–20%) [3]
Myelitis [2]

Neuromuscular/Skeletal
Asthenia (fatigue) (4–24%) [3]
Myalgia/Myopathy (3–7%) [3]

Gastrointestinal/Hepatic
Abdominal pain (6%) [2]
Diarrhea (<3%)
Nausea (2–8%)
Vomiting (2%)

Local
Injection-site edema [3]
Injection-site erythema (4–5%) [2]
Injection-site induration (5–15%)
Injection-site pain (27–41%) [5]

Other
Adverse effects [4]
Death [2]

UMECLIDINIUM

Trade name: Incruse (GSK)
Indications: Chronic obstructive pulmonary disease (COPD)
Class: Anticholinergic, Muscarinic antagonist
Half-life: 11 hours
Clinically important, potentially hazardous interactions with: anticholinergics
Pregnancy category: C
Important contra-indications noted in the prescribing guidelines for: nursing mothers; pediatric patients

---

Mucosal
Oropharyngeal pain [2]

Cardiovascular
Angina [2]
Arrhythmias [2]
Extrasystoles [3]
Hypertension [3]
Supraventricular tachycardia [2]
Tachycardia [2]

Central Nervous System
Dysgeusia (taste perversion) [3]
Headache [12]

Neuromuscular/Skeletal
Arthralgia (2%) [2]
Back pain [5]

Gastrointestinal/Hepatic
Constipation [2]

Respiratory
Bronchitis [2]
COPD (exacerbation) [5]
Cough (3%) [6]
Dysphonia [4]
Influenza [2]
Nasopharyngitis (8%) [12]
Pharyngitis [2]
Pneumonia [4]
Sinusitis [3]
Upper respiratory tract infection [5]

Genitourinary
Urinary tract infection [2]

Other
Adverse effects [4]

URSODIOL

Synonyms: ursodeoxycholic acid; UDCA
Trade names: Actigall (Watson), Destolit (Norgine), Urdox (Wockhardt), Urso 250 (Aptalis), Urso Forte (Aptalis), Ursogal (Galen)
Indications: The dissolution of radiolucent (i.e. non-radio opaque) cholesterol gallstones in patients with a functioning gallbladder, primary biliary cirrhosis, biliary calculus, cholelithiasis
Class: Cholesterol antagonist, Urolithic
Half-life: 100 hours
Clinically important, potentially hazardous interactions with: aluminum based antacids, aluminum hydroxide, charcoal, cholestyramine, clofibrate, colestimide, colestipol, cyclosporine, dapsone, estradiol, estrogens, nitrendipine, oral contraceptives, P4503A substrates
Pregnancy category: B
Important contra-indications noted in the prescribing guidelines for: the elderly; nursing mothers; pediatric patients

---

Skin
Lichenoid eruption [3]
Pruritus [3]
Rash (3%)

Hair
Alopecia (<5%)

Cardiovascular
Chest pain (3%)

Central Nervous System
Headache (18–25%)
Insomnia (2%)
Vertigo (dizziness) (17%)

Neuromuscular/Skeletal
Arthralgia (7%)
Asthenia (fatigue) (3–7%)
Back pain (7–12%)
Bone or joint pain (6%)
Myalgia/Myopathy (5%)

Gastrointestinal/Hepatic
Abdominal pain (43%)
Cholecystitis (5%)
Constipation (26%)
Diarrhea (27%) [4]
Dyspepsia (16%) [2]
Flatulence (7%)
Nausea (14%) [4]
Vomiting (9–14%) [3]

Respiratory
Bronchitis (6%)
Cough (7%)
Flu-like syndrome (6%)
Pharyngitis (8%)
Rhinitis (5%)
Sinusitis (5–11%)
Upper respiratory tract infection (12–15%)

Endocrine/Metabolic
Weight gain [2]

Genitourinary
Dysmenorrhea (5%)
Urinary tract infection (6%)

Hematologic
Leukopenia (3%)

Other
Adverse effects [3]
Allergic reactions (5%)
Infection (viral) (9–19%)

USTEKINUMAB

Trade name: Stelara (Centocor)
Indications: Plaque psoriasis (moderate to severe), active psoriatic arthritis, active Crohn's disease (moderate to severe)
Class: Interleukin-12/23 antagonist, Monoclonal antibody
Half-life: 15–32 days
Clinically important, potentially hazardous interactions with: live vaccines
Pregnancy category: B
Important contra-indications noted in the prescribing guidelines for: nursing mothers; pediatric patients

---

Skin
Cellulitis (<10%)
Herpes zoster [2]
Malignancies [2]
Pruritus (<10%)
Psoriasis [2]

Mucosal
Nasal congestion (<10%)

Cardiovascular
Cardiotoxicity [3]

Central Nervous System
Depression (<10%)
Headache (<10%) [5]
Leukoencephalopathy [2]
Vertigo (dizziness) (<10%)

Neuromuscular/Skeletal
Arthralgia [3]
Asthenia (fatigue) (<10%) [2]
Back pain (<10%)
Myalgia/Myopathy (<10%)
Psoriatic arthralgia [2]

Gastrointestinal/Hepatic
Diarrhea (<10%)
Hepatotoxicity [2]

Respiratory
Nasopharyngitis (10%) [4]
Pharyngolaryngeal pain (<10%)
Upper respiratory tract infection (10%) [5]

Local
Injection-site reactions [3]

Other
Adverse effects [11]
Infection [8]

VALACYCLOVIR

Trade name: Valtrex (GSK)
Indications: Genital herpes, herpes simplex, herpes zoster
Class: Antiviral, Guanine nucleoside analog
Half-life: 3 hours
Clinically important, potentially hazardous interactions with: cobicistat/elvitegravir/emtricitabine/tenofovir disoproxil, immunosuppressants, meperidine, tenofovir disoproxil
Pregnancy category: B
Important contra-indications noted in the prescribing guidelines for: the elderly; pediatric patients

---

Central Nervous System
Hallucinations [2]
Headache [5]
Neurotoxicity [4]

Gastrointestinal/Hepatic
Abdominal pain [2]
Nausea [4]
Vomiting [3]

VALGANCICLOVIR

Trade name: Valcyte (Roche)
Indications: Cytomegalovirus retinitis (CMV) in patients with AIDS, prevention of CMV disease in high-risk transplant patients
Class: Antiviral, Guanine nucleoside analog
Half-life: 4 hours (in severe renal impairment up to 68%)
Clinically important, potentially hazardous interactions with: abacavir, cobicistat/elvitegravir/emtricitabine/tenofovir disoproxil, emtricitabine, tenofovir disoproxil
Pregnancy category: N/A (May cause fetal toxicity based on findings in animal studies)
Important contra-indications noted in the prescribing guidelines for: nursing mothers
Note: Valganciclovir is rapidly converted to ganciclovir in the body.
Black Box Warning: HEMATOLOGIC TOXICITY, IMPAIRMENT OF FERTILITY, FETAL TOXICITY, MUTAGENESIS AND CARCINOGENESIS

Mucosal
Oral candidiasis [2]

Central Nervous System
Fever [3]
Headache [2]
Neurotoxicity [2]
Paresthesias (8%)

Hematologic
Neutropenia [8]

Other
Allergic reactions (<5%)
Infection (<5%)

VALPROIC ACID

Synonyms: valproate sodium; divalproex
Trade names: Depacon (AbbVie), Depakene (AbbVie), Depakote (AbbVie)
Indications: Seizures, migraine
Class: Anticonvulsant, Antipsychotic
Half-life: 6–16 hours
Clinically important, potentially hazardous interactions with: amitriptyline, aspirin, ceftobiprole, cholestyramine, clobazam, clozapine, doripenem, eslicarbazepine, ethosuximide, indinavir, ivermectin, lesinurad, levomepromazine, olanzapine, oxcarbazepine, paliperidone, risperidone, rufinamide, temozolomide, tipranavir, vorinostat, zidovudine, zinc, zuclopenthixol
Pregnancy category: D
Black Box Warning: LIFE THREATENING ADVERSE REACTIONS

Skin
Anticonvulsant hypersensitivity syndrome [6]
DRESS syndrome [7]
Ecchymoses (<5%) [4]
Edema [2]
Erythema multiforme [3]
Erythroderma [3]
Exanthems (5%) [3]
Facial edema (>5%)
Furunculosis (<5%)
Hypersensitivity [5]
Lupus erythematosus [5]
Peripheral edema (<5%)
Petechiae (<5%)
Pruritus (>5%)
Pseudolymphoma [2]
Purpura [2]
Rash (>5%) [7]
Stevens–Johnson syndrome [10]
Toxic epidermal necrolysis [7]
Vasculitis [3]

Hair
Alopecia (7%) [20]
Curly hair [6]
Hirsutism [2]

Mucosal
Gingival hyperplasia/hypertrophy [7]
Glossitis (<5%)
Stomatitis (<5%)
Xerostomia (<5%) [2]

Central Nervous System
Cerebral edema [2]
Cognitive impairment [2]
Coma [3]
Confusion [2]
Delirium [2]
Dysgeusia (taste perversion) (<5%)
Encephalopathy [13]
Neurotoxicity [4]
Paresthesias (<5%)
Parkinsonism [15]
Sedation [2]
Seizures [10]
Somnolence (drowsiness) [10]
Tremor [12]
Vertigo (dizziness) [5]

Neuromuscular/Skeletal
Asthenia (fatigue) [4]
Osteoporosis [3]
Rhabdomyolysis [3]

Gastrointestinal/Hepatic
Constipation [2]
Dyspepsia [2]
Hepatic steatosis [2]
Hepatotoxicity [17]
Nausea [2]
Pancreatitis [32]
Vomiting [2]

Respiratory
Pleural effusion [2]
Pneumonitis [2]

Endocrine/Metabolic
Acute intermittent porphyria [2]
Hyperammonemia [7]
Hyponatremia [2]
Metabolic syndrome [3]
Porphyria [2]
SIADH [6]
Weight gain [21]

Genitourinary
Vaginitis (<5%)

Renal
Enuresis [2]
Fanconi syndrome [4]

Hematologic
Bone marrow suppression [4]
Coagulopathy [2]
Eosinophilia [2]
Hemotoxicity [3]
Neutropenia [2]
Thrombocytopenia [4]

Other
Adverse effects [7]
Allergic reactions (<5%)
Congenital malformations [4]
Death [8]
Teratogenicity [31]

VALSARTAN

Trade names: Byvalson (Forest), Diovan (Novartis), Diovan HCT (Novartis), Exforge (Novartis), Valturna (Novartis)
Indications: Hypertension
Class: Angiotensin II receptor antagonist (blocker), Antihypertensive
Half-life: 9 hours
Clinically important, potentially hazardous interactions with: none known
Pregnancy category: D
Important contra-indications noted in the prescribing guidelines for: nursing mothers; pediatric patients
Note: Byvalson is valsartan and nebivolol; Exforge is valsartan and amlodipine; Valturna is valsartan and aliskiren; Diovan HCT is valsartan and hydrochlorothiazide. Hydrochlorothiazide is a sulfonamide and can be absorbed systemically. Sulfonamides can produce severe, possibly fatal, reactions such as toxic epidermal necrolysis and Stevens-Johnson syndrome.
See also separate profile for Sacubitril/Valsartan.

Black Box Warning: FETAL TOXICITY

Skin
Angioedema (>2%) [9]
Edema [5]
Peripheral edema [3]
Photosensitivity [2]
Pruritus (>2%)
Pseudolymphoma [2]
Rash (>2%)

Mucosal
Aphthous stomatitis (<10%)
Xerostomia (>10%)

Central Nervous System
Dysgeusia (taste perversion) (>10%)
Headache [6]
Paresthesias (>2%)
Vertigo (dizziness) [8]

Neuromuscular/Skeletal
Arthralgia (<10%)
Myalgia/Myopathy (10–29%)

Gastrointestinal/Hepatic
Enteropathy [2]

Respiratory
Cough [2]
Nasopharyngitis [3]
Upper respiratory tract infection [2]

Endocrine/Metabolic
Hyperkalemia [3]

Other
Adverse effects [5]
Allergic reactions (>2%)

VANCOMYCIN

Trade name: Vancocin (Lilly)
Indications: Various infections caused by susceptible organisms
Class: Antibiotic, glycopeptide
Half-life: 5–11 hours
Clinically important, potentially hazardous interactions with: meloxicam, metformin, pentamidine, rocuronium, succinylcholine, teicoplanin, trospium
Pregnancy category: C

Skin
AGEP [8]
Anaphylactoid reactions/Anaphylaxis [13]
Angioedema [3]
Bullous dermatitis [5]
DRESS syndrome [17]
Erythema multiforme [5]
Exanthems [16]
Exfoliative dermatitis [4]
Fixed eruption [2]
Hypersensitivity [8]
Leukocytoclastic vasculitis [3]
Linear IgA bullous dermatosis [48]
Lupus erythematosus [2]
Pruritus [11]
Rash [17]
Red man syndrome (<14%) [49]
Red neck syndrome [2]
Stevens–Johnson syndrome [10]
Toxic epidermal necrolysis [10]
Urticaria [8]
Vasculitis [2]

Cardiovascular
Extravasation [2]
Flushing (<10%)
Hypotension [3]
Phlebitis (14–23%) [6]

Central Nervous System
Chills (>10%) [2]
Dysgeusia (taste perversion) (>10%)
Fever [7]
Headache [2]

Gastrointestinal/Hepatic
Constipation [2]
Diarrhea [5]
Gastrointestinal disorder [2]
Nausea [7]
Vomiting [2]

Renal
Nephrotoxicity [30]
Renal failure [2]

Hematologic
Anemia [2]
Eosinophilia [3]
Leukopenia [2]
Neutropenia [7]
Thrombocytopenia [16]

Otic
Ototoxicity [5]
Tinnitus [2]

Local
Infusion-related reactions [2]

Other
Adverse effects [5]
Allergic reactions (<5%) [5]
Death [5]

VANDETANIB

Trade name: Caprelsa (AstraZeneca)
Indications: Medullary thyroid cancer
Class: Tyrosine kinase inhibitor
Half-life: 19 days
Clinically important, potentially hazardous interactions with: amiodarone, amoxapine, antiarrhythmics, arsenic, carbamazepine, chloroquine, clarithromycin, CYP3A4 inducers, dexamethasone, disopyramide, dofetilide, dolasetron, efavirenz, granisetron, haloperidol, methadone, moxifloxacin, pazopanib, phenobarbital, phenytoin, pimozide, procainamide, QT prolonging agents, rifabutin, rifampin, rifapentine, sotalol, St John's wort, telavancin
Pregnancy category: D
Important contra-indications noted in the prescribing guidelines for: nursing mothers; pediatric patients
Note: Contraindicated in patients with congenital long QT syndrome.
Black Box Warning: QT PROLONGATION, TORSADES DE POINTES, AND SUDDEN DEATH

Skin
Acneform eruption (35%) [3]
Folliculitis [4]
Hand–foot syndrome [3]
Photosensitivity (13%) [6]
Phototoxicity [2]
Pigmentation [4]
Pruritus (11%) [2]
Rash (53%) [33]
Stevens–Johnson syndrome [2]
Toxicity [9]
Xerosis (15%) [2]

Nails
Paronychia [3]

Mucosal
Mucositis [2]
Stomatitis [2]

Cardiovascular
Hypertension (33%) [23]
QT prolongation (14%) [24]

Central Nervous System
Anorexia [3]
Depression (10%)
Headache (26%) [4]
Insomnia (13%)
Neurotoxicity [2]

Neuromuscular/Skeletal
Asthenia (fatigue) (15–24%) [16]

Gastrointestinal/Hepatic
Abdominal pain (21%)
Constipation [2]
Diarrhea (57%) [43]
Dyspepsia (11%)
Hepatotoxicity [4]
Nausea (33%) [13]
Vomiting (15%) [5]

Respiratory
Cough (11%)
Dyspnea [3]
Nasopharyngitis (11%)

Endocrine/Metabolic
ALT increased (51%) [2]
Appetite decreased (21%) [2]
Hypocalcemia (11%)
Hypothyroidism [2]
Thyroid dysfunction [2]
Weight loss (10%) [2]

Renal
Proteinuria (10%) [2]

Hematologic
Anemia [3]
Hemorrhage [2]
Hemotoxicity [2]
Myelosuppression [2]
Neutropenia [5]
Platelets decreased (9%)

Other
Adverse effects [6]
Death [3]

VARDENAFIL

Trade name: Levitra (Bayer)
Indications: Erectile dysfunction
Class: Phosphodiesterase type 5 (PDE5) inhibitor
Half-life: 4–5 hours
Clinically important, potentially hazardous interactions with: alfuzosin, alpha blockers, amyl nitrite, antifungals, antihypertensives, atazanavir, boceprevir, bosentan, cobicistat/elvitegravir/emtricitabine/tenofovir disoproxil, conivaptan, CYP3A4 inhibitors, darunavir, dasatinib, disopyramide, doxazosin, erythromycin, etravirine, fosamprenavir, grapefruit juice, high-fat foods, indinavir, itraconazole, ketoconazole, lopinavir, macrolide antibiotics, nelfinavir, nicorandil, nifedipine, nitrates, nitroglycerin, phosphodiesterase 5 inhibitors, protease inhibitors, riociguat, ritonavir, sapropterin, saquinavir, tamsulosin, telaprevir, terazosin, tipranavir
Pregnancy category: B (not indicated for use in women)
Important contra-indications noted in the prescribing guidelines for: pediatric patients

---

Skin
Anaphylactoid reactions/Anaphylaxis (<2%)
Angioedema (<2%)
Diaphoresis (<2%)
Erythema (<2%)
Facial edema (<2%)
Photosensitivity (<2%)
Pruritus (<2%)
Rash (<2%)

Mucosal
Nasal congestion [4]
Xerostomia (<2%)

Cardiovascular
Angina (<2%)
Chest pain (<2%)
Flushing (11%) [14]
Hypotension (<2%)
Myocardial infarction (<2%)
Palpitation (<2%)
QT prolongation [2]
Tachycardia (<2%)
Ventricular arrhythmia (<2%)

Central Nervous System
Amnesia (<2%)
Dysesthesia (<2%)
Headache (7–15%) [16]
Pain (<2%)
Paresthesias (<2%)
Seizures (<2%)
Sleep related disorder (<2%)
Somnolence (drowsiness) (<2%)
Syncope (<2%)
Vertigo (dizziness) (2%) [3]

Neuromuscular/Skeletal
Arthralgia (<2%)
Back pain (<2%)
Cramps (<2%)
Myalgia/Myopathy (<2%)

Gastrointestinal/Hepatic
Abdominal pain (<2%)
Diarrhea (<2%)
Dyspepsia [3]
Gastritis (<2%)
Gastroesophageal reflux (<2%)
Nausea (<2%)
Vomiting (<2%)

Respiratory
Dyspnea (<2%)
Flu-like syndrome (3%)
Rhinitis (9%) [10]
Sinusitis (3%)

Endocrine/Metabolic
ALT increased (<2%)
Creatine phosphokinase increased (<2%)

Genitourinary
Erection (<2%)
Priapism (<2%)

Otic
Hearing loss [2]
Tinnitus (<2%)

Ocular
Conjunctivitis (<2%)
Dyschromatopsia (<2%)
Intraocular pressure increased (<2%)
Ocular hyperemia (<2%)
Ocular pain (<2%)
Photophobia (<2%)
Visual disturbances (<2%)

Other
Allergic reactions (<2%)

VARENICLINE

Trade names: Champix (Pfizer), Chantix (Pfizer)
Indications: Smoking deterrent
Class: Nicotinic antagonist
Half-life: 24 hours
Clinically important, potentially hazardous interactions with: none known
Pregnancy category: C
Important contra-indications noted in the prescribing guidelines for: nursing mothers; pediatric patients
Black Box Warning: SERIOUS NEUROPSYCHIATRIC EVENTS

Skin
AGEP [3]
Rash (<3%)

Mucosal
Xerostomia (4–6%)

Cardiovascular
Cardiotoxicity [4]

Central Nervous System
Abnormal dreams (9–13%) [16]
Aggression [3]
Anorexia (<2%)
Anxiety [5]
Depression [9]
Dysgeusia (taste perversion) (5–8%)
Hallucinations [2]
Headache (15–19%) [12]
Insomnia (18–19%) [15]
Mania [5]
Mood changes [4]
Neuropsychiatric disturbances [2]
Nightmares (<2%)
Psychosis [7]
Sleep disturbances [7]
Sleep related disorder (2–5%) [3]
Somnolence (drowsiness) (3%) [2]
Suicidal ideation [7]

Neuromuscular/Skeletal
Asthenia (fatigue) (<7%) [5]

Gastrointestinal/Hepatic
Abdominal pain (5–7%) [3]
Constipation (5–8%) [4]
Dyspepsia (5%) [2]
Flatulence (6–9%)
Hepatotoxicity [2]
Nausea (16–30%) [29]
Vomiting (<5%) [2]

Respiratory
Dyspnea (<2%)
Upper respiratory tract infection (5–7%)

Endocrine/Metabolic
Appetite decreased (<2%)
Appetite increased (3–4%)

Ocular
Hallucinations, visual [2]

Other
Adverse effects [10]
Death [3]

VARICELLA VACCINE

Trade names: Varilrix (GSK), Varivax (Merck)
Indications: Immunization, varicella
Class: Vaccine
Half-life: N/A
Clinically important, potentially hazardous interactions with: none known
Pregnancy category: C

Skin
Herpes zoster [10]
Rash [10]
Stevens-Johnson syndrome [2]

Central Nervous System
Fever (15%) [3]

Ocular
Uveitis [2]

Local
Injection-site edema (19%)
Injection-site erythema (19%)
Injection-site hematoma (19%)
Injection-site induration (19%)
Injection-site pain (19%)
Injection-site pruritus (19%)
Injection-site reactions [4]

VASOPRESSIN

Trade name: Vasostrict (Par)
Indications: Diabetes insipidus, prevention and treatment of postoperative abdominal distension, hypotension in adults with vasodilatory shock (Vasostrict)
Class: Antidiuretic hormone
Half-life: 10–20 minutes
Clinically important, potentially hazardous interactions with: none known

Pregnancy category: C
Important contra-indications noted in the prescribing guidelines for: pediatric patients

Skin
Bullous dermatitis [4]
Diaphoresis (<10%)
Ecchymoses [2]
Pallor (<10%)
Purpura [2]
Urticaria (<10%)

Central Nervous System
Tremor (<10%)

Neuromuscular/Skeletal
Rhabdomyolysis [6]

Endocrine/Metabolic
SIADH [2]

Local
Injection-site inflammation [7]

Other
Death [3]

VEDOLIZUMAB

Trade name: Entyvio (Takeda)
Indications: Ulcerative colitis, Crohn's disease
Class: Integrin receptor antagonist, Monoclonal antibody
Half-life: 25 days
Clinically important, potentially hazardous interactions with: live vaccines, natalizumab, TNF blockers
Pregnancy category: B
Important contra-indications noted in the prescribing guidelines for: nursing mothers; pediatric patients

Skin
Pruritus (3%)
Rash (3%)

Mucosal
Oropharyngeal pain (3%)

Central Nervous System
Fever (9%) [4]
Headache (12%) [10]

Neuromuscular/Skeletal
Arthralgia (12%) [7]
Asthenia (fatigue) (6%) [6]
Back pain (4%) [3]
Pain in extremities (3%)

Gastrointestinal/Hepatic
Abdominal pain [6]
Colitis [5]
Crohn's disease (exacerbation) [2]
Nausea (9%) [8]
Vomiting [3]

Respiratory
Bronchitis (4%)
Cough (5%) [3]
Influenza (4%)
Nasopharyngitis (13%) [9]
Sinusitis (3%)
Upper respiratory tract infection (7%) [6]

Hematologic
Anemia [3]

Local
Infusion-related reactions (4%) [4]

Other
Adverse effects [6]
Cancer [2]
Infection [5]

VEMURAFENIB

Trade name: Zelboraf (Roche)
Indications: Melanoma (metastatic or unresectable)
Class: BRAF inhibitor
Half-life: 57 hours
Clinically important, potentially hazardous interactions with: amoxapine, arsenic, atazanavir, carbamazepine, clarithromycin, CYP substrates, dolasetron, efavirenz, indinavir, itraconazole, ketoconazole, nefazodone, nelfinavir, pazopanib, phenobarbital, phenytoin, rifabutin, rifampin, rifapentine, ritonavir, saquinavir, telavancin, telithromycin, voriconazole, warfarin
Pregnancy category: D
Important contra-indications noted in the prescribing guidelines for: nursing mothers; pediatric patients

Skin
Acneform eruption [5]
Actinic keratoses [3]
DRESS syndrome [4]
Eccrine squamous syringometaplasia [2]
Erythema (14%)
Exanthems [6]
Granulomas [2]
Grover's disease [4]
Hand–foot syndrome [8]
Hyperkeratosis (24%) [13]
Keratoacanthoma [24]
Keratoses [4]
Keratosis pilaris [9]
Lymphoma [2]
Melanoma [2]
Milia [2]
Neoplasms [2]
Nevi [6]
Panniculitis [8]
Papillomas (21%)
Papular lesions (5%)
Peripheral edema (17%)
Photosensitivity (33%) [24]
Pruritus (23%) [8]
Radiation recall dermatitis [2]
Rash (37%) [22]
Squamous cell carcinoma (24%) [31]
Stevens–Johnson syndrome [4]
Sunburn (10%)
Toxic epidermal necrolysis [4]
Toxicity [9]
Verrucous lesions [3]
Vitiligo [2]
Warts [2]
Xerosis [3]

Hair
Alopecia (45%) [16]
Hair changes [2]

Nails
Paronychia [2]

Mucosal
Gingival hyperplasia/hypertrophy [2]

Cardiovascular
QT prolongation [2]

Central Nervous System
Dysgeusia (taste perversion) (14%)
Fever (19%) [3]
Headache (23%)
Paralysis [2]

Neuromuscular/Skeletal
Arthralgia (53%) [16]
Asthenia (fatigue) (38%) [17]
Back pain (8%)
Bone or joint pain (8%)
Myalgia/Myopathy (8–13%)
Pain in extremities (18%)

Gastrointestinal/Hepatic
Constipation (12%)
Diarrhea (28%) [6]
Hepatotoxicity [4]
Nausea (35%) [7]
Vomiting (18%) [2]

Respiratory
Cough (8%)

Endocrine/Metabolic
ALT increased [4]
Appetite decreased (18%)
AST increased [4]

Ocular
Uveitis [3]

Other
Adverse effects [10]

VENETOCLAX *

Trade name: Venclexta (AbbVie)
Indications: <p>Chronic lymphocytic leukemia in patients with 17p deletion, as detected by an FDA approved test, who have received at least one prior therapy

Class: BCL-2 inhibitor
Half-life: 26 hours
Clinically important, potentially hazardous interactions with: amiodarone, azithromycin, bosentan, captopril, carbamazepine, carvedilol, ciprofloxacin, clarithromycin, conivaptan, cyclosporine, digoxin, diltiazem, dronedarone, efavirenz, erythromycin, etravirine, everolimus, felodipine, fluconazole, grapefruit juice, indinavir, itraconazole, ketoconazole, live vaccines, lopinavir, modafinil, nafcillin, phenytoin, posaconazole, quercetin, quinidine, ranolazine, rifampin, ritonavir, sirolimus, St John's wort, stong or moderate P-gp inhibitors or substrates, strong or moderate CYP3A inducers or inhibitors, telaprevir, ticagrelor, verapamil, voriconazole
Pregnancy category: N/A (May cause fetal harm)
Important contra-indications noted in the prescribing guidelines for: nursing mothers; pediatric patients

Note: Concomitant use of strong CYP3A inhibitors during initiation and ramp-up phase is contraindicated.

Skin
Peripheral edema (11%)
Tumor lysis syndrome (6%) [3]

Central Nervous System
Fever (16%)
Headache (15%)

Neuromuscular/Skeletal
Asthenia (fatigue) (21%)
Back pain (10%)

Gastrointestinal/Hepatic
Constipation (14%)
Diarrhea (35%) [2]
Nausea (33%) [2]
Vomiting (15%)

Respiratory
Cough (13%)
Pneumonia (8%)
Upper respiratory tract infection (22%)

Endocrine/Metabolic
Hyperkalemia (20%)
Hyperphosphatemia (15%)
Hyperuricemia (6%)
Hypocalcemia (9%)
Hypokalemia (12%)

Hematologic
Anemia (29%)
Neutropenia (45%) [3]
Thrombocytopenia (22%)

VENLAFAXINE

Trade names: Effexor (Wyeth), Effexor XL (Wyeth)
Indications: Major depressive disorder
Class: Antidepressant, Serotonin-norepinephrine reuptake inhibitor
Half-life: 3–7 hours
Clinically important, potentially hazardous interactions with: 5HT1 agonists, artemether/lumefantrine, aspirin, atomoxetine, clozapine, desvenlafaxine, dexibuprofen, diclofenac, duloxetine, entacapone, haloperidol, indinavir, isocarboxazid, ketoconazole, linezolid, lithium, MAO inhibitors, meloxicam, metoclopramide, metoprolol, mirtazapine, moclobemide, naratriptan, NSAIDs, phenelzine, selegiline, sibutramine, SNRIs, SSRIs, St John's wort, sumatriptan, tramadol, tranylcypromine, trazodone, trimipramine, triptans, voriconazole, warfarin
Pregnancy category: C
Important contra-indications noted in the prescribing guidelines for: the elderly; nursing mothers; pediatric patients
Black Box Warning: SUICIDALITY AND ANTIDEPRESSANT DRUGS

Skin
Diaphoresis [7]
Ecchymoses [2]
Hyperhidrosis [2]
Pruritus (<10%)
Rash (3%)

Hair
Alopecia [2]

Mucosal
Xerostomia (22%) [9]

Cardiovascular
Cardiac failure [2]
Cardiomyopathy [3]
Hypertension [7]
Myocardial infarction [2]
Orthostatic hypotension [2]
Preeclampsia [2]
QT prolongation [6]
Tachycardia [2]

Central Nervous System
Akathisia [2]
Delirium [2]
Dysgeusia (taste perversion) (2%)
Headache [7]
Insomnia [4]
Mania [10]
Paresthesias (3%)
Psychosis [3]
Restless legs syndrome [3]
Seizures [7]
Serotonin syndrome [22]
Somnolence (drowsiness) [7]
Tremor (<10%) [3]
Vertigo (dizziness) [9]
Yawning [2]

Neuromuscular/Skeletal
Asthenia (fatigue) [5]
Dystonia [2]
Rhabdomyolysis [3]

Gastrointestinal/Hepatic
Constipation [6]
Hepatotoxicity [8]
Nausea [15]
Vomiting [2]

Respiratory
Pneumonitis [3]

Endocrine/Metabolic
Appetite decreased [2]
Galactorrhea [3]
Hyponatremia [4]
Libido increased [2]
Mastodynia [2]
SIADH [6]
Weight gain [2]

Genitourinary
Ejaculatory dysfunction [2]
Sexual dysfunction [8]
Urinary incontinence [2]

Ocular
Glaucoma [2]
Hallucinations, visual [3]

Other
Adverse effects [3]
Bruxism [7]

VERAPAMIL

Trade names: Calan (Pfizer), Covera-HS (Pfizer), Isoptin (AbbVie), Tarka (AbbVie), Verelan (Schwarz)
Indications: Angina, arrhythmias, hypertension
Class: Antiarrhythmic class IV, Calcium channel blocker, CYP3A4 inhibitor
Half-life: 2–8 hours
Clinically important, potentially hazardous interactions with: acebutolol, afatinib, aliskiren, amiodarone, amitriptyline, amprenavir, aspirin, atazanavir, atenolol, atorvastatin, avanafil, betaxolol, bisoprolol, carbamazepine, carteolol, celiprolol, clonidine, cobicistat/elvitegravir/emtricitabine/tenofovir disoproxil, colchicine, dabigatran, dantrolene, darifenacin, delavirdine, digoxin, dofetilide, dronedarone, dutasteride, epirubicin, eplerenone, erythromycin, esmolol, everolimus, fingolimod, flibanserin, indacaterol, lovastatin, metoprolol, mifepristone, nadolol, nevirapine, oxprenolol, oxtriphylline, penbutolol, pindolol, posaconazole, propranolol, quinidine, ranolazine, sibutramine, silodosin, simvastatin, telaprevir, telithromycin, timolol, trabectedin, venetoclax
Pregnancy category: C
Important contra-indications noted in the prescribing guidelines for: nursing mothers; pediatric patients
Note: Tarka is verapamil and trandolapril.

Skin
Angioedema [3]
Diaphoresis [2]
Edema (2%)
Erythema multiforme [4]
Exanthems [8]
Exfoliative dermatitis [2]
Hyperkeratosis (palms) [2]
Lupus erythematosus [2]
Peripheral edema (<10%)
Photosensitivity [4]
Pruritus [6]
Rash [2]
Stevens–Johnson syndrome [5]
Urticaria [5]
Vasculitis [2]

Hair
Alopecia [5]

Mucosal
Gingival hyperplasia/hypertrophy (19%) [10]

Cardiovascular
Atrial fibrillation [2]
Atrioventricular block [2]
Bradycardia [10]
Congestive heart failure [2]
Flushing (<7%) [4]
Hypotension [2]
Torsades de pointes [2]

Central Nervous System
Parkinsonism [2]
Seizures [3]

Neuromuscular/Skeletal
Rhabdomyolysis [2]

Endocrine/Metabolic
Gynecomastia [8]

Other
Side effects [2]

VERTEPORFIN

Trade name: Visudyne (Novartis)
Indications: Neovascular (wet) age-related macular degeneration
Class: Photosensitizer
Half-life: 5–6 hours
Clinically important, potentially hazardous interactions with: none known
Pregnancy category: C
Important contra-indications noted in the prescribing guidelines for: nursing mothers; pediatric patients

Skin
Eczema (<10%)
Photosensitivity (<10%) [2]

Mucosal
Burning mouth syndrome (<10%)

Cardiovascular
Atrial fibrillation (<10%)
Chest pain [2]
Hypertension (<10%)

Central Nervous System
Fever (<10%)
Hypoesthesia (<10%)
Sleep related disorder (<10%)
Vertigo (dizziness) (<10%)

Neuromuscular/Skeletal
Arthralgia (<10%)
Asthenia (fatigue) (<10%)
Back pain (<10%)
Myasthenia gravis (<10%)

Gastrointestinal/Hepatic
Constipation (<10%)
Nausea (<10%)

Respiratory
Flu-like syndrome (<10%)
Pharyngitis (<10%)

Endocrine/Metabolic
Creatine phosphokinase increased (<10%)

Genitourinary
Albuminuria (<10%)

Hematologic
Anemia (<10%)
Leukocytosis (<10%)
Leukopenia (<10%)

Otic
Hearing loss (<10%)

Ocular
Blepharitis (<10%)
Cataract (<10%)
Conjunctivitis (<10%)
Diplopia (<10%)
Endophthalmitis [2]
Intraocular inflammation [2]
Lacrimation (<10%)
Ocular itching (<10%)
Vision loss (severe) (<5%)
Visual disturbances (10–30%)
Xerophthalmia (<10%)

Local
Infusion-site pain (<10%)
Injection-site reactions (10–30%)

Other
Cancer (gastrointestinal) (<10%)

VIGABATRIN

Trade name: Sabril (Lundbeck)
Indications: Epilepsy, infantile spasms (West's syndrome)
Class: Anticonvulsant, Antiepileptic
Half-life: 7.5 hours
Clinically important, potentially hazardous interactions with: antipsychotics, chloroquine, hydroxychloroquine, MAO inhibitors, mefloquine, orlistat, phenytoin, rufinamide, SSRIs, St John's wort, tricyclic antidepressants
Pregnancy category: C
Important contra-indications noted in the prescribing guidelines for: nursing mothers; pediatric patients
Black Box Warning: VISION LOSS

Skin
Peripheral edema (5–7%)
Rash (6%) [2]

Cardiovascular
Chest pain (<5%)

Central Nervous System
Abnormal dreams (<5%)
Anxiety (4%)
Confusion (4–14%)
Depression (8%) [4]
Dysarthria (2%)
Encephalopathy [4]
Fever (4–7%)
Gait instability (6–12%)
Headache (18%)
Hypoesthesia (4–5%)
Hyporeflexia (4–5%)
Impaired concentration (9%)
Incoordination (7%)
Insomnia (7%)
Irritability (7%)
Memory loss (7%)
Nervousness (2–5%)
Peripheral neuropathy (4%)
Psychosis [2]
Sedation (4%)
Seizures (11%) [4]
Somnolence (drowsiness) (17%) [3]
Status epilepticus (2–5%)
Tremor (7%)
Vertigo (dizziness) (15%)

Neuromuscular/Skeletal
Arthralgia (5–10%)
Asthenia (fatigue) (16%) [2]
Back pain (4–7%)
Muscle spasm (3%)
Myalgia/Myopathy (3–5%)
Pain in extremities (2–6%)

Gastrointestinal/Hepatic
Abdominal distension (2%)
Abdominal pain (2–3%)
Constipation (5–8%)
Diarrhea (7%)
Dyspepsia (4–5%)
Nausea (7%)
Vomiting (6%)

Respiratory
Bronchitis (5%)
Cough (2–14%)
Influenza (5–7%)
Nasopharyngitis (10%)
Pharyngolaryngeal pain (7–14%)
Upper respiratory tract infection (10%)

Endocrine/Metabolic
Appetite increased (<5%)
Weight gain (10%) [4]

Genitourinary
Dysmenorrhea (5–9%)
Erectile dysfunction (5%)
Urinary tract infection (4–5%)

Hematologic
Anemia (6%)

Otic
Tinnitus (2%)

Ocular
Diplopia (6%)
Nystagmus (7%)
Ocular pain (5%)
Optic atrophy [2]
Retinopathy [12]
Vision blurred (6%)
Vision impaired [20]

Other
Adverse effects [2]
Dipsia (thirst) (2%)
Toothache (2–5%)

VILAZODONE

Trade name: Viibryd (Merck KGaA)
Indications: Major depressive disorder
Class: Antidepressant, Serotonin-norepinephrine reuptake inhibitor
Half-life: 25 hours
Clinically important, potentially hazardous interactions with: anticoagulants, aspirin, buspirone, CNS-active agents, CYP3A4 inhibitors or inducers, efavirenz, erythromycin, ketoconazole, MAO inhibitors, NSAIDs, SNRIs, SSRIs, tramadol, triptans, tryptophan, warfarin
Pregnancy category: C
Important contra-indications noted in the prescribing guidelines for: nursing mothers; pediatric patients
Black Box Warning: SUICIDALITY AND ANTIDEPRESSANT DRUGS

Mucosal
Xerostomia (8%)

Cardiovascular
Palpitation (2%)

Central Nervous System
Abnormal dreams (4%)
Headache [3]
Insomnia (6%) [3]
Paresthesias (3%)
Restlessness (3%)
Somnolence (drowsiness) (3%)
Tremor (2%)

Vertigo (dizziness) (9%)

Neuromuscular/Skeletal
Arthralgia (3%)
Asthenia (fatigue) (4%)

Gastrointestinal/Hepatic
Diarrhea (28%) [12]
Dyspepsia (3%)
Flatulence (3%)
Gastroenteritis (3%)
Nausea (23%) [12]
Vomiting (5%) [3]

Endocrine/Metabolic
Appetite increased (2%)
Libido decreased (4–5%)

Genitourinary
Ejaculatory dysfunction (2%)
Erectile dysfunction (2%)
Sexual dysfunction (3%) [2]

Other
Adverse effects [3]

VINBLASTINE

Trade names: Velban (Lilly), Velbe (Lilly), Velsar (Lilly)
Indications: Lymphomas, melanoma, carcinomas
Class: Antimitotic, Vinca alkaloid
Half-life: initial: 3.7 minutes; terminal: 24.8 hours
Clinically important, potentially hazardous interactions with: aldesleukin, aprepitant, erythromycin, fluconazole, itraconazole, ketoconazole, lopinavir, miconazole, posaconazole
Pregnancy category: D
Important contra-indications noted in the prescribing guidelines for: nursing mothers

---

Skin
Acral necrosis [2]
Dermatitis (<10%)
Photosensitivity (<10%) [2]
Pigmentation [3]
Radiation recall dermatitis [2]
Rash (<10%)
Raynaud's phenomenon (<10%) [17]

Hair
Alopecia (>10%)

Mucosal
Mucositis [2]
Oral lesions (<5%)
Stomatitis (>10%)

Central Nervous System
Dysgeusia (taste perversion) (metallic taste) (>10%)
Paresthesias (<10%)

Neuromuscular/Skeletal
Myalgia/Myopathy (<10%)

Endocrine/Metabolic
SIADH [4]

Renal
Nephrotoxicity [2]

Hematologic
Hemolytic uremic syndrome [2]
Neutropenia [2]

Otic
Tinnitus [2]

Local
Injection-site necrosis [2]

Other
Adverse effects [2]

VINCRISTINE

Synonym: oncovin
Trade name: Vincasar (Teva)
Indications: Leukemias, lymphomas, neuroblastoma, Wilm's tumor
Class: Antimitotic, Vinca alkaloid
Half-life: 24 hours
Clinically important, potentially hazardous interactions with: aldesleukin, aprepitant, bromelain, fluconazole, gadobenate, influenza vaccine, itraconazole, ketoconazole, lopinavir, miconazole, nifedipine, posaconazole, thalidomide
Pregnancy category: D
Important contra-indications noted in the prescribing guidelines for: nursing mothers

---

Skin
Erythroderma [2]
Exanthems [3]
Hand–foot syndrome [2]
Rash (<10%)
Raynaud's phenomenon [2]

Hair
Alopecia (20–70%) [9]

Nails
Beau's lines (transverse nail bands) [2]
Leukonychia (Mees' lines) [5]

Mucosal
Oral lesions (<10%) [2]
Oral ulceration (<10%)

Cardiovascular
Hypertension [2]
Phlebitis (<10%)

Central Nervous System
Anorexia [2]
Dysgeusia (taste perversion) (<10%)
Neurotoxicity [14]
Paresthesias (<10%)
Peripheral neuropathy [7]
Seizures [6]

Neuromuscular/Skeletal
Asthenia (fatigue) [2]
Myalgia/Myopathy (<10%)

Gastrointestinal/Hepatic
Abdominal pain [2]

Endocrine/Metabolic
Hyponatremia [2]
SIADH [10]

Hematologic
Febrile neutropenia [5]
Hemolytic uremic syndrome [4]
Hemotoxicity [2]
Leukopenia [2]
Neutropenia [8]
Thrombocytopenia [8]

Ocular
Ptosis [3]

Local
Injection-site cellulitis (>10%)
Injection-site necrosis (>10%)

Other
Adverse effects [7]
Death [4]
Infection [3]

VINORELBINE

Trade name: Navelbine (Kyowa)
Indications: Non-small cell lung cancer
Class: Antimitotic, Vinca alkaloid
Half-life: 28–44 hours
Clinically important, potentially hazardous interactions with: aldesleukin, itraconazole
Pregnancy category: D
Important contra-indications noted in the prescribing guidelines for: nursing mothers; pediatric patients
Black Box Warning: MYELOSUPPRESSION

Skin
Acneform eruption [3]
Hand–foot syndrome [6]
Rash (<5%) [2]
Recall reaction [2]

Hair
Alopecia (12%) [5]

Mucosal
Mucositis [2]
Stomatitis (>10%) [6]

Cardiovascular
Hypertension [2]
Phlebitis (7%)

Central Nervous System
Anorexia [7]
Dysgeusia (taste perversion) (metallic taste) (>10%)
Hyperesthesia (<10%)
Neurotoxicity [4]
Paresthesias (<10%)

Neuromuscular/Skeletal
Asthenia (fatigue) [13]
Bone or joint pain [2]
Myalgia/Myopathy (<5%)

Gastrointestinal/Hepatic
Constipation [4]
Diarrhea [11]
Hepatotoxicity [2]
Nausea [8]
Vomiting [6]

Endocrine/Metabolic
ALT increased [2]
AST increased [2]
SIADH [3]

Hematologic
Anemia [7]
Febrile neutropenia [5]
Leukopenia [8]
Myelotoxicity [2]
Neutropenia [22]
Thrombocytopenia [4]

Local
Injection-site irritation (<10%)
Injection-site necrosis (<10%)
Injection-site phlebitis (12%) [2]

Other
Death [2]
Infection [4]

VISMODEGIB

Trade name: Erivedge (Genentech)
Indications: Basal cell carcinoma
Class: Hedgehog (Hh) signaling pathway inhibitor
Half-life: 4–12 days
Clinically important, potentially hazardous interactions with: none known
Pregnancy category: D
Important contra-indications noted in the prescribing guidelines for: nursing mothers; pediatric patients
Note: Patients should not donate blood or blood products while receiving vismodegib and for at least 7 months after the last dose.
Black Box Warning: EMBRYO-FETAL TOXICITY

Skin
Squamous cell carcinoma [2]
Toxicity [2]

Hair
Alopecia (64%) [22]

Central Nervous System
Ageusia (taste loss) (11%) [6]
Anorexia [2]
Dysgeusia (taste perversion) (55%) [19]

Neuromuscular/Skeletal
Arthralgia (16%) [2]
Asthenia (fatigue) (40%) [15]
Muscle spasm (72%) [19]
Myalgia/Myopathy [5]

Gastrointestinal/Hepatic
Constipation (21%)
Diarrhea (29%) [7]
Hepatotoxicity [2]
Nausea (30%) [7]
Vomiting (14%) [2]

Endocrine/Metabolic
Amenorrhea [2]
Appetite decreased (25%) [6]
Hyperglycemia [2]
Hyponatremia (4%) [3]
Weight loss (45%) [15]

Genitourinary
Azotemia (2%)

Other
Adverse effects [9]
Death [2]

VITAMIN A

Trade name: Aquasol A (aaiPharma)
Indications: Vitamin A deficiency
Class: Vitamin
Half-life: N/A
Clinically important, potentially hazardous interactions with: acitretin, alitretinoin, bexarotene, cholestyramine, fish oil supplements, isotretinoin, minocycline, orlistat, prednisone, tetracycline, warfarin
Pregnancy category: A (the pregnancy category will be X if used in doses above the RDA)

Skin
Dermatitis [7]
Pruritus [2]
Xerosis (<10%)

Hair
Alopecia [11]

Mucosal
Oral mucosal eruption [2]

VITAMIN E

Synonym: alpha tocopherol
Trade name: Aquasol E (aaiPharma)
Indications: Vitamin E deficiency
Class: Vitamin
Half-life: N/A
Clinically important, potentially hazardous interactions with: amprenavir, cholestyramine, orlistat, tipranavir, warfarin
Pregnancy category: A (the pregnancy category will be C if used in doses above the RDA)

Skin
Dermatitis [13]
Erythema multiforme [3]
Sclerosing lipogranuloma [2]

Genitourinary
Prostate cancer (increased risk) [4]

VORAPAXAR

Trade name: Zontivity (Merck)
Indications: Reduction of thrombotic cardiovascular events in patients with a history of myocardial infarction or with peripheral arterial disease
Class: Protease-activated receptor-1 (PAR-1) antagonist
Half-life: 3–4 days
Clinically important, potentially hazardous interactions with: boceprevir, carbamazepine, clarithromycin, conivaptan, indinavir, itraconazole, ketoconazole, nefazodone, nelfinavir, phenytoin, posaconazole, rifampin, ritonavir, saquinavir, St John's wort, strong CYP3A inhibitors or inducers, telaprevir, telithromycin
Pregnancy category: B
Important contra-indications noted in the prescribing guidelines for: nursing mothers; pediatric patients
Note: Contraindicated in patients with a history of stroke, transient ischemic attack, or intracranial hemorrhage, or with active pathological bleeding.
Black Box Warning: BLEEDING RISK

Skin
Exanthems (2%)
Rash (2%)

Cardiovascular
Cardiotoxicity [2]

Central Nervous System
Depression (2%)
Intracranial hemorrhage [5]

Hematologic
Anemia (5%)
Bleeding (25%) [10]

Ocular
Diplopia (<2%)
Retinopathy (<2%)

Other
Adverse effects [3]

VORICONAZOLE

Trade name: Vfend (Pfizer)
Indications: Invasive aspergillosis
Class: Antibiotic, triazole, Antifungal, azole, CYP3A4 inhibitor
Half-life: 6–24 hours (dose dependent)
Clinically important, potentially hazardous interactions with: abiraterone, alfentanil, alfuzosin, almotriptan, alosetron, amphotericin B, antineoplastics, apixaban, aprepitant, artemether/lumefantrine, astemizole, atazanavir, atorvastatin, barbiturates, benzodiazepines, boceprevir, bortezomib, bosentan, brinzolamide, buspirone, busulfan, cabazitaxel, cabozantinib, calcium channel blockers, carbamazepine, carvedilol, chloramphenicol, chloroquine, ciclesonide, cilostazol, cinacalcet, ciprofloxacin, cisapride, clopidogrel, cobicistat/elvitegravir/emtricitabine/tenofovir disoproxil, colchicine, conivaptan, coumarins, crizotinib, cyclosporine, CYP2C19 inhibitors and inducers, CYP2C9 inhibitors and substrates, CYP3A4 substrates, darunavir, diazepam, diclofenac, didanosine, dienogest, docetaxel, dofetilide, dronedarone, dutasteride, efavirenz, eletriptan, eplerenone, ergot alkaloids, ergotamine, erlotinib, esomeprazole, estrogens, eszopiclone, etravirine, everolimus, fentanyl, fesoterodine, food, gadobutrol, gefitinib, grapefruit juice, guanfacine, halofantrine, HMG-CoA reductase inhibitors, ibrutinib, ibuprofen, imatinib, irinotecan, ixabepilone, lapatinib, lomitapide, lopinavir, losartan, macrolide antibiotics, maraviroc, meloxicam, methadone, methylergonovine, methylprednisolone, methysergide, midazolam, mifepristone, mometasone, nilotinib, nisoldipine, ombitasvir/paritaprevir/ritonavir, omeprazole, oxycodone, pantoprazole, paricalcitol, pazopanib, PEG-interferon, phenobarbital, phenytoin, phosphodiesterase 5 inhibitors, pimecrolimus, pimozide, ponatinib, prasugrel, progestins, progestogens, protease inhibitors, proton pump inhibitors, QT prolonging agents, quetiapine, quinidine, quinine, ramelteon, ranolazine, reboxetine, regorafenib, repaglinide, rifabutin, rifampin, rifapentine, rilpivirine, ritonavir,

rivaroxaban, romidepsin, ruxolitinib, salmeterol, saquinavir, saxagliptin, silodosin, simeprevir, simvastatin, sirolimus, solifenacin, sorafenib, St John's wort, sucralfate, sulfonylureas, sunitinib, tacrolimus, tadalafil, tamsulosin, telaprevir, temsirolimus, tetrabenazine, thioridazine, ticagrelor, tolterodine, tolvaptan, vemurafenib, venetoclax, venlafaxine, vitamin K antagonists, ziprasidone, zolpidem

Pregnancy category: D

Important contra-indications noted in the prescribing guidelines for: nursing mothers; pediatric patients

Note: Safety and effectiveness in pediatric patients <12 years of age have not been established.

Skin

Actinic keratoses [2]
Anaphylactoid reactions/Anaphylaxis (<2%)
Angioedema (<2%)
Cellulitis (<2%)
Contact dermatitis (<2%)
Cyanosis (<2%)
Dermatitis (<2%)
Diaphoresis (<2%) [2]
Ecchymoses (<2%)
Eczema (<2%)
Edema (<2%)
Erythema [5]
Erythema multiforme (<2%)
Exfoliative dermatitis (<2%)
Facial edema (<2%)
Fixed eruption (<2%)
Furunculosis (<2%)
Graft-versus-host reaction (<2%)
Granulomas (<2%)
Herpes simplex (<2%)
Lentigo [2]
Lupus erythematosus (<2%) [4]
Lymphadenopathy (<2%)
Malignancies [2]
Melanoma (<2%)
Melanosis (<2%)
Peripheral edema (<2%)
Petechiae (<2%)
Photosensitivity (8%) [17]
Phototoxicity [13]
Pigmentation (<2%)
Pruritus (8%)
Psoriasis (<2%)
Purpura (<2%)
Rash (5%) [6]
Squamous cell carcinoma (<2%) [7]
Stevens–Johnson syndrome (<2%) [4]
Toxic epidermal necrolysis (<2%) [4]
Urticaria (<2%)
Xerosis (<2%) [2]

Hair

Alopecia (<2%) [4]

Nails

Nail changes [3]

Mucosal

Cheilitis (<2%) [4]
Gingival bleeding (<2%)
Gingival hyperplasia/hypertrophy (<2%)
Gingivitis (<2%)
Glossitis (<2%)
Rectal hemorrhage (<2%)
Stomatitis (<2%)
Tongue edema (<2%)
Xerostomia (<2%)

Cardiovascular

Arrhythmias (<2%)
Atrial fibrillation (<2%)
Atrioventricular block (<2%)
Bradycardia (<2%)
Bundle branch block (<2%)
Cardiac arrest (<2%)
Cardiomyopathy (<2%)
Chest pain (<2%)
Congestive heart failure (<2%)
Extrasystoles (<2%)
Hypertension (<2%)
Hypotension (<2%)
Myocardial infarction (<2%)
Palpitation (<2%)
Phlebitis (<2%)
Postural hypotension (<2%)
QT prolongation (<2%) [9]
Supraventricular tachycardia (<2%)
Tachycardia (2%) [2]
Thrombophlebitis (<2%)
Torsades de pointes [7]
Vasodilation (<2%)
Ventricular arrhythmia (<2%)
Ventricular fibrillation (<2%)
Ventricular tachycardia (<2%)

Central Nervous System

Abnormal dreams (<2%)
Ageusia (taste loss) (<2%)
Agitation (<2%)
Akathisia (<2%)
Amnesia (<2%)
Anorexia (<2%)
Anxiety (<2%)
Cerebral edema (<2%)
Cerebral hemorrhage (<2%)
Cerebral ischemia (<2%)
Cerebrovascular accident (<2%)
Chills (4%)
Coma (<2%)
Confusion (<2%) [2]
Delirium (<2%) [2]
Dementia (<2%)
Depersonalization (<2%)
Depression (<2%)
Dysgeusia (taste perversion) (<2%)
Encephalitis (<2%)
Encephalopathy (<2%) [3]
Euphoria (<2%)
Extrapyramidal symptoms (<2%)
Fever (6%)
Guillain–Barré syndrome (<2%)
Hallucinations (2%) [8]
Headache (3%) [3]
Hypoesthesia (<2%)
Insomnia (<2%)
Intracranial pressure increased (<2%)
Neurotoxicity [5]
Paresthesias (<2%)
Peripheral neuropathy [4]
Psychosis (<2%) [2]
Seizures (<2%)
Somnolence (drowsiness) (<2%)
Status epilepticus (<2%)
Suicidal ideation (<2%)
Syncope (<2%)
Tremor (<2%)
Vertigo (dizziness) (<2%)

Neuromuscular/Skeletal

Arthralgia (<2%) [2]
Asthenia (fatigue) (<2%) [2]
Ataxia (<2%)
Back pain (<2%)
Bone or joint pain (<2%)
Hypertonia (<2%)
Leg cramps (<2%)
Myalgia/Myopathy (<2%)
Osteomalacia (<2%)
Osteoporosis (<2%)
Periostitis deformans [19]
Skeletal fluorosis [2]

Gastrointestinal/Hepatic

Abdominal pain (<2%)
Ascites (<2%)
Black stools (<2%)
Cholecystitis (<2%)
Cholelithiasis (gallstones) (<2%)
Constipation (<2%)
Diarrhea (<2%) [2]
Duodentitis (<2%)
Dyspepsia (<2%)
Dysphagia (<2%)
Esophagitis (<2%)
Flatulence (<2%)
Gastroenteritis (<2%)
Gastrointestinal bleeding (<2%)
Gastrointestinal perforation (<2%)
Gastrointestinal ulceration (<2%)
Hematemesis (<2%)
Hepatic failure (<2%)
Hepatotoxicity [15]
Nausea (5%) [2]
Pancreatitis (<2%)
Peritonitis (<2%)
Pseudomembranous colitis (<2%)
Vomiting (4%) [2]

Respiratory

Cough (<2%)
Dysphonia (<2%)
Dyspnea (<2%)
Flu-like syndrome (<2%)
Hemoptysis (<2%)
Hypoxia (<2%)
Pharyngitis (<2%)
Pleural effusion (<2%)
Pneumonia (<2%)
Pneumonitis [2]
Pulmonary embolism (<2%)
Respiratory distress (<2%)
Rhinitis (<2%)
Sinusitis (<2%)
Upper respiratory tract infection (<2%)

Endocrine/Metabolic

ALP increased (4%)
ALT increased [2]
AST increased [2]
Creatine phosphokinase increased (<2%)
Diabetes insipidus (<2%)
GGT increased (<2%)
Hypercalcemia (<2%)
Hypercholesterolemia (<2%)
Hyperglycemia (<2%)
Hyperkalemia (<2%)
Hypermagnesemia (<2%)
Hypernatremia (<2%)
Hyperthyroidism (<2%)

Hyperuricemia (<2%)
Hypervolemia (<2%)
Hypocalcemia (<2%)
Hypoglycemia (<2%)
Hypokalemia (2%) [2]
Hypomagnesemia (<2%)
Hyponatremia (<2%)
Hypophosphatemia (<2%)
Hypothyroidism (<2%)
Libido decreased (<2%)
Pseudoporphyria [6]

Genitourinary
Anuria (<2%)
Cystitis (<2%)
Dysmenorrhea (<2%)
Dysuria (<2%)
Epididymitis (<2%)
Glycosuria (<2%)
Hematuria (<2%)
Impotence (<2%)
Oliguria (<2%)
Urinary incontinence (<2%)
Urinary retention (<2%)
Urinary tract infection (<2%)
Uterine bleeding (<2%)
Vaginal bleeding (<2%)

Renal
Nephrotoxicity (<2%) [2]
Renal tubular necrosis (<2%)

Hematologic
Agranulocytosis (<2%)
Anemia (<2%)
Bone marrow suppression (<2%)
Eosinophilia (<2%)
Hemolytic anemia (<2%)
Leukopenia (<2%)
Pancytopenia (<2%)
Prothrombin time increased (<2%)
Sepsis (<2%)
Thrombocytopenia (<2%)

Otic
Ear pain (<2%)
Hearing loss (<2%)
Hypoacusis (<2%)
Tinnitus (<2%)

Ocular
Abnormal vision (19%)
Accommodation disorder (<2%)
Blepharitis (<2%)
Conjunctivitis (<2%)
Corneal opacity (<2%)
Diplopia (<2%)
Hallucinations, visual [4]
Keratitis (<2%)
Keratoconjunctivitis (<2%)
Mydriasis (<2%)
Night blindness (<2%)
Nystagmus (<2%)
Ocular hemorrhage (<2%)
Ocular pain (<2%)
Oculogyric crisis (<2%)
Optic atrophy (<2%)
Optic neuritis (<2%)
Papilledema (<2%)
Photophobia (2%)
Retinitis (<2%)
Scleritis (<2%)
Uveitis (<2%)
Visual disturbances (19%) [13]
Xerophthalmia (<2%)

Local
Injection-site infection (<2%)
Injection-site inflammation (<2%)
Injection-site pain (<2%)

Other
Adverse effects (20%) [11]
Infection (<2%)
Multiorgan failure (<2%)
Periodontal infection (<2%)

VORINOSTAT

Trade name: Zolinza (Merck)
Indications: Cutaneous T-cell lymphoma
Class: Antineoplastic, Histone deacetylase (HDAC) inhibitor
Half-life: ~2 hours
Clinically important, potentially hazardous interactions with: alfuzosin, artemether/lumefantrine, chloroquine, ciprofloxacin, coumarins, dronedarone, gadobutrol, nilotinib, pimozide, QT prolonging agents, quinine, tetrabenazine, thioridazine, valproic acid, vitamin K antagonists, ziprasidone
Pregnancy category: D
Important contra-indications noted in the prescribing guidelines for: nursing mothers; pediatric patients

---

Skin
Exanthems [2]
Peripheral edema (13%)
Pruritus (12%)

Hair
Alopecia (19%) [2]

Mucosal
Mucositis [2]
Xerostomia (16%)

Cardiovascular
QT prolongation [3]

Central Nervous System
Anorexia [5]
Chills (16%)
Dysgeusia (taste perversion) (28%)
Fever (10%)
Headache (12%)
Vertigo (dizziness) (15%)

Neuromuscular/Skeletal
Asthenia (fatigue) (52%) [10]

Gastrointestinal/Hepatic
Abdominal pain [2]
Constipation [2]
Diarrhea [7]
Nausea [9]
Vomiting [4]

Respiratory
Cough (11%)
Upper respiratory tract infection (10%)

Endocrine/Metabolic
Creatine phosphokinase increased [2]
Dehydration [2]
Hyperglycemia [3]
Weight loss [4]

Renal
Renal failure [2]

Hematologic
Anemia (14%) [7]
Febrile neutropenia [2]
Hemotoxicity [2]
Leukopenia [2]
Lymphopenia [5]
Neutropenia [9]
Thrombocytopenia [15]

Other
Adverse effects [2]

VORTIOXETINE

Trade name: Trintellix (formerly Brintellix) (Takeda)
Indications: Major depressive disorder
Class: Antidepressant, Serotonin receptor agonist, Serotonin receptor antagonist, Serotonin reuptake inhibitor
Half-life: ~66 hours
Clinically important, potentially hazardous interactions with: bupropion, carbamazepine, fluoxetine, MAO inhibitors, paroxetine hydrochloride, phenytoin, quinidine, rifampin
Pregnancy category: C
Important contra-indications noted in the prescribing guidelines for: nursing mothers; pediatric patients
Black Box Warning: SUICIDAL THOUGHTS AND BEHAVIORS

Skin
Hyperhidrosis [6]
Pruritus (<3%)

Mucosal
Xerostomia (6–8%) [13]

Central Nervous System
Abnormal dreams (<3%)
Headache [23]
Insomnia [4]
Somnolence (drowsiness) [3]
Vertigo (dizziness) (6–9%) [13]

Neuromuscular/Skeletal
Asthenia (fatigue) [6]

Gastrointestinal/Hepatic
Constipation (3–6%) [9]
Diarrhea (7–10%) [11]
Flatulence (<3%)
Nausea (21–32%) [28]
Vomiting (3–6%) [13]

Respiratory
Nasopharyngitis [5]
Upper respiratory tract infection [2]

Endocrine/Metabolic
Weight gain [2]

Genitourinary
Sexual dysfunction (<5%) [10]

Other
Adverse effects [2]

WARFARIN

Trade name: Coumadin (Bristol-Myers Squibb)
Indications: Thromboembolic disease, pulmonary embolism
Class: Anticoagulant, Coumarin
Half-life: 1.5–2.5 days (highly variable)
Clinically important, potentially hazardous interactions with: acemetacin, amiodarone, amobarbital, amprenavir, antithyroid agents, aprepitant, aprobarbital, aspirin, atazanavir, atorvastatin, azathioprine, azithromycin, barbiturates, beclomethasone, betamethasone, bezafibrate, bismuth, bivalirudin, boceprevir, bosentan, butabarbital, capecitabine, cefixime, celecoxib, chondroitin, cimetidine, ciprofloxacin, clarithromycin, clofibrate, clopidogrel, clorazepate, co-trimoxazole, cobicistat/elvitegravir/emtricitabine/tenofovir disoproxil, colesevelam, cyclosporine, danazol, daptomycin, darunavir, delavirdine, desvenlafaxine, dexamethasone, dexibuprofen, dexlansoprazole, diclofenac, dicloxacillin, dirithromycin, disulfiram, dronedarone, duloxetine, econazole, efavirenz, enzalutamide, ergotamine, erlotinib, erythromycin, eslicarbazepine, etoricoxib, exenatide, fenofibrate, fluconazole, flunisolide, fluoxymesterone, fosamprenavir, gefitinib, gemfibrozil, glucagon, grapefruit juice, heparin, imatinib, influenza vaccine, itraconazole, ketoconazole, leflunomide, lepirudin, levofloxacin, levothyroxine, liothyronine, liraglutide, lomitapide, lopinavir, menadione, mephobarbital, methimazole, methyl salicylate, methylprednisolone, methyltestosterone, metronidazole, miconazole, mifepristone, moricizine, moxifloxacin, nafcillin, nalidixic acid, nandrolone, nilutamide, norfloxacin, obeticholic acid, ofloxacin, omeprazole, orlistat, pantoprazole, PEG-interferon, penicillin G, penicillin V, penicillins, pentobarbital, phenobarbital, phenylbutazones, phytonadione, piperacillin, piroxicam, prasugrel, primidone, propoxyphene, propranolol, propylthiouracil, quinidine, quinine, rabeprazole, resveratrol, rifampin, rifapentine, rofecoxib, romidepsin, ropinirole, rosuvastatin, roxithromycin, salicylates, secobarbital, simvastatin, sitaxentan, sorafenib, St John's wort, stanozolol, sulfamethoxazole, sulfinpyrazone, sulfisoxazole, sulfonamides, sulindac, tamsulosin, tegafur/gimeracil/oteracil, telaprevir, telithromycin, teriflunomide, testosterone, tibolone, tigecycline, tinidazole, tolmetin, tolterodine, triamcinolone, troleandomycin, uracil/tegafur, valdecoxib, vemurafenib, venlafaxine, vilazodone, vitamin A, vitamin E, zafirlukast, zileuton
Pregnancy category: X (category D for women with mechanical heart valves)
Note: Alternative remedies, including herbals, may potentially increase the risk of bleeding or potentiate the effects of warfarin therapy. Some of these include the following: angelica root, arnica flower, anise, asafetida, bogbean, borage seed oil, bromelain, dan-shen, devil's claw, fenugreek, feverfew, garlic, ginger, ginkgo biloba, ginseng, horse chestnut, lovage root, meadowsweet, onion, parsley, passionflower herb, poplar, quassia, red clover, rue, turmeric and willow bark.

Black Box Warning: BLEEDING RISK

Skin
- Bullous dermatitis [2]
- Calcification [3]
- Dermatitis [2]
- Ecchymoses [2]
- Exanthems [7]
- Gangrene [6]
- Hematoma [2]
- Hypersensitivity [3]
- Necrosis (>10%) [115]
- Pruritus [2]
- Purplish erythema (feet and toes) [8]
- Purpura [3]
- Rash [2]
- Urticaria [3]
- Vasculitis [7]

Hair
- Alopecia (>10%) [6]

Central Nervous System
- Headache [2]
- Intracranial hemorrhage [2]
- Vertigo (dizziness) [2]

Neuromuscular/Skeletal
- Rhabdomyolysis [2]

Gastrointestinal/Hepatic
- Black stools [2]
- Gastrointestinal bleeding [5]
- Hematemesis [2]

Genitourinary
- Priapism [4]

Renal
- Nephrotoxicity [2]

Hematologic
- Anticoagulation [3]
- Bleeding [17]
- Hemorrhage [8]
- Prothrombin time increased [5]

Other
- Adverse effects [7]
- Death [2]

XYLOMETAZOLINE

Trade name: Otrivine (Novartis)
Indications: Nasal congestion, perennial and allergic rhinitis, sinusitis
Class: Alpha 1 adrenoreceptor antagonist, Sympathomimetic
Half-life: N/A
Clinically important, potentially hazardous interactions with: none known
Pregnancy category: C
Important contra-indications noted in the prescribing guidelines for: nursing mothers

Mucosal
- Epistaxis (nosebleed) [2]
- Mucosal bleeding [2]

YELLOW FEVER VACCINE

Trade names: Stamaril (Sanofi Pasteur), YF-VAX (Sanofi Pasteur)
Indications: Immunization against yellow fever
Class: Vaccine
Half-life: N/A
Clinically important, potentially hazardous interactions with: azathioprine, belimumab, corticosteroids, fingolimod, hydroxychloroquine, immunosuppressants, interferon-gamma, leflunomide, mercaptopurine, prednisone, tocilizumab, ustekinumab
Pregnancy category: C
Important contra-indications noted in the prescribing guidelines for: the elderly; nursing mothers; pediatric patients
Note: Contraindicated in patients with hypersensitivity to egg or chick embryo protein.

Skin
Anaphylactoid reactions/Anaphylaxis [8]
Hypersensitivity [2]
Rash (3%)
Urticaria [2]

Central Nervous System
Encephalopathy [4]
Fever (low-grade) (<5%) [3]
Headache (<30%) [2]
Myelitis [2]
Neurotoxicity [11]

Neuromuscular/Skeletal
Asthenia (fatigue) (10–30%) [2]
Myalgia/Myopathy (10–30%) [2]

Gastrointestinal/Hepatic
Diarrhea (<10%) [2]
Hepatitis [2]
Nausea (<10%)
Vomiting (<10%) [2]

Respiratory
Influenza [2]

Local
Infusion-site erythema (<5%)
Infusion-site pain (<5%)

Other
Adverse effects [14]
Death [13]
Multiorgan failure [3]
Viscerotropic disease [20]

ZAFIRLUKAST

Trade name: Accolate (AstraZeneca)
Indications: Asthma
Class: Leukotriene receptor antagonist
Half-life: 10 hours
Clinically important, potentially hazardous interactions with: aminophylline, aspirin, carvedilol, CYP2C9 substrates, CYP3A4 substrates, erythromycin, high protein foods, interferon alfa, primidone, vitamin K antagonists, warfarin
Pregnancy category: B
Important contra-indications noted in the prescribing guidelines for: nursing mothers; pediatric patients
Note: Safety and effectiveness for pediatric patients <5 years of age has not been established. Contraindicated in patients with hepatic impairment including hepatic cirrhosis.

Skin
Churg-Strauss syndrome [6]

Central Nervous System
Fever (2%)
Headache (13%)
Pain (generalized) (2%)
Vertigo (dizziness) (2%)

Neuromuscular/Skeletal
Asthenia (fatigue) (2%)
Back pain (2%)
Myalgia/Myopathy (2%)

Gastrointestinal/Hepatic
Abdominal pain (2%)
Diarrhea (3%)
Nausea (3%)
Vomiting (2%)

Respiratory
Cough [2]

Other
Infection (4%)

ZALCITABINE

Synonyms: dideoxycytidine; ddC
Trade name: Hivid (Roche)
Indications: Advanced HIV infection
Class: Antiretroviral, Nucleoside analog reverse transcriptase inhibitor
Half-life: 2.9 hours
Clinically important, potentially hazardous interactions with: none known
Pregnancy category: C
Important contra-indications noted in the prescribing guidelines for: the elderly; nursing mothers; pediatric patients

---

Skin
Edema [3]
Exanthems [9]
Pruritus (3–5%)
Rash (2–11%) [2]
Urticaria (3%)

Mucosal
Aphthous stomatitis [6]
Oral lesions (40–73%) [3]
Oral ulceration (3–64%) [4]
Stomatitis (3%)

Central Nervous System
Neurotoxicity [2]

Neuromuscular/Skeletal
Myalgia/Myopathy (<6%)

Other
Side effects [2]

ZALEPLON

Trade name: Sonata (Wyeth)
Indications: Insomnia
Class: Hypnotic, non-benzodiazepine
Half-life: 1 hour
Clinically important, potentially hazardous interactions with: alcohol, cimetidine, erythromycin, imipramine, ketoconazole, promethazine, rifampin, rifapentine, thioridazine
Pregnancy category: C
Important contra-indications noted in the prescribing guidelines for: nursing mothers; pediatric patients

---

Cardiovascular
Tachycardia [2]

Central Nervous System
Amnesia (2–4%)
Anorexia (<2%)
Confusion [2]
Depersonalization (<2%)
Hallucinations [3]
Headache (30–42%) [3]
Hypoesthesia (<2%)
Paresthesias (3%)
Parosmia (<2%)
Slurred speech [2]
Somnambulism [2]
Somnolence (drowsiness) (5–6%) [4]
Tremor (2%)
Vertigo (dizziness) (7–9%) [4]

Neuromuscular/Skeletal
Asthenia (fatigue) (5–7%)
Ataxia [2]

Gastrointestinal/Hepatic
Abdominal pain (6%)
Nausea (6–8%)
Vomiting [2]

Genitourinary
Dysmenorrhea (3–4%)

Otic
Hyperacusis (<2%)

Ocular
Ocular pain (3–4%)

Other
Adverse effects [2]
Viscerotropic disease [2]

ZANAMIVIR

Trade name: Relenza (GSK)
Indications: Influenza A and B
Class: Antiviral, Neuraminidase inhibitor
Half-life: 2.5–5.1 hours
Clinically important, potentially hazardous interactions with: live attenuated influenza vaccine
Pregnancy category: C
Important contra-indications noted in the prescribing guidelines for: nursing mothers

Skin
- Urticaria (<2%)

Mucosal
- Nasal discomfort (12%)

Central Nervous System
- Anorexia (4%)
- Chills (5–9%)
- Fever (5–9%)
- Headache (13–24%) [2]
- Vertigo (dizziness) (<2%)

Neuromuscular/Skeletal
- Arthralgia (<2%)
- Asthenia (fatigue) (5–8%)
- Bone or joint pain (6%)
- Myalgia/Myopathy (<8%)

Gastrointestinal/Hepatic
- Abdominal pain (<2%)
- Diarrhea (3%)
- Nausea (3%) [2]

Respiratory
- Bronchitis (2%)
- Bronchospasm [3]
- Cough (7–17%)
- Sinusitis (2%)
- Upper respiratory tract infection (3–13%) [2]

Endocrine/Metabolic
- Appetite decreased (4%)
- Appetite increased (4%)

Other
- Infection (2%)

ZICONOTIDE

Trade name: Prialt (Jazz)
Indications: Analgesic, severe chronic pain
Class: Neuronal calcium channel blocker
Half-life: 4.6 hours
Clinically important, potentially hazardous interactions with: CNS depressants
Pregnancy category: C
Important contra-indications noted in the prescribing guidelines for: the elderly; nursing mothers; pediatric patients
Note: Ziconotide is a synthetic analog of a substance isolated from the venom of carnivorous oceanic snails that sting their prey with a cocktail of neurotoxins injected through a harpoon-like tube. Ziconotide is 100 to 1,000 times more powerful than morphine.
Black Box Warning: NEUROPSYCHIATRIC ADVERSE REACTIONS

Skin
- Cellulitis (~2%)
- Diaphoresis (5%)
- Ecchymoses (~2%)
- Edema (~2%)
- Pruritus (7%)
- Xerosis (~2%)

Mucosal
- Xerostomia (~2%)

Cardiovascular
- Atrial fibrillation (~2%)
- Chest pain (~2%)
- Hypertension (~2%)
- Hypotension (~2%)
- Tachycardia (~2%)

Central Nervous System
- Amnesia (8%)
- Anorexia (6%)
- Anxiety (8%)
- Chills (~2%)
- Confusion (15%) [4]
- Depression (~2%)
- Dysarthria (7%)
- Dysesthesia (7%)
- Dysgeusia (taste perversion) (5%)
- Fever (5%)
- Hallucinations [3]
- Headache (13%)
- Hyperesthesia (~2%)
- Insomnia (6%)
- Pain (11%)
- Paresthesias (7%)
- Rigors (7%)
- Seizures (<2%)
- Somnolence (drowsiness) (17%) [3]
- Suicidal ideation (<2%)
- Tremor (7%)
- Twitching (~2%)
- Vertigo (dizziness) (47%) [7]

Neuromuscular/Skeletal
- Arthralgia (~2%)
- Asthenia (fatigue) (18%)
- Ataxia (14%)
- Back pain (~2%)
- Muscle spasm (6%)
- Myalgia/Myopathy (~2%)
- Rhabdomyolysis (<2%)

Gastrointestinal/Hepatic
- Abdominal pain (~2%)
- Diarrhea (18%)
- Nausea (40%) [2]
- Vomiting (16%) [2]

Respiratory
- Flu-like syndrome (~2%)
- Sinusitis (5%)

Genitourinary
- Urinary retention (9%) [3]

Otic
- Tinnitus (~2%)

Ocular
- Diplopia (~2%)
- Nystagmus (8%) [2]
- Periorbital edema (~2%)
- Photophobia (~2%)
- Vision blurred (12%) [2]
- Visual disturbances (10%)

Other
- Adverse effects [3]
- Infection (~2%)

ZIDOVUDINE

Synonyms: azidothymidine; AZT
Trade names: Combivir (ViiV), Retrovir (ViiV), Trizivir (ViiV)
Indications: HIV infection
Class: Antiretroviral, Nucleoside analog reverse transcriptase inhibitor
Half-life: 0.5–3 hours
Clinically important, potentially hazardous interactions with: atovaquone, bone marrow suppressives, clarithromycin, darunavir, diclofenac, doxorubicin, fluconazole, ganciclovir, indinavir, interferon alfa, interferon beta, lopinavir, meloxicam, methadone, NSAIDs, PEG-interferon, phenytoin, probenecid, pyrimethamine, ribavirin, rifampin, rifapentine, stavudine, tipranavir, valproic acid
Pregnancy category: C
Important contra-indications noted in the prescribing guidelines for: the elderly; nursing mothers
Note: Combivir is zidovudine and lamivudine; Trizivir is zidovudine, abacavir and lamivudine.
Black Box Warning: HEMATOLOGICAL TOXICITY, MYOPATHY, LACTIC ACIDOSIS AND SEVERE HEPATOMEGALY, and EXACERBATIONS OF HEPATITIS B

Skin
- Acneform eruption (<5%)
- Bromhidrosis (<5%)
- Diaphoresis (5–19%)
- Edema of lip (<5%)
- Erythema multiforme [2]
- Exanthems (<5%) [6]
- Lipoatrophy [2]
- Lipodystrophy [2]
- Pigmentation [10]
- Pruritus [4]
- Rash (17%) [8]
- Stevens-Johnson syndrome [4]
- Toxic epidermal necrolysis [3]
- Urticaria (<5%) [2]
- Vasculitis [2]

Hair
- Alopecia [2]
- Hypertrichosis (eyelashes) [2]

Nails
- Nail pigmentation [27]

Mucosal
- Oral lichenoid eruption [2]
- Oral pigmentation [7]
- Oral ulceration (<5%)
- Tongue edema (<5%)
- Tongue pigmentation [4]

Central Nervous System
- Dysgeusia (taste perversion) (5–19%) [2]
- Headache [3]
- Paresthesias (<8%)

Neuromuscular/Skeletal
- Asthenia (fatigue) [3]
- Myalgia/Myopathy [5]

Gastrointestinal/Hepatic
- Abdominal pain [3]
- Diarrhea [2]
- Hepatotoxicity [2]
- Nausea [3]
- Pancreatitis [3]
- Vomiting [2]

Endocrine/Metabolic
- Acidosis [6]

Hematologic
- Anemia [13]
- Neutropenia [3]

Other
- Adverse effects [9]
- Teratogenicity [2]

ZILEUTON

Trade name: Zyflo (AbbVie)
Indications: Asthma
Class: Leukotriene receptor antagonist
Half-life: 2.5 hours
Clinically important, potentially hazardous interactions with: anisindione, anticoagulants, astemizole, dicumarol, methylergonovine, pimozide, propranolol, warfarin
Pregnancy category: C
Important contra-indications noted in the prescribing guidelines for: nursing mothers; pediatric patients

---

Neuromuscular/Skeletal
- Myalgia/Myopathy (3%)

ZIPRASIDONE

Trade name: Geodon (Pfizer)
Indications: Schizophrenia, bipolar I disorder
Class: Antipsychotic
Half-life: 7 hours
Clinically important, potentially hazardous interactions with: acetylcholinesterase inhibitors, alcohol, alfuzosin, amitriptyline, amoxapine, amphetamines, antifungals, arsenic, artemether/lumefantrine, asenapine, astemizole, carbamazepine, chloroquine, ciprofloxacin, citalopram, CNS depressants, conivaptan, dasatinib, degarelix, dolasetron, dopamine agonists, dopamine agonists, dronedarone, food, gadobutrol, ketoconazole, lapatinib, levodopa, levofloxacin, lithium, methylphenidate, metoclopramide, moxifloxacin, nilotinib, pazopanib, pimozide, QT prolonging agents, quinagolide, quinine, ranolazine, St John's wort, telavancin, telithromycin, tetrabenazine, thioridazine, voriconazole, vorinostat
Pregnancy category: C
Important contra-indications noted in the prescribing guidelines for: the elderly; nursing mothers; pediatric patients
Note: Ziprasidone should be avoided in patients with congenital long QT syndrome or a history of cardiac arrhythmias.
Black Box Warning: INCREASED MORTALITY IN ELDERLY PATIENTS WITH DEMENTIA-RELATED PSYCHOSIS

Skin
- Angioedema [2]
- Diaphoresis (2%)
- DRESS syndrome [2]
- Fungal dermatitis (2%)
- Furunculosis (2%)
- Lupus erythematosus [2]
- Rash (4%)
- Urticaria (5%)

Mucosal
- Rectal hemorrhage (2%)
- Sialorrhea (4%)
- Tongue edema (3%)
- Xerostomia (<5%)

Cardiovascular
- Bradycardia (2%)
- Chest pain (3%)
- Hypertension (2–3%)
- Postural hypotension (5%)
- QT prolongation [22]
- Tachycardia (2%) [2]
- Torsades de pointes [6]

Central Nervous System
- Agitation (2%) [2]
- Akathisia (2–10%) [5]
- Anorexia (2%)
- Anxiety (2–5%)
- Dyskinesia (<10%) [2]
- Extrapyramidal symptoms (2–31%) [5]
- Headache (3–18%) [3]
- Hyperesthesia (<2%)
- Hypokinesia (<5%)
- Insomnia (3%) [4]
- Mania [2]
- Neuroleptic malignant syndrome [6]
- Paralysis (<10%)
- Paresthesias (<2%)
- Sedation [3]
- Somnolence (drowsiness) (8–31%) [10]
- Speech disorder (2%)
- Tardive dyskinesia [4]
- Tremor (<10%) [2]
- Twitching (<10%)
- Vertigo (dizziness) (3–16%) [2]

Neuromuscular/Skeletal
- Asthenia (fatigue) (2–6%) [2]
- Dystonia (<10%) [5]
- Hypertonia (<10%)
- Myalgia/Myopathy (2%)
- Rhabdomyolysis [2]

Gastrointestinal/Hepatic
- Abdominal pain (<2%)
- Constipation (2–9%)
- Diarrhea (3–5%)
- Dyspepsia (<8%)
- Dysphagia (2%)
- Nausea (4–12%) [2]
- Vomiting (3–5%)

Respiratory
- Cough (increased) (3%)
- Dyspnea (2%)
- Pharyngitis (3%)
- Respiratory tract infection (8%)
- Rhinitis (<4%)
- Upper respiratory tract infection (8%)

Endocrine/Metabolic
- Galactorrhea [3]
- Weight gain [6]

Genitourinary
- Dysmenorrhea (2%)
- Priapism [4]

Ocular
- Abnormal vision (3–6%)

Local
- Infusion-site pain (7–9%)

Other
- Adverse effects [8]
- Death [2]

ZOLEDRONATE

Synonym: zoledronic acid
Trade names: Aclasta (Novartis), Reclast (Novartis), Zometa (Novartis)
Indications: Hypercalcemia of malignancy, Paget's disease, osteoporosis
Class: Bisphosphonate
Half-life: 7 days
Clinically important, potentially hazardous interactions with: aminoglycosides, bisphosphonates, loop diuretics, nephrotoxics
Pregnancy category: D
Important contra-indications noted in the prescribing guidelines for: the elderly; nursing mothers; pediatric patients

---

Skin
- Candidiasis (12%)
- Dermatitis (11%)
- Dermatomyositis [3]
- Edema [3]
- Neoplasms (malignant / aggrevated) (20%)
- Peripheral edema (5–21%)
- Rash [3]

Hair
- Alopecia (12%)

Mucosal
- Mucositis (5–10%)
- Stomatitis (8%)

Cardiovascular
- Atrial fibrillation [3]
- Chest pain (5–10%)
- Hypotension (11%)

Central Nervous System
- Agitation (13%)
- Anorexia (9–22%)
- Anxiety (11–14%)
- Chills [2]
- Confusion (7–13%)
- Depression (14%)
- Fever (32–44%) [20]
- Headache (5–19%) [4]
- Hypoesthesia (12%)
- Insomnia (15–16%)
- Paresthesias (15%)
- Rigors (11%)
- Seizures [2]
- Somnolence (drowsiness) (5–10%)
- Vertigo (dizziness) (18%)

Neuromuscular/Skeletal
- Arthralgia (5–10%) [9]
- Asthenia (fatigue) (5–39%) [11]
- Back pain (15%)
- Bone or joint pain (12–55%) [15]

Fractures [4]
Myalgia/Myopathy (23%) [7]
Osteonecrosis [52]
Pain in extremities (14%)

Gastrointestinal/Hepatic
Abdominal pain (14–16%)
Constipation (27–31%) [3]
Diarrhea (17–24%)
Dyspepsia (10%)
Dysphagia (5–10%)
Hepatotoxicity [3]
Nausea (29–46%) [12]
Vomiting (14–32%) [2]

Respiratory
Cough (12–22%)
Dyspnea (22–27%)
Flu-like syndrome [8]
Pharyngolaryngeal pain (8%)
Upper respiratory tract infection (10%)

Endocrine/Metabolic
Appetite decreased (13%)
Creatine phosphokinase increased [2]
Dehydration (5–14%)
Hyperparathyroidism [2]
Hypocalcemia (5–10%) [24]
Hypokalemia (12%)
Hypomagnesemia (11%)
Hypophosphatemia (13%) [3]
Weight loss (16%)

Genitourinary
Urinary tract infection (12–14%)

Renal
Fanconi syndrome [2]
Nephrotoxicity [13]
Renal failure [4]
Renal function abnormal [2]

Hematologic
Anemia (22–33%) [8]
Granulocytopenia (5–10%)
Neutropenia (12%)
Pancytopenia (5–10%)
Thrombocytopenia (5–10%)

Ocular
Ocular adverse effects [2]
Ocular inflammation [3]
Scleritis [2]
Uveitis [9]

Other
Adverse effects [6]
Infection (5–10%)

ZOLMITRIPTAN

Trade name: Zomig (AstraZeneca)
Indications: Migraine attacks
Class: 5-HT1 agonist, Serotonin receptor agonist, Triptan
Half-life: 3 hours
Clinically important, potentially hazardous interactions with: cimetidine, ciprofloxacin, dihydroergotamine, ergot-containing drugs, fluoxetine, fluvoxamine, isocarboxazid, levofloxacin, MAO inhibitors, methysergide, moclobemide, moxifloxacin, naratriptan, norfloxacin, ofloxacin, oral contraceptives, phenelzine, propranolol, rizatriptan, sertraline, sibutramine, SNRIs, SSRIs, St John's wort, sumatriptan, tranylcypromine
Pregnancy category: C
Important contra-indications noted in the prescribing guidelines for: nursing mothers; pediatric patients

---

Skin
Diaphoresis (2–3%)
Hot flashes (>10%)

Mucosal
Xerostomia (3–5%)

Cardiovascular
Chest pain (2–4%)
Myocardial infarction [4]

Central Nervous System
Dysgeusia (taste perversion) [4]
Headache [2]
Neurotoxicity [2]
Paresthesias (5–9%) [5]
Somnolence (drowsiness) (5–8%)
Vertigo (dizziness) (2–10%) [2]
Warm feeling (5–7%)

Neuromuscular/Skeletal
Jaw pain (4–10%)
Myalgia/Myopathy (2%) [2]
Neck pain (4–10%)

Gastrointestinal/Hepatic
Dyspepsia (<3%)
Dysphagia (<2%)
Nausea (4–9%)

Renal
Nephrotoxicity [2]

Other
Adverse effects [6]

ZOLPIDEM

Trade name: Ambien (Sanofi-Aventis)
Indications: Insomnia
Class: Hypnotic, non-benzodiazepine
Half-life: 2.6 hours
Clinically important, potentially hazardous interactions with: alcohol, antihistamines, azatadine, azelastine, brompheniramine, buclizine, chlorpheniramine, chlorpromazine, cimetidine, clemastine, cobicistat/elvitegravir/emtricitabine/tenofovir disoproxil, dexchlorpheniramine, erythromycin, imipramine, ketoconazole, meclizine, pizotifen, ramelteon, rifampin, rifapentine, ritonavir, telaprevir, voriconazole
Pregnancy category: C
Important contra-indications noted in the prescribing guidelines for: nursing mothers; pediatric patients

---

Skin
Rash (2%)

Mucosal
Xerostomia (3%) [3]

Cardiovascular
Palpitation (2%)
Tachycardia [2]
Torsades de pointes [2]

Central Nervous System
Amnesia [16]
Anxiety [2]
Compulsions [2]
Confusion [3]
Delirium [5]
Depression (2%)
Dysgeusia (taste perversion) [4]
Gait instability [3]
Hallucinations [13]
Headache (7%) [11]
Nightmares [2]
Seizures [7]
Sleep related disorder [19]
Slurred speech [2]
Somnambulism [15]
Somnolence (drowsiness) (2–8%) [10]
Vertigo (dizziness) (<5%) [12]

Neuromuscular/Skeletal
Asthenia (fatigue) (3%) [4]
Ataxia [3]
Back pain (3%)
Fractures [2]
Myalgia/Myopathy (7%)

Gastrointestinal/Hepatic
Abdominal pain (2%)
Constipation (2%)
Diarrhea (<3%)
Hepatotoxicity [2]
Nausea [5]
Vomiting [2]

Respiratory
Flu-like syndrome (2%)
Pharyngitis (3%)
Sinusitis (4%)

Ocular
Hallucinations, visual [8]

Other
Adverse effects [8]
Allergic reactions (4%)

ZONISAMIDE

Trade name: Zonegran (Concordia)
Indications: Epilepsy
Class: Anticonvulsant, Antiepileptic, sulfonamide
Half-life: 63 hours
Clinically important, potentially hazardous interactions with: caffeine, metformin
Pregnancy category: C
Important contra-indications noted in the prescribing guidelines for: nursing mothers; pediatric patients
Note: Zonisamide is a sulfonamide and can be absorbed systemically. Sulfonamides can produce severe, possibly fatal, reactions such as toxic epidermal necrolysis and Stevens-Johnson syndrome.

Skin
DRESS syndrome [3]
Ecchymoses (2%)
Hypersensitivity [4]
Oligohydrosis [8]
Purpura (2%)
Rash (3%) [6]
Stevens-Johnson syndrome [3]

Mucosal
Xerostomia (2%)

Central Nervous System
Agitation (9%) [4]
Anorexia (13%) [9]
Anxiety (3%)
Cognitive impairment (6%) [4]
Confusion (6%)
Depression (6%) [4]
Dysgeusia (taste perversion) (2%)
Fever [2]
Headache (10%) [7]
Insomnia (6%)
Irritability (9%) [3]
Mania [2]
Nervousness (2%)
Neuroleptic malignant syndrome [2]
Paresthesias (4%)
Psychosis [3]
Restless legs syndrome [3]
Schizophrenia (2%)
Somnolence (drowsiness) (17%) [21]
Speech disorder (2–5%)
Suicidal ideation [2]
Vertigo (dizziness) (13%) [17]

Neuromuscular/Skeletal
Asthenia (fatigue) (7–8%) [8]
Ataxia (6%) [2]

Gastrointestinal/Hepatic
Abdominal pain (6%)
Constipation (2%)
Diarrhea (5%)
Dyspepsia (3%)
Nausea (9%) [2]
Vomiting [2]

Respiratory
Flu-like syndrome (4%)
Pneumonitis [2]
Rhinitis (2%)

Endocrine/Metabolic
Appetite decreased [6]
Weight loss (3%) [19]

Renal
Nephrolithiasis [4]
Nephrotoxicity [2]

Ocular
Diplopia (6%)
Nystagmus (4%)

Other
Adverse effects [12]
Side effects [4]
Teratogenicity [2]

ZOSTER VACCINE

Trade name: Zostavax (Oka/Merck)
Indications: To reduce the risk of developing herpes zoster (in people over 60)
Class: Vaccine
Half-life: N/A
Clinically important, potentially hazardous interactions with: none known
Pregnancy category: C

Skin
Herpes zoster [7]
Rash [2]

Central Nervous System
Fever (<2%)
Headache [4]

Respiratory
Flu-like syndrome (<2%)

Local
Injection-site edema [2]
Injection-site erythema [2]
Injection-site pain [2]
Injection-site reactions [8]

Other
Adverse effects [2]
Death [2]

ZOTAROLIMUS

Trade names: Endeavor (Medtronic), ZoMaxx Drug-Eluting Coronary Stent (AbbVie)
Indications: Ischemic heart disease, restenosis
Class: Angiogenesis inhibitor, Macrolide immunosuppressant (derivative of sirolimus), mTOR inhibitor
Half-life: 33–36 hours
Clinically important, potentially hazardous interactions with: ketoconazole, sirolimus
Pregnancy category: C
Important contra-indications noted in the prescribing guidelines for: nursing mothers; pediatric patients

---

Skin
Rash (<6%)
Xerosis (<13%)

Cardiovascular
Cardiotoxicity [4]
Myocardial infarction [3]
Subacute thrombosis [2]

Central Nervous System
Headache (4–13%)
Pain (13–63%)

Gastrointestinal/Hepatic
Abdominal pain (<6%)
Diarrhea (<6%)

Genitourinary
Hematuria (<13%)

Local
Application-site reactions (13–63%)
Injection-site reactions (13–38%)

Descriptions of Important Reactions

Acanthosis nigricans

Acanthosis nigricans (AN) is a process characterized by a soft, velvety, brown or grayish-black thickening of the skin that is symmetrically distributed over the axillae, neck, inguinal areas and other body folds.

While most cases of AN are seen in obese and prepubertal children, it can occur as a marker for various endocrinopathies as well as in female patients with elevated testosterone levels, irregular menses, and hirsutism.

It is frequently a concomitant of an underlying malignant condition, principally an adenocarcinoma of the intestinal tract.

Acneform lesions

Acneform eruptions are inflammatory follicular reactions that resemble acne vulgaris and that are manifested clinically as papules or pustules. They are monomorphic reactions, have a monomorphic appearance, and are found primarily on the upper parts of the body. Unlike acne vulgaris, there are rarely comedones present. Consider a drug-induced acneform eruption if:

- The onset is sudden
- There is a worsening of existing acne lesions
- The extent is considerable from the outset
- The appearance is monomorphic
- The localization is unusual for acne as, for example, when the distal extremities are involved
- The patient's age is unusual for regular acne
- There is an exposure to a potentially responsible drug.

The most common drugs responsible for acneform eruptions are: ACTH, androgenic hormones, anticonvulsants (hydantoin derivatives, phenobarbital, trimethadione), corticosteroids, danazol, disulfiram, halogens (bromides, chlorides, iodides), lithium, oral contraceptives, tuberculostatics (ethionamide, isoniazid, rifampin), vitamins B_2, B_6 and B_{12}.

Acute febrile neutrophilic dermatosis

Acute febrile neutrophilic dermatosis is a disorder that appears more frequently in females and has several characteristic features.

The lesions - tender, erythematous or purple, annular plaques or nodules - appear suddenly and are most prominent on the face, neck and upper extremities. Pain and fever often accompany the eruption.

While the cause is unknown, about 15% of the patients have some type of myeloproliferative disorder, primarily leukemias.

Drugs commonly reported to cause Sweet's syndrome are clofazimine, co-trimoxazole, furosemide, granulocyte-colony stimulating factor and minocycline.

Acute generalized exanthematous pustulosis

Arising on the face or intertriginous areas, acute generalized exanthematous pustulosis (AGEP) is characterized by a rapidly evolving, widespread, scarlatiniform eruption covered with hundreds of small superficial pustules.

Often accompanied by a high fever, AGEP is most frequently associated with acetaminophen, carbamazepine, penicillin and macrolide antibiotics, and usually occurs within 24 hours of the drug exposure.

Ageusia

Ageusia is the loss of taste functions of the tongue, essentially the inability to detect sweet, sour, bitter, or salty substances, and umami (the taste of monosodium glutamate).

Atorvastatin, captopril, enalapril, indomethacin, and paroxetine are some of the drugs that can occasion ageusia.

Alopecia

Many drugs have been reported to occasion hair loss. Commonly appearing as a diffuse alopecia, it affects women more frequently than men and is limited in most instances to the scalp. Axillary and pubic hairs are rarely affected except with anticoagulants.

The hair loss from cytostatic agents, which is dose-dependent and begins about 2 weeks after the onset of therapy, is a result of the interruption of the anagen (growing) cycle of hair. With other drugs the hair loss does not begin until 2–5 months after the medication has been begun. With cholesterol-lowering drugs, diffuse alopecia is a result of interference with normal keratinization.

The scalp is normal and the drug-induced alopecia is almost always reversible within 1–3 months after the therapy has been discontinued. The regrown hair is frequently depigmented and occasionally more curly

The most frequent offenders are cytostatic agents and anticoagulants, but hair loss can occur with a variety of common drugs, including hormones, anticonvulsants, amantadine, amiodarone, captopril, cholesterol-lowering drugs, cimetidine, colchicine, etretinate, isotretinoin, ketoconazole, heavy metals, lithium, penicillamine, valproic acid, and propranolol.

Angioedema

Angioedema is a term applied to a variant of urticaria in which the subcutaneous tissues, rather than the dermis, are mainly involved.

Also known as Quincke's edema, giant urticaria, and angioneurotic edema, this acute, evanescent, skin-colored, circumscribed edema usually affects the most distensible tissues: the lips, eyelids, earlobes, and genitalia. It can also affect the mucous membranes of the tongue, mouth, and larynx.

Symptoms of angioedema, frequently unilateral, asymmetrical and non-pruritic, last for an hour or two but can persist for 2–5 days.

The etiological factors associated with angioedema are as varied as that of urticaria (see separate entry).

Anosmia

Anosmia, or odor blindness, is the total absence of the sense of smell. It can be either temporary or permanent.

Some of the drugs that can cause anosmia are ciprofloxacin, doxycycline, enalapril, paroxetine and sparfloxacin.

Aphthous stomatitis

Aphthous stomatitis – also known as canker sores – is a common disease of the oral mucous membranes.

Arising as tiny, discrete or grouped, papules or vesicles, these painful lesions develop into small (2–5 mm in diameter), round, shallow ulcerations having a grayish, yellow base surrounded by a thin red border.

Located predominantly over the labial and buccal mucosae, these aphthae heal without scarring in 10–14 days. Recurrences are common.

Baboon syndrome (SDRIFE)

Baboon syndrome or symmetric drug-related intertriginous and flexural exanthema (SDRIFE) is an unusual presentation of a drug eruption with a characteristic intertriginous distribution pattern. Several drugs have been implicated, notably mercury, nickel, heparin, aminophylline, pseudoephedrine, terbinafine, IVIG, various antibiotics (amoxicillin, ampicillin), and food additives.

Originally described as a type of systemic contact dermatitis characterized by a pruritic exanthems involving the buttocks and major flexures – groins and axillae, some investigators believe that this entity is a form of recall phenomenon. In children, it is important in the differential diagnosis of viral exanthems.

Black tongue (lingua villosa nigra)

Black hairy tongue (BHT) represents a benign hyperplasia of the filiform papillae of the anterior two-thirds of the tongue.

These papillary elongations, usually associated with black, brown, or yellow pigmentation attributed to the overgrowth of pigment-producing bacteria, may be as long as 2 cm.

Occurring only in adults, BHT has been associated with the administration of oral antibiotics, poor dental hygiene, and excessive smoking.

Bullous dermatitis

Bullous and vesicular drug eruptions are diseases in which blisters and vesicles occur as a complication of the administration of drugs. Blisters are a well-known manifestation of cutaneous reactions to drugs.

In many types of drug reactions, bullae and vesicles may be found in addition to other manifestations. Bullae are usually noted in: erythema multiforme; Stevens–Johnson syndrome; toxic epidermal necrolysis; fixed eruptions when very intense; urticaria; vasculitis; porphyria cutanea tarda; and phototoxic reactions (from furosemide and nalidixic acid). Tense, thick-walled bullae can be seen in bromoderma and iododerma as well as in barbiturate overdosage.

Common drugs that cause bullous eruptions and bullous pemphigoid are: nadalol, penicillamine, piroxicam, psoralens, rifampin, clonidine, furosemide, diclofenac, mefenamic acid, and bleomycin.

DRESS syndrome

The DRESS syndrome is an acronym for Drug Rash with Eosinophilia and Systemic Symptoms. It is also known as the Drug-Induced Pseudolymphoma and Drug Hypersensitivity Syndrome.

The symptoms of DRESS syndrome usually begin 1 to 8 weeks after exposure to the offending drug. Common causes include carbamazepine, phenobarbital, phenytoin, terbinafine, and valproic acid.

Erythema multiforme

Erythema multiforme is a relatively common, acute, self-limited, inflammatory reaction pattern that is often associated with a preceding herpes simplex or mycoplasma infection. Other causes are associated with connective tissue disease, physical agents, X-ray therapy, pregnancy and internal malignancies, to mention a few. In 50% of the cases, no cause can be found. In a recent prospective study of erythema multiforme, only 10% were drug related.

The eruption rapidly occurs over a period of 12 to 24 hours. In about half the cases there are prodromal symptoms of an upper respiratory infection accompanied by fever, malaise, and varying degrees of muscular and joint pains.

Clinically, bluish-red, well-demarcated, macular, papular, or urticarial lesions, as well as the classical 'iris' or 'target lesions', sometimes with central vesicles, bullae, or purpura, are distributed preferentially over the distal extremities, especially over the dorsa of the hands and extensor aspects of the forearms. Lesions tend to spread peripherally and may involve the palms and trunk as well as the mucous membranes of the mouth and genitalia. Central healing and overlapping lesions often lead to arciform, annular and gyrate patterns. Lesions appear over the course of a week or 10 days and resolve over the next two weeks.

The following drugs have been most often associated with erythema multiforme: allopurinol, barbiturates, carbamazepine, estrogens/progestins, gold, lamotrigine, NSAIDs, penicillamine, phenytoin, sulfonamides, tetracycline, tolbutamide and valproic acid.

Erythema nodosum

Erythema nodosum is a cutaneous reaction pattern characterized by erythematous, tender or painful subcutaneous nodules commonly distributed over the anterior aspect of the lower legs, and occasionally elsewhere.

More common in young women, erythema nodosum is often associated with increased estrogen levels as occurs during pregnancy and with the ingestion of oral contraceptives. It is also an occasional manifestation of streptococcal infection, sarcoidosis, secondary syphilis, tuberculosis, certain deep fungal infections, Hodgkin's disease, leukemia, ulcerative colitis, and radiation therapy and is often preceded by fever, fatigue, arthralgia, vomiting, and diarrhea.

The incidence of erythema nodosum due to drugs is low and it is impossible to distinguish clinically between erythema nodosum due to drugs and that caused by other factors.

Some of the drugs that are known to occasion erythema nodosum are: antibiotics, estrogens, amiodarone, gold, NSAIDs, oral contraceptives, sulfonamides, and opiates.

Exanthems

Exanthems, commonly resembling viral rashes, represent the most common type of cutaneous drug eruption. Described as maculopapular or morbilliform eruptions, these flat, barely raised, erythematous patches, from one to several millimeters in diameter, are usually bilateral and symmetrical. They commonly begin on the head and neck or upper torso and progress downward to the limbs. They may present or develop into confluent areas and may be accompanied by pruritus and a mild fever.

The exanthems caused by drugs can be classified as:

- Morbilliform eruptions: fingernail-sized erythematous patches
- Scarlatiniform eruptions: punctate, pinpoint, or pinhead-sized lesions in erythematous areas that have a tendency to coalesce. Circumoral pallor and the subsequent appearance of scaling may also be noted.

Maculopapular drug eruptions usually fade with desquamation and, occasionally, postinflammatory hyperpigmentation, in about 2 weeks. They invariably recur on rechallenge.

Exanthems often have a sudden onset during the first 2 weeks of administration, except in cases of semisynthetic penicillin administration, when the exanthems frequently develop after the first 2 weeks following the initial dose.

The drugs most commonly associated with exanthems are: amoxicillin, ampicillin, bleomycin, captopril, carbamazepine, chlorpromazine, cotrimoxazole, gold, nalidixic acid, naproxen, phenytoin, penicillamine, and piroxicam.

Exfoliative dermatitis

Exfoliative dermatitis is a rare but serious reaction pattern that is characterized by erythema, pruritus and scaling over the entire body (erythroderma).

Drug-induced exfoliative dermatitis usually begins a few weeks or longer following the administration of a culpable drug. Beginning as erythematous, edematous patches, often on the face, it spreads to involve the entire integument. The skin becomes swollen and scarlet and may ooze a straw-colored fluid; this is followed in a few days by desquamation.

High fever, severe malaise and chills, along with enlargement of lymph nodes, often coexist with the cutaneous changes.

One of the most dangerous of all reaction patterns, exfoliative dermatitis can be accompanied by any or all of the following: hypothermia, fluid and electrolyte loss, cardiac failure, and gastrointestinal hemorrhage. Death may supervene if the drug is continued after the onset of the eruption. Secondary infection often complicates the course of the disease. Once the active dermatitis has receded, hyperpigmentation as well as loss of hair and nails may ensue.

The following drugs, among others, can bring about exfoliative dermatitis: barbiturates, captopril, carbamazepine, cimetidine, furosemide, gold, isoniazid, lithium, nitrofurantoin, NSAIDs, penicillamine, phenytoin, pyrazolons, quinidine, streptomycin, sulfonamides, and thiazides.

Fixed eruption

A fixed eruption is an unusual hypersensitivity reaction characterized by one or more well-demarcated erythematous plaques that recur at the same cutaneous (or mucosal) site or sites each time exposure to the offending agent occurs. The sizes of the lesions vary from a few millimeters to as much as 20 centimeters in diameter. Almost any drug that is ingested, injected, inhaled, or inserted into the body can trigger this skin reaction.

The eruption typically begins as a sharply marginated, solitary edematous papule or plaque – occasionally surmounted by a large bulla – which usually develops 30 minutes to 8 hours following the administration of a drug. If the offending agent is not promptly eliminated, the inflammation intensifies, producing a dusky red, violaceous or brown patch that may crust, desquamate, or blister within 7 to 10 days. The lesions are rarely pruritic. Favored sites are the hands, feet, face, and genitalia – especially the glans penis.

The reason for the specific localization of the skin lesions in a fixed drug eruption is unknown. The offending drug cannot be detected at the skin site. Certain drugs cause a fixed eruption at specific sites, for example, tetracycline and ampicillin often elicit a fixed eruption on the penis, whereas aspirin usually causes skin lesions on the face, limbs and trunk.

Common causes of fixed eruptions are: ampicillin, aspirin, barbiturates, dapsone, metronidazole, NSAIDs, oral contraceptives, phenolphthalein, phenytoin, quinine, sulfonamides, and tetracyclines.

Gingival hyperplasia/hypertrophy

Gingival hyperplasia, a common, undesirable, non-allergic drug reaction begins as a diffuse swelling of the interdental papillae.

Particularly prevalent with phenytoin therapy, gingival hyperplasia begins about 3 months after the onset of therapy, and occurs in 30 to 70% of patients receiving it. The severity of the reaction is dose-dependent and children and young adults are more frequently affected. The most severe cases are noted in young women.

In many cases, gingival hyperplasia is accompanied by painful and bleeding gums. There is often superimposed secondary bacterial gingivitis. This can be so extensive that the teeth of the maxilla and mandible are completely overgrown.

While it is characteristically a side effect of hydantoin derivatives, it may occur during the administration of phenobarbital, nifedipine, diltiazem and other medications.

Hand-foot syndrome

Hand-foot syndrome (also known as acral erythema, palmar-plantar erythrodysesthesia, palmoplantar erythrodysesthesia, palmar-plantar erythema, and Bergdorf's reaction) is a syndrome that is characterized by well-demarcated painful erythema, edema, numbness and desquamation over the palms and soles that may develop following treatment with a variety of chemotherapeutic agents including bleomycin, cisplatin, cyclophosphamide, hydroxyurea, idarubicin, methotrexate, sorafenib, sunitinib, and others. Tenderness involving the skin overlying the fingers and toes, followed by bulla formation and subsequent desquamation, often supervenes.

This side effect results when a small amount of the culpable drug leaks out of the blood vessels, damaging tissues. This reaction predominates over the palms and soles, where eccrine glands are more numerous, and also as a result of the increased friction and heat that extremities are exposed to through daily activities.

Lichenoid (lichen planus-like) eruptions

Lichenoid eruptions are so called because of their resemblance to lichen planus, a papulosquamous disorder that characteristically presents as multiple, discrete, violaceous, flat-topped papules, often polygonal in shape and which are extremely pruritic.

Not infrequently, lichenoid lesions appear weeks or months following exposure to the responsible drug. As a rule, the symptoms begin to recede a few weeks following the discontinuation of the drug.

Common drug causes of lichenoid eruptions are: antimalarials, beta-blockers, chlorpropamide, furosemide, gold, methyldopa, phenothiazines, quinidine, thiazides, and tolazamide.

Lupus erythematosus

A reaction, clinically and pathologically resembling idiopathic systemic lupus erythematosus (SLE), has been reported in association with a large variety of drugs. There is some evidence that drug-induced SLE, invariably accompanied by a positive ANA reaction with 90% having antihistone antibodies, may have a genetically determined basis. These symptoms of SLE, a relatively benign form of lupus, recede within days or weeks following the discontinuation of the responsible drug. Skin lesions occur in about 20% of cases. Drugs cause fewer than 8% of all cases of SLE.

The following drugs have been commonly associated with inducing, aggravating or unmasking SLE: beta-blockers, carbamazepine, chlorpromazine, estrogens, griseofulvin, hydralazine, isoniazid (INH), lithium, methyldopa, minoxidil, oral contraceptives, penicillamine, phenytoin (diphenylhydantoin), procainamide, propylthiouracil, quinidine, and testosterone.

Onycholysis

Onycholysis, the painless separation of the nail plate from the nail bed, is one of the most common nail disorders.

The unattached portion, which is white and opaque, usually begins at the free margin and proceeds proximally, causing part or most of the nail plate to become separated. The attached, healthy portion of the nail, by contrast, is pink and translucent.

Paresthesias

Paresthesias are abnormal neurological sensations such as burning, prickling, numbness, pruritus, formication, or tingling, often described as 'pins and needles' or of a limb being 'asleep'. It is a symptom of partial damage to a peripheral nerve, as occurs from a head or spinal injury, lack of blood supply to a nerve, or in many cases medications.

Paresthesias can affect various parts of the body; hands, fingers, and feet are common sites but all areas are possibilities.

Scores of generic drugs have been reported to occasion paresthesias including alprazolam, allopurinol, buspirone, celecoxib, ciprofloxacin, cyclosporine, enalapril, glipizine and many others.

Pemphigus vulgaris

Pemphigus vulgaris (PV) is a rare, serious, acute or chronic, blistering disease involving the skin and mucous membranes.

Characterized by thin-walled, easily ruptured, flaccid bullae that are seen to arise on normal or erythematous skin and over mucous membranes, the lesions of PV appear initially in the mouth (in about 60% of the cases) and then spread, after weeks or months, to involve the axillae and groin, scalp, face and neck. The lesions may become generalized.

Because of their fragile roofs, the bullae rupture leaving painful erosions and crusts may develop principally over the scalp.

Peyronie's disease

First described in 1743 by the French surgeon, Francois de la Peyronie, Peyronie's disease is a rare, benign connective tissue disorder involving the growth of fibrous plaques in the soft tissue of the penis. Beginning as a localized inflammation, it often develops into a hardened scar. Affecting as many as 1% of men, it may cause deformity, pain, cord-like lesions, or abnormal curvature of the penis when erect.

It has been associated with several drugs, including all the adrenergic blocking agents (beta-blockers), methotrexate, colchicine and others.

Photosensitivity

A photosensitive reaction is a chemically induced change in the skin that makes an individual unusually sensitive to electromagnetic radiation (light). On absorbing light of a specific wavelength, an oral, injected or topical drug may be chemically altered to produce a reaction ranging from macules and papules, vesicles and bullae, edema, urticaria, or an acute eczematous reaction.

Any eruption that is prominent on the face, the dorsa of the hands, the 'V' of the neck, and the presternal area should suggest an adverse reaction to light. The distribution is the key to the diagnosis.

Initially the eruption, which consists of erythema, edema, blisters, weeping and desquamation, involves the forehead, rims of the ears, the nose, the malar eminences and cheeks, the sides and back of the neck, the extensor surfaces of the forearms and the dorsa of the hands. These reactions commonly spare the shaded areas: those under the chin, under the nose, behind the ears and inside the fold of the upper eyelids. There is usually a sharp cut-off at the site of jewelry and at clothing margins. All light-exposed areas need not be affected equally.

There are two main types of photosensitive reactions: the phototoxic and the photoallergic reaction.

Phototoxic reactions, the most common type of drug-induced photosensitivity, resemble an exaggerated sunburn and occur within 5 to 20 hours after the skin has been exposed to a photosensitizing substance and light of the proper wavelength and intensity. It is not a form of allergy – prior sensitization is not required – and, theoretically, could occur in anyone given enough drug and light. Phototoxic reactions are dose-dependent both for drug and sunlight. Patients with phototoxicity reactions are commonly sensitive to ultraviolet A (UVA radiation), the so-called 'tanning rays' at 320–400 nm. Phototoxic reactions may cause onycholysis, as the nailbed is particularly susceptible because of its lack of melanin protection.

Patients with a true photoallergy (the interaction of drug, light and the immune system), a less common form of drug-induced photosensitivity, are often sensitive to UVB radiation, the so-called 'burning rays' at 290–320 nm. Photoallergic reactions, unlike phototoxic responses, represent an immunologic change and require a latent period of from 24 to 48 hours during which sensitization occurs. They are not dose-related.

If the photosensitizer acts internally, it is a photodrug reaction; if it acts externally, it is photocontact dermatitis.

Drugs that are likely to cause phototoxic reactions are: amiodarone, nalidixic acid, various NSAIDs, phenothiazines (especially chlorpromazine), and tetracyclines (particularly demeclocycline).

Photoallergic reactions may occur as a result of exposure to systemically-administered drugs such as griseofulvin, NSAIDs, phenothiazines, quinidine, sulfonamides, sulfonylureas, and thiazide diuretics as well as to external agents such as para-aminobenzoic acid (found in sunscreens), bithionol (used in soaps and cosmetics), paraphenylenediamine, and others.

Pigmentation

Drug-induced pigmentation on the skin, hair, nails, and mucous membranes is a result of either melanin synthesis, increased lipofuscin synthesis, or post-inflammatory pigmentation.

Color changes, which can be localized or widespread, can also be a result of a deposition of bile pigments (jaundice), exogenous metal compounds, and direct deposition of elements such as carotene or quinacrine.

Post-inflammatory pigmentation can follow a variety of drug-induced inflammatory cutaneous reactions; fixed eruptions are known to leave a residual pigmentation that can persist for months.

The following is a partial list of those drugs that can cause various pigmentary changes: anticonvulsants, antimalarials, cytostatics, hormones, metals, tetracyclines, phenothiazine tranquilizers, psoralens and amiodarone.

Pityriasis rosea-like eruption

Pityriasis rosea, commonly mistaken for ringworm, is a unique disorder that usually begins as a single, large, round or oval pinkish patch known as the 'mother' or 'herald' patch. The most common sites for this solitary lesion are the chest, the back, or the abdomen. This is followed in about 2 weeks by a blossoming of small, flat, round or oval, scaly patches of similar color, each with a central collarette scale, usually distributed in a Christmas tree pattern over the trunk and, to a lesser degree, the extremities. This eruption seldom itches and usually limits itself to areas from the neck to the knees.

While the etiology of idiopathic pityriasis rosea is unknown, various medications have been reported to give rise to this disorder. These include: barbiturates, beta-blockers, bismuth, captopril, clonidine, gold, griseofulvin, isotretinoin, labetalol, meprobamate, metronidazole, penicillin, and tripelennamine.

In drug-induced pityriasis rosea, the 'herald patch' is usually absent, and the eruption will often not follow the classic pattern.

Pruritus

Generalized itching, without any visible signs, is one of the least common adverse reactions to drugs. More frequently than not, drug-induced itching – moderate or severe – is fairly generalized.

For most drugs it is not known in what way they elicit pruritus; some drugs can cause itching directly or indirectly through cholestasis. Pruritus may develop by different pathogenetic mechanisms: allergic, pseudoallergic (histamine release), neurogenic, by vasodilatation, cholestatic effect, and others.

A partial list of those drugs that can cause pruritus are as follows: aspirin, NSAIDs, penicillins, sulfonamides, chloroquine, ACE-inhibitors, amiodarone, nicotinic acid derivatives, lithium, bleomycin, tamoxifen, interferons, gold, penicillamine, methoxsalen and isotretinoin.

Pseudolymphoma

Pseudolymphoma is not a specific disease. It is an inflammatory response to various stimuli – known or unknown – that results in a lymphomatous-appearing, but benign, accumulation of inflammatory cells. It may resemble true lymphoma clinically and histologically. Localized, nodular pseudolymphomas typically mimic B-cell lymphoma.

The following drugs, among others, are known to occasion pseudolymphoma: alprazolam, carbamazepine, co-trimoxazole, gold, lamotrigine, lithium, methotrexate, etc.

Pseudoporphyria

Pseudoporphyria is an uncommon, reversible, photoinduced, cutaneous bullous disorder with clinical, histologic and immunofluorescent similarities to porphyria cutanea tarda but without the accompanying biochemical porphyrin abnormalities.

It is commonly seen as localized bullae and skin fragility on sun-exposed skin, often on the dorsum of the hands and fingers. While pseudoporphyria has been linked with numerous causes, including chronic renal failure, dialysis, and ultraviolet radiation, several medications, primarily naproxen and other nonsteroidal inflammatory drugs, have been reported to trigger this reaction pattern. Blue/gray eye color appears to be an independent risk factor for the development of pseudoporphyria.

Psoriasis

Many drugs, as a result of their pharmacological action, have been implicated in the precipitation or exacerbation of psoriasis or psoriasiform eruptions.

Psoriasis is a common, chronic, papulosquamous disorder of unknown etiology with characteristic histopathological features and many biochemical, physiological, and immunological abnormalities.

Drugs that can precipitate psoriasis are, among others, beta-blockers and lithium. Drugs that are reported to aggravate psoriasis are antimalarials, beta-blockers, lithium, NSAIDs, quinidine, and photosensitizing drugs. The effect and extent of these drug-induced psoriatic eruptions are dose-dependent.

Purpura

Purpura, a result of hemorrhage into the skin, can be divided into thrombocytopenic purpura and non-thrombocytopenic purpura (vascular purpura). Both thrombocytopenic and vascular purpura may be due to drugs, and most of the drugs producing purpura may do so by giving rise to vascular damage and thrombocytopenia. In both types of purpura, allergic or toxic (nonallergic) mechanisms may be involved.

Some drugs combine with platelets to form an antigen, stimulating formation of antibody to the platelet–drug combination. Thus, the drug appears to act as a hapten; subsequent antigen–antibody reaction causes platelet destruction leading to thrombocytopenia.

The purpuric lesions are usually more marked over the lower portions of the body, notably the legs and dorsal aspects of the feet in ambulatory patients.

Other drug-induced cutaneous reactions – erythema multiforme, erythema nodosum, fixed eruption, necrotizing vasculitis, and others – can have a prominent purpuric component.

A whole host of drugs can give rise to purpura, the most common being: NSAIDs, thiazide diuretics, phenothiazines, cytostatics, gold, penicillamine, hydantoins, thiouracils, and sulfonamides.

Raynaud's phenomenon

Raynaud's phenomenon is the paroxysmal, cold-induced constriction of small arteries and arterioles of the fingers and, less often, the toes.

Although estimates vary, recent surveys show that Raynaud's phenomenon may affect 5 to 10 percent of the general population in the United States. Occurring more frequently in women, Raynaud's phenomenon is characterized by blanching, pallor, and cyanosis. In severe cases, secondary changes may occur: thinning and ridging of the nails, telangiectases of the nail folds, and, in the later stages, sclerosis and atrophy of the digits.

Rhabdomyolysis

Rhabdomyolysis is the breakdown of muscle fibers, the result of skeletal muscle injury, that leads to the release of potentially toxic intracellular contents into the plasma. The causes are diverse: muscle trauma from vigorous exercise, electrolyte imbalance, extensive thermal burns, crush injuries, infections, various toxins and drugs, and a host of other factors.

Rhabdomyolysis can result from direct muscle injury by myotoxic drugs such as cocaine, heroin and alcohol. About 10–40% of patients with rhabdomyolysis develop acute renal failure.

The classic triad of symptoms of rhabdomyolysis is muscle pain, weakness and dark urine. Most frequently, the involved muscle groups are those of the back and lower calves. The primary diagnostic indicator of this syndrome is significantly elevated serum creatine phosphokinase.

Some of the drugs that have been reported to cause rhabdomyolysis are salicylates, amphotericin, quinine, statin drugs, SSRIs, theophylline, and amphetamines.

Stevens–Johnson syndrome

The Stevens–Johnson syndrome (erythema multiforme major), a severe and occasionally fatal variety of erythema multiforme, has an abrupt onset and is accompanied by any or all of the following: fever, myalgia, malaise, headache, arthralgia, ocular involvement, with occasional bullae and erosions covering less than 10% of the body surface. Painful stomatitis is an early and conspicuous symptom. Hemorrhagic bullae may appear over the lips, mouth and genital mucous membranes. Patients are often acutely ill with high fever. The course from eruption to the healing of the lesions may extend up to six weeks.

The following drugs have been most often associated with Stevens-Johnson syndrome: allopurinol, barbiturates, carbamazepine, estrogens/progestins, gold, lamotrigine, NSAIDs, penicillamine, phenytoin, sulfonamides, tetracycline, tolbutamide, and valproic acid.

Tinnitus

Tinnitus (from the Latin word to tinkle or ring like a bell) is the perception of sound—ringing, buzzing, hissing, humming, whistling, whining, roaring, or ticking, clicking, banging, beeping, pulsating—in the human ear, when none exists. It has also been described as a 'whooshing' sound, like wind or waves, 'crickets' or 'tree frogs' or 'locusts.' To some it's a chirping, clanging, sizzling, rumbling, or a dreadful shrieking noise. And it can be like rushing water, breaking glass or chain saws running. Nearly 40 million Americans suffer from this disorder.

There are more than 200 drugs listed in the Litt's Drug Eruption & Reaction Database that have been reported to trigger tinnitus, the more common being aspirin, quinine, aminoglycoside antibiotics, cytotoxic drugs, diuretics, and NSAIDs.

Toxic epidermal necrolysis (TEN)

Also known as Lyell's syndrome, toxic epidermal necrolysis is a rare, serious, acute exfoliative, bullous eruption of the skin and mucous membranes that usually develops as a reaction to diverse drugs. TEN can also be a result of a bacterial or viral infection and can develop after radiation therapy or vaccinations.

In the drug-induced form of TEN, a morbilliform eruption accompanied by large red, tender areas of the skin will develop shortly after the drug has been administered. This progresses rapidly to blistering, and a widespread exfoliation of the epidermis develops dramatically over a very short period accompanied by high fever. The hairy parts of the body are usually spared. The mucous membranes and eyes are often involved.

The clinical picture resembles an extensive second-degree burn; the patient is acutely ill. Fatigue, vomiting, diarrhea and angina are prodromal symptoms. In a few hours the condition becomes grave.

TEN is a medical emergency and unless the offending agent is discontinued immediately, the outcome may be fatal in the course of a few days.

Drugs that are the most common cause of TEN are: allopurinol, ampicillin, amoxicillin, carbamazepine, NSAIDs, phenobarbital, pentamidine, phenytoin (diphenylhydantoin), pyrazolons, and sulfonamides.

Urticaria

Urticaria induced by drugs is, after exanthems, the second most common type of drug reaction. Urticaria, or hives, is a vascular reaction of the skin characterized by pruritic, erythematous wheals. These welts – or wheals – caused by localized edema, can vary in size from one millimeter in diameter to large palm-sized swellings, favor the covered areas (trunk, buttocks, chest), and are, more often than not, generalized. Urticaria usually develops within 36 hours following the administration of the responsible drug. Individual lesions rarely persist for more than 24 hours.

Urticaria may be the only symptom of drug sensitivity, or it may be a concomitant or followed by the manifestations of serum sickness. Urticaria may be accompanied by angioedema of the lips or eyelids. It may, on rare occasions, progress to anaphylactoid reactions or to anaphylaxis.

The following are the most common causes of drug-induced urticaria: antibiotics, notably penicillin (more commonly following parenteral administration than by ingestion), barbiturates, captopril, levamisole, NSAIDs, quinine, rifampin, sulfonamides, thiopental, and vancomycin.

Vasculitis

Drug-induced cutaneous necrotizing vasculitis, a clinicopathologic process characterized by inflammation and necrosis of blood vessels, often presents with a variety of small, palpable purpuric lesions most frequently distributed over the lower extremities: urticaria-like lesions, small ulcerations, and occasional hemorrhagic vesicles and pustules. The basic process involves an immunologically mediated response to antigens that result in vessel wall damage.

Beginning as small macules and papules, they ultimately eventuate into purpuric lesions and, in the more severe cases, into hemorrhagic blisters and frank ulcerations. A polymorphonuclear infiltrate and fibrinoid changes in the small dermal vessels characterize the vasculitic reaction.

Drugs that are commonly associated with vasculitis are: ACE-inhibitors, amiodarone, ampicillin, cimetidine, coumadin, furosemide, hydantoins, hydralazine, NSAIDs, pyrazolons, quinidine, sulfonamides, thiazides, and thiouracils.

Vertigo

Vertigo, a specific type of dizziness, is a feeling of unsteadiness. It is the sensation of spinning or swaying while actually remaining stationary with respect to the surroundings. It is a result of either motion sickness, a viral infection of the organs of balance, low blood sugar, or medications. It is a symptom of multiple sclerosis, carbon monoxide poisoning, and Meniere's disease.

Vertigo is one of the most common health problems in adults. According to the National Institutes of Health, about 40% of people in the United States experience vertigo at least once during their lifetime. Prevalence is higher in women and increases with age.

Classes of drugs that have been reported to trigger vertigo include, aminoglycoside antibiotics, antihypertensives, diuretics, vasodilators, phenothiazines, tranquilizers, antidepressants, anticonvulsants, hypnotics, analgesics, alcohol, caffeine, and tobacco.

Xerostomia

Xerostomia is a dryness of the oral cavity that makes speaking, chewing and swallowing difficult. Some people also experience changes in taste and salivary gland enlargement. Lack of saliva may predispose one to oral infection, such as candidiasis, and increase the risk of dental caries.

Resulting from a partial or complete absence of saliva production, xerostomia can be caused by more than 400 generic drugs.

Drugs that cause important reactions

Acanthosis nigricans
- Amprenavir
- Azathioprine
- Diethylstilbestrol
- Estrogens
- Fusidic Acid
- Heroin
- Insulin
- Mechlorethamine
- Methsuximide
- Methyltestosterone
- Niacin
- Niacinamide
- Oral Contraceptives
- Palifermin
- Prednisolone
- Prednisone
- Somatropin
- Thioridazine
- Tryptophan

Acneform lesions
- Acamprosate
- Acyclovir
- Adalimumab
- Adapalene
- Afatinib
- Alosetron
- Alprazolam
- Aminolevulinic Acid
- Androstenedione
- Aprepitant
- Aripiprazole
- Atorvastatin
- Azathioprine
- Basiliximab
- Bedaquiline
- Belatacept
- Betamethasone
- Bevacizumab
- Bexarotene
- Bosutinib
- Brimonidine
- Budesonide
- Bupropion
- Buserelin
- Buspirone
- Cabergoline
- Capecitabine
- Carbamazepine
- Ceritinib
- Cetirizine
- Cetuximab
- Chloral Hydrate
- Chlorotrianisene
- Cidofovir
- Ciprofloxacin
- Cisplatin
- Clobetasol
- Clofazimine
- Clomipramine
- Cobimetinib
- Crofelemer
- Cyanocobalamin
- Cyclophosphamide
- Cyclosporine
- Dabrafenib
- Daclizumab
- Dactinomycin
- Danazol
- Dantrolene
- Dapsone
- Dasatinib
- Demeclocycline
- Dexamethasone
- Dexlansoprazole
- Diazepam
- Diltiazem
- Disulfiram
- Doxycycline
- Duloxetine
- Efalizumab
- Eflornithine
- Epoetin Alfa
- Erlotinib
- Erythromycin
- Escitalopram
- Esmolol
- Esomeprazole
- Estazolam
- Estramustine
- Estrogens
- Eszopiclone
- Etanercept
- Ethionamide
- Everolimus
- Famotidine
- Felbamate
- Fenoprofen
- Finasteride
- Fluconazole
- Fluorides
- Fluorouracil
- Fluoxetine
- Fluoxymesterone
- Fluvoxamine
- Folic Acid
- Follitropin Alfa/Beta
- Fosphenytoin
- Gabapentin
- Ganciclovir
- Gefitinib
- Gemcitabine
- Gestrinone
- Glatiramer
- Gold & Gold Compounds
- Goserelin
- Granulocyte Colony-Stimulating Factor (G-CSF)
- Grepafloxacin
- Halothane
- Heroin
- Histrelin
- Hyaluronic Acid
- Hydroquinone
- Imatinib
- Infliximab
- Interferon Alfa
- Interferon Beta
- Irinotecan
- Isoniazid
- Isotretinoin
- Ivacaftor
- Ixazomib
- Lamotrigine
- Lansoprazole
- Lapatinib
- Leflunomide
- Lenalidomide
- Letrozole
- Leucovorin
- Levonorgestrel
- Lisdexamfetamine
- Lithium
- Lopinavir
- Maprotiline
- MDMA
- Medroxyprogesterone
- Mephenytoin
- Mesalamine
- Methotrexate
- Methoxsalen
- Methyltestosterone
- Minoxidil
- Mometasone
- Mycophenolate
- Nabumetone
- Nadolol
- Nafarelin
- Naltrexone
- Nandrolone
- Naratriptan
- Necitumumab
- Nefazodone
- Nicotine
- Nilotinib
- Nimodipine
- Nisoldipine
- Nitrofurantoin
- Nivolumab
- Nizatidine
- Olsalazine
- Oral Contraceptives
- Osimertinib
- Oxcarbazepine
- Paclitaxel
- Panitumumab
- Panobinostat
- Pantoprazole
- Paroxetine Hydrochloride
- Pentostatin
- Phenobarbital
- Phenylbutazone
- Phenytoin
- Pimecrolimus
- Ponatinib
- Potassium Iodide
- Prednisolone
- Prednisone
- Progestins
- Propafenone
- Propranolol
- Propylthiouracil
- Psoralens
- Pyrazinamide
- Pyridoxine
- Quinidine
- Quinine
- Ramipril
- Riboflavin
- Rifampin
- Rifapentine
- Risperidone
- Ritonavir
- Rufinamide
- Saquinavir
- Sertraline
- Sibutramine
- Simvastatin
- Sirolimus
- Smallpox Vaccine
- Sodium Oxybate
- Sorafenib
- Sparfloxacin
- Stanozolol
- Sunitinib
- Tacrine
- Temsirolimus
- Teriflunomide
- Testosterone
- Tetracycline
- Tiagabine
- Tibolone
- Tizanidine
- Topiramate
- Trametinib
- Trastuzumab
- Tretinoin
- Trioxsalen
- Triptorelin
- Ulipristal
- Valdecoxib
- Vandetanib
- Vemurafenib
- Venlafaxine
- Verapamil
- Vinblastine
- Vinorelbine
- Vorinostat
- Zalcitabine
- Zaleplon
- Zidovudine
- Zolpidem
- Zonisamide

Acute febrile neutrophilic dermatosis
- Abacavir
- Aceclofenac
- Aldesleukin
- Allopurinol
- Amoxapine
- Azacitidine
- Azathioprine
- BCG Vaccine
- Bortezomib
- Celecoxib
- Chloroquine

Ciprofloxacin
Citalopram
Clindamycin
Clofazimine
Clozapine
Co-Trimoxazole
Cytarabine
Dasatinib
Diazepam
Doxycycline
Esomeprazole
Furosemide
Glucagon
Granulocyte Colony-Stimulating Factor (G-CSF)
Hydralazine
Imatinib
Infliximab
Influenza Vaccine
Ipilimumab
Isotretinoin
Ixazomib
Lenalidomide
Minocycline
Mitoxantrone
Nilotinib
Nitrofurantoin
Norfloxacin
Ofloxacin
Omeprazole
Oral Contraceptives
Pandemic Influenza Vaccine (H1N1)
PEG-Interferon
Perphenazine
Phenylbutazone
Pneumococcal Vaccine
Propylthiouracil
Quinupristin/Dalfopristin
Ribavirin
Sulfamethoxazole
Sulfasalazine
Ticagrelor
Tretinoin
Verapamil
Vorinostat

Acute generalized exanthematous pustulosis

Acarbose
Acetaminophen
Acetazolamide
Aldesleukin
Allopurinol
Amoxapine
Amoxicillin
Amphotericin B
Ampicillin
Aspirin
Atovaquone/Proguanil
Azathioprine
Azithromycin
Bacampicillin
Bupropion
Carbamazepine
Carbimazole
Cefaclor
Cefazolin
Cefepime
Cefotaxime
Ceftazidime
Ceftriaxone
Cefuroxime
Celecoxib
Cephalexin
Cephradine
Cetirizine
Chloramphenicol
Chloroquine
Chlorzoxazone
Ciprofloxacin
Clindamycin
Clopidogrel
Cloxacillin
Clozapine
Co-Trimoxazole
Codeine
Cytarabine
Dalteparin
Dapsone
Daptomycin
Dexamethasone
Dextromethorphan
Dihydrocodeine
Diltiazem
Diphenhydramine
Docetaxel
Doripenem
Doxycycline
Epoetin Alfa
Erlotinib
Ertapenem
Erythromycin
Etanercept
Etodolac
Famotidine
Fenofibrate
Fexofenadine
Finasteride
Flucloxacillin
Fluconazole
Furosemide
Galantamine
Gefitinib
Hydrochlorothiazide
Hydroxychloroquine
Hydroxyzine
Ibuprofen
Icodextrin
Imatinib
Imipenem/Cilastatin
Immune Globulin IV
Infliximab
Influenza Vaccine
Iodixanol
Iohexol
Ioversol
Isoniazid
Isotretinoin
Itraconazole
Ketoconazole
Lamivudine
Lamotrigine
Lansoprazole
Levofloxacin
Lincomycin
Lindane
Lopinavir
Meloxicam
Meropenem
Metamizole
Methimazole
Methoxsalen
Methylphenidate
Methylprednisolone
Metronidazole
Mexiletine
Midodrine
Mifepristone
Minocycline
Morphine
Moxifloxacin
Nifedipine
Nimesulide
Nystatin
Olanzapine
Omeprazole
Pemetrexed
Phenobarbital
Phenytoin
Piperacillin/Tazobactam
Piroxicam
Prednisolone
Pristinamycin
Progestins
Propafenone
Propoxyphene
Pseudoephedrine
Pyrazinamide
Pyrimethamine
Quetiapine
Quinidine
Ranibizumab
Ranitidine
Ranolazine
Rifabutin
Rifampin
Ritodrine
Sertraline
Simvastatin
Sorafenib
Streptomycin
Sulfamethoxazole
Sulfasalazine
Teicoplanin
Telavancin
Terazosin
Terbinafine
Tetrazepam
Thalidomide
Thallium
Ticlopidine
Tigecycline
Tocilizumab
Valdecoxib
Vancomycin
Varenicline
Vemurafenib
Zidovudine

Ageusia

Acarbose
Aspirin
Atorvastatin
Azelastine
Betaxolol
Candesartan
Captopril
Carbamazepine
Cetirizine
Chlorhexidine
Clindamycin
Clopidogrel
Cocaine
Cyclobenzaprine
Doxorubicin
Enalapril
Eslicarbazepine
Etidronate
Fluoxetine
Fluvoxamine
Fosinopril
Grepafloxacin
Hydroxychloroquine
Indomethacin
Interferon Alfa
Isotretinoin
Losartan
Methimazole
Nefazodone
Nitroglycerin
Paroxetine Hydrochloride
Penicillamine
Phenylbutazone
Phenytoin
Propylthiouracil
Ramipril
Rifabutin
Rifaximin
Rimantadine
Ritonavir
Rivastigmine
Sonidegib
Sulindac
Terbinafine
Tiagabine
Tiopronin
Topiramate
Valrubicin
Venlafaxine
Vismodegib
Voriconazole
Zalcitabine

Alopecia

Acetohexamide
Acitretin
Acyclovir
Adalimumab
Ado-Trastuzumab Emtansine
Afatinib
Aflibercept
Albendazole
Aldesleukin
Alectinib
Allopurinol
Altretamine
Amantadine
Amiloride
Aminolevulinic Acid
Aminosalicylate Sodium
Amiodarone
Amitriptyline
Amlodipine
Amoxapine
Anagrelide
Anastrozole
Androstenedione
Anidulafungin
Aprepitant
Arsenic
Aspirin
Astemizole
Atenolol
Atorvastatin
Atovaquone/Proguanil
Atropine Sulfate

Axitinib
Azathioprine
Belatacept
Belinostat
Bendamustine
Betamethasone
Betaxolol
Bevacizumab
Bexarotene
Bezafibrate
Bicalutamide
Bismuth
Bleomycin
Botulinum Toxin (A & B)
Brentuximab Vedotin
Brinzolamide
Bromocriptine
Budesonide
Bupropion
Buspirone
Busulfan
Cabazitaxel
Cabergoline
Cabozantinib
Calcipotriol
Capecitabine
Captopril
Carbamazepine
Carboplatin
Carmustine
Carvedilol
Celecoxib
Certolizumab
Cetirizine
Cetuximab
Cevimeline
Chlorambucil
Chloramphenicol
Chlordiazepoxide
Chlorpropamide
Cidofovir
Cimetidine
Cisplatin
Citalopram
Clarithromycin
Clofibrate
Clomiphene
Clomipramine
Clonazepam
Clonidine
Cobimetinib
Colchicine
Cyclophosphamide
Cyclosporine
Cytarabine
Dabrafenib
Dacarbazine
Daclatasvir
Daclizumab
Dactinomycin
Dalteparin
Danazol
Dasatinib
Daunorubicin
Decitabine
Deferasirox
Degarelix
Delavirdine
Desipramine
Dexamethasone
Diazoxide
Diclofenac
Dicumarol
Didanosine
Diethylpropion
Diflunisal
Diltiazem
Docetaxel
Donepezil
Doxazosin
Doxepin
Doxorubicin
Duloxetine
Eculizumab
Efavirenz
Eflornithine
Eltrombopag
Enalapril
Enoxaparin
Entecavir
Epinephrine
Epirubicin
Epoetin Alfa
Eribulin
Erlotinib
Erythromycin
Escitalopram
Eslicarbazepine
Estramustine
Estrogens
Eszopiclone
Etanercept
Ethambutol
Ethionamide
Etoposide
Everolimus
Exemestane
Febuxostat
Fenofibrate
Fenoprofen
Fingolimod
Flecainide
Fluconazole
Fludarabine
Fluorouracil
Fluoxetine
Fluoxymesterone
Flurbiprofen
Fluvoxamine
Foscarnet
Fulvestrant
Gabapentin
Gadodiamide
Ganciclovir
Gefitinib
Gemcitabine
Gentamicin
Glatiramer
Gold & Gold Compounds
Goserelin
Granisetron
Granulocyte Colony-Stimulating Factor (G-CSF)
Grepafloxacin
Haloperidol
Halothane
Heparin
Hepatitis B Vaccine
Human Papillomavirus Vaccine (Bivalent)
Hydroxychloroquine
Hydroxyurea
Hyoscyamine
Ibandronate
Ibritumomab
Ibuprofen
Idarubicin
Ifosfamide
Imatinib
Imipramine
Imiquimod
Immune Globulin IV
Indinavir
Indomethacin
Infliximab
Interferon Alfa
Interferon Beta
Ipilimumab
Ipratropium
Irinotecan
Isavuconazonium Sulfate
Isoniazid
Isotretinoin
Itraconazole
Ixabepilone
Ixazomib
Ketoconazole
Ketoprofen
Ketorolac
Labetalol
Lamivudine
Lamotrigine
Lanreotide
Lansoprazole
Lapatinib
Leflunomide
Lenvatinib
Letrozole
Leucovorin
Leuprolide
Levamisole
Levobetaxolol
Levobunolol
Levodopa
Levothyroxine
Liothyronine
Lisinopril
Lithium
Lomustine
Lopinavir
Loratadine
Losartan
Lovastatin
Maprotiline
Mebendazole
Mechlorethamine
Meclofenamate
Medroxyprogesterone
Mefloquine
Meloxicam
Melphalan
Memantine
Mercaptopurine
Mesalamine
Metformin
Methimazole
Methotrexate
Methyltestosterone
Methysergide
Metoprolol
Mexiletine
Minocycline
Minoxidil
Mirtazapine
Mitomycin
Mitotane
Mitoxantrone
Mizoribine
Moexipril
Mycophenolate
Nabumetone
Nadolol
Nalidixic Acid
Naltrexone
Naproxen
Naratriptan
Nefazodone
Nifedipine
Nilotinib
Nimodipine
Nintedanib
Nisoldipine
Nitisinone
Nitrofurantoin
Nortriptyline
Octreotide
Olanzapine
Olaparib
Olaratumab
Omacetaxine
Omalizumab
Omeprazole
Oral Contraceptives
Oxaliplatin
Oxerutins
Paclitaxel
Palbociclib
Panitumumab
Panobinostat
Pantoprazole
Paricalcitol
Paroxetine Hydrochloride
Pasireotide
Pazopanib
PEG-Interferon
Pegvisomant
Pembrolizumab
Pemetrexed
Penicillamine
Pentosan
Pentostatin
Peplomycin
Pergolide
Pertuzumab
Phentermine
Phenytoin
Piroxicam
Pramipexole
Prazosin
Prednisolone
Prednisone
Procarbazine
Propafenone
Propranolol
Propylthiouracil
Protriptyline
Pyridostigmine
Quetiapine
Quinacrine
Quinapril
Quinidine
Rabeprazole
Raltitrexed
Ramipril

Regorafenib
Ribavirin
Riluzole
Risperidone
Ritonavir
Rituximab
Rivastigmine
Rofecoxib
Ropinirole
Selenium
Sertraline
Sodium Oxybate
Sonidegib
Sorafenib
Sotalol
Sparfloxacin
Spinosad
Spironolactone
Strontium Ranelate
Sulfasalazine
Sulfisoxazole
Sulindac
Sunitinib
Tacrine
Tacrolimus
Tamoxifen
Tegafur/Gimeracil/Oteracil
Temozolomide
Temsirolimus
Teniposide
Terbinafine
Terfenadine
Teriflunomide
Testosterone
Thalidomide
Thallium
Thioguanine
Thiotepa
Tiagabine
Timolol
Tinzaparin
Tiopronin
Tizanidine
Tocainide
Tolcapone
Topiramate
Topotecan
Trabectedin
Trametinib
Trastuzumab
Trazodone
Trifluridine & Tipiracil
Trimethadione
Trimipramine
Triptorelin
Ursodiol
Valdecoxib
Valproic Acid
Vandetanib
Vasopressin
Vemurafenib
Venlafaxine
Verapamil
Vinblastine
Vincristine
Vinorelbine
Vismodegib
Vitamin A
Voriconazole
Vorinostat
Warfarin
Zaleplon
Zidovudine
Ziprasidone
Zoledronate
Zonisamide
Zoster Vaccine

Angioedema

Acetaminophen
Acetylcysteine
Acitretin
Acyclovir
Adalimumab
Albendazole
Aldesleukin
Alefacept
Alemtuzumab
Alendronate
Aliskiren
Allopurinol
Alogliptin
Alprazolam
Alteplase
Aminoglutethimide
Aminosalicylate Sodium
Amiodarone
Amitriptyline
Amlodipine
Amodiaquine
Amoxicillin
Ampicillin
Ampicillin/Sulbactam
Anidulafungin
Anthrax Vaccine
Ascorbic Acid
Asenapine
Asparaginase
Aspartame
Aspirin
Atorvastatin
Atracurium
Azatadine
Azathioprine
Azithromycin
Aztreonam
Benazepril
Bevacizumab
Bezafibrate
Bismuth
Bleomycin
Brivaracetam
Brompheniramine
Budesonide
Bupropion
Butabarbital
Canagliflozin
Candesartan
Captopril
Carbamazepine
Carisoprodol
Carvedilol
Cefaclor
Cefadroxil
Cefixime
Cefoxitin
Cefprozil
Ceftazidime
Ceftriaxone
Cefuroxime
Celecoxib
Cephalexin
Certolizumab
Cetirizine
Chloral Hydrate
Chlorambucil
Chloramphenicol
Chlordiazepoxide
Chloroquine
Chlorpheniramine
Chlorpromazine
Chlorpropamide
Chlorthalidone
Chlorzoxazone
Cilazapril
Cimetidine
Cinoxacin
Ciprofloxacin
Cisplatin
Clarithromycin
Clemastine
Clonazepam
Clonidine
Clopidogrel
Cloxacillin
Clozapine
Co-Trimoxazole
Cocaine
Codeine
Cromolyn
Cyanocobalamin
Cyclamate
Cyclobenzaprine
Cyclophosphamide
Cyclosporine
Cyproheptadine
Dacarbazine
Danazol
Darunavir
Dasabuvir/Ombitasvir/Paritaprevir/Ritonavir
Daunorubicin
Deferoxamine
Delavirdine
Desipramine
Dexchlorpheniramine
Diazepam
Diclofenac
Dicumarol
Diethylstilbestrol
Diflunisal
Dihydrocodeine
Diltiazem
Dimenhydrinate
Diphenhydramine
Dipyridamole
Disulfiram
Dofetilide
Doxazosin
Doxorubicin
Doxycycline
Droperidol
Dutasteride
Efalizumab
Enalapril
Enoxaparin
Epoetin Alfa
Erythromycin
Esomeprazole
Estramustine
Estrogens
Etanercept
Ethambutol
Etidronate
Etodolac
Etomidate
Etoricoxib
Everolimus
Ezetimibe
Famotidine
Febuxostat
Felodipine
Fenoprofen
Fentanyl
Fluconazole
Fluorouracil
Fluoxetine
Fluphenazine
Flurbiprofen
Fluvoxamine
Fosinopril
Fulvestrant
Glatiramer
Glucagon
Gold & Gold Compounds
Griseofulvin
Haloperidol
Halothane
Heparin
Hepatitis B Vaccine
Heroin
Histrelin
Hyaluronic Acid
Hydralazine
Hydrochlorothiazide
Hydrocortisone
Hydromorphone
Hydroxychloroquine
Hydroxyzine
Ibritumomab
Ibuprofen
Icatibant
Iloperidone
Imidapril
Imiglucerase
Imipenem/Cilastatin
Imipramine
Imiquimod
Indapamide
Indomethacin
Infliximab
Insulin
Interferon Alfa
Iothalamate
Irbesartan
Isoniazid
Isotretinoin
Itraconazole
Ivacaftor
Ivermectin
Ixekizumab
Ketoconazole
Ketoprofen
Ketorolac
Labetalol
Lacosamide
Lamivudine
Lamotrigine
Ledipasvir & Sofosbuvir
Lepirudin
Levamisole
Levothyroxine
Lidocaine
Linezolid
Lisinopril

Lithium
Lixisenatide
Loratadine
Losartan
Lurasidone
MDMA
Mebendazole
Mebeverine
Mechlorethamine
Meclizine
Meclofenamate
Mefenamic Acid
Meloxicam
Melphalan
Meperidine
Mephenytoin
Mephobarbital
Mepivacaine
Meprobamate
Mesna
Metformin
Methohexital
Methotrexate
Methylphenidate
Metoclopramide
Metoprolol
Metronidazole
Miconazole
Midazolam
Minocycline
Mirtazapine
Mitotane
Moexipril
Montelukast
Nabumetone
Nalidixic Acid
Naloxone
Naproxen
Neomycin
Nevirapine
Nicardipine
Nifedipine
Nimesulide
Nitrofurantoin
Ofloxacin
Olanzapine
Olmesartan
Omalizumab
Omeprazole
Oral Contraceptives
Oritavancin
Oxaliplatin
Oxaprozin
Paclitaxel
Pamidronate
Panitumumab
Pantoprazole
Paroxetine Hydrochloride
PEG-Interferon
Pegaptanib
Pegaspargase
Penicillin G
Penicillin V
Pentagastrin
Pentobarbital
Pentoxifylline
Perflutren
Perindopril
Phenelzine
Phenobarbital
Phenolphthalein
Phenylbutazone
Phenytoin
Pioglitazone
Piroxicam
Potassium Iodide
Prasugrel
Praziquantel
Prazosin
Prilocaine
Primaquine
Pristinamycin
Procainamide
Procarbazine
Progestins
Promethazine
Propafenone
Propofol
Propranolol
Propylthiouracil
Protamine Sulfate
Pseudoephedrine
Pyrimethamine
Quinapril
Quinestrol
Quinidine
Quinine
Ramipril
Ranitidine
Riboflavin
Rifampin
Risperidone
Rituximab
Rofecoxib
Ropinirole
Sacubitril/Valsartan
Saxagliptin
Secobarbital
Sertraline
Sirolimus
Sitagliptin
Sorafenib
Sparfloxacin
Streptokinase
Streptomycin
Sulfadoxine
Sulfamethoxazole
Sulfasalazine
Sulfisoxazole
Sulindac
Sumatriptan
Tacrolimus
Tartrazine
Telithromycin
Telmisartan
Tenecteplase
Terbinafine
Terfenadine
Teriflunomide
Tetracycline
Thiamine
Thiopental
Thioridazine
Thiotepa
Ticlopidine
Tinidazole
Tiopronin
Tiotropium
Tolmetin
Tositumomab & Iodine[131]
Tosufloxacin
Tramadol
Trandolapril
Trastuzumab
Trazodone
Trifluoperazine
Trimeprazine
Trimetrexate
Tripelennamine
Triprolidine
Triptorelin
Troleandomycin
Trospium
Trovafloxacin
Urokinase
Valsartan
Vancomycin
Vardenafil
Vedolizumab
Venlafaxine
Verapamil
Vildagliptin
Vinblastine
Vincristine
Voriconazole
Vorinostat
Warfarin
Yellow Fever Vaccine
Zalcitabine
Zidovudine
Ziprasidone
Zofenopril

Anosmia

Amikacin
Aspirin
Cocaine
Dorzolamide
Doxycycline
Enalapril
Interferon Alfa
Levodopa
Methazolamide
Methoxsalen
Midodrine
Nifedipine
Pyrazinamide
Terbinafine
Uracil/Tegafur
Zinc

Aphthous stomatitis

Afatinib
Aldesleukin
Amodiaquine
Amoxicillin
Anagrelide
Artesunate
Asparaginase
Aspirin
Azathioprine
Azelastine
Aztreonam
Belatacept
Bupropion
Candesartan
Captopril
Cefaclor
Certolizumab
Cetuximab
Cisplatin
Co-Trimoxazole
Cyclophosphamide
Cyclosporine
Delavirdine
Diclofenac
Docetaxel
Doxepin
Doxorubicin
Epirubicin
Erlotinib
Everolimus
Exemestane
Fenoprofen
Fluorides
Fluorouracil
Fluoxetine
Gold & Gold Compounds
Hepatitis B Vaccine
Imatinib
Imiquimod
Indinavir
Interferon Alfa
Ipilimumab
Ketorolac
Labetalol
Ledipasvir & Sofosbuvir
Lenvatinib
Losartan
Methotrexate
Mycophenolate
Naproxen
Nicorandil
Olanzapine
Omacetaxine
Orlistat
Paclitaxel
Pantoprazole
Paroxetine Hydrochloride
Pemetrexed
Penicillamine
Piroxicam
Prednisone
Pyrimethamine
Rifabutin
Rofecoxib
Sertraline
Siltuximab
Sirolimus
Sorafenib
Sulfadoxine
Sulfamethoxazole
Sulfasalazine
Sulfisoxazole
Tegafur/Gimeracil/Oteracil
Temsirolimus
Tocilizumab
Tosufloxacin
Trametinib
Valsartan
Vedolizumab
Zalcitabine

Baboon syndrome (SDRIFE)

Acetaminophen
Allopurinol
Aminophylline
Amoxicillin
Ampicillin
Aspirin
Betamethasone
Cefadroxil
Cefuroxime
Celecoxib
Cephalexin
Cetuximab
Cimetidine

Cisplatin
Clarithromycin
Cloxacillin
Clozapine
Erythromycin
Everolimus
Fluorouracil
Gemcitabine
Heparin
Hydrochlorothiazide
Hydroxyurea
Immune Globulin IV
Infliximab
Iomeprol
Iopromide
Mesalamine
Mitomycin
Naproxen
Nystatin
Omeprazole
Oral Contraceptives
Oxycodone
Penicillin V
Pseudoephedrine
Ranitidine
Risperidone
Rivastigmine
Roxithromycin
Telmisartan
Terbinafine

Black tongue (lingua villosa nigra)

Amoxicillin
Benztropine
Ceftriaxone
Chloramphenicol
Clarithromycin
Clonazepam
Co-Trimoxazole
Cocaine
Doxycycline
Fluoxetine
Griseofulvin
Lansoprazole
Methyldopa
Minocycline
Nicotine
Nortriptyline
Olanzapine
Oxytetracycline
PEG-Interferon
Ribavirin
Streptomycin
Sulfamethoxazole
Tetracycline
Thiothixene

Bullous dermatitis

Acetazolamide
Acitretin
Afatinib
Aldesleukin
Alemtuzumab
Amifostine
Aminocaproic Acid
Aminophylline
Aminosalicylate Sodium
Amitriptyline
Ampicillin
Anthrax Vaccine
Argatroban
Arsenic
Aspirin
Atropine Sulfate
Bleomycin
Bumetanide
Buspirone
Busulfan
Butabarbital
Butalbital
Captopril
Carbamazepine
Celecoxib
Cetirizine
Cevimeline
Chloral Hydrate
Chloramphenicol
Chlorpromazine
Chlorpropamide
Ciprofloxacin
Clonazepam
Clopidogrel
Co-Trimoxazole
Cocaine
Codeine
Colchicine
Cyanocobalamin
Cyclamate
Cyclosporine
Cytarabine
Dalteparin
Dapsone
Desoximetasone
Dextromethorphan
Diazepam
Diclofenac
Dicumarol
Diethylstilbestrol
Diflunisal
Digoxin
Disulfiram
Enoxaparin
Entacapone
Ephedrine
Erlotinib
Estrogens
Ethambutol
Ethchlorvynol
Felbamate
Fluconazole
Fluorouracil
Fluoxetine
Fluvoxamine
Fondaparinux
Fosphenytoin
Frovatriptan
Furosemide
Ganciclovir
Gemcitabine
Glyburide
Gold & Gold Compounds
Griseofulvin
Heparin
Hydralazine
Hydrochlorothiazide
Hydroxychloroquine
Ibuprofen
Ibutilide
Imipramine
Imiquimod
Indomethacin
Infliximab
Influenza Vaccine
Insulin
Interferon Alfa
Isoniazid
Ivermectin
Ketoprofen
Lamotrigine
Leflunomide
Lindane
Lisinopril
Lithium
Lomefloxacin
Mechlorethamine
Meloxicam
Mephenytoin
Meprobamate
Methicillin
Methotrexate
Methoxsalen
Miconazole
Minoxidil
Mitomycin
Mometasone
Moxifloxacin
Mycophenolate
Nabumetone
Nalidixic Acid
Naproxen
Nifedipine
Norfloxacin
Omeprazole
Oral Contraceptives
Oxacillin
Penicillamine
Pentamidine
Pentobarbital
Pentostatin
Phenobarbital
Phenolphthalein
Phenytoin
Piroxicam
Prednicarbate
Promethazine
Propranolol
Propyphenazone
Pyridoxine
Pyrimethamine
Quinethazone
Reserpine
Rifampin
Risperidone
Ritonavir
Rituximab
Rivastigmine
Rofecoxib
Sertraline
Smallpox Vaccine
Sparfloxacin
Streptomycin
Sulfadoxine
Sulfamethoxazole
Sulfisoxazole
Sunitinib
Temazepam
Tetracycline
Thalidomide
Thiopental
Tinzaparin
Tolbutamide
Tranexamic Acid
Tretinoin
Trioxsalen
Urokinase
Ustekinumab
Valproic Acid
Vancomycin
Vasopressin
Vinblastine
Warfarin
Zalcitabine
Zidovudine
Zolpidem

DRESS syndrome

Abacavir
Acenocoumarol
Acetaminophen
Allopurinol
Amikacin
Amitriptyline
Amoxicillin
Ampicillin
Aspirin
Atenolol
Atorvastatin
Azithromycin
Boceprevir
Bosentan
Bupropion
Captopril
Carbamazepine
Cefadroxil
Cefixime
Cefotaxime
Ceftriaxone
Celecoxib
Chlorambucil
Cidofovir
Cilostazol
Ciprofloxacin
Clindamycin
Clomipramine
Clonazepam
Clopidogrel
Co-Trimoxazole
Codeine
Cyclobenzaprine
Daclatasvir
Dapsone
Darunavir
Dextromethorphan
Diclofenac
Doxycycline
Efalizumab
Efavirenz
Emtricitabine
Erlotinib
Esomeprazole
Ethambutol
Fenofibrate
Fluoxetine
Hydroxychloroquine
Ibuprofen
Imatinib
Isoniazid
Lamotrigine
Leflunomide
Lenalidomide
Leucovorin
Levetiracetam
Linezolid
Metamizole
Metformin
Minocycline

Mitoxantrone
Naproxen
Nelfinavir
Nevirapine
Nitrofurantoin
Olanzapine
Oxazepam
Oxcarbazepine
Pandemic Influenza Vaccine (H1N1)
PEG-Interferon
Penicillin V
Perampanel
Phenobarbital
Phenylbutazone
Phenytoin
Piperacillin/Tazobactam
Piroxicam
Promethazine
Propylthiouracil
Pyrazinamide
Pyrimethamine
Quinine
Raltegravir
Ramipril
Ribavirin
Rifampin
Ritonavir
Rivaroxaban
Sorafenib
Spironolactone
Streptomycin
Strontium Ranelate
Sulfadiazine
Sulfamethoxazole
Sulfasalazine
Teicoplanin
Telaprevir
Tenofovir Disoproxil
Tenoxicam
Terbinafine
Teriflunomide
Thiamine
Torsemide
Trimethoprim
Valproic Acid
Vancomycin
Vemurafenib
Ziprasidone
Zonisamide

Erythema multiforme

Acamprosate
Acarbose
Acebutolol
Acetaminophen
Acetazolamide
Adalimumab
Aldesleukin
Alendronate
Allopurinol
Amifostine
Aminosalicylate Sodium
Amiodarone
Amlodipine
Amoxicillin
Amphotericin B
Ampicillin
Anthrax Vaccine
Arsenic
Aspirin
Atovaquone/Proguanil
Atropine Sulfate
Azathioprine
Aztreonam
Bezafibrate
Bortezomib
Bosutinib
Bumetanide
Bupropion
Busulfan
Butabarbital
Butalbital
Candesartan
Carbamazepine
Carisoprodol
Cefaclor
Cefadroxil
Cefamandole
Cefixime
Cefotaxime
Cefpodoxime
Cefprozil
Ceftazidime
Ceftriaxone
Cefuroxime
Celecoxib
Cephalexin
Cephalothin
Chloral Hydrate
Chlorambucil
Chloramphenicol
Chlordiazepoxide
Chloroquine
Chlorpromazine
Chlorpropamide
Chlorzoxazone
Cimetidine
Ciprofloxacin
Cisplatin
Clindamycin
Clofibrate
Clonazepam
Clozapine
Co-Trimoxazole
Codeine
Collagen (Bovine)
Crizotinib
Cyclobenzaprine
Cyclophosphamide
Danazol
Dapsone
Delavirdine
Desoximetasone
Dexamethasone
Diclofenac
Dicloxacillin
Didanosine
Diflunisal
Dihydrocodeine
Diltiazem
Dimenhydrinate
Docetaxel
Dorzolamide
Doxycycline
Elotuzumab
Enalapril
Enoxacin
Enoxaparin
Erythromycin
Estrogens
Ethambutol
Ethosuximide
Etodolac
Etoposide
Etoricoxib
Famotidine
Fenbufen
Fenoprofen
Flucloxacillin
Fluconazole
Fluorouracil
Fluoxetine
Flurbiprofen
Fosphenytoin
Furazolidone
Furosemide
Gadoversetamide
Gemfibrozil
Glucagon
Glyburide
Gold & Gold Compounds
Griseofulvin
Hepatitis B Vaccine
Human Papillomavirus (HPV) Vaccine
Hyaluronic Acid
Hydrochlorothiazide
Hydroxychloroquine
Hydroxyurea
Hydroxyzine
Ibuprofen
Icodextrin
Imatinib
Imipenem/Cilastatin
Imiquimod
Indapamide
Indomethacin
Infliximab
Interferon Beta
Iomeprol
Ipilimumab
Isoniazid
Isotretinoin
Ixazomib
Ketoprofen
Lamotrigine
Lansoprazole
Leflunomide
Lenalidomide
Levamisole
Levetiracetam
Levofloxacin
Lidocaine
Lithium
Loracarbef
Loratadine
Lorazepam
Maprotiline
Mechlorethamine
Meclofenamate
Mefenamic Acid
Meloxicam
Mephenytoin
Meprobamate
Metamizole
Methenamine
Methicillin
Methotrexate
Methyldopa
Minocycline
Minoxidil
Misoprostol
Mitomycin
Mitotane
Nabumetone
Nalidixic Acid
Naproxen
Neomycin
Nifedipine
Nilotinib
Nitrofurantoin
Nitroglycerin
Nivolumab
Nystatin
Omeprazole
Oral Contraceptives
Oritavancin
Oxaprozin
Oxazepam
Oxybutynin
Paclitaxel
Pancreatin
Pandemic Influenza Vaccine (H1N1)
Pantoprazole
Paramethadione
Pemetrexed
Penicillamine
Pentobarbital
Permethrin
Phenobarbital
Phenolphthalein
Phensuximide
Phenylbutazone
Phenytoin
Piroxicam
Pravastatin
Prednicarbate
Prednisolone
Primidone
Probenecid
Progestins
Promethazine
Propranolol
Pseudoephedrine
Pyrazinamide
Pyrimethamine
Quetiapine
Quinidine
Quinine
Ramipril
Regorafenib
Ribavirin
Rifampin
Ritodrine
Roxatidine
Saquinavir
Scopolamine
Sertraline
Simvastatin
Smallpox Vaccine
Sorafenib
Spironolactone
Streptomycin
Sulfacetamide
Sulfadiazine
Sulfadoxine
Sulfamethoxazole
Sulfasalazine
Sulfisoxazole
Sulindac
Tamsulosin
Telithromycin
Telmisartan

- Terbinafine
- Tetracycline
- Tetrazepam
- Thalidomide
- Thiabendazole
- Thiopental
- Thioridazine
- Ticlopidine
- Tiopronin
- Tobramycin
- Tocainide
- Tolbutamide
- Tolcapone
- Tolmetin
- Trazodone
- Trihexyphenidyl
- Trimethadione
- Valproic Acid
- Vancomycin
- Vandetanib
- Verapamil
- Vinblastine
- Vitamin A
- Vitamin E
- Voriconazole
- Zalcitabine
- Zidovudine

Erythema nodosum

- Abatacept
- Acetaminophen
- Acyclovir
- Aldesleukin
- Amiodarone
- Anastrozole
- Arsenic
- Aspartame
- Aspirin
- Azathioprine
- Busulfan
- Carbamazepine
- Carbimazole
- Certolizumab
- Chlordiazepoxide
- Chlorpropamide
- Ciprofloxacin
- Clomiphene
- Co-Trimoxazole
- Codeine
- Colchicine
- Dapsone
- Dasatinib
- Diclofenac
- Disopyramide
- Estrogens
- Etanercept
- Fluoxetine
- Furosemide
- Glucagon
- Gold & Gold Compounds
- Granulocyte Colony-Stimulating Factor (G-CSF)
- Hepatitis B Vaccine
- Human Papillomavirus (HPV) Vaccine
- Hydralazine
- Hydroxychloroquine
- Ibuprofen
- Indomethacin
- Interferon Alfa
- Isotretinoin
- Ixazomib
- Levofloxacin
- Lidocaine
- Meclofenamate
- Medroxyprogesterone
- Meprobamate
- Metamizole
- Methyldopa
- Minocycline
- Montelukast
- Naproxen
- Nifedipine
- Nitrofurantoin
- Omeprazole
- Oral Contraceptives
- Paroxetine Hydrochloride
- Penicillamine
- Ponatinib
- Propylthiouracil
- Quinacrine
- Smallpox Vaccine
- Streptomycin
- Sulfamethoxazole
- Sulfasalazine
- Sulfisoxazole
- Terbinafine
- Thalidomide
- Ticlopidine
- Tretinoin
- Trimethoprim
- Verapamil
- Zileuton

Exanthems

- Abacavir
- Acamprosate
- Acebutolol
- Acenocoumarol
- Acetaminophen
- Acetazolamide
- Acetohexamide
- Acitretin
- Acyclovir
- Aldesleukin
- Allopurinol
- Alprazolam
- Amantadine
- Amcinonide
- Amikacin
- Amiloride
- Aminocaproic Acid
- Aminoglutethimide
- Aminophylline
- Aminosalicylate Sodium
- Amiodarone
- Amlodipine
- Amoxapine
- Amoxicillin
- Amphotericin B
- Ampicillin
- Amprenavir
- Anastrozole
- Anidulafungin
- Anistreplase
- Anthrax Vaccine
- Aprotinin
- Arsenic
- Aspartame
- Aspirin
- Astemizole
- Atovaquone
- Atovaquone/Proguanil
- Azacitidine
- Azathioprine
- Azelastine
- Azithromycin
- Aztreonam
- Bacampicillin
- Baclofen
- Benactyzine
- Benazepril
- Bendamustine
- Bendroflumethiazide
- Betamethasone
- Bevacizumab
- Bexarotene
- Bicalutamide
- Bismuth
- Bleomycin
- Bortezomib
- Bosentan
- Brompheniramine
- Budesonide
- Bupropion
- Buserelin
- Busulfan
- Butabarbital
- Butalbital
- Candesartan
- Captopril
- Carbamazepine
- Carboplatin
- Carisoprodol
- Carmustine
- Carvedilol
- Cefaclor
- Cefadroxil
- Cefamandole
- Cefazolin
- Cefdinir
- Cefepime
- Cefoperazone
- Cefotaxime
- Cefoxitin
- Cefpodoxime
- Ceftazidime
- Ceftriaxone
- Cefuroxime
- Celecoxib
- Cephalexin
- Cephalothin
- Cephapirin
- Cephradine
- Ceritinib
- Cetirizine
- Cetuximab
- Cevimeline
- Chloral Hydrate
- Chlorambucil
- Chloramphenicol
- Chlordiazepoxide
- Chlormezanone
- Chloroquine
- Chlorothiazide
- Chlorpromazine
- Chlorpropamide
- Cimetidine
- Ciprofloxacin
- Cisplatin
- Citalopram
- Cladribine
- Clarithromycin
- Clemastine
- Clindamycin
- Clofibrate
- Clomiphene
- Clonazepam
- Clopidogrel
- Clorazepate
- Cloxacillin
- Clozapine
- Co-Trimoxazole
- Codeine
- Colchicine
- Colestipol
- Cyanocobalamin
- Cyclamate
- Cyclophosphamide
- Cycloserine
- Cyclosporine
- Cyclothiazide
- Cyproheptadine
- Cytarabine
- Dabigatran
- Dabrafenib
- Dacarbazine
- Daclizumab
- Dalteparin
- Danazol
- Dantrolene
- Dapsone
- Daunorubicin
- Deferasirox
- Delavirdine
- Denosumab
- Desipramine
- Dexamethasone
- Diazepam
- Diclofenac
- Dicloxacillin
- Dicumarol
- Dicyclomine
- Diethylpropion
- Diethylstilbestrol
- Diflunisal
- Digoxin
- Diltiazem
- Dimenhydrinate
- Diphenhydramine
- Dipyridamole
- Disopyramide
- Disulfiram
- Docetaxel
- Docusate
- Doxazosin
- Doxepin
- Doxorubicin
- Doxycycline
- Dronedarone
- Efavirenz
- Eletriptan
- Elotuzumab
- Emtricitabine
- Enalapril
- Enoxacin
- Enoxaparin
- Entecavir
- Ephedrine
- Epoetin Alfa
- Eprosartan
- Erlotinib
- Erythromycin
- Esomeprazole
- Estramustine
- Estrogens

Etanercept
Ethacrynic Acid
Ethambutol
Ethionamide
Ethosuximide
Etodolac
Etoposide
Etoricoxib
Etravirine
Everolimus
Felodipine
Fenofibrate
Fenoprofen
Flecainide
Fluconazole
Flucytosine
Fludarabine
Fluorouracil
Fluoxetine
Flurazepam
Flurbiprofen
Flutamide
Folic Acid
Foscarnet
Fosfomycin
Furazolidone
Furosemide
Gabapentin
Galantamine
Ganciclovir
Gatifloxacin
Gefitinib
Gemcitabine
Gemfibrozil
Gemifloxacin
Gentamicin
Glimepiride
Glipizide
Glucagon
Glyburide
Gold & Gold Compounds
Granulocyte Colony-Stimulating Factor (G-CSF)
Grepafloxacin
Griseofulvin
Halothane
Heparin
Heroin
Hydralazine
Hydrochlorothiazide
Hydromorphone
Hydroxychloroquine
Hydroxyurea
Hydroxyzine
Ibuprofen
Icodextrin
Idarubicin
Imatinib
Imipenem/Cilastatin
Imipramine
Imiquimod
Indapamide
Indinavir
Indomethacin
Infliximab
Insulin
Interferon Alfa
Iobenguane
Ipilimumab
Irbesartan
Irinotecan
Isocarboxazid
Isoniazid
Isosorbide Dinitrate
Isotretinoin
Isradipine
Itraconazole
Ivermectin
Ixazomib
Ketoconazole
Ketoprofen
Ketorolac
Labetalol
Lamivudine
Lamotrigine
Lapatinib
Lenalidomide
Lenvatinib
Letrozole
Levamisole
Levetiracetam
Levodopa
Levofloxacin
Lidocaine
Lincomycin
Linezolid
Lisinopril
Lithium
Loracarbef
Lovastatin
Maprotiline
Mebendazole
Mechlorethamine
Meclofenamate
Mefenamic Acid
Mefloquine
Meloxicam
Melphalan
Memantine
Mephenytoin
Meprobamate
Mercaptopurine
Meropenem
Mesalamine
Mesna
Metamizole
Methazolamide
Methenamine
Methicillin
Methimazole
Methohexital
Methotrexate
Methoxsalen
Methsuximide
Methyldopa
Methylphenidate
Metoclopramide
Metoprolol
Metronidazole
Mexiletine
Miconazole
Minocycline
Minoxidil
Misoprostol
Mitomycin
Mitotane
Moexipril
Moricizine
Morphine
Nabumetone
Nadolol
Nafarelin
Nafcillin
Nalidixic Acid
Naltrexone
Naproxen
Naratriptan
Nefazodone
Nelfinavir
Neomycin
Nevirapine
Niacin
Nifedipine
Nilotinib
Nimesulide
Nimodipine
Nisoldipine
Nitisinone
Nitrofurantoin
Nivolumab
Norfloxacin
Nystatin
Octreotide
Ofloxacin
Olanzapine
Olmesartan
Olsalazine
Omeprazole
Oral Contraceptives
Oxacillin
Oxaliplatin
Oxaprozin
Oxcarbazepine
Paclitaxel
Paliperidone
Pamidronate
Panobinostat
Pantoprazole
Paromomycin
Paroxetine Hydrochloride
PEG-Interferon
Pembrolizumab
Pemoline
Penbutolol
Penicillamine
Penicillin V
Pentagastrin
Pentamidine
Pentazocine
Pentobarbital
Pentostatin
Perflutren
Perphenazine
Phenazopyridine
Phenobarbital
Phenolphthalein
Phenylbutazone
Phenytoin
Phytonadione
Piperacillin/Tazobactam
Piroxicam
Potassium Iodide
Prazosin
Prednisolone
Primaquine
Primidone
Pristinamycin
Procainamide
Procarbazine
Prochlorperazine
Promazine
Promethazine
Propafenone
Propofol
Propoxyphene
Propranolol
Propylthiouracil
Protamine Sulfate
Pseudoephedrine
Pyrazinamide
Pyrimethamine
Quinacrine
Quinapril
Quinethazone
Quinidine
Quinine
Quinupristin/Dalfopristin
Ramipril
Ranitidine
Rapacuronium
Regorafenib
Repaglinide
Ribavirin
Rifampin
Ritodrine
Ritonavir
Rituximab
Rivastigmine
Rofecoxib
Ropinirole
Saccharin
Saquinavir
Scopolamine
Sertraline
Simvastatin
Smallpox Vaccine
Sorafenib
Sparfloxacin
Spironolactone
Streptokinase
Streptomycin
Streptozocin
Succimer
Sucralfate
Sulfadiazine
Sulfadoxine
Sulfamethoxazole
Sulfasalazine
Sulfinpyrazone
Sulfisoxazole
Sulindac
Tacrine
Tacrolimus
Tamoxifen
Teicoplanin
Telaprevir
Telmisartan
Temozolomide
Temsirolimus
Terazosin
Terbinafine
Terfenadine
Testosterone
Tetracycline
Tetrazepam
Thalidomide
Thiabendazole
Thiamine
Thimerosal
Thioguanine
Thiopental
Thioridazine
Thiothixene
Tiagabine

Ticarcillin
Ticlopidine
Tinzaparin
Tiopronin
Tipranavir
Tizanidine
Tobramycin
Tocainide
Tolazamide
Tolazoline
Tolbutamide
Tolmetin
Topiramate
Tramadol
Trametinib
Trazodone
Triamcinolone
Trimeprazine
Trimethadione
Trimetrexate
Troleandomycin
Uracil/Tegafur
Valdecoxib
Valproic Acid
Valsartan
Vancomycin
Vardenafil
Vemurafenib
Venlafaxine
Verapamil
Vincristine
Vitamin A
Vorapaxar
Vorinostat
Warfarin
Zalcitabine
Zidovudine
Ziprasidone
Zoledronate
Zonisamide

Exfoliative dermatitis

Acamprosate
Acetaminophen
Acitretin
Afatinib
Aldesleukin
Alitretinoin
Allopurinol
Aminoglutethimide
Aminolevulinic Acid
Aminophylline
Aminosalicylate Sodium
Amiodarone
Amobarbital
Amoxicillin
Amphotericin B
Ampicillin
Arsenic
Aspirin
Azathioprine
Aztreonam
Benzyl Alcohol
Bexarotene
Bismuth
Bosutinib
Bumetanide
Butabarbital
Butalbital
Capecitabine
Captopril
Carbamazepine
Carvedilol
Cefoxitin
Cefpodoxime
Celecoxib
Chlorambucil
Chloroquine
Chlorpropamide
Cimetidine
Ciprofloxacin
Cisplatin
Clofazimine
Clofibrate
Clonazepam
Co-Trimoxazole
Codeine
Cytarabine
Dapsone
Daunorubicin
Demeclocycline
Desipramine
Dexamethasone
Diazepam
Diclofenac
Dicloxacillin
Diethylstilbestrol
Diflunisal
Diltiazem
Doxorubicin
Efavirenz
Eletriptan
Enalapril
Enoxacin
Ephedrine
Esmolol
Esomeprazole
Estrogens
Ethambutol
Ethosuximide
Fenoprofen
Flecainide
Fluconazole
Flurbiprofen
Fluvoxamine
Fosphenytoin
Furosemide
Gefitinib
Gemcitabine
Gemfibrozil
Gentamicin
Gold & Gold Compounds
Granulocyte Colony-Stimulating Factor (G-CSF)
Grepafloxacin
Griseofulvin
Hydroxychloroquine
Ibuprofen
Icodextrin
Imatinib
Imipramine
Indomethacin
Irinotecan
Isavuconazonium Sulfate
Isoniazid
Isotretinoin
Ixabepilone
Ixazomib
Ketoconazole
Ketoprofen
Ketorolac
Lansoprazole
Lapatinib
Leflunomide
Lenalidomide
Lidocaine
Lisinopril
Lithium
Lomefloxacin
Meclofenamate
Mefenamic Acid
Mefloquine
Mephenytoin
Mephobarbital
Methicillin
Methsuximide
Methylphenidate
Mexiletine
Mezlocillin
Minocycline
Mitomycin
Nalidixic Acid
Nifedipine
Nilotinib
Nisoldipine
Nitisinone
Nitrofurantoin
Nitroglycerin
Nivolumab
Omacetaxine
Ombitasvir/Paritaprevir/Ritonavir
Omeprazole
Oxaprozin
Oxcarbazepine
Oxytetracycline
Panitumumab
Pantoprazole
Paramethadione
Pazopanib
Pembrolizumab
Pentobarbital
Pentostatin
Phenobarbital
Phenolphthalein
Phenylbutazone
Phenytoin
Piroxicam
Procarbazine
Propranolol
Propylthiouracil
Pseudoephedrine
Pyrimethamine
Quinacrine
Quinapril
Quinidine
Quinine
Raltitrexed
Rifampin
Risperidone
Rivastigmine
Romidepsin
Secobarbital
Sildenafil
Smallpox Vaccine
Sorafenib
Sparfloxacin
Streptomycin
Strontium Ranelate
Sulfacetamide
Sulfadoxine
Sulfamethoxazole
Sulfasalazine
Sulfisoxazole
Sulindac
Sunitinib
Tacrolimus
Teicoplanin
Terfenadine
Tetracycline
Thalidomide
Tiagabine
Ticlopidine
Tizanidine
Tobramycin
Tocainide
Trazodone
Tretinoin
Trimethadione
Trimethoprim
Trovafloxacin
Vancomycin
Venlafaxine
Verapamil
Vitamin A
Voriconazole
Vorinostat
Zalcitabine
Ziprasidone

Fixed eruption

Aceclofenac
Acetaminophen
Acyclovir
Adalimumab
Albendazole
Alendronate
Allopurinol
Aminosalicylate Sodium
Amitriptyline
Amlexanox
Amodiaquine
Amoxicillin
Amphotericin B
Ampicillin
Arsenic
Aspirin
Atenolol
Atorvastatin
Atropine Sulfate
Azathioprine
Bacampicillin
BCG Vaccine
Bisacodyl
Bismuth
Bisoprolol
Bleomycin
Bucillamine
Butabarbital
Butalbital
Carbamazepine
Carisoprodol
Cefaclor
Cefazolin
Cefixime
Ceftriaxone
Celecoxib
Cephalexin
Cetirizine
Chloral Hydrate
Chloramphenicol
Chlordiazepoxide
Chlorhexidine
Chlormezanone
Chloroquine
Chlorothiazide

Chlorpromazine
Chlorpropamide
Cimetidine
Ciprofloxacin
Clarithromycin
Clindamycin
Clioquinol
Clopidogrel
Co-Trimoxazole
Cocaine
Codeine
Colchicine
Cyproterone
Dacarbazine
Danazol
Dapsone
Demeclocycline
Dextromethorphan
Diazepam
Diclofenac
Diflunisal
Dimenhydrinate
Diphenhydramine
Disulfiram
Docetaxel
Doxorubicin
Doxycycline
Ephedrine
Erythromycin
Esomeprazole
Estrogens
Etanercept
Ethchlorvynol
Etodolac
Etoricoxib
Finasteride
Flavoxate
Flecainide
Fluconazole
Flurbiprofen
Foscarnet
Furosemide
Gabapentin
Ganciclovir
Glipizide
Griseofulvin
Guanethidine
Heparin
Heroin
Hydralazine
Hydrochlorothiazide
Hydroxychloroquine
Hydroxyurea
Hydroxyzine
Ibuprofen
Imipramine
Indapamide
Indomethacin
Infliximab
Influenza Vaccine
Iohexol
Iopromide
Isotretinoin
Itraconazole
Ketoconazole
Lamotrigine
Leuprolide
Levamisole
Levocetirizine
Lidocaine
Loperamide
Loratadine
Lorazepam
Meclofenamate
Mefenamic Acid
Meloxicam
Meprobamate
Mesna
Metamizole
Metformin
Methenamine
Methimazole
Methyldopa
Methylphenidate
Metronidazole
Miconazole
Minocycline
Modafinil
Nabumetone
Naproxen
Neomycin
Niacin
Nifedipine
Nimesulide
Nitrofurantoin
Norfloxacin
Nystatin
Ofloxacin
Olopatadine
Omeprazole
Ondansetron
Oral Contraceptives
Orphenadrine
Oxazepam
Oxcarbazepine
Oxybutynin
Oxytetracycline
Paclitaxel
Papaverine
Paroxetine Hydrochloride
PEG-Interferon
Pentobarbital
Phenobarbital
Phenolphthalein
Phenylbutazone
Phenylephrine
Phenylpropanolamine
Phenytoin
Piperacillin/Tazobactam
Piroxicam
Procarbazine
Prochlorperazine
Promethazine
Propofol
Propranolol
Pseudoephedrine
Pyrazinamide
Pyridoxine
Pyrimethamine
Quinacrine
Quinidine
Quinine
Ranitidine
Ribavirin
Rifampin
Rofecoxib
Roxithromycin
Rupatadine
Saccharin
Saquinavir
Scopolamine
Sorafenib
Streptomycin
Sulfadiazine
Sulfadoxine
Sulfamethoxazole
Sulfasalazine
Sulfisoxazole
Sulindac
Tartrazine
Temazepam
Terbinafine
Terfenadine
Tetracycline
Thiabendazole
Thiopental
Ticlopidine
Tinidazole
Tolbutamide
Topiramate
Topotecan
Tosufloxacin
Tranexamic Acid
Triamcinolone
Trifluoperazine
Trimethoprim
Tripelennamine
Triprolidine
Ursodiol
Valproic Acid
Vancomycin
Voriconazole
Zolmitriptan

Gingival hyperplasia/ hypertrophy

Amlodipine
Basiliximab
Cevimeline
Clarithromycin
Co-Trimoxazole
Cycloserine
Cyclosporine
Diltiazem
Erythromycin
Eslicarbazepine
Felodipine
Fosphenytoin
Isradipine
Ketoconazole
Lamotrigine
Levonorgestrel
Lithium
Marihuana
Metoprolol
Mycophenolate
Nicardipine
Nifedipine
Nisoldipine
Oral Contraceptives
Palifermin
Penicillamine
Phenobarbital
Phenytoin
Propranolol
Sertraline
Sirolimus
Tacrolimus
Tartrazine
Tiagabine
Topiramate
Valproic Acid
Vemurafenib
Verapamil
Vigabatrin
Voriconazole
Zonisamide

Hand-foot syndrome

Afatinib
Aflibercept
Axitinib
Bevacizumab
Bleomycin
Bosutinib
Brentuximab Vedotin
Cabazitaxel
Cabozantinib
Capecitabine
Carboplatin
Cetuximab
Cisplatin
Clofarabine
Co-Trimoxazole
Cobimetinib
Cyclophosphamide
Cytarabine
Dabrafenib
Daunorubicin
Docetaxel
Doxorubicin
Epirubicin
Erlotinib
Etoposide
Everolimus
Fluorouracil
Gefitinib
Gemcitabine
Ibandronate
Idarubicin
Imatinib
Infliximab
Interferon Alfa
Ipilimumab
Irinotecan
Ixabepilone
Ketoconazole
Lapatinib
Lenvatinib
Letrozole
Leucovorin
Mercaptopurine
Mesalamine
Mitomycin
Nintedanib
Oxaliplatin
Paclitaxel
Palifermin
Panitumumab
Pazopanib
PEG-Interferon
Phenytoin
Regorafenib
Sorafenib
Sunitinib
Tegafur/Gimeracil/Oteracil
Temozolomide
Temsirolimus
Trabectedin
Trametinib
Trastuzumab
Uracil/Tegafur
Valproic Acid
Vandetanib
Varenicline
Vemurafenib

Vincristine
Vinorelbine
Vorinostat

Lichenoid (lichen planus-like) eruptions

Acebutolol
Acyclovir
Adalimumab
Alendronate
Allopurinol
Aminosalicylate Sodium
Amoxicillin
Anakinra
Aspirin
Atenolol
Atorvastatin
Azathioprine
BCG Vaccine
Captopril
Carbamazepine
Carvedilol
Ceftriaxone
Chloral Hydrate
Chloroquine
Chlorothiazide
Chlorpromazine
Chlorpropamide
Cinnarizine
Clopidogrel
Co-Trimoxazole
Colchicine
Cycloserine
Cyclosporine
Dactinomycin
Demeclocycline
Diazoxide
Diflunisal
Diltiazem
Dorzolamide
Enalapril
Etanercept
Ethambutol
Fluoxymesterone
Flurbiprofen
Fluvastatin
Furosemide
Glimepiride
Glyburide
Gold & Gold Compounds
Granulocyte Colony-Stimulating Factor (G-CSF)
Griseofulvin
Hepatitis B Vaccine
Hydrochlorothiazide
Hydroxychloroquine
Hydroxyurea
Ibuprofen
Imatinib
Imiquimod
Immune Globulin IV
Indomethacin
Infliximab
Interferon Alfa
Irbesartan
Isoniazid
Isotretinoin
Ketoconazole
Labetalol
Lansoprazole
Leflunomide
Levamisole
Lisinopril
Lorazepam
Lovastatin
Mercaptopurine
Mesalamine
Metformin
Methamphetamine
Methyldopa
Methyltestosterone
Metoprolol
Nadolol
Naproxen
Nebivolol
Nelfinavir
Nifedipine
Nivolumab
Obinutuzumab
Olanzapine
Omeprazole
Oral Contraceptives
Orlistat
Pantoprazole
PEG-Interferon
Pembrolizumab
Penicillamine
Phenytoin
Pindolol
Piroxicam
Pneumococcal Vaccine
Pravastatin
Propranolol
Propylthiouracil
Pyrimethamine
Quinacrine
Quinidine
Quinine
Ranitidine
Ribavirin
Rifampin
Risperidone
Roxatidine
Salsalate
Sildenafil
Simeprevir
Simvastatin
Sofosbuvir
Solifenacin
Sotalol
Sparfloxacin
Spironolactone
Streptomycin
Sulfadoxine
Sulfamethoxazole
Sulindac
Temazepam
Tenofovir Disoproxil
Terazosin
Terbinafine
Testosterone
Tetracycline
Thimerosal
Thioridazine
Timolol
Tiopronin
Tiotropium
Tolazamide
Tolbutamide
Torsemide
Trichlormethiazide
Tripelennamine
Triprolidine
Ursodiol
Venlafaxine
Zidovudine

Lupus erythematosus

Acebutolol
Acetazolamide
Adalimumab
Albuterol
Aldesleukin
Allopurinol
Aminoglutethimide
Aminosalicylate Sodium
Amiodarone
Amitriptyline
Anastrozole
Anthrax Vaccine
Atenolol
Atorvastatin
Betaxolol
Bevacizumab
Bortezomib
Bupropion
Butabarbital
Butalbital
Capecitabine
Captopril
Carbamazepine
Carbimazole
Cefepime
Cefuroxime
Celecoxib
Celiprolol
Chlorambucil
Chlordiazepoxide
Chlorothiazide
Chlorpromazine
Chlorpropamide
Chlorthalidone
Cilazapril
Cimetidine
Cinnarizine
Citalopram
Clobazam
Clofibrate
Clonidine
Clozapine
Co-Trimoxazole
Cyclophosphamide
Cyclosporine
Cysteamine
Danazol
Dapsone
Dasatinib
Denosumab
Diethylstilbestrol
Diltiazem
Disopyramide
Docetaxel
Domperidone
Doxazosin
Doxorubicin
Doxycycline
Efalizumab
Enalapril
Esomeprazole
Estrogens
Etanercept
Ethambutol
Ethionamide
Ethosuximide
Fluorouracil
Fluoxymesterone
Fluphenazine
Flutamide
Fluvastatin
Fosphenytoin
Furosemide
Gemcitabine
Gold & Gold Compounds
Golimumab
Granulocyte Colony-Stimulating Factor (G-CSF)
Griseofulvin
Hepatitis B Vaccine
Human Papillomavirus (HPV) Vaccine
Hydralazine
Hydrochlorothiazide
Hydroxyurea
Ibandronate
Ibuprofen
Imipramine
Imiquimod
Infliximab
Interferon Alfa
Interferon Beta
Isoniazid
Labetalol
Lamotrigine
Lansoprazole
Leflunomide
Leuprolide
Levodopa
Lidocaine
Lisinopril
Lithium
Lovastatin
Mephenytoin
Meprobamate
Mercaptopurine
Mesalamine
Methimazole
Methoxsalen
Methsuximide
Methyldopa
Methyltestosterone
Methysergide
Metoprolol
Mexiletine
Minocycline
Minoxidil
Mitotane
Nafcillin
Nalidixic Acid
Naproxen
Nifedipine
Nitrofurantoin
Olsalazine
Omeprazole
Oral Contraceptives
Paclitaxel
Pantoprazole
PEG-Interferon
Penicillamine
Pentobarbital
Perphenazine
Phenelzine
Phenobarbital
Phenolphthalein
Phenylbutazone
Phenytoin
Pindolol

Piroxicam
Potassium Iodide
Pravastatin
Prazosin
Prednicarbate
Primidone
Procainamide
Promethazine
Propafenone
Propranolol
Propylthiouracil
Psoralens
Quinidine
Quinine
Ranitidine
Reserpine
Ribavirin
Rifabutin
Rifampin
Rituximab
Sertraline
Simvastatin
Smallpox Vaccine
Somatropin
Spironolactone
Streptomycin
Sulfadiazine
Sulfamethoxazole
Sulfasalazine
Sulfisoxazole
Tamoxifen
Terbinafine
Terfenadine
Testosterone
Tetracycline
Thioridazine
Ticlopidine
Timolol
Tiopronin
Tiotropium
Tocainide
Triamterene
Trichlormethiazide
Trientine
Trimethadione
Trimethoprim
Trioxsalen
Uracil/Tegafur
Valproic Acid
Vancomycin
Verapamil
Vitamin E
Voriconazole
Zafirlukast
Zinc
Ziprasidone
Zonisamide

Onycholysis

Acitretin
Adalimumab
Allopurinol
Bleomycin
Capecitabine
Captopril
Chloramphenicol
Chlorpromazine
Clofazimine
Clorazepate
Dabrafenib
Demeclocycline
Diclofenac
Docetaxel
Doxorubicin
Doxycycline
Estrogens
Etoposide
Gold & Gold Compounds
Griseofulvin
Hydroxyurea
Ibuprofen
Indapamide
Irinotecan
Isotretinoin
Ketoprofen
Methotrexate
Methoxsalen
Minocycline
Mitoxantrone
Mycophenolate
Nintedanib
Nitrofurantoin
Norfloxacin
Ofloxacin
Oral Contraceptives
Paclitaxel
Pemetrexed
Propranolol
Psoralens
Quinine
Roxithromycin
Sparfloxacin
Tasonermin
Tetracycline
Trioxsalen
Vemurafenib
Voriconazole

Paresthesias

Acamprosate
Acetazolamide
Acitretin
Acyclovir
Adalimumab
Adenosine
Afamelanotide
Agalsidase
Alitretinoin
Allopurinol
Almotriptan
Alprazolam
Altretamine
Amikacin
Amiloride
Amiodarone
Amlodipine
Amoxapine
Amphotericin B
Amprenavir
Anagrelide
Apraclonidine
Arbutamine
Arformoterol
Aripiprazole
Arsenic
Artemether/Lumefantrine
Articaine
Aspirin
Astemizole
Atorvastatin
Avanafil
Azatadine
Azithromycin
Baclofen
Basiliximab
Benazepril
Benzthiazide
Bepridil
Betaxolol
Bicalutamide
Blinatumomab
Bortezomib
Brivaracetam
Bromocriptine
Brompheniramine
Bupivacaine
Bupropion
Buspirone
Cabergoline
Cabozantinib
Calcitonin
Candesartan
Capecitabine
Captopril
Carboplatin
Carfilzomib
Carisoprodol
Carteolol
Carvedilol
Caspofungin
Ceftazidime
Ceftibuten
Ceftizoxime
Ceftolozane & Tazobactam
Celecoxib
Cephapirin
Ceritinib
Cetirizine
Cevimeline
Chloramphenicol
Chlorothiazide
Chlorpheniramine
Chlorthalidone
Cidofovir
Cilostazol
Cinacalcet
Cinoxacin
Ciprofloxacin
Cisplatin
Citalopram
Clemastine
Clonazepam
Clopidogrel
Clozapine
Coagulation Factor IX (Recombinant)
Colistin
Cyclamate
Cyclobenzaprine
Cyclophosphamide
Cyclosporine
Cyproheptadine
Dalfampridine
Daptomycin
Dasatinib
Delavirdine
Demeclocycline
Denileukin
Desvenlafaxine
Dexamethasone
Dexchlorpheniramine
Dichlorphenamide
Diclofenac
Diflunisal
Dihydroergotamine
Diltiazem
Dimenhydrinate
Diphenhydramine
Dipyridamole
Dirithromycin
Disopyramide
Dobutamine
Docetaxel
Dofetilide
Donepezil
Doxycycline
Duloxetine
Efavirenz
Eflornithine
Eletriptan
Eltrombopag
Emtricitabine
Enalapril
Enoxacin
Entecavir
Enzalutamide
Epirubicin
Epoetin Alfa
Epoprostenol
Eprosartan
Ergotamine
Ertapenem
Escitalopram
Esmolol
Esomeprazole
Estazolam
Eszopiclone
Etanercept
Ethoxzolamide
Etravirine
Evolocumab
Exemestane
Ezetimibe
Ezogabine
Famciclovir
Famotidine
Febuxostat
Felbamate
Felodipine
Fentanyl
Ferric Gluconate
Ferumoxsil
Ferumoxytol
Fingolimod
Flecainide
Fluconazole
Flucytosine
Fludarabine
Flumazenil
Fluorouracil
Fluoxetine
Flurbiprofen
Flutamide
Fosamprenavir
Foscarnet
Fosfomycin
Fosinopril
Fosphenytoin
Frovatriptan
Fulvestrant
Gabapentin
Gadobenate
Gadobutrol
Gadodiamide
Gadofosveset
Gadopentetate

Gadoteridol
Gadoversetamide
Gadoxetate
Galantamine
Ganciclovir
Gatifloxacin
Gemcitabine
Gemfibrozil
Gentamicin
Glatiramer
Glipizide
Glucarpidase
Glyburide
Grepafloxacin
Griseofulvin
Guanadrel
Guanethidine
Guanfacine
Halofantrine
Histrelin
Human Papillomavirus Vaccine (Bivalent)
Hydrocodone
Hydroflumethiazide
Imatinib
Imipenem/Cilastatin
Indapamide
Indinavir
Indomethacin
Infliximab
Insulin
Interferon Alfa
Interferon Beta
Iodixanol
Iohexol
Iopromide
Ioversol
Ipilimumab
Ipratropium
Irbesartan
Isavuconazonium Sulfate
Isoniazid
Isradipine
Ixazomib
Ketoconazole
Ketoprofen
Ketorolac
Labetalol
Lamivudine
Lamotrigine
Lansoprazole
Laronidase
Leflunomide
Leuprolide
Levalbuterol
Levamisole
Levetiracetam
Levobupivacaine
Levofloxacin
Levomilnacipran
Lidocaine
Lisinopril
Lomefloxacin
Loratadine
Lorcainide
Losartan
Lovastatin
Lubiprostone
Maraviroc
MDMA
Meclizine
Meclofenamate
Medroxyprogesterone
Meloxicam
Menadione
Methazolamide
Methimazole
Methyclothiazide
Methyldopa
Metoclopramide
Metolazone
Metronidazole
Mexiletine
Midodrine
Miglustat
Milnacipran
Miltefosine
Minocycline
Mirtazapine
Mitomycin
Modafinil
Moricizine
Moxifloxacin
Nabumetone
Nadolol
Nafarelin
Naproxen
Naratriptan
Nebivolol
Nefazodone
Nelarabine
Nelfinavir
Nesiritide
Nevirapine
Niacin
Niacinamide
Nicardipine
Nifedipine
Nilotinib
Nilutamide
Nisoldipine
Nitrofurantoin
Nivolumab
Nizatidine
Ofloxacin
Omacetaxine
Omalizumab
Omeprazole
Ondansetron
Oseltamivir
Oxaliplatin
Oxilan
Oxprenolol
Oxycodone
Oxytetracycline
Paclitaxel
Palifermin
Pandemic Influenza Vaccine (HINI)
Pantoprazole
Paricalcitol
Paroxetine Hydrochloride
Pegaspargase
Pegvisomant
Pembrolizumab
Pentamidine
Pentostatin
Pentoxifylline
Perampanel
Perflutren
Pergolide
Perindopril
Phentermine
Phenytoin
Pindolol
Pirbuterol
Piroxicam
Pizotifen
Plasma (Human) Blood Product
Posaconazole
Pramipexole
Pravastatin
Prazosin
Prednicarbate
Pregabalin
Prilocaine
Procarbazine
Promethazine
Propafenone
Propylthiouracil
Pyridoxine
Quetiapine
Quinapril
Quinupristin/Dalfopristin
Rabeprazole
Ramipril
Ranolazine
Rasagiline
Rasburicase
Reboxetine
Repaglinide
Rifabutin
Rifampin
Riluzole
Rimantadine
Risedronate
Risperidone
Ritonavir
Rivaroxaban
Rivastigmine
Rizatriptan
Rofecoxib
Romiplostim
Ropinirole
Ropivacaine
Rosuvastatin
Rotigotine
Saquinavir
Sertraline
Sibutramine
Sildenafil
Siltuximab
Sincalide
Sipuleucel-T
Sirolimus
Smallpox Vaccine
Sodium Oxybate
Somatropin
Sotalol
Sparfloxacin
Stavudine
Streptomycin
Succimer
Sufentanil
Sugammadex
Sulfasalazine
Sulindac
Sumatriptan
Tacrine
Tacrolimus
Tadalafil
Taliglucerase
Tartrazine
Tegafur/Gimeracil/Oteracil
Telaprevir
Telbivudine
Telithromycin
Telmisartan
Temozolomide
Terazosin
Terfenadine
Teriflunomide
Teriparatide
Tesamorelin
Testosterone
Tetrabenazine
Tetracycline
Thalidomide
Thallium
Thiamine
Thyrotropin Alfa
Tiagabine
Tibolone
Tiludronate
Timolol
Tinidazole
Tiotropium
Tizanidine
Tobramycin
Tocainide
Tofacitinib
Tolcapone
Tolterodine
Topiramate
Topotecan
Torsemide
Trabectedin
Tramadol
Trandolapril
Trastuzumab
Travoprost
Trazodone
Tretinoin
Triazolam
Trihexyphenidyl
Trimeprazine
Tripelennamine
Triprolidine
Triptorelin
Trovafloxacin
Unoprostone
Valacyclovir
Valdecoxib
Valganciclovir
Valproic Acid
Valsartan
Vardenafil
Venlafaxine
Verapamil
Vernakalant
Vilazodone
Vinblastine
Vincristine
Vinorelbine
Voriconazole
Zaleplon
Ziconotide
Zidovudine
Zileuton
Ziprasidone
Zoledronate
Zolmitriptan
Zolpidem

Zonisamide
Zuclopenthixol

Pemphigus vulgaris

Acetaminophen
Acetazolamide
Aldesleukin
Amoxicillin
Ampicillin
Aspirin
Atorvastatin
Benazepril
Bucillamine
Captopril
Carbamazepine
Carbimazole
Cefaclor
Cefadroxil
Cefazolin
Cefixime
Ceftazidime
Ceftriaxone
Cefuroxime
Cephalexin
Chloroquine
Cilazapril
Clonidine
Cocaine
Cyclophosphamide
Diclofenac
Enalapril
Epinephrine
Famotidine
Fludarabine
Fosinopril
Glyburide
Gold & Gold Compounds
Haloperidol
Hepatitis B Vaccine
Heroin
Hydroxychloroquine
Ibuprofen
Imiquimod
Influenza Vaccine
Ingenol Mebutate
Interferon Alfa
Interferon Beta
Isotretinoin
Ketoprofen
Latanoprost
Levamisole
Levodopa
Meprobamate
Metamizole
Metformin
Methoxsalen
Moexipril
Montelukast
Mycophenolate
Nifedipine
Omeprazole
Pembrolizumab
Penicillamine
Phenobarbital
Phenylbutazone
Phenytoin
Piroxicam
Propranolol
Psoralens
Quinapril
Ramipril
Rifampin
Rituximab
Spironolactone
Timolol
Tiopronin
Trandolapril
Trioxsalen
Typhoid Vaccine

Peyronie's disease

Acebutolol
Betaxolol
Carvedilol
Labetalol
Methotrexate
Metoprolol
Nadolol
Papaverine
Pindolol
Propranolol
Ropinirole
Timolol

Photosensitivity

Acamprosate
Aceclofenac
Acetohexamide
Acetylcysteine
Acitretin
Acyclovir
Aldesleukin
Alectinib
Allopurinol
Almotriptan
Alprazolam
Amantadine
Amiloride
Aminolevulinic Acid
Aminosalicylate Sodium
Amiodarone
Amitriptyline
Amoxapine
Anagrelide
Arsenic
Astemizole
Atorvastatin
Atropine Sulfate
Azatadine
Azathioprine
Azithromycin
Benazepril
Bendroflumethiazide
Benztropine
Bezafibrate
Bicalutamide
Brompheniramine
Bumetanide
Bupropion
Butabarbital
Butalbital
Calcipotriol
Canagliflozin
Candesartan
Capecitabine
Captopril
Carbamazepine
Carisoprodol
Carvedilol
Cefazolin
Ceftazidime
Celecoxib
Cetirizine
Cevimeline
Chlorambucil
Chlordiazepoxide
Chlorhexidine
Chloroquine
Chlorothiazide
Chlorpheniramine
Chlorpromazine
Chlorpropamide
Chlortetracycline
Chlorthalidone
Ciprofloxacin
Clemastine
Clofazimine
Clofibrate
Clomipramine
Clopidogrel
Clorazepate
Clozapine
Co-Trimoxazole
Cobimetinib
Colchicine
Crizotinib
Cyclamate
Cyproheptadine
Dabrafenib
Dacarbazine
Danazol
Dapsone
Dasatinib
Demeclocycline
Desipramine
Desoximetasone
Dexamethasone
Dexchlorpheniramine
Diazoxide
Diclofenac
Diflunisal
Diltiazem
Dimenhydrinate
Diphenhydramine
Disopyramide
Docetaxel
Doxepin
Doxycycline
Dronedarone
Duloxetine
Eculizumab
Efavirenz
Enalapril
Enoxacin
Epoetin Alfa
Erlotinib
Esomeprazole
Estrogens
Eszopiclone
Ethambutol
Ethionamide
Etodolac
Febuxostat
Felbamate
Fenofibrate
Flucytosine
Fluorouracil
Fluoxetine
Flurbiprofen
Flutamide
Fluvoxamine
Fosinopril
Furazolidone
Furosemide
Ganciclovir
Gatifloxacin
Gemifloxacin
Gentamicin
Glimepiride
Glipizide
Glyburide
Glycopyrrolate
Gold & Gold Compounds
Grepafloxacin
Griseofulvin
Haloperidol
Heroin
Hydralazine
Hydrochlorothiazide
Hydroflumethiazide
Hydroxychloroquine
Hydroxyurea
Hydroxyzine
Hyoscyamine
Ibuprofen
Imatinib
Imipramine
Indapamide
Indomethacin
Interferon Alfa
Interferon Beta
Irbesartan
Irinotecan
Isocarboxazid
Isoniazid
Isotretinoin
Itraconazole
Kanamycin
Ketoconazole
Ketoprofen
Ketorolac
Lamotrigine
Levofloxacin
Lisinopril
Lomefloxacin
Loratadine
Losartan
Loxapine
Maprotiline
Meclizine
Meclofenamate
Meloxicam
Meprobamate
Mercaptopurine
Mesalamine
Mesoridazine
Metformin
Methenamine
Methotrexate
Methoxsalen
Methyclothiazide
Methyldopa
Methylphenidate
Metolazone
Minocycline
Minoxidil
Mitomycin
Moexipril
Molindone
Moxifloxacin
Nabumetone
Nalidixic Acid
Naproxen
Naratriptan
Nefazodone
Nifedipine
Nimesulide

Nivolumab
Norfloxacin
Nortriptyline
Ofloxacin
Olanzapine
Olmesartan
Omalizumab
Ombitasvir/Paritaprevir/Ritonavir
Oral Contraceptives
Oxaprozin
Oxerutins
Oxytetracycline
Paclitaxel
Pantoprazole
Paroxetine Hydrochloride
PEG-Interferon
Pentobarbital
Pentosan
Pentostatin
Phenelzine
Phenobarbital
Phenytoin
Pilocarpine
Pimozide
Pirfenidone
Piroxicam
Polythiazide
Porfimer
Pravastatin
Procainamide
Prochlorperazine
Procyclidine
Promazine
Promethazine
Propranolol
Propylthiouracil
Protriptyline
Psoralens
Pyrazinamide
Pyridoxine
Pyrimethamine
Quetiapine
Quinacrine
Quinapril
Quinethazone
Quinidine
Quinine
Rabeprazole
Ramipril
Ranitidine
Regorafenib
Ribavirin
Rifaximin
Risperidone
Ritonavir
Ropinirole
Saccharin
Saquinavir
Scopolamine
Sertraline
Sildenafil
Simeprevir
Simvastatin
Sitagliptin
Smallpox Vaccine
Sotalol
Sparfloxacin
Streptomycin
Sulfadiazine
Sulfadoxine
Sulfamethoxazole
Sulfasalazine
Sulfisoxazole
Sulindac
Sumatriptan
Tacrolimus
Tartrazine
Tegafur/Gimeracil/Oteracil
Telmisartan
Terfenadine
Tetracycline
Thimerosal
Thioguanine
Thioridazine
Thiothixene
Tiagabine
Tiopronin
Tiotropium
Tocilizumab
Tolazamide
Tolbutamide
Tolmetin
Topiramate
Torsemide
Tranylcypromine
Trastuzumab
Trazodone
Tretinoin
Triamterene
Triazolam
Trichlormethiazide
Trifluoperazine
Trihexyphenidyl
Trimeprazine
Trimethadione
Trimipramine
Trioxsalen
Tripelennamine
Triprolidine
Trovafloxacin
Uracil/Tegafur
Valdecoxib
Valproic Acid
Valsartan
Vandetanib
Vardenafil
Vemurafenib
Venlafaxine
Verapamil
Verteporfin
Vinblastine
Voriconazole
Xipamide
Zalcitabine
Zaleplon
Ziprasidone
Zolmitriptan
Zolpidem

Pigmentation

Acitretin
Adapalene
Afamelanotide
Alitretinoin
Amantadine
Amifostine
Aminolevulinic Acid
Amiodarone
Amitriptyline
Amlodipine
Amoxicillin
Apomorphine
Arformoterol
Arsenic
Asfotase Alfa
Azacitidine
Azathioprine
Betaxolol
Bevacizumab
Bimatoprost
Bismuth
Bleomycin
Bortezomib
Bupropion
Busulfan
Cabozantinib
Calcipotriol
Capecitabine
Captopril
Carboplatin
Carmustine
Ceftriaxone
Cetirizine
Cevimeline
Chlorhexidine
Chloroquine
Chlorotrianisene
Chlorpromazine
Cidofovir
Ciprofloxacin
Cisplatin
Citalopram
Clobetasol
Clofazimine
Clomipramine
Clonazepam
Clonidine
Clozapine
Co-Trimoxazole
Cobicistat/Elvitegravir/Emtricitabine/Tenofovir Disoproxil
Collagen (Bovine)
Cyclophosphamide
Dactinomycin
Dapsone
Dasatinib
Daunorubicin
Deferasirox
Degarelix
Deoxycholic Acid
Desipramine
Dexamethasone
Diazepam
Dicumarol
Diethylstilbestrol
Diltiazem
Docetaxel
Donepezil
Doxorubicin
Doxycycline
Eletriptan
Elotuzumab
Eltrombopag
Emtricitabine
Enoxacin
Epirubicin
Erythromycin
Esmolol
Estradiol
Estramustine
Estrogens
Eszopiclone
Etoposide
Ezogabine
Fentanyl
Finasteride
Fluconazole
Fluorouracil
Fluoxetine
Fluphenazine
Fluvoxamine
Foscarnet
Ganciclovir
Gefitinib
Glyburide
Gold & Gold Compounds
Goserelin
Grepafloxacin
Griseofulvin
Halobetasol
Haloperidol
Heroin
Human Papillomavirus (HPV) Vaccine
Hyaluronic Acid
Hydrochlorothiazide
Hydroquinone
Hydroxychloroquine
Hydroxyurea
Ifosfamide
Imatinib
Imipramine
Imiquimod
Indapamide
Indinavir
Insulin
Interferon Alfa
Irinotecan
Isotretinoin
Ixabepilone
Ixazomib
Ketoconazole
Ketoprofen
Labetalol
Lamivudine
Lapatinib
Latanoprost
Leflunomide
Lenalidomide
Leuprolide
Levobupivacaine
Levodopa
Levofloxacin
Levonorgestrel
Levothyroxine
Lidocaine
Linezolid
Lithium
Lomefloxacin
Loxapine
Mechlorethamine
Medroxyprogesterone
Mephenytoin
Mercaptopurine
Mesoridazine
Methamphetamine
Methotrexate
Methoxsalen
Methyldopa
Methysergide
Metoclopramide
Minocycline
Minoxidil

Mirtazapine
Mitomycin
Mitotane
Molindone
Naratriptan
Niacin
Nicotine
Nifedipine
Nisoldipine
Nitazoxanide
Nitisinone
Olanzapine
Omacetaxine
Omeprazole
Oral Contraceptives
Orphenadrine
Oxytetracycline
Paclitaxel
Palifermin
Panitumumab
Pantoprazole
Paroxetine Hydrochloride
Pazopanib
PEG-Interferon
Pemetrexed
Pentazocine
Pentostatin
Perphenazine
Phenazopyridine
Phenobarbital
Phenolphthalein
Phenytoin
Pimozide
Polidocanol
Porfimer
Prilocaine
Procarbazine
Prochlorperazine
Promazine
Propofol
Propranolol
Psoralens
Pyridoxine
Pyrimethamine
Quinacrine
Quinestrol
Quinidine
Quinine
Rabeprazole
Regorafenib
Ribavirin
Rifabutin
Rifapentine
Risperidone
Ropinirole
Saquinavir
Sertraline
Sildenafil
Siltuximab
Smallpox Vaccine
Sorafenib
Sparfloxacin
Spironolactone
Stanozolol
Sulfadiazine
Sulfasalazine
Sunitinib
Tacrolimus
Tafluprost
Tamoxifen
Tegafur/Gimeracil/Oteracil
Telithromycin
Telmisartan
Terbinafine
Tetracycline
Thioridazine
Thiotepa
Thiothixene
Tiagabine
Tigecycline
Tinidazole
Tolcapone
Topiramate
Trastuzumab
Travoprost
Tretinoin
Triamcinolone
Trifluoperazine
Trioxsalen
Triptorelin
Unoprostone
Uracil/Tegafur
Vandetanib
Venlafaxine
Verapamil
Vinblastine
Vincristine
Vinorelbine
Vitamin A
Voriconazole
Warfarin
Zidovudine
Zinc

Pityriasis rosea-like eruption

Acetaminophen
Acyclovir
Allopurinol
Ampicillin
Arsenic
Asenapine
Aspirin
Atenolol
BCG Vaccine
Bismuth
Captopril
Clonidine
Clozapine
Codeine
Everolimus
Gold & Gold Compounds
Hydrochlorothiazide
Imatinib
Isotretinoin
Ketotifen
Lamotrigine
Lisinopril
Meprobamate
Metronidazole
Mitomycin
Naproxen
Nimesulide
Nortriptyline
Omeprazole
Pneumococcal Vaccine
Terbinafine
Tiopronin
Tripelennamine

Pruritus

Abacavir
Abatacept
Abciximab
Acamprosate
Acebutolol
Acetaminophen
Acetohexamide
Acetylcysteine
Acitretin
Acyclovir
Adalimumab
Adapalene
Adefovir
Ado-Trastuzumab Emtansine
Afatinib
Albendazole
Albuterol
Alcaftadine
Aldesleukin
Alefacept
Alemtuzumab
Alendronate
Alfentanil
Alglucerase
Alitretinoin
Allopurinol
Almotriptan
Alogliptin
Alpha-Lipoic Acid
Alprazolam
Alprostadil
Altretamine
Alvimopan
Amantadine
Amcinonide
Amikacin
Amiloride
Aminoglutethimide
Aminolevulinic Acid
Aminophylline
Aminosalicylate Sodium
Amiodarone
Amitriptyline
Amlodipine
Amodiaquine
Amoxapine
Amoxicillin
Amphotericin B
Ampicillin
Anagrelide
Anastrozole
Anidulafungin
Anthrax Vaccine
Anti-Thymocyte Immunoglobulin (Rabbit)
Apomorphine
Apraclonidine
Aprepitant
Arsenic
Artemether/Lumefantrine
Artesunate
Asfotase Alfa
Asparaginase
Aspartame
Aspirin
Astemizole
Atazanavir
Atenolol
Atezolizumab
Atomoxetine
Atorvastatin
Atovaquone
Atovaquone/Proguanil
Atracurium
Axitinib
Azacitidine
Azathioprine
Azithromycin
Aztreonam
Bacampicillin
Bacitracin
Baclofen
Basiliximab
Becaplermin
Belinostat
Benazepril
Bendamustine
Bendroflumethiazide
Benzalkonium
Benzyl Alcohol
Besifloxacin
Betamethasone
Betaxolol
Bevacizumab
Bexarotene
Bezafibrate
Bicalutamide
Bimatoprost
Bismuth
Bleomycin
Boceprevir
Bortezomib
Bosentan
Bosutinib
Botulinum Toxin (A & B)
Brentuximab Vedotin
Brimonidine
Brinzolamide
Bromfenac
Budesonide
Bumetanide
Bupivacaine
Buprenorphine
Bupropion
Buspirone
Butorphanol
Cabergoline
Calcipotriol
Calcium Hydroxylapatite
Canagliflozin
Capecitabine
Captopril
Carbamazepine
Carbetocin
Carboplatin
Carisoprodol
Carmustine
Carvedilol
Caspofungin
Cefaclor
Cefadroxil
Cefamandole
Cefazolin
Cefdinir
Cefditoren
Cefepime
Cefixime
Cefmetazole
Cefonicid
Cefoperazone
Cefotaxime
Cefotetan
Cefoxitin
Cefpodoxime
Cefprozil
Ceftaroline Fosamil

Ceftazidime
Ceftibuten
Ceftizoxime
Ceftobiprole
Ceftolozane & Tazobactam
Ceftriaxone
Cefuroxime
Celecoxib
Cephalexin
Cephalothin
Cephapirin
Cephradine
Certolizumab
Cetirizine
Cetrorelix
Cetuximab
Cevimeline
Chloral Hydrate
Chlorambucil
Chloramphenicol
Chlordiazepoxide
Chlorhexidine
Chlormezanone
Chloroquine
Chlorothiazide
Chlorpheniramine
Chlorpromazine
Chlorpropamide
Cholestyramine
Ciclopirox
Cidofovir
Cimetidine
Cinoxacin
Ciprofloxacin
Cisplatin
Citalopram
Cladribine
Clarithromycin
Clindamycin
Clobetasol
Clofarabine
Clofazimine
Clofibrate
Clomiphene
Clomipramine
Clonidine
Clopidogrel
Clotrimazole
Cloxacillin
Clozapine
Co-Trimoxazole
Coagulation Factor IX (Recombinant)
Codeine
Colchicine
Collagen (Bovine)
Conivaptan
Cromolyn
Cyanocobalamin
Cyclamate
Cyclobenzaprine
Cyclophosphamide
Cyclosporine
Cytarabine
Dabrafenib
Dacarbazine
Daclatasvir
Daclizumab
Dactinomycin
Dalbavancin
Dalteparin
Danaparoid
Danazol
Dapsone
Daptomycin
Darbepoetin Alfa
Darifenacin
Darunavir
Dasabuvir/Ombitasvir/Paritaprevir/Ritonavir
Dasatinib
Daunorubicin
Decitabine
Deferasirox
Deferoxamine
Defibrotide
Delavirdine
Demeclocycline
Denileukin
Denosumab
Deoxycholic Acid
Desipramine
Desonide
Desoximetasone
Dexamethasone
Dexlansoprazole
Diatrizoate
Diazepam
Diclofenac
Dicloxacillin
Dicumarol
Dicyclomine
Didanosine
Diethylpropion
Diethylstilbestrol
Diflunisal
Difluprednate
Digoxin
Dihydrocodeine
Dihydrotachysterol
Diltiazem
Dimethyl Fumarate
Diphenhydramine
Diphenoxylate
Dipyridamole
Dirithromycin
Disopyramide
Dobutamine
Docetaxel
Dolasetron
Dolutegravir
Donepezil
Doripenem
Dorzolamide
Doxapram
Doxazosin
Doxepin
Doxercalciferol
Doxorubicin
Doxycycline
Dronedarone
Droperidol
Duloxetine
Ecallantide
Econazole
Eculizumab
Efavirenz
Eflornithine
Eletriptan
Emtricitabine
Enalapril
Enfuvirtide
Enoxacin
Enoxaparin
Enzalutamide
Epinastine
Epinephrine
Epirubicin
Epoetin Alfa
Epoprostenol
Eprosartan
Ergocalciferol
Erlotinib
Ertapenem
Erythromycin
Escitalopram
Esomeprazole
Estazolam
Estramustine
Estrogens
Eszopiclone
Etanercept
Ethambutol
Etidronate
Etodolac
Everolimus
Evolocumab
Exemestane
Exenatide
Ezetimibe
Factor VIII - von Willebrand Factor
Famciclovir
Famotidine
Febuxostat
Felbamate
Felodipine
Fenofibrate
Fenoprofen
Fentanyl
Ferric Gluconate
Ferumoxytol
Fidaxomicin
Finafloxacin
Finasteride
Fingolimod
Flecainide
Fluconazole
Fludarabine
Fluocinonide
Fluorides
Fluorouracil
Fluoxetine
Fluphenazine
Flurbiprofen
Fluticasone Propionate
Folic Acid
Follitropin Alfa/Beta
Fondaparinux
Formoterol
Fosamprenavir
Foscarnet
Fosfomycin
Fosinopril
Fosphenytoin
Frovatriptan
Fulvestrant
Furazolidone
Furosemide
Gabapentin
Gadobenate
Gadobutrol
Gadodiamide
Gadofosveset
Gadopentetate
Gadoteridol
Gadoversetamide
Gadoxetate
Ganciclovir
Gatifloxacin
Gefitinib
Gemcitabine
Gemfibrozil
Gemifloxacin
Gemtuzumab
Gentamicin
Glatiramer
Gliclazide
Glimepiride
Glipizide
Glucosamine
Glyburide
Gold & Gold Compounds
Golimumab
Goserelin
Granulocyte Colony-Stimulating Factor (G-CSF)
Grepafloxacin
Griseofulvin
Guanabenz
Guanfacine
Halcinonide
Halobetasol
Halofantrine
Halometasone
Haloperidol
Heparin
Heroin
Histrelin
Human Papillomavirus (HPV) Vaccine
Human Papillomavirus Vaccine (Bivalent)
Hyaluronic Acid
Hydralazine
Hydrochlorothiazide
Hydrocodone
Hydrocortisone
Hydromorphone
Hydroquinone
Hydroxychloroquine
Hydroxyurea
Ibandronate
Ibritumomab
Ibuprofen
Icatibant
Icodextrin
Idursulfase
Imatinib
Imidapril
Imiglucerase
Imipenem/Cilastatin
Imipramine
Imiquimod
Immune Globulin IV
Immune Globulin SC
Indapamide
Indinavir
Indomethacin
Infliximab
Ingenol Mebutate
Insulin
Insulin Glulisine
Interferon Alfa

Iobenguane
Iodixanol
Iohexol
Iomeprol
Iopromide
Ioversol
Ipilimumab
Ipratropium
Irbesartan
Irinotecan
Isavuconazonium Sulfate
Isocarboxazid
Isoniazid
Isosorbide Mononitrate
Isotretinoin
Isradipine
Itraconazole
Ivermectin
Ixabepilone
Ixazomib
Japanese Encephalitis Vaccine
Kanamycin
Ketamine
Ketoconazole
Ketoprofen
Ketorolac
Ketotifen
Labetalol
Lacosamide
Lamivudine
Lamotrigine
Lanreotide
Lansoprazole
Lapatinib
Latanoprost
Ledipasvir & Sofosbuvir
Leflunomide
Lenalidomide
Lepirudin
Letrozole
Leucovorin
Leuprolide
Levalbuterol
Levamisole
Levetiracetam
Levobunolol
Levobupivacaine
Levofloxacin
Levomilnacipran
Levothyroxine
Lidocaine
Lifitegrast
Linagliptin
Lincomycin
Lindane
Linezolid
Liraglutide
Lisinopril
Lithium
Lixisenatide
Lodoxamide
Lomefloxacin
Loracarbef
Loratadine
Losartan
Lovastatin
Loxapine
Luliconazole
Lurasidone
Mafenide
Maraviroc
Mebendazole
Mechlorethamine
Meclofenamate
Medroxyprogesterone
Mefenamic Acid
Mefloquine
Meloxicam
Melphalan
Memantine
Meperidine
Mephenytoin
Mepivacaine
Mepolizumab
Meprobamate
Meropenem
Mesalamine
Mesna
Metamizole
Metformin
Methadone
Methenamine
Methimazole
Methotrexate
Methoxsalen
Methyl salicylate
Methyldopa
Methylprednisolone
Metolazone
Metoprolol
Metronidazole
Mexiletine
Micafungin
Miconazole
Midazolam
Midodrine
Mifepristone
Milnacipran
Miltefosine
Minocycline
Minoxidil
Mirabegron
Mitomycin
Mitotane
Modafinil
Moexipril
Molindone
Mometasone
Moricizine
Morphine
Moxifloxacin
Mupirocin
Muromonab-CD3
Mycophenolate
Nabumetone
Nadolol
Nafarelin
Nalbuphine
Nalidixic Acid
Nalmefene
Naloxone
Naltrexone
Naproxen
Naratriptan
Natalizumab
Necitumumab
Nefazodone
Nelfinavir
Neostigmine
Nepafenac
Nesiritide
Nevirapine
Niacin
Niacinamide
Nicotine
Nifedipine
Nilotinib
Nilutamide
Nimesulide
Nimodipine
Nintedanib
Nisoldipine
Nitazoxanide
Nitisinone
Nitrofurantoin
Nitrofurazone
Nitroglycerin
Nivolumab
Nizatidine
Norfloxacin
Nystatin
Obeticholic Acid
Octreotide
Ofatumumab
Ofloxacin
Olanzapine
Olaparib
Olsalazine
Omacetaxine
Omalizumab
Ombitasvir/Paritaprevir/Ritonavir
Omeprazole
Ondansetron
Oral Contraceptives
Oritavancin
Oxacillin
Oxaliplatin
Oxaprozin
Oxerutins
Oxilan
Oxybutynin
Oxycodone
Oxymorphone
Oxytetracycline
Paclitaxel
Palifermin
Paliperidone
Palonosetron
Pancrelipase
Panitumumab
Pantoprazole
Papaverine
Paricalcitol
Paromomycin
Paroxetine Hydrochloride
Paroxetine Mesylate
Pasireotide
Pazopanib
PEG-Interferon
Pegaspargase
Pegvisomant
Pembrolizumab
Pemetrexed
Penicillamine
Penicillin V
Pentagastrin
Pentamidine
Pentazocine
Pentosan
Pentostatin
Pentoxifylline
Perflutren
Perindopril
Permethrin
Pertuzumab
Phenelzine
Phenobarbital
Phenolphthalein
Phenytoin
Pimecrolimus
Pindolol
Pirfenidone
Piroxicam
Plasma (Human) Blood Product
Pneumococcal Vaccine
Podophyllotoxin
Polidocanol
Pomalidomide
Posaconazole
Pralatrexate
Pramipexole
Pravastatin
Praziquantel
Prazosin
Prednicarbate
Prednisolone
Prednisone
Pregabalin
Prilocaine
Primaquine
Pristinamycin
Probenecid
Procainamide
Procarbazine
Prochlorperazine
Propafenone
Propofol
Propranolol
Propylthiouracil
Protriptyline
Psoralens
Pyrazinamide
Pyrimethamine
Quazepam
Quinacrine
Quinapril
Quinethazone
Quinidine
Quinine
Quinupristin/Dalfopristin
Rabeprazole
Raltegravir
Raltitrexed
Ramipril
Ranibizumab
Ranitidine
Rasburicase
Regorafenib
Remifentanil
Repaglinide
Retapamulin
Ribavirin
Rifampin
Rifapentine
Rifaximin
Risedronate
Risperidone
Ritonavir
Rituximab
Rivaroxaban
Rivastigmine
Rizatriptan

Rocuronium
Rofecoxib
Romidepsin
Ropinirole
Ropivacaine
Rosuvastatin
Rotigotine
Rufinamide
Saccharin
Sacubitril/Valsartan
Saquinavir
Saxagliptin
Scopolamine
Secukinumab
Sertaconazole
Sertraline
Sevelamer
Sevoflurane
Sibutramine
Sildenafil
Siltuximab
Simeprevir
Simvastatin
Sirolimus
Smallpox Vaccine
Sodium Iodide I-131
Sodium Oxybate
Sofosbuvir
Sonidegib
Sorafenib
Sotalol
Sparfloxacin
Spectinomycin
Spinosad
Spironolactone
Streptokinase
Streptomycin
Streptozocin
Succimer
Succinylcholine
Sucralfate
Sufentanil
Sugammadex
Sulfadiazine
Sulfadoxine
Sulfamethoxazole
Sulfasalazine
Sulfisoxazole
Sulindac
Sumatriptan
Sunitinib
Tacrine
Tacrolimus
Tadalafil
Tafluprost
Taliglucerase
Tamoxifen
Tartrazine
Tazarotene
Tedizolid
Tegafur/Gimeracil/Oteracil
Tegaserod
Teicoplanin
Telaprevir
Telavancin
Telbivudine
Telithromycin
Telmisartan
Temozolomide
Temsirolimus
Terazosin
Terbinafine
Terbutaline
Terconazole
Teriflunomide
Tesamorelin
Testosterone
Tetracycline
Thalidomide
Thiabendazole
Thiamine
Thioguanine
Thiopental
Thiotepa
Thyrotropin Alfa
Tiagabine
Tibolone
Ticlopidine
Tigecycline
Tiludronate
Timolol
Tinidazole
Tinzaparin
Tiopronin
Tipranavir
Tizanidine
Tobramycin
Tocainide
Tocilizumab
Tofacitinib
Tolazamide
Tolbutamide
Tolcapone
Tolmetin
Tolterodine
Tolvaptan
Topiramate
Tositumomab & Iodine[131]
Tosufloxacin
Tramadol
Trametinib
Trandolapril
Trastuzumab
Travoprost
Trazodone
Treprostinil
Tretinoin
Triamcinolone
Triazolam
Trimeprazine
Trimethadione
Trimethoprim
Trimetrexate
Trioxsalen
Triprolidine
Triptorelin
Troleandomycin
Trovafloxacin
Typhoid Vaccine
Ulipristal
Unoprostone
Ursodiol
Ustekinumab
Valdecoxib
Valganciclovir
Valproic Acid
Valrubicin
Valsartan
Vancomycin
Vandetanib
Vardenafil
Varenicline
Varicella Vaccine
Vedolizumab
Vemurafenib
Venlafaxine
Verapamil
Vernakalant
Vincristine
Vitamin A
Voriconazole
Vorinostat
Vortioxetine
Warfarin
Zalcitabine
Zaleplon
Ziconotide
Zidovudine
Zileuton
Zolmitriptan
Zolpidem
Zonisamide
Zoster Vaccine
Zuclopenthixol

Pseudolymphoma

Adalimumab
Aldesleukin
Allopurinol
Alprazolam
Amitriptyline
Amlodipine
Aspirin
Atenolol
Bromocriptine
Captopril
Carbamazepine
Cefixime
Cefuroxime
Chlorpromazine
Cimetidine
Clarithromycin
Clonazepam
Clonidine
Co-Trimoxazole
Cyclosporine
Dapsone
Desipramine
Diclofenac
Diflunisal
Diltiazem
Doxepin
Estrogens
Etanercept
Ethosuximide
Ethotoin
Fluorouracil
Fluoxetine
Fosinopril
Furosemide
Gemcitabine
Gemfibrozil
Glatiramer
Gold & Gold Compounds
Hepatitis A Vaccine
Hepatitis B Vaccine
Hydrochlorothiazide
Ibuprofen
Imatinib
Indomethacin
Infliximab
Interferon Alfa
Ketoprofen
Lamotrigine
Leucovorin
Lisinopril
Lithium
Lorazepam
Losartan
Lovastatin
Methotrexate
Methylphenidate
Metoprolol
Mexiletine
Nabumetone
Naproxen
Nitrofurantoin
Nizatidine
Oxaliplatin
Oxaprozin
Perphenazine
Phenobarbital
Phenytoin
Procainamide
Ranitidine
Sulfamethoxazole
Sulfasalazine
Sulindac
Tamoxifen
Terfenadine
Thioridazine
Valproic Acid
Valsartan
Zoledronate

Pseudoporphyria

Acitretin
Amiodarone
Ampicillin
Ampicillin/Sulbactam
Aspirin
Bumetanide
Carisoprodol
Cefepime
Celecoxib
Chlorthalidone
Ciprofloxacin
Cyclosporine
Diclofenac
Diflunisal
Fluorouracil
Flutamide
Hydrochlorothiazide
Ibuprofen
Imatinib
Indomethacin
Isotretinoin
Ketoprofen
Mefenamic Acid
Metformin
Nabumetone
Nalidixic Acid
Naproxen
Oral Contraceptives
Oxaprozin
Piroxicam
Pyridoxine
Quinidine
Rofecoxib
Tetracycline
Torsemide
Triamterene
Voriconazole

Psoriasis

Abatacept
Acebutolol

Aceclofenac
Acetazolamide
Acitretin
Adalimumab
Aldesleukin
Aminoglutethimide
Amiodarone
Amoxicillin
Ampicillin
Anakinra
Apremilast
Arsenic
Aspirin
Atenolol
BCG Vaccine
Betamethasone
Bisoprolol
Bupropion
Calcipotriol
Candesartan
Captopril
Carbamazepine
Carvedilol
Certolizumab
Cetuximab
Chlorambucil
Chloroquine
Chlorthalidone
Cimetidine
Clarithromycin
Clonidine
Clopidogrel
Co-Trimoxazole
Cyclosporine
Dabrafenib
Daclizumab
Diclofenac
Digoxin
Diltiazem
Dipyridamole
Docetaxel
Donepezil
Doxorubicin
Doxycycline
Efalizumab
Eletriptan
Enalapril
Esmolol
Etanercept
Fexofenadine
Flecainide
Fluorouracil
Fluoxetine
Fluoxymesterone
Foscarnet
Gemfibrozil
Glyburide
Gold & Gold Compounds
Golimumab
Granulocyte Colony-Stimulating Factor (G-CSF)
Human Papillomavirus (HPV) Vaccine
Hydroxychloroquine
Hydroxyurea
Ibuprofen
Imatinib
Imiquimod
Indomethacin
Infliximab
Interferon Alfa
Interferon Beta
Ketoprofen
Labetalol
Lapatinib
Letrozole
Levamisole
Levetiracetam
Levobetaxolol
Lisinopril
Lithium
Losartan
MDMA
Meclofenamate
Mefloquine
Meloxicam
Mesalamine
Methicillin
Methotrexate
Methyltestosterone
Metipranolol
Metoprolol
Modafinil
Morphine
Mycophenolate
Nadolol
Nilotinib
Nivolumab
Olanzapine
Ombitasvir/Paritaprevir/Ritonavir
Omeprazole
Oral Contraceptives
Oxprenolol
Paroxetine Hydrochloride
PEG-Interferon
Pembrolizumab
Penicillamine
Pentostatin
Perindopril
Phenylbutazone
Pindolol
Potassium Iodide
Prednisolone
Primaquine
Propafenone
Propranolol
Quinacrine
Quinidine
Rabeprazole
Ramipril
Ranitidine
Ribavirin
Risperidone
Ritonavir
Rituximab
Rivastigmine
Rofecoxib
Ropinirole
Saquinavir
Secukinumab
Sertraline
Siltuximab
Sitagliptin
Sorafenib
Sotalol
Sulfamethoxazole
Sulfasalazine
Sulfisoxazole
Tacrine
Tazarotene
Telmisartan
Terbinafine
Terfenadine
Testosterone
Tetracycline
Thalidomide
Thioguanine
Tiagabine
Timolol
Tocilizumab
Tofacitinib
Trazodone
Urapidil
Ustekinumab
Valdecoxib
Venlafaxine
Voriconazole

Purpura

Acenocoumarol
Acetaminophen
Acetazolamide
Acitretin
Adalimumab
Aldesleukin
Alemtuzumab
Allopurinol
Alteplase
Aminocaproic Acid
Aminoglutethimide
Aminolevulinic Acid
Aminosalicylate Sodium
Amiodarone
Amitriptyline
Amlodipine
Amphotericin B
Ampicillin
Anastrozole
Anti-Thymocyte Globulin (Equine)
Arsenic
Artemether/Lumefantrine
Aspartame
Aspirin
Azacitidine
Aztreonam
Bendamustine
Beta-Carotene
Betaxolol
Bevacizumab
Bortezomib
Botulinum Toxin (A & B)
Buspirone
Busulfan
Butabarbital
Butalbital
Capecitabine
Captopril
Carbamazepine
Carbenicillin
Carteolol
Carvedilol
Cefaclor
Cefoxitin
Celecoxib
Cephalothin
Cetirizine
Chloral Hydrate
Chlorambucil
Chloramphenicol
Chlordiazepoxide
Chlorothiazide
Chlorpromazine
Chlorpropamide
Chlorthalidone
Cilostazol
Cinacalcet
Ciprofloxacin
Citalopram
Cladribine
Clarithromycin
Clidinium
Clofibrate
Clomiphene
Clomipramine
Clonazepam
Clopidogrel
Clozapine
Co-Trimoxazole
Cocaine
Codeine
Cycloserine
Cyclosporine
Cytarabine
Danazol
Dapsone
Deferiprone
Delavirdine
Desipramine
Diazepam
Diclofenac
Dicumarol
Diethylpropion
Diethylstilbestrol
Digoxin
Diltiazem
Diphenhydramine
Dipyridamole
Disopyramide
Disulfiram
Donepezil
Doxazosin
Doxepin
Doxorubicin
Doxycycline
Drotrecogin Alfa
Duloxetine
Enalapril
Enoxacin
Enoxaparin
Entacapone
Ephedrine
Eprosartan
Erlotinib
Escitalopram
Estazolam
Estramustine
Estrogens
Etanercept
Ethacrynic Acid
Ethambutol
Ethchlorvynol
Ethionamide
Ethosuximide
Ethotoin
Famotidine
Febuxostat
Felodipine
Fenoprofen
Fentanyl
Flucloxacillin
Fluconazole
Fluoxetine
Fluvoxamine

Fondaparinux
Frovatriptan
Furosemide
Gabapentin
Galantamine
Gefitinib
Gentamicin
Glatiramer
Glipizide
Glyburide
Gold & Gold Compounds
Griseofulvin
Guanfacine
Heparin
Hepatitis B Vaccine
Heroin
Histrelin
Hyaluronic Acid
Hydralazine
Hydrochlorothiazide
Hydrocortisone
Hydroxyurea
Hydroxyzine
Ibritumomab
Ibuprofen
Imatinib
Imipramine
Indomethacin
Infliximab
Influenza Vaccine
Insulin
Interferon Alfa
Interferon Beta
Iohexol
Ipodate
Isoniazid
Isotretinoin
Itraconazole
Ketoconazole
Ketoprofen
Ketorolac
Labetalol
Lamotrigine
Leflunomide
Lenalidomide
Leuprolide
Levamisole
Levobupivacaine
Levodopa
Levofloxacin
Lidocaine
Lincomycin
Lindane
Linezolid
Lisinopril
Lithium
Lomefloxacin
Loratadine
Losartan
Lovastatin
Maprotiline
Measles, Mumps & Rubella (MMR) Virus Vaccine
Mecasermin
Mechlorethamine
Meclofenamate
Medroxyprogesterone
Mefloquine
Meloxicam
Meningococcal Groups C & Y & Haemophilus B Tetanus Toxoid Conjugate Vaccine
Mephenytoin
Meprobamate
Metformin
Methimazole
Methoxsalen
Methyldopa
Methylphenidate
Metoclopramide
Metolazone
Miconazole
Minocycline
Mirabegron
Mitomycin
Mitoxantrone
Montelukast
Nalidixic Acid
Naproxen
Naratriptan
Natalizumab
Nifedipine
Nimesulide
Nitrofurantoin
Nitroglycerin
Octreotide
Olanzapine
Omacetaxine
Oral Contraceptives
Oxaliplatin
Oxcarbazepine
Oxytetracycline
Pandemic Influenza Vaccine (H1N1)
Paroxetine Hydrochloride
Pegaspargase
Penicillamine
Pentagastrin
Pentobarbital
Pentosan
Pentostatin
Perindopril
Phenobarbital
Phensuximide
Phenytoin
Pirbuterol
Piroxicam
Plicamycin
Pravastatin
Prednisone
Prilocaine
Procainamide
Prochlorperazine
Promethazine
Propafenone
Propranolol
Propylthiouracil
Pyrimethamine
Quinidine
Quinine
Ramipril
Ranitidine
Rapacuronium
Rifampin
Rifapentine
Risperidone
Rituximab
Rivastigmine
Ropinirole
Rosuvastatin
Rotigotine
Ruxolitinib
Sertraline
Sildenafil
Simvastatin
Sirolimus
Smallpox Vaccine
Streptokinase
Streptomycin
Sulfadoxine
Sulfamethoxazole
Sulfasalazine
Sulfisoxazole
Sulindac
Tacrine
Tacrolimus
Tadalafil
Tamoxifen
Tartrazine
Teicoplanin
Tetracycline
Thalidomide
Thiamine
Thiopental
Ticlopidine
Tinzaparin
Tizanidine
Tolbutamide
Tolmetin
Topiramate
Topotecan
Torsemide
Tosufloxacin
Trichlormethiazide
Trimethadione
Tripelennamine
Valacyclovir
Valproic Acid
Vancomycin
Varicella Vaccine
Vasopressin
Verapamil
Voriconazole
Warfarin
Zolpidem
Zonisamide

Raynaud's phenomenon

Acebutolol
Amphotericin B
Aripiprazole
Arsenic
Atenolol
Bisoprolol
Bleomycin
Bromocriptine
Carboplatin
Carteolol
Cisplatin
Clonidine
Cocaine
Cyclosporine
Dextroamphetamine
Dopamine
Doxorubicin
Estrogens
Ethosuximide
Fluoxetine
Gemcitabine
Gemfibrozil
Hepatitis B Vaccine
Human Papillomavirus (HPV) Vaccine
Iloprost
Interferon Alfa
Interferon Beta
Labetalol
Lamotrigine
Methotrexate
Methylphenidate
Metoprolol
Minocycline
Nadolol
Octreotide
Phentermine
Pindolol
Propofol
Propranolol
Quinine
Sotalol
Spironolactone
Sulfasalazine
Sulindac
Sumatriptan
Tegafur/Gimeracil/Oteracil
Tegaserod
Thiothixene
Timolol
Uracil/Tegafur
Vinblastine
Vincristine

Rhabdomyolysis

Abacavir
Abiraterone
Acetaminophen
Aldesleukin
Allopurinol
Alprazolam
Aminocaproic Acid
Aminophylline
Amiodarone
Amisulpride
Amitriptyline
Amlodipine
Amobarbital
Amoxicillin
Amphotericin B
Aprobarbital
Aspirin
Atorvastatin
Atropine Sulfate
Azacitidine
Azathioprine
Azithromycin
Baclofen
Benztropine
Bezafibrate
Buprenorphine
Bupropion
Butabarbital
Butalbital
Carbamazepine
Chlorpromazine
Cholestyramine
Ciprofibrate
Ciprofloxacin
Cisplatin
Citalopram
Clarithromycin
Clofibrate
Clopidogrel
Clozapine
Co-Trimoxazole

Cobicistat/Elvitegravir/ Emtricitabine/Tenofovir Disoproxil
Cocaine
Colchicine
Colistin
Cyclosporine
Cytarabine
Dacarbazine
Danazol
Daptomycin
Dasatinib
Deferasirox
Delavirdine
Desipramine
Dexketoprofen
Dextroamphetamine
Diatrizoate
Diazepam
Diclofenac
Didanosine
Digoxin
Diltiazem
Diphenhydramine
Distigmine
Dolutegravir
Domperidone
Doxepin
Droperidol
Enflurane
Enoxacin
Epinephrine
Erlotinib
Erythromycin
Esomeprazole
Fenbufen
Fenofibrate
Fluconazole
Fluorouracil
Fluoxetine
Fluphenazine
Fluprednisolone
Fluvastatin
Fusidic Acid
Gabapentin
Gatifloxacin
Gemcitabine
Gemfibrozil
Haloperidol
Halothane
Heroin
Hydroxychloroquine
Ibuprofen
Imatinib
Infliximab
Influenza Vaccine
Interferon Alfa
Interferon Beta
Ipilimumab
Isoflurane
Isoniazid
Isotretinoin
Itraconazole
Ketoconazole
Labetalol
Lamivudine
Lamotrigine
Leflunomide
Lenalidomide
Leuprolide
Levetiracetam
Levodopa
Levofloxacin
Levomepromazine
Lindane
Linezolid
Lithium
Lorazepam
Lovastatin
Loxapine
Lurasidone
Maraviroc
MDMA
Meloxicam
Melphalan
Mephobarbital
Meprobamate
Metformin
Methadone
Methamphetamine
Methohexital
Metoprolol
Minocycline
Mirtazapine
Mizoribine
Molindone
Morphine
Moxifloxacin
Naltrexone
Naproxen
Nefazodone
Nelarabine
Nelfinavir
Nitrazepam
Nivolumab
Norfloxacin
Ofloxacin
Olanzapine
Omeprazole
Paclitaxel
Paliperidone
Pancuronium
Pantoprazole
PEG-Interferon
Pembrolizumab
Pemetrexed
Pemoline
Pentamidine
Pentobarbital
Perphenazine
Phendimetrazine
Phenelzine
Phenobarbital
Phenylpropanolamine
Phenytoin
Pioglitazone
Pravastatin
Pregabalin
Primidone
Propofol
Protamine Sulfate
Protriptyline
Pyrazinamide
Quetiapine
Quinacrine
Quinine
Rabeprazole
Raltegravir
Ranolazine
Ribavirin
Risperidone
Ritodrine
Ritonavir
Rosuvastatin
Secobarbital
Sertraline
Sevoflurane
Sildenafil
Simeprevir
Simvastatin
Sirolimus
Sitagliptin
Sonidegib
Sotalol
Stanozolol
Streptokinase
Streptomycin
Succinylcholine
Sulfamethoxazole
Sulfasalazine
Sulpiride
Sunitinib
Tacrolimus
Tasonermin
Tenecteplase
Tenofovir Disoproxil
Terbinafine
Terbutaline
Teriflunomide
Terlipressin
Thiopental
Ticagrelor
Tolcapone
Tolvaptan
Trabectedin
Trametinib
Trandolapril
Tranylcypromine
Trifluoperazine
Trimethoprim
Trospium
Valproic Acid
Vasopressin
Venlafaxine
Verapamil
Vinblastine
Warfarin
Ziconotide
Ziprasidone

Stevens–Johnson syndrome

Abacavir
Aceclofenac
Acetaminophen
Acetazolamide
Acyclovir
Adalimumab
Adefovir
Afatinib
Albendazole
Albuterol
Aldesleukin
Allopurinol
Alogliptin
Amifostine
Aminophylline
Amiodarone
Amlodipine
Amobarbital
Amoxicillin
Ampicillin
Amprenavir
Anthrax Vaccine
Aripiprazole
Arsenic
Aspirin
Astemizole
Atovaquone
Atovaquone/Proguanil
Atropine Sulfate
Azathioprine
Azithromycin
Bendamustine
Bezafibrate
Bleomycin
Bromfenac
Bupropion
Butabarbital
Butalbital
Captopril
Carbamazepine
Carvedilol
Cefaclor
Cefadroxil
Cefamandole
Cefazolin
Cefdinir
Cefepime
Cefixime
Cefmetazole
Cefonicid
Cefoperazone
Cefotaxime
Cefotetan
Cefoxitin
Cefpodoxime
Cefprozil
Ceftazidime
Ceftibuten
Ceftizoxime
Ceftriaxone
Cefuroxime
Celecoxib
Cephalexin
Cephalothin
Cephapirin
Cephradine
Cetuximab
Chloramphenicol
Chlordiazepoxide
Chlormezanone
Chloroquine
Chlorpropamide
Cimetidine
Ciprofloxacin
Cisplatin
Clarithromycin
Clindamycin
Clobazam
Clofibrate
Clopidogrel
Cloxacillin
Clozapine
Co-Trimoxazole
Cocaine
Cyclophosphamide
Cycloserine
Dapsone
Darunavir
Delavirdine
Dexamethasone
Diclofenac
Dicloxacillin
Didanosine
Diflunisal

Diltiazem
Dimenhydrinate
Dipyridamole
Docetaxel
Doxycycline
Duloxetine
Efavirenz
Enalapril
Enoxacin
Erythromycin
Ethambutol
Ethosuximide
Etodolac
Etoposide
Etoricoxib
Felbamate
Fenbufen
Fenoprofen
Flucloxacillin
Fluconazole
Fluoxetine
Flurbiprofen
Furosemide
Gabapentin
Galantamine
Gemcitabine
Glipizide
Griseofulvin
Human Papillomavirus (HPV) Vaccine
Hydrochlorothiazide
Hydroxychloroquine
Ibuprofen
Imatinib
Immune Globulin IV
Indapamide
Indinavir
Indomethacin
Infliximab
Iohexol
Ipilimumab
Isoniazid
Itraconazole
Ixazomib
Ketoprofen
Ketorolac
Lacosamide
Lamivudine
Lamotrigine
Lansoprazole
Leflunomide
Lenalidomide
Levamisole
Levetiracetam
Levofloxacin
Lidocaine
Lincomycin
Lomefloxacin
Loracarbef
Lorazepam
Lovastatin
Lymecycline
Maprotiline
Mebendazole
Mechlorethamine
Meclofenamate
Mefenamic Acid
Mefloquine
Meloxicam
Mephenytoin
Mephobarbital
Meprobamate
Metamizole
Methazolamide
Methimazole
Methotrexate
Methsuximide
Methyldopa
Methylprednisolone
Metronidazole
Mexiletine
Miltefosine
Minocycline
Minoxidil
Mizoribine
Nabumetone
Naproxen
Nevirapine
Nifedipine
Nimesulide
Nitrofurantoin
Norfloxacin
Nystatin
Ofloxacin
Omeprazole
Oral Contraceptives
Oxacillin
Oxaprozin
Oxcarbazepine
Paclitaxel
Pantoprazole
PEG-Interferon
Pentamidine
Pentobarbital
Peplomycin
Phenobarbital
Phenolphthalein
Phenylbutazone
Phenytoin
Piroxicam
Prednisolone
Pristinamycin
Promethazine
Propranolol
Pyrimethamine
Quinine
Raltegravir
Ramipril
Ranitidine
Regorafenib
Ribavirin
Rifampin
Risedronate
Rituximab
Rofecoxib
Secobarbital
Sertraline
Sibutramine
Sitagliptin
Smallpox Vaccine
Sorafenib
Stavudine
Streptomycin
Strontium Ranelate
Sulfacetamide
Sulfadiazine
Sulfadoxine
Sulfamethoxazole
Sulfasalazine
Sulfisoxazole
Sulindac
Tamoxifen
Tegafur/Gimeracil/Oteracil
Teicoplanin
Telaprevir
Temozolomide
Tenofovir Disoproxil
Terbinafine
Teriflunomide
Tetracycline
Tetrazepam
Thalidomide
Thiabendazole
Thiopental
Ticlopidine
Tigecycline
Tiludronate
Tocainide
Tolmetin
Torsemide
Trimethadione
Trimethoprim
Trovafloxacin
Valdecoxib
Valproic Acid
Vancomycin
Vandetanib
Varicella Vaccine
Vemurafenib
Venlafaxine
Verapamil
Vitamin A
Voriconazole
Zidovudine
Zoledronate
Zonisamide

Tinnitus

Acamprosate
Acetaminophen
Acetazolamide
Acitretin
Adalimumab
Almotriptan
Amikacin
Amitriptyline
Anagrelide
Aprepitant
Arsenic
Artemether/Lumefantrine
Artesunate
Aspirin
Atorvastatin
Azithromycin
Betaxolol
Bismuth
Bleomycin
Bortezomib
Botulinum Toxin (A & B)
Bupropion
Carbimazole
Carboplatin
Carvedilol
Cefpodoxime
Chlorambucil
Chloramphenicol
Chloroquine
Chlorpromazine
Cilostazol
Ciprofloxacin
Cisplatin
Citalopram
Clarithromycin
Clindamycin
Clomipramine
Colistin
Cyclobenzaprine
Cycloserine
Cyclosporine
Dasatinib
Daunorubicin
Deferoxamine
Degarelix
Desvenlafaxine
Dexamethasone
Dexlansoprazole
Doxepin
Doxycycline
Dronabinol
Duloxetine
Eletriptan
Elotuzumab
Eprosartan
Erlotinib
Erythromycin
Escitalopram
Eslicarbazepine
Esomeprazole
Eszopiclone
Etanercept
Ethambutol
Etoposide
Febuxostat
Frovatriptan
Gadodiamide
Gadoteridol
Gadoversetamide
Gentamicin
Glatiramer
Halofantrine
Hepatitis B Vaccine
Ibuprofen
Imipramine
Indomethacin
Interferon Alfa
Isavuconazonium Sulfate
Isoniazid
Kanamycin
Ketorolac
Lapatinib
Lenalidomide
Levobetaxolol
Lidocaine
Mefloquine
Meloxicam
Mesalamine
Methyl salicylate
Metronidazole
Minocycline
Moexipril
Muromonab-CD3
Nabumetone
Nadolol
Naproxen
Nitroprusside
Omacetaxine
Pamidronate
Paromomycin
PEG-Interferon
Perflutren
Phenelzine
Piroxicam
Propylthiouracil
Quinine
Rabeprazole

Ranitidine
Ranolazine
Ribavirin
Rifaximin
Rivastigmine
Ropivacaine
Rotigotine
Salsalate
Sertraline
Sildenafil
Sirolimus
Sodium Oxybate
Sorafenib
Sumatriptan
Tacrolimus
Tadalafil
Teicoplanin
Tetracycline
Tiagabine
Tobramycin
Tramadol
Triptorelin
Valdecoxib
Valproic Acid
Vancomycin
Vardenafil
Venlafaxine
Vigabatrin
Vinblastine
Vincristine
Voriconazole
Zaleplon
Ziconotide
Ziprasidone
Zolpidem
Zonisamide

Toxic epidermal necrolysis (TEN)

Abacavir
Aceclofenac
Acetaminophen
Acetazolamide
Adefovir
Aldesleukin
Alfuzosin
Allopurinol
Alprostadil
Amifostine
Aminosalicylate Sodium
Amiodarone
Amlodipine
Amobarbital
Amoxapine
Amoxicillin
Ampicillin
Anthrax Vaccine
Arsenic
Asparaginase
Aspirin
Atorvastatin
Atovaquone
Azathioprine
Aztreonam
BCG Vaccine
Bendamustine
Bezafibrate
Bucillamine
Busulfan
Butabarbital
Butalbital
Captopril
Carbamazepine
Carbenicillin
Caspofungin
Cefaclor
Cefamandole
Cefazolin
Cefixime
Cefotaxime
Cefoxitin
Ceftazidime
Ceftriaxone
Cefuroxime
Celecoxib
Cephalexin
Cephalothin
Cephradine
Cetuximab
Chlorambucil
Chloramphenicol
Chlormezanone
Chloroquine
Chlorpromazine
Chlorpropamide
Chlorthalidone
Cilostazol
Cimetidine
Ciprofloxacin
Cisplatin
Cladribine
Clarithromycin
Clindamycin
Clobazam
Co-Trimoxazole
Codeine
Colchicine
Cyclophosphamide
Cyclosporine
Cytarabine
Dapsone
Darunavir
Demeclocycline
Denileukin
Dexamethasone
Dextroamphetamine
Diatrizoate
Diclofenac
Diflunisal
Diltiazem
Diphenhydramine
Dipyridamole
Disulfiram
Docetaxel
Dorzolamide
Doxycycline
Dronedarone
Efavirenz
Enalapril
Enoxacin
Ephedrine
Erythromycin
Eslicarbazepine
Ethambutol
Etidronate
Etodolac
Etoricoxib
Famotidine
Felbamate
Fenbufen
Fenofibrate
Fenoprofen
Flucloxacillin
Fluconazole
Fludarabine
Fluoxetine
Fluphenazine
Flurazepam
Flurbiprofen
Fluvoxamine
Foscarnet
Furosemide
Gefitinib
Gemcitabine
Gemeprost
Gentamicin
Gold & Gold Compounds
Grepafloxacin
Griseofulvin
Heparin
Heroin
Hydralazine
Hydrochlorothiazide
Hydroxychloroquine
Ibandronate
Ibuprofen
Imatinib
Imipenem/Cilastatin
Immune Globulin IV
Indapamide
Indomethacin
Infliximab
Iohexol
Ipilimumab
Isoniazid
Isotretinoin
Ketoprofen
Ketorolac
Lacosamide
Lamivudine
Lamotrigine
Lansoprazole
Latanoprost
Leflunomide
Lenalidomide
Letrozole
Levetiracetam
Levofloxacin
Lincomycin
Lomefloxacin
Lomustine
Meclofenamate
Mefenamic Acid
Mefloquine
Meloxicam
Meperidine
Mephenytoin
Meprobamate
Mercaptopurine
Meropenem
Mesna
Metamizole
Methamphetamine
Methazolamide
Methimazole
Methotrexate
Metolazone
Metronidazole
Minocycline
Minoxidil
Moxifloxacin
Mupirocin
Nabumetone
Nalidixic Acid
Naproxen
Neomycin
Nevirapine
Nifedipine
Nitrofurantoin
Norfloxacin
Ofloxacin
Omeprazole
Ondansetron
Oseltamivir
Oxaprozin
Oxazepam
Oxcarbazepine
Pantoprazole
Papaverine
PEG-Interferon
Pemetrexed
Penicillamine
Penicillin V
Pentamidine
Pentazocine
Pentobarbital
Phenobarbital
Phenolphthalein
Phenylbutazone
Phenytoin
Piroxicam
Plicamycin
Prednisolone
Primidone
Pristinamycin
Procarbazine
Prochlorperazine
Promethazine
Propranolol
Propylthiouracil
Pyridoxine
Pyrimethamine
Quinidine
Quinine
Ranitidine
Regorafenib
Reserpine
Ribavirin
Rifampin
Rifaximin
Ritodrine
Rituximab
Rofecoxib
Smallpox Vaccine
Stavudine
Streptomycin
Streptozocin
Strontium Ranelate
Sulfacetamide
Sulfadiazine
Sulfadoxine
Sulfamethoxazole
Sulfasalazine
Sulfisoxazole
Sulindac
Tegafur/Gimeracil/Oteracil
Telaprevir
Temozolomide
Terbinafine
Terconazole
Teriflunomide
Tetracycline
Tetrazepam
Thalidomide
Thiabendazole

Thiopental
Thioridazine
Timolol
Tolbutamide
Tolmetin
Trimethoprim
Trovafloxacin
Valdecoxib
Valproic Acid
Vancomycin
Vemurafenib
Vinorelbine
Voriconazole
Zidovudine
Zonisamide

Urticaria

Abatacept
Acamprosate
Acarbose
Acebutolol
Aceclofenac
Acetaminophen
Acetohexamide
Acetylcysteine
Acyclovir
Adalimumab
Albendazole
Albiglutide
Albuterol
Alclometasone
Aldesleukin
Alefacept
Alemtuzumab
Alendronate
Alfentanil
Alglucerase
Alglucosidase Alfa
Allopurinol
Alpha-Lipoic Acid
Alprazolam
Alprostadil
Alteplase
Amcinonide
Aminolevulinic Acid
Aminophylline
Aminosalicylate Sodium
Amiodarone
Amlodipine
Amobarbital
Amodiaquine
Amoxapine
Amoxicillin
Amphotericin B
Ampicillin
Anagrelide
Anakinra
Anidulafungin
Anistreplase
Anthrax Vaccine
Anti-Thymocyte Globulin (Equine)
Aprepitant
Arsenic
Artemether/Lumefantrine
Artesunate
Asfotase Alfa
Asparaginase
Asparaginase *Erwinia chrysanthemi*
Aspartame
Aspirin
Astemizole
Atenolol
Atorvastatin
Atovaquone/Proguanil
Atracurium
Atropine Sulfate
Azacitidine
Azathioprine
Azithromycin
Aztreonam
Bacitracin
BCG Vaccine
Benazepril
Bepotastine
Betamethasone
Bezafibrate
Bosutinib
Brinzolamide
Bumetanide
Bupropion
Buspirone
Busulfan
Butorphanol
Calcipotriol
Calcitonin
Canagliflozin
Captopril
Carbamazepine
Carbenicillin
Carboplatin
Carisoprodol
Caspofungin
Cefaclor
Cefadroxil
Cefamandole
Cefazolin
Cefdinir
Cefditoren
Cefepime
Cefixime
Cefmetazole
Cefonicid
Cefoperazone
Cefotaxime
Cefotetan
Cefpodoxime
Cefprozil
Ceftaroline Fosamil
Ceftazidime
Ceftibuten
Ceftizoxime
Ceftolozane & Tazobactam
Ceftriaxone
Cefuroxime
Celecoxib
Cephalexin
Cephalothin
Cephapirin
Cephradine
Certolizumab
Cetirizine
Chloral Hydrate
Chlorambucil
Chloramphenicol
Chlordiazepoxide
Chlorhexidine
Chloroquine
Chlorothiazide
Chlorpromazine
Chlorpropamide
Chlorthalidone
Chlorzoxazone
Cidofovir
Cilostazol
Cimetidine
Cinoxacin
Ciprofloxacin
Cisplatin
Clarithromycin
Clemastine
Clindamycin
Clioquinol
Clofibrate
Clomiphene
Clomipramine
Clonidine
Clopidogrel
Clorazepate
Cloxacillin
Clozapine
Co-Trimoxazole
Coagulation Factor IX (Recombinant)
Cocaine
Codeine
Colchicine
Colestipol
Cromolyn
Cyanocobalamin
Cyclamate
Cyclobenzaprine
Cyclophosphamide
Cycloserine
Cyclosporine
Cysteamine
Cytarabine
Dacarbazine
Daclizumab
Dalbavancin
Dapagliflozin
Dapsone
Darunavir
Dasatinib
Daunorubicin
Decitabine
Deferasirox
Deferoxamine
Degarelix
Delavirdine
Deoxycholic Acid
Desipramine
Desloratadine
Dexamethasone
Dexlansoprazole
Dextroamphetamine
Diazepam
Diclofenac
Dicloxacillin
Dicumarol
Diethylstilbestrol
Diflunisal
Digoxin
Dihydrocodeine
Diltiazem
Dimenhydrinate
Dimethyl Fumarate
Dinutuximab
Diphenoxylate
Dipyridamole
Dirithromycin
Disulfiram
Docetaxel
Donepezil
Doxacurium
Doxazosin
Doxorubicin
Doxycycline
Efalizumab
Efavirenz
Eletriptan
Emtricitabine
Enalapril
Enfuvirtide
Enoxacin
Enoxaparin
Ephedrine
Ertapenem
Erythromycin
Esomeprazole
Estazolam
Estrogens
Eszopiclone
Etanercept
Ethambutol
Ethionamide
Ethosuximide
Etodolac
Etoricoxib
Evolocumab
Exenatide
Famotidine
Febuxostat
Felbamate
Felodipine
Fenofibrate
Fenoprofen
Fentanyl
Ferumoxytol
Fexofenadine
Finasteride
Flecainide
Flucloxacillin
Flumazenil
Fluorides
Fluoxetine
Flurbiprofen
Fluvoxamine
Folic Acid
Foscarnet
Fosinopril
Fulvestrant
Furazolidone
Furosemide
Gadobenate
Gadodiamide
Gadopentetate
Gadoteridol
Gadoversetamide
Ganciclovir
Gefitinib
Gemfibrozil
Gemifloxacin
Gentamicin
Glatiramer
Glimepiride
Glipizide
Glucagon
Glyburide
Gold & Gold Compounds
Golimumab
Granulocyte Colony-Stimulating Factor (G-CSF)
Grepafloxacin

Griseofulvin
Halothane
Heparin
Hepatitis B Vaccine
Heroin
Histrelin
Human Papillomavirus Vaccine (Bivalent)
Hydrochlorothiazide
Hydrocodone
Hydrocortisone
Hydromorphone
Hydroxychloroquine
Hydroxyzine
Ibritumomab
Ibuprofen
Idarubicin
Idursulfase
Imatinib
Imiglucerase
Imipenem/Cilastatin
Imipramine
Indapamide
Indinavir
Indomethacin
Infliximab
Insulin
Insulin Glulisine
Interferon Alfa
Interferon Beta
Iodixanol
Iohexol
Iomeprol
Iopromide
Ioversol
Ipilimumab
Ipratropium
Irbesartan
Isavuconazonium Sulfate
Isoniazid
Isotretinoin
Isradipine
Itraconazole
Ivacaftor
Ivermectin
Ixazomib
Ixekizumab
Japanese Encephalitis Vaccine
Ketoconazole
Ketoprofen
Ketorolac
Labetalol
Lamivudine
Lamotrigine
Lansoprazole
Leflunomide
Lenalidomide
Lepirudin
Lesinurad
Leucovorin
Leuprolide
Levamisole
Levetiracetam
Levocetirizine
Levofloxacin
Levomilnacipran
Levonorgestrel
Levothyroxine
Lidocaine
Linaclotide
Linagliptin
Lincomycin
Lindane
Linezolid
Liothyronine
Liraglutide
Lisinopril
Lithium
Lixisenatide
Lomefloxacin
Loracarbef
Loratadine
Losartan
Lubiprostone
Maprotiline
Measles, Mumps & Rubella (MMR) Virus Vaccine
Mebeverine
Mechlorethamine
Meclofenamate
Medroxyprogesterone
Mefenamic Acid
Mefloquine
Meloxicam
Melphalan
Memantine
Meperidine
Mephenytoin
Meprobamate
Mercaptopurine
Meropenem
Mesna
Metamizole
Metformin
Methadone
Methamphetamine
Methazolamide
Methimazole
Methohexital
Methotrexate
Methoxsalen
Methsuximide
Methyldopa
Methylphenidate
Methylprednisolone
Metoclopramide
Metolazone
Metronidazole
Mexiletine
Micafungin
Miconazole
Midazolam
Miltefosine
Minocycline
Mirabegron
Mitomycin
Mitotane
Mivacurium
Moexipril
Montelukast
Moricizine
Moxifloxacin
Mycophenolate
Nabumetone
Nafarelin
Nalbuphine
Nalidixic Acid
Naloxone
Naproxen
Naratriptan
Nefazodone
Nelfinavir
Neomycin
Neostigmine
Nevirapine
Niacin
Nicardipine
Nifedipine
Nilotinib
Nimesulide
Nisoldipine
Nitrofurantoin
Nitroglycerin
Nivolumab
Nizatidine
Norfloxacin
Obeticholic Acid
Octreotide
Ofatumumab
Ofloxacin
Olanzapine
Olsalazine
Omalizumab
Ombitasvir/Paritaprevir/Ritonavir
Omeprazole
Ondansetron
Oral Contraceptives
Oritavancin
Oxacillin
Oxaliplatin
Oxaprozin
Oxerutins
Oxilan
Oxprenolol
Oxycodone
Oxymorphone
Paclitaxel
Pantoprazole
Pantothenic Acid
Paroxetine Hydrochloride
PEG-Interferon
Pegaptanib
Pegaspargase
Pemetrexed
Penicillamine
Penicillin G
Penicillin V
Pentamidine
Pentosan
Pentostatin
Perflutren
Permethrin
Perphenazine
Phenobarbital
Phenolphthalein
Phenylbutazone
Phenytoin
Phytonadione
Pilocarpine
Pipecuronium
Piroxicam
Pitavastatin
Pizotifen
Plasma (Human) Blood Product
Pneumococcal Vaccine
Polidocanol
Pomalidomide
Porfimer
Potassium Iodide
Praziquantel
Prazosin
Prednicarbate
Prednisolone
Prednisone
Prilocaine
Primaquine
Primidone
Pristinamycin
Probenecid
Procainamide
Procarbazine
Progestins
Promethazine
Propafenone
Propofol
Propoxyphene
Propranolol
Propylthiouracil
Propyphenazone
Protamine Sulfate
Psoralens
Quinacrine
Quinapril
Quinestrol
Quinidine
Quinine
Quinupristin/Dalfopristin
Rabeprazole
Ramipril
Ranitidine
Rapacuronium
Remifentanil
Ribavirin
Riboflavin
Rifampin
Rifapentine
Rifaximin
Risedronate
Risperidone
Ritonavir
Rituximab
Rivaroxaban
Rivastigmine
Rofecoxib
Ropinirole
Roxithromycin
Rupatadine
Saccharin
Salmeterol
Salsalate
Saquinavir
Sebelipase Alfa
Secretin
Secukinumab
Sertraline
Sildenafil
Simvastatin
Smallpox Vaccine
Sodium Oxybate
Sorafenib
Sparfloxacin
Spectinomycin
Spironolactone
Streptokinase
Streptomycin
Sufentanil
Sulfadiazine
Sulfamethoxazole
Sulfasalazine
Sulfisoxazole
Sulindac
Sulpiride

Sumatriptan
Tacrine
Tacrolimus
Tartrazine
Tedizolid
Teicoplanin
Telithromycin
Telmisartan
Tenecteplase
Teniposide
Tenofovir Disoproxil
Terbinafine
Terfenadine
Teriflunomide
Tesamorelin
Tetracycline
Thalidomide
Thiabendazole
Thimerosal
Thiopental
Thiotepa
Thyrotropin Alfa
Tiagabine
Ticlopidine
Tigecycline
Tinidazole
Tinzaparin
Tirofiban
Tizanidine
Tocilizumab
Tolazamide
Tolbutamide
Tolcapone
Tolmetin
Topiramate
Torsemide
Tosufloxacin
Tramadol
Trazodone
Triamcinolone
Trimethadione
Trimethoprim
Tripelennamine
Troleandomycin
Trovafloxacin
Urofollitropin
Valdecoxib
Valsartan
Vancomycin
Vardenafil
Varicella Vaccine
Vasopressin
Vedolizumab
Velaglucerase Alfa
Venlafaxine
Verapamil
Voriconazole
Warfarin
Yellow Fever Vaccine
Zalcitabine
Zaleplon
Zanamivir
Zidovudine
Ziprasidone
Zolmitriptan
Zolpidem
Zonisamide

Vasculitis

Abatacept
Acebutolol
Aceclofenac
Acenocoumarol
Acetaminophen
Acyclovir
Adalimumab
Ado-Trastuzumab Emtansine
Aldesleukin
Allopurinol
Aminosalicylate Sodium
Amiodarone
Amitriptyline
Amlodipine
Amoxapine
Amoxicillin
Amphotericin B
Ampicillin
Anastrozole
Anistreplase
Anthrax Vaccine
Asparaginase
Aspartame
Aspirin
Atenolol
Atorvastatin
Azacitidine
Azatadine
Azathioprine
Azithromycin
BCG Vaccine
Bendamustine
Bexarotene
Bortezomib
Bosentan
Bromocriptine
Busulfan
Captopril
Carbamazepine
Carbimazole
Carvedilol
Caspofungin
Celecoxib
Certolizumab
Cevimeline
Chloramphenicol
Chlordiazepoxide
Chloroquine
Chlorothiazide
Chlorpromazine
Chlorpropamide
Chlorthalidone
Chlorzoxazone
Cimetidine
Cinacalcet
Ciprofloxacin
Citalopram
Cladribine
Clarithromycin
Clindamycin
Clorazepate
Clozapine
Co-Trimoxazole
Cocaine
Colchicine
Cromolyn
Cyclophosphamide
Cyclosporine
Cyproheptadine
Cytarabine
Delavirdine
Diazepam
Diclofenac
Didanosine
Diflunisal
Digoxin
Diltiazem
Diphenhydramine
Disulfiram
Doxycycline
Efavirenz
Enalapril
Enfuvirtide
Ephedrine
Epirubicin
Erlotinib
Erythromycin
Estrogens
Etanercept
Ethacrynic Acid
Etodolac
Etoposide
Everolimus
Exemestane
Ezetimibe
Famciclovir
Famotidine
Fenbufen
Flucloxacillin
Fluorouracil
Fluoxetine
Flurbiprofen
Fluticasone Propionate
Furosemide
Gabapentin
Gefitinib
Gemcitabine
Gemfibrozil
Gentamicin
Glatiramer
Glimepiride
Glucagon
Glyburide
Gold & Gold Compounds
Golimumab
Granulocyte Colony-Stimulating Factor (G-CSF)
Griseofulvin
Guanethidine
Heparin
Hepatitis B Vaccine
Heroin
Hydralazine
Hydrochlorothiazide
Hydroxychloroquine
Hydroxyurea
Ibuprofen
Icodextrin
Imatinib
Imipenem/Cilastatin
Imipramine
Imiquimod
Immune Globulin IV
Indapamide
Indinavir
Indomethacin
Infliximab
Influenza Vaccine
Insulin
Insulin Aspart
Interferon Alfa
Interferon Beta
Isoniazid
Isotretinoin
Itraconazole
Ixazomib
Ketoconazole
Ketorolac
Leflunomide
Leuprolide
Levamisole
Levetiracetam
Levofloxacin
Lisinopril
Lithium
Maprotiline
MDMA
Meclofenamate
Mefenamic Acid
Mefloquine
Meloxicam
Melphalan
Meperidine
Meprobamate
Mercaptopurine
Mesalamine
Metformin
Methimazole
Methocarbamol
Methotrexate
Methoxsalen
Methyldopa
Methylphenidate
Metolazone
Minocycline
Mitotane
Nabumetone
Naproxen
Nelfinavir
Nicotine
Nifedipine
Nimesulide
Nizatidine
Ofloxacin
Olanzapine
Omeprazole
Oxacillin
Oxaliplatin
Pantoprazole
Paroxetine Hydrochloride
PEG-Interferon
Pemetrexed
Penicillamine
Penicillin V
Pergolide
Phenobarbital
Phenylbutazone
Phenytoin
Phytonadione
Piroxicam
Potassium Iodide
Pramipexole
Pregabalin
Procainamide
Propylthiouracil
Psoralens
Pyridoxine
Quinapril
Quinidine
Quinine
Ramipril
Ranitidine
Ribavirin
Rifampin
Risedronate
Ritodrine

Rituximab
Rivastigmine
Rofecoxib
Simvastatin
Sirolimus
Sorafenib
Sotalol
Spironolactone
Streptokinase
Streptomycin
Sulfadiazine
Sulfamethoxazole
Sulfasalazine
Sulfisoxazole
Sulindac
Tacrolimus
Tamoxifen
Tartrazine
Telithromycin
Telmisartan
Terbutaline
Tetracycline
Thalidomide
Thiamine
Thioridazine
Ticlopidine
Tinidazole
Tocainide
Torsemide
Trazodone
Tretinoin
Trichlormethiazide
Trimethadione
Trioxsalen
Triptorelin
Valproic Acid
Vancomycin
Vemurafenib
Verapamil
Vinorelbine
Warfarin
Zafirlukast
Zidovudine

Vertigo

Abacavir
Abarelix
Abatacept
Abiraterone
Acamprosate
Acebutolol
Aceclofenac
Acetaminophen
Acetohexamide
Acitretin
Adalimumab
Adenosine
Ado-Trastuzumab Emtansine
Afatinib
Aflibercept
Agalsidase
Albendazole
Albiglutide
Aldesleukin
Alefacept
Alemtuzumab
Alfuzosin
Alirocumab
Aliskiren
Allopurinol
Almotriptan
Alogliptin
Alosetron
Alpha-Lipoic Acid
Alprazolam
Alprostadil
Amantadine
Amiloride
Amiodarone
Amitriptyline
Amlodipine
Amodiaquine
Amoxapine
Amoxicillin
Anagrelide
Anidulafungin
Anti-Thymocyte Immunoglobulin (Rabbit)
Antihemophilic Factor
Apixaban
Apomorphine
Apremilast
Aprepitant
Arformoterol
Aripiprazole
Armodafinil
Arsenic
Artemether/Lumefantrine
Artesunate
Articaine
Asenapine
Atazanavir
Atenolol
Atomoxetine
Atorvastatin
Atovaquone/Proguanil
Avanafil
Axitinib
Azacitidine
Azathioprine
Azilsartan
Azithromycin
Baclofen
Basiliximab
Bedaquiline
Belatacept
Belinostat
Benazepril
Bendamustine
Benzphetamine
Bepridil
Betaxolol
Bezafibrate
Biperiden
Bismuth
Bisoprolol
Bleomycin
Blinatumomab
Bortezomib
Bosentan
Bosutinib
Botulinum Toxin (A & B)
Brentuximab Vedotin
Brexpiprazole
Brinzolamide
Brivaracetam
Bromocriptine
Bupivacaine
Buprenorphine
Bupropion
Butorphanol
C1-Esterase Inhibitor
Cabazitaxel
Cabergoline
Cabozantinib
Canagliflozin
Canakinumab
Candesartan
Capecitabine
Carbamazepine
Carbetocin
Carboplatin
Carfilzomib
Cariprazine
Carisoprodol
Carvedilol
Caspofungin
Cefditoren
Cefepime
Cefpodoxime
Ceftaroline Fosamil
Ceftazidime & Avibactam
Ceftolozane & Tazobactam
Ceftriaxone
Cefuroxime
Celecoxib
Celiprolol
Certolizumab
Cevimeline
Chloroquine
Chlorpromazine
Chlorzoxazone
Cholera Vaccine
Choline Fenofibrate
Cilazapril
Cilostazol
Cinacalcet
Cinnarizine
Ciprofloxacin
Cisplatin
Citalopram
Clevidipine
Clobazam
Clofarabine
Clofazimine
Clomipramine
Clonidine
Clozapine
Co-Trimoxazole
Coagulation Factor IX (Recombinant)
Cobicistat/Elvitegravir/Emtricitabine/Tenofovir Disoproxil
Codeine
Colesevelam
Crizotinib
Crofelemer
Cyclobenzaprine
Cycloserine
Cyclosporine
Cysteamine
Cytarabine
Dabigatran
Daclizumab
Dalbavancin
Dalfampridine
Dantrolene
Dapagliflozin
Dapsone
Daptomycin
Darbepoetin Alfa
Darifenacin
Dasatinib
Daunorubicin
Decitabine
Deferasirox
Degarelix
Denileukin
Denosumab
Desvenlafaxine
Dexamethasone
Dexketoprofen
Dextroamphetamine
Dextromethorphan
Diatrizoate
Diazepam
Diazoxide
Diclofenac
Dicyclomine
Diethylpropion
Dihydrocodeine
Dihydroergotamine
Diltiazem
Diphenhydramine
Disopyramide
Disulfiram
Docetaxel
Dofetilide
Dolasetron
Dolutegravir
Donepezil
Doxazosin
Doxepin
Doxercalciferol
Doxorubicin
Doxycycline
Dronabinol
Dronedarone
Droxidopa
Duloxetine
Dutasteride
Eculizumab
Edrophonium
Efavirenz
Eflornithine
Eletriptan
Eliglustat
Elotuzumab
Eluxadoline
Empagliflozin
Emtricitabine
Enalapril
Entacapone
Entecavir
Enzalutamide
Eplerenone
Epoetin Alfa
Eprosartan
Eribulin
Escitalopram
Eslicarbazepine
Esomeprazole
Estramustine
Eszopiclone
Etanercept
Etravirine
Everolimus
Evolocumab
Exenatide
Ezetimibe
Ezogabine
Factor VIII - von Willebrand Factor
Famotidine

Febuxostat
Felbamate
Fentanyl
Ferric Gluconate
Ferumoxytol
Fesoterodine
Finasteride
Fingolimod
Flecainide
Flibanserin
Flumazenil
Fluorouracil
Fluoxetine
Fluphenazine
Flurbiprofen
Fluticasone Furoate
Fluticasone Propionate
Fluvoxamine
Follitropin Alfa/Beta
Fomepizole
Fomivirsen
Formoterol
Fosfomycin
Fosphenytoin
Frovatriptan
Fulvestrant
Furazolidone
Gabapentin
Gadobenate
Gadobutrol
Gadodiamide
Gadofosveset
Gadopentetate
Gadoteridol
Gadoversetamide
Gadoxetate
Galantamine
Gatifloxacin
Gefitinib
Gemifloxacin
Gentamicin
Glatiramer
Gliclazide
Glimepiride
Glipizide
Glycopyrrolate
Golimumab
Goserelin
Granisetron
Granulocyte Colony-Stimulating Factor (G-CSF)
Guanabenz
Guanadrel
Guanethidine
Guanfacine
Halofantrine
Haloperidol
Human Papillomavirus (HPV) Vaccine
Human Papillomavirus Vaccine (Bivalent)
Hydrochlorothiazide
Hydrocodone
Hydromorphone
Ibandronate
Ibritumomab
Ibrutinib
Icatibant
Icodextrin
Idebenone
Iloperidone
Iloprost
Imatinib
Imidapril
Imiglucerase
Imipramine
Imiquimod
Indapamide
Indinavir
Indoramin
Infliximab
Influenza Vaccine
Insulin
Insulin Detemir
Interferon Alfa
Interferon Beta
Iobenguane
Iodixanol
Iohexol
Iomeprol
Iopromide
Ioversol
Irinotecan
Isavuconazonium Sulfate
Isocarboxazid
Isosorbide Mononitrate
Isradipine
Itraconazole
Ivabradine
Ivacaftor
Ivermectin
Ixabepilone
Japanese Encephalitis Vaccine
Kanamycin
Ketamine
Ketoconazole
Ketorolac
Lacosamide
Lamivudine
Lamotrigine
Lansoprazole
Lapatinib
Latanoprost
Ledipasvir & Sofosbuvir
Leflunomide
Lenalidomide
Lenvatinib
Lesinurad
Letrozole
Levetiracetam
Levodopa
Levofloxacin
Levomepromazine
Levomilnacipran
Levonorgestrel
Lidocaine
Linagliptin
Linezolid
Liothyronine
Liraglutide
Lisdexamfetamine
Lisinopril
Lithium
Lixisenatide
Lomitapide
Lopinavir
Loratadine
Lorazepam
Lorcainide
Lorcaserin
Losartan
Lovastatin
Loxapine
Lubiprostone
Lumiracoxib
Lurasidone
Maraviroc
Mazindol
MDMA
Mebendazole
Mefloquine
Meloxicam
Memantine
Meperidine
Mepolizumab
Meptazinol
Mesalamine
Metamizole
Metaxalone
Metformin
Methocarbamol
Methotrexate
Methoxyflurane
Methylnaltrexone
Methylphenidate
Methylprednisolone
Metronidazole
Micafungin
Midazolam
Mifepristone
Miglustat
Milnacipran
Miltefosine
Minocycline
Minoxidil
Mirabegron
Mirtazapine
Mivacurium
Moclobemide
Modafinil
Moexipril
Montelukast
Morphine
Moxifloxacin
Moxonidine
Mupirocin
Muromonab-CD3
Mycophenolate
Nabilone
Nabumetone
Nadolol
Nalbuphine
Nalmefene
Naloxegol
Naltrexone
Naproxen
Naratriptan
Nateglinide
Nebivolol
Nefazodone
Nelarabine
Nelfinavir
Nesiritide
Netupitant & Palonosetron
Niacin
Nicorandil
Nifedipine
Nilotinib
Nilutamide
Nisoldipine
Nitazoxanide
Nivolumab
Nizatidine
Norfloxacin
Nortriptyline
Obeticholic Acid
Octreotide
Ofloxacin
Olanzapine
Olmesartan
Olodaterol
Omacetaxine
Omalizumab
Ombitasvir/Paritaprevir/Ritonavir
Omeprazole
Ondansetron
Oral Contraceptives
Oritavancin
Orlistat
Oxaliplatin
Oxcarbazepine
Oxerutins
Oxilan
Oxprenolol
Oxybutynin
Oxycodone
Oxymorphone
Paclitaxel
Palbociclib
Paliperidone
Palonosetron
Pancrelipase
Pandemic Influenza Vaccine (H1N1)
Panitumumab
Panobinostat
Pantoprazole
Paricalcitol
Paroxetine Hydrochloride
Paroxetine Mesylate
Pasireotide
PEG-Interferon
Pegaptanib
Pegaspargase
Peginesatide
Pegloticase
Pegvisomant
Pembrolizumab
Pemetrexed
Pentamidine
Pentazocine
Perampanel
Perflutren
Pergolide
Perindopril
Pertuzumab
Phendimetrazine
Phenelzine
Phenobarbital
Phenoxybenzamine
Phentermine
Pilocarpine
Pioglitazone
Piracetam
Pirfenidone
Piroxicam
Pizotifen
Pomalidomide
Ponatinib
Posaconazole
Pramipexole
Pramlintide
Pranlukast

Prasugrel
Pravastatin
Praziquantel
Prazosin
Prednicarbate
Prednisolone
Pregabalin
Prenylamine
Promazine
Promethazine
Propafenone
Propoxyphene
Propranolol
Pseudoephedrine
Pyrimethamine
Quetiapine
Quinagolide
Quinapril
Quinidine
Quinine
Rabeprazole
Radium-223 Dichloride
Raltegravir
Ramelteon
Ramipril
Ranolazine
Rasagiline
Reboxetine
Regadenoson
Remifentanil
Repaglinide
Ribavirin
Rifabutin
Rifampin
Rifapentine
Rifaximin
Rilpivirine
Riluzole
Rimantadine
Rimonabant
Riociguat
Risedronate
Risperidone
Ritonavir
Rituximab
Rivaroxaban
Rivastigmine
Rizatriptan
Rofecoxib
Roflumilast
Rolapitant
Romiplostim
Ropinirole
Ropivacaine
Rosuvastatin
Rotigotine
Roxatidine
Rufinamide
Rupatadine
Ruxolitinib
Sacubitril/Valsartan
Salmeterol
Saxagliptin
Scopolamine
Selegiline
Selenium
Selexipag
Sertraline
Sibutramine
Sildenafil
Silodosin
Simvastatin
Sincalide
Sipuleucel-T
Sitaxentan
Sodium Oxybate
Sofosbuvir
Solifenacin
Sonidegib
Sorafenib
Spectinomycin
Streptomycin
Strontium Ranelate
Sucralfate
Sugammadex
Sulfadoxine
Sulfasalazine
Sumatriptan
Sunitinib
Suvorexant
Tacrine
Tacrolimus
Tadalafil
Taliglucerase
Talimogene Laherparepvec
Tamoxifen
Tamsulosin
Tapentadol
Tedizolid
Tegafur/Gimeracil/Oteracil
Tegaserod
Teicoplanin
Telavancin
Telbivudine
Telithromycin
Telmisartan
Temozolomide
Tenofovir Disoproxil
Terazosin
Terbutaline
Teriparatide
Tetrabenazine
Thalidomide
Thiabendazole
Thyrotropin Alfa
Tiagabine
Tianeptine
Ticagrelor
Tigecycline
Tiludronate
Timolol
Tinidazole
Tiotropium
Tipranavir
Tizanidine
Tocainide
Tocilizumab
Tofacitinib
Tolcapone
Tolterodine
Tolvaptan
Topiramate
Toremifene
Torsemide
Tositumomab & Iodine[131]
Tosufloxacin
Trabectedin
Tramadol
Trametinib
Trandolapril
Tranylcypromine
Trastuzumab
Trazodone
Treprostinil
Trimipramine
Triptorelin
Troglitazone
Trospium
Trovafloxacin
Typhoid Vaccine
Ulipristal
Unoprostone
Urapidil
Ursodiol
Ustekinumab
Valproic Acid
Valrubicin
Valsartan
Vardenafil
Varenicline
Varicella Vaccine
Velaglucerase Alfa
Venlafaxine
Verapamil
Verteporfin
Vigabatrin
Vilazodone
Vildagliptin
Vismodegib
Voriconazole
Vorinostat
Vortioxetine
Warfarin
Zafirlukast
Zaleplon
Zanamivir
Ziconotide
Zidovudine
Ziprasidone
Zofenopril
Zoledronate
Zolmitriptan
Zolpidem
Zonisamide
Zoster Vaccine
Zuclopenthixol

Xerostomia

Acamprosate
Acebutolol
Acetaminophen
Acetazolamide
Acitretin
Aclidinium
Ado-Trastuzumab Emtansine
Afatinib
Aflibercept
Albendazole
Albuterol
Aldesleukin
Almotriptan
Alprazolam
Alprostadil
Amantadine
Amifostine
Amiloride
Amisulpride
Amitriptyline
Amlodipine
Amoxapine
Amoxicillin
Apraclonidine
Aprepitant
Arbutamine
Aripiprazole
Armodafinil
Arsenic
Asenapine
Astemizole
Atomoxetine
Atropine Sulfate
Azatadine
Azelastine
Baclofen
Balsalazide
Bendamustine
Bendroflumethiazide
Benzphetamine
Benztropine
Bepridil
Betaxolol
Bexarotene
Bicalutamide
Bisacodyl
Bismuth
Bisoprolol
Botulinum Toxin (A & B)
Brexpiprazole
Brimonidine
Brinzolamide
Bromocriptine
Brompheniramine
Bumetanide
Buprenorphine
Bupropion
Buspirone
Butorphanol
Cabergoline
Canagliflozin
Captopril
Cariprazine
Carisoprodol
Carvedilol
Cefditoren
Cefixime
Ceftibuten
Celecoxib
Cetirizine
Cetuximab
Cevimeline
Chlordiazepoxide
Chlormezanone
Chlorpheniramine
Chlorpromazine
Ciprofloxacin
Cisplatin
Citalopram
Clarithromycin
Clemastine
Clindamycin
Clomipramine
Clonazepam
Clonidine
Clorazepate
Clozapine
Codeine
Conivaptan
Crofelemer
Cromolyn
Cyclobenzaprine
Cyproheptadine
Dapagliflozin
Darifenacin
Dasatinib
Daunorubicin

Degarelix
Delavirdine
Desipramine
Desloratadine
Desvenlafaxine
Dexchlorpheniramine
Dexketoprofen
Dexlansoprazole
Dexmedetomidine
Dexmethylphenidate
Dextroamphetamine
Diazepam
Diclofenac
Dicyclomine
Didanosine
Diethylpropion
Diflunisal
Dihydrocodeine
Dihydroergotamine
Diltiazem
Dimenhydrinate
Diphenhydramine
Diphenoxylate
Dirithromycin
Disopyramide
Domperidone
Donepezil
Doxazosin
Doxepin
Dronabinol
Duloxetine
Dutasteride
Efavirenz
Eletriptan
Eltrombopag
Enalapril
Enfuvirtide
Enoxacin
Entacapone
Ephedrine
Epinephrine
Eprosartan
Eribulin
Escitalopram
Eslicarbazepine
Esmolol
Estazolam
Eszopiclone
Etravirine
Everolimus
Exemestane
Ezogabine
Famotidine
Felbamate
Felodipine
Fenoprofen
Fentanyl
Fesoterodine
Flavoxate
Flecainide
Flibanserin
Fluconazole
Flumazenil
Fluorides
Fluoxetine
Fluphenazine
Flurazepam
Flurbiprofen
Fluvoxamine
Formoterol
Fosfomycin
Fosinopril
Fosphenytoin
Frovatriptan
Furosemide
Gabapentin
Gadobenate
Gadodiamide
Gadopentetate
Gadoteridol
Gadoversetamide
Gadoxetate
Ganciclovir
Gemifloxacin
Glatiramer
Glycopyrrolate
Goserelin
Granisetron
Grepafloxacin
Griseofulvin
Guanabenz
Guanadrel
Guanethidine
Guanfacine
Haloperidol
Hydrocodone
Hydromorphone
Hydroxyzine
Hyoscyamine
Ibuprofen
Iloperidone
Imatinib
Imipramine
Indapamide
Indinavir
Insulin
Interferon Alfa
Ioversol
Ipratropium
Isocarboxazid
Isoetharine
Isoproterenol
Isotretinoin
Isradipine
Itraconazole
Ketoprofen
Ketorolac
Ketotifen
Lamivudine
Lamotrigine
Lansoprazole
Leflunomide
Lenalidomide
Lenvatinib
Letrozole
Levocetirizine
Levodopa
Levofloxacin
Levomilnacipran
Lisdexamfetamine
Lisinopril
Lithium
Lomefloxacin
Loperamide
Loratadine
Lorazepam
Lorcaserin
Losartan
Lovastatin
Loxapine
Lubiprostone
Maprotiline
Marihuana
Mazindol
MDMA
Meclizine
Meloxicam
Meperidine
Mesalamine
Metamizole
Methadone
Methamphetamine
Methantheline
Methazolamide
Methyldopa
Methylphenidate
Metoclopramide
Metolazone
Metronidazole
Mexiletine
Midodrine
Mifepristone
Miglustat
Milnacipran
Minocycline
Mirabegron
Mirtazapine
Mizolastine
Modafinil
Moexipril
Molindone
Moricizine
Morphine
Moxifloxacin
Moxisylyte
Moxonidine
Mupirocin
Nabilone
Nabumetone
Nadolol
Nalbuphine
Nalmefene
Naloxone
Naltrexone
Naproxen
Nedocromil
Nefazodone
Nevirapine
Nicardipine
Nicotine
Nifedipine
Nilotinib
Nilutamide
Nisoldipine
Nitrofurantoin
Nitroglycerin
Nivolumab
Nizatidine
Norfloxacin
Nortriptyline
Ofloxacin
Olanzapine
Olaparib
Omacetaxine
Omeprazole
Ondansetron
Orlistat
Oxaliplatin
Oxazepam
Oxcarbazepine
Oxprenolol
Oxybutynin
Oxycodone
Oxymorphone
Oxytocin
Paliperidone
Palonosetron
Panobinostat
Pantoprazole
Papaverine
Paricalcitol
Paromomycin
Paroxetine Hydrochloride
Pembrolizumab
Pemetrexed
Pentamidine
Pentazocine
Pentoxifylline
Perflutren
Pergolide
Perindopril
Phendimetrazine
Phenelzine
Phenobarbital
Phenoxybenzamine
Phentermine
Pilocarpine
Pimozide
Pirfenidone
Piroxicam
Pizotifen
Posaconazole
Pramipexole
Prazepam
Prazosin
Pregabalin
Prochlorperazine
Procyclidine
Promethazine
Propafenone
Propantheline
Propofol
Propoxyphene
Propranolol
Protriptyline
Pseudoephedrine
Pyridostigmine
Pyrimethamine
Quazepam
Quetiapine
Quinapril
Rabeprazole
Raltitrexed
Ramipril
Ranolazine
Rasagiline
Reboxetine
Regadenoson
Regorafenib
Remifentanil
Reserpine
Rifaximin
Riluzole
Rimantadine
Risperidone
Ritonavir
Rivaroxaban
Rivastigmine
Rizatriptan
Rofecoxib
Ropinirole
Rotigotine
Rupatadine
Salmeterol

Saquinavir
Scopolamine
Selegiline
Sertindole
Sertraline
Sevoflurane
Sibutramine
Sildenafil
Solifenacin
Sorafenib
Sotalol
Sparfloxacin
Spironolactone
Sucralfate
Sugammadex
Sulfamethoxazole
Sulfasalazine
Sulindac
Sulpiride
Sumatriptan
Sunitinib
Suvorexant
Tacrine
Tadalafil
Tamoxifen
Tamsulosin
Tapentadol
Tasimelteon
Tedizolid
Telithromycin
Telmisartan
Temazepam
Terazosin
Terbutaline
Terfenadine
Thalidomide
Thiabendazole
Thioguanine
Thioridazine
Thiothixene
Tiagabine
Tianeptine
Tigecycline
Tiludronate
Timolol
Tinidazole
Tiotropium
Tizanidine
Tocainide
Tolcapone
Tolterodine
Tolvaptan
Topiramate
Toremifene
Tosufloxacin
Tramadol
Trametinib
Trandolapril
Tranylcypromine
Trazodone
Tretinoin
Triamcinolone
Triamterene
Triazolam
Trihexyphenidyl
Trimeprazine
Trimipramine
Tripelennamine
Triprolidine
Trospium
Trovafloxacin
Tryptophan
Ulipristal
Umeclidinium
Unoprostone
Valdecoxib
Valproic Acid
Valsartan
Vardenafil
Varenicline
Vemurafenib
Venlafaxine
Verapamil
Vilazodone
Vitamin A
Voriconazole
Vorinostat
Vortioxetine
Zalcitabine
Zaleplon
Ziconotide
Zidovudine
Ziprasidone
Zolmitriptan
Zolpidem
Zonisamide
Zuclopenthixol

Main Classes of Drugs

5-HT1 agonist
- Almotriptan
- Eletriptan
- Frovatriptan
- Naratriptan
- Rizatriptan
- Sumatriptan
- Zolmitriptan

5-HT3 antagonist
- Alosetron
- Dolasetron
- Granisetron
- Ondansetron
- Palonosetron

ACE inhibitor
- Benazepril
- Captopril
- Cilazapril
- Enalapril
- Fosinopril
- Imidapril
- Lisinopril
- Moexipril
- Perindopril
- Quinapril
- Ramipril
- Trandolapril
- Zofenopril

Adrenergic alpha-receptor agonist
- Clonidine
- Dexmedetomidine
- Dopamine
- Ephedrine
- Guanabenz
- Guanadrel
- Guanethidine
- Guanfacine
- Methyldopa
- Midodrine
- Mirtazapine
- Phenylephrine
- Phenylpropanolamine
- Polythiazide
- Pseudoephedrine

Adrenergic alpha-receptor antagonist
- Alfuzosin
- Doxazosin
- Phenoxybenzamine
- Phentolamine
- Prazosin
- Silodosin
- Tamsulosin
- Terazosin
- Urapidil

Adrenergic alpha2-receptor agonist
- Apraclonidine
- Brimonidine
- Tizanidine

Adrenergic beta-receptor agonist
- Arbutamine
- Dobutamine
- Isoetharine
- Isoproterenol
- Isoxsuprine
- Metoprolol

Adrenergic beta-receptor antagonist
- Betaxolol
- Carteolol
- Carvedilol
- Esmolol
- Labetalol
- Levobetaxolol
- Levobunolol
- Metipranolol
- Nadolol
- Nebivolol
- Penbutolol
- Pindolol
- Timolol

Alkylating agent
- Altretamine
- Bendamustine
- Busulfan
- Carboplatin
- Carmustine
- Chlorambucil
- Cisplatin
- Cyclophosphamide
- Dacarbazine
- Estramustine
- Ifosfamide
- Lomustine
- Mechlorethamine
- Melphalan
- Mitomycin
- Oxaliplatin
- Procarbazine
- Streptozocin
- Temozolomide
- Thiotepa

Amphetamine
- Benzphetamine
- Dextroamphetamine
- Diethylpropion
- MDMA
- Methamphetamine
- Methylphenidate
- Pemoline
- Phendimetrazine
- Phentermine
- Prenylamine

Analeptic
- Doxapram
- Modafinil

Analgesic

narcotic
- Dextromethorphan

non-narcotic
- Acetaminophen

non-opioid
- Ketorolac

opioid
- Alfentanil
- Dihydrocodeine
- Fentanyl
- Meptazinol
- Tapentadol

urinary
- Pentosan
- Phenazopyridine

Anesthetic
- Alfentanil
- Edrophonium
- Fentanyl
- Ketamine

general
- Chloral Hydrate
- Propofol
- Sodium Oxybate
- Sufentanil

inhalation
- Desflurane
- Enflurane
- Halothane
- Isoflurane
- Methoxyflurane
- Sevoflurane

local
- Articaine
- Bupivacaine
- Cocaine
- Levobupivacaine
- Lidocaine
- Mepivacaine
- Ropivacaine

Angiotensin II receptor antagonist (blocker)
- Azilsartan
- Candesartan
- Eprosartan
- Irbesartan
- Losartan
- Olmesartan
- Telmisartan
- Valsartan

Anti-inflammatory
- Amlexanox
- Amodiaquine
- Clofazimine
- Colchicine
- Fluprednisolone
- Roflumilast

Antiarrhythmic

class Ia
- Disopyramide
- Procainamide
- Quinidine

class Ib
- Lidocaine
- Mexiletine
- Phenytoin
- Tocainide

class Ic
- Flecainide
- Lorcainide
- Moricizine
- Propafenone

class II
- Acebutolol
- Atenolol
- Esmolol
- Labetalol
- Metoprolol
- Nadolol
- Propranolol
- Sotalol

class III
- Amiodarone
- Bretylium
- Dofetilide
- Dronedarone
- Ibutilide
- Sotalol
- Vernakalant

class IV
- Adenosine
- Amlodipine
- Bepridil
- Digoxin
- Diltiazem
- Verapamil

Antibiotic
- Doripenem
- Ertapenem
- Imipenem/Cilastatin
- Meropenem

aminoglycoside
- Amikacin
- Gentamicin
- Kanamycin
- Neomycin
- Paromomycin
- Streptomycin
- Tobramycin

anthracycline
- Bleomycin
- Dactinomycin
- Daunorubicin
- Doxorubicin
- Epirubicin
- Idarubicin
- Mitomycin
- Mitoxantrone
- Peplomycin
- Valrubicin

beta-lactam
- Ampicillin/Sulbactam
- Aztreonam
- Ceftazidime & Avibactam
- Ceftolozane & Tazobactam
- Flucloxacillin

fluoroquinolone
Besifloxacin
Ciprofloxacin
Enoxacin
Finafloxacin
Gatifloxacin
Gemifloxacin
Levofloxacin
Lomefloxacin
Moxifloxacin
Norfloxacin
Ofloxacin
Sparfloxacin
Tosufloxacin
glycopeptide
Daptomycin
Teicoplanin
Vancomycin
imidazole
Clotrimazole
Ketoconazole
Mebendazole
Miconazole
Sertaconazole
Thiabendazole
lincosamide
Clindamycin
Clindamycin/Tretinoin
Lincomycin
macrolide
Azithromycin
Clarithromycin
Dirithromycin
Erythromycin
Fidaxomicin
Roxithromycin
Telithromycin
Troleandomycin
nitrofuran
Furazolidone
Nitrofurazone
nitroimidazole
Metronidazole
Tinidazole
oxazolidinone
Linezolid
Tedizolid
penicillin
Amoxicillin
Ampicillin
Ampicillin/Sulbactam
Bacampicillin
Carbenicillin
Cloxacillin
Dicloxacillin
Methicillin
Mezlocillin
Nafcillin
Oxacillin
Penicillin G
Penicillin V
Piperacillin
Ticarcillin
quinolone
Cinoxacin
Grepafloxacin
Nalidixic Acid
Trovafloxacin
rifamycin
Rifabutin
Rifampin
Rifapentine
Rifaximin
streptogramin
Pristinamycin
Quinupristin/Dalfopristin
sulfonamide
Co-Trimoxazole
Sulfacetamide
Sulfadiazine
Sulfadoxine
Sulfamethoxazole
Sulfisoxazole
tetracycline
Chlortetracycline
Demeclocycline
Doxycycline
Lymecycline
Minocycline
Oxytetracycline
Tetracycline
Tigecycline
topical
Mupirocin
Retapamulin
triazole
Fluconazole
Itraconazole
Posaconazole
Terconazole
Voriconazole
miscellaneous
Aminosalicylate Sodium
Bacitracin
Capreomycin
Ceftriaxone
Chloramphenicol
Cycloserine
Dapsone
Ethionamide
Fosfomycin
Isoniazid
Methenamine
Nitrofurantoin
Plicamycin
Pyrazinamide
Quinacrine
Spectinomycin
Tigecycline
Trimethoprim

Anticonvulsant
Brivaracetam
Carbamazepine
Ezogabine
Felbamate
Gabapentin
Lacosamide
Lamotrigine
Levetiracetam
Mephenytoin
Oxcarbazepine
Perampanel
Phenacemide
Phenobarbital
Phensuximide
Phenytoin
Pregabalin
Primidone
Tetrazepam
Tiagabine
Topiramate
Valproic Acid
Vigabatrin
Zonisamide
antiepileptic
Brivaracetam
Clobazam
Eslicarbazepine
Lacosamide
Lamotrigine
Perampanel
Rufinamide
Vigabatrin
hydantoin
Ethotoin
Fosphenytoin
Mephenytoin
Phenytoin
oxazolidinedione
Paramethadione
Trimethadione
succinimide
Ethosuximide
Methsuximide

Antidepressant
Bupropion
Citalopram
Desvenlafaxine
Duloxetine
Escitalopram
Fluoxetine
Fluvoxamine
Isocarboxazid
Levomilnacipran
Milnacipran
Moclobemide
Nefazodone
Paroxetine Hydrochloride
Phenelzine
Reboxetine
Selegiline
Sertraline
Tianeptine
Tranylcypromine
Tryptophan
Venlafaxine
Vilazodone
Vortioxetine
tetracyclic
Maprotiline
Mianserin
Mirtazapine
tricyclic
Amitriptyline
Amoxapine
Clomipramine
Desipramine
Doxepin
Imipramine
Nortriptyline
Protriptyline
Trazodone
Trimipramine

Antiemetic
Aprepitant
Chlorpromazine
Dexamethasone
Dimenhydrinate
Diphenhydramine
Domperidone
Dronabinol
Droperidol
Granisetron
Haloperidol
Marihuana
Meclizine
Metoclopramide
Nabilone
Ondansetron
Palonosetron
Perphenazine
Prochlorperazine
Rolapitant
Scopolamine
Trimethobenzamide

Antifungal
Amphotericin B
Caspofungin
Ciclopirox
Clioquinol
Econazole
Efinaconazole
Griseofulvin
Micafungin
Nystatin
Terbinafine
azole
Clotrimazole
Fluconazole
Isavuconazonium Sulfate
Itraconazole
Ketoconazole
Luliconazole
Miconazole
Posaconazole
Voriconazole
oxaborole
Tavaborole

Antimalarial
Amodiaquine
Artemether/Lumefantrine
Artesunate
Atovaquone
Atovaquone/Proguanil
Chloroquine
Halofantrine
Hydroxychloroquine
Mefloquine
Primaquine
Pyrimethamine
Quinacrine
Quinidine
Quinine
Sulfadoxine

Antimycobacterial
Bedaquiline
Clofazimine
Dapsone
Ethambutol
Flucytosine
Isoniazid
Potassium Iodide
echinocandin
Anidulafungin

Antineoplastic
Anastrozole
Arsenic
Asparaginase
Asparaginase *Erwinia chrysanthemi*

Azacitidine
Bexarotene
Cabazitaxel
Capecitabine
Carboplatin
Cetuximab
Cisplatin
Cladribine
Cytarabine
Dacarbazine
Dasatinib
Decitabine
Denileukin
Docetaxel
Eribulin
Erlotinib
Everolimus
Floxuridine
Fludarabine
Fluorouracil
Gefitinib
Gemcitabine
Gemtuzumab
Hydroxyurea
Ibritumomab
Imatinib
Irinotecan
Ixabepilone
Lapatinib
Levamisole
Mercaptopurine
Mitotane
Mitoxantrone
Nelarabine
Nilotinib
Nilutamide
Oxaliplatin
Paclitaxel
Panitumumab
Pazopanib
Pegaspargase
Pentostatin
Porfimer
Raltitrexed
Sorafenib
Streptozocin
Sunitinib
Tegafur/Gimeracil/Oteracil
Temozolomide
Temsirolimus
Teniposide
Testolactone
Thioguanine
Topotecan
Tositumomab & Iodine^{131}
Trabectedin
Trastuzumab
Tretinoin
Trifluridine & Tipiracil
Vorinostat

Antiplatelet

Abciximab
Aspirin
Cangrelor
Cilostazol
Clopidogrel
Dipyridamole
Eptifibatide
Ticagrelor
Tirofiban

CPTP

Cangrelor
Ticagrelor

thienopyridine

Clopidogrel
Prasugrel
Ticlopidine

Antiprotozoal

Atovaquone
Chloroquine
Hydroxychloroquine
Mefloquine
Nitazoxanide
Pentamidine
Primaquine
Pyrimethamine
Quinidine
Quinine

Antipsychotic

Amisulpride
Aripiprazole
Asenapine
Brexpiprazole
Carbamazepine
Cariprazine
Chlorpromazine
Clozapine
Droperidol
Fluphenazine
Iloperidone
Levomepromazine
Lithium
Lurasidone
Mesoridazine
Molindone
Olanzapine
Paliperidone
Perphenazine
Pimavanserin
Pimozide
Prochlorperazine
Promazine
Quetiapine
Risperidone
Sertindole
Thioridazine
Thiothixene
Trifluoperazine
Trimeprazine
Valproic Acid
Ziprasidone
Zuclopenthixol
Zuclopenthixol Acetate
Zuclopenthixol Decanoate
Zuclopenthixol Dihydrochloride

butyrophenone

Haloperidol

tricyclic

Loxapine

Antiretroviral

Adefovir
Amprenavir
Atazanavir
Cobicistat/Elvitegravir/Emtricitabine/Tenofovir Alafenamide
Cobicistat/Elvitegravir/Emtricitabine/Tenofovir Disoproxil
Darunavir
Delavirdine
Didanosine
Dolutegravir
Efavirenz
Emtricitabine
Enfuvirtide
Fosamprenavir
Hydroxyurea
Indinavir
Lamivudine
Lopinavir
Maraviroc
Nelfinavir
Nevirapine
Raltegravir
Rilpivirine
Ritonavir
Saquinavir
Stavudine
Tenofovir Disoproxil
Zalcitabine
Zidovudine

Antiviral

Acyclovir
Amantadine
Cytarabine
Entecavir
Famciclovir
Foscarnet
Ganciclovir
Imiquimod
Oseltamivir
Penciclovir
Peramivir
Podophyllotoxin
Rimantadine
Simeprevir
Telaprevir
Tenofovir Alafenamide
Trifluridine
Valacyclovir
Valganciclovir
Zanamivir

nucleoside analog

Ribavirin
Vidarabine

nucleotide analog

Cidofovir

topical

Acyclovir
Docosanol

Anxiolytic

Buspirone
Chlormezanone
Meprobamate
Tetrazepam

Barbiturate

Amobarbital
Aprobarbital
Butabarbital
Butalbital
Mephobarbital
Methohexital
Pentobarbital
Phenobarbital
Primidone
Secobarbital
Thiopental

Benzodiazepine

Alprazolam
Chlordiazepoxide
Clobazam
Clonazepam
Clorazepate
Diazepam
Estazolam
Flurazepam
Lorazepam
Midazolam
Nitrazepam
Oxazepam
Prazepam
Quazepam
Temazepam
Tetrazepam
Triazolam

Bisphosphonate

Alendronate
Etidronate
Ibandronate
Pamidronate
Risedronate
Tiludronate
Zoledronate

Calcium channel blocker

Amlodipine
Bepridil
Clevidipine
Diltiazem
Felodipine
Isradipine
Nicardipine
Nifedipine
Nimodipine
Nisoldipine
Prenylamine
Verapamil

Carbonic anhydrase inhibitor

Acetazolamide
Brinzolamide
Dichlorphenamide
Dorzolamide
Ethoxzolamide
Methazolamide

CB1 Cannabinoid receptor antagonist

Rimonabant

Central muscle relaxant

Carisoprodol
Chlormezanone
Chlorzoxazone
Cyclobenzaprine
Meprobamate
Metaxalone
Methocarbamol
Orphenadrine

Cephalosporin

1st generation

Cefadroxil
Cefazolin
Cephalexin
Cephalothin

Cephapirin
Cephradine
2nd generation
Cefaclor
Cefamandole
Cefmetazole
Cefonicid
Cefotetan
Cefoxitin
Cefprozil
Cefuroxime
Loracarbef
3rd generation
Cefdinir
Cefditoren
Cefixime
Cefoperazone
Cefotaxime
Cefpodoxime
Ceftazidime
Ceftazidime & Avibactam
Ceftibuten
Ceftizoxime
Ceftriaxone
4th generation
Cefepime
5th generation
Ceftaroline Fosamil
Ceftobiprole
Ceftolozane & Tazobactam

Cholinesterase inhibitor
Donepezil
Edrophonium
Galantamine
Neostigmine
Physostigmine
Rivastigmine
Succinylcholine
Tacrine

CNS stimulant
Cocaine
Dexmethylphenidate
Dextroamphetamine
Lisdexamfetamine
Modafinil

Corticosteroid
Alclometasone
Amcinonide
Beclomethasone
Betamethasone
Budesonide
Ciclesonide
Clobetasol
Cortisone
Desonide
Desoximetasone
Dexamethasone
Difluprednate
Fludrocortisone
Flumetasone
Flunisolide
Fluocinolone
Fluocinonide
Fluprednisolone
Fluticasone Furoate
Fluticasone Propionate
Halcinonide
Halobetasol
Halometasone
Hydrocortisone
Loteprednol
Methylprednisolone
Mometasone
Prednicarbate
Prednisolone
Prednisone
Tixocortol
Triamcinolone
antagonist
Mifepristone
Misoprostol

COX-2 inhibitor
Celecoxib
Etodolac
Etoricoxib
Meloxicam
Nimesulide
Rofecoxib
Valdecoxib

CYP3A4 inhibitor
Amiodarone
Aprepitant
Boceprevir
Chloramphenicol
Cimetidine
Ciprofloxacin
Clarithromycin
Conivaptan
Dasabuvir/Ombitasvir/Paritaprevir/Ritonavir
Delavirdine
Diltiazem
Erythromycin
Fluconazole
Fluvoxamine
Imatinib
Indinavir
Itraconazole
Ketoconazole
Mifepristone
Nefazodone
Nelfinavir
Norfloxacin
Ombitasvir/Paritaprevir/Ritonavir
Ritonavir
Saquinavir
Telaprevir
Telithromycin
Verapamil
Voriconazole

Dermal filler
Azficel-T
Calcium Hydroxylapatite

Disease-modifying antirheumatic drug (DMARD)
Abatacept
Adalimumab
Azathioprine
Bucillamine
Certolizumab
Chloroquine
Cyclosporine
Etanercept
Gold & Gold Compounds
Golimumab
Hydroxychloroquine
Infliximab
Leflunomide
Methotrexate
Minocycline
Penicillamine
Rituximab
Sulfasalazine
Tocilizumab

Diuretic
Acetazolamide
Brinzolamide
Dorzolamide
Eplerenone
Isosorbide
Methazolamide
Spironolactone
loop
Bumetanide
Ethacrynic Acid
Furosemide
Torsemide
potassium-sparing
Amiloride
Triamterene
thiazide
Bendroflumethiazide
Benzthiazide
Chlorothiazide
Chlorthalidone
Cyclothiazide
Hydrochlorothiazide
Hydroflumethiazide
Indapamide
Methyclothiazide
Metolazone
Polythiazide
Quinethazone
Trichlormethiazide

Dopamine receptor agonist
Apomorphine
Bromocriptine
Cabergoline
Dopexamine
Fenoldopam
Pergolide
Pramipexole
Quinagolide
Ropinirole
Rotigotine

Dopamine receptor antagonist
Amisulpride
Domperidone
Metoclopramide
Sulpiride

Endothelin receptor (ETR) antagonist
Ambrisentan
Bosentan
Macitentan
Sitaxentan

Epidermal growth factor receptor (EGFR) inhibitor
Cetuximab
Erlotinib
Gefitinib
Lapatinib
Necitumumab
Nilotinib
Panitumumab
Pazopanib
Sorafenib
Sunitinib

Eugeroic
Armodafinil

Fibrinolytic
Alteplase
Anistreplase
Reteplase
Streptokinase
Tenecteplase
Urokinase

Gonadotropin-releasing hormone (GnRH)
agonist
Buserelin
Goserelin
Histrelin
Leuprolide
Nafarelin
Triptorelin
antagonist
Abarelix
Cetrorelix
Degarelix
Ganirelix

Histamine
H1 receptor antagonist
Alcaftadine
Astemizole
Azatadine
Azelastine
Bepotastine
Brompheniramine
Buclizine
Carbinoxamine
Cetirizine
Chlorpheniramine
Cinnarizine
Clemastine
Cyproheptadine
Desloratadine
Dexchlorpheniramine
Diphenhydramine
Epinastine
Fexofenadine
Hydroxyzine
Ketotifen
Levocetirizine
Loratadine
Meclizine
Mizolastine
Olopatadine
Phenindamine
Promethazine
Pyrilamine
Rupatadine
Terfenadine
Trimeprazine
Tripelennamine
Triprolidine
H2 receptor antagonist
Cimetidine
Famotidine
Nizatidine
Ranitidine
Roxatidine

Histone deacetylase (HDAC) inhibitor
Belinostat
Panobinostat
Romidepsin
Vorinostat

HMG-CoA reductase inhibitor
Atorvastatin
Fluvastatin
Lovastatin
Pravastatin
Rosuvastatin
Simvastatin

Hormone
Estradiol
Levonorgestrel
Oral Contraceptives
Sincalide

polypeptide
Glucagon
Insulin
Insulin Aspart
Mecasermin
Nesiritide
Secretin

Immunomodulator
Aldesleukin
Efalizumab
Glatiramer
Imiquimod
Immune Globulin IV
Immune Globulin SC
Interferon Alfa
Interferon Beta
Lenalidomide
Levamisole
Natalizumab
Palivizumab
PEG-Interferon
Pimecrolimus
Pomalidomide
Sinecatechins

Immunosuppressant
Alefacept
Alemtuzumab
Anti-Thymocyte Globulin (Equine)
Anti-Thymocyte Immunoglobulin (Rabbit)
Azathioprine
Belatacept
Belimumab
Cyclosporine
Daclizumab
Everolimus
Fingolimod
Mizoribine
Muromonab-CD3
Mycophenolate
Pirfenidone
Rituximab
Sirolimus
Tacrolimus
Thalidomide

Mast cell stabilizer
Cromolyn
Lodoxamide
Nedocromil
Pemirolast

Monoamine oxidase (MAO) inhibitor
Isocarboxazid
Phenelzine
Tranylcypromine

Monoclonal antibody
Abciximab
Adalimumab
Alemtuzumab
Alirocumab
Atezolizumab
Basiliximab
Belimumab
Bevacizumab
Bezlotoxumab
Blinatumomab
Brentuximab Vedotin
Canakinumab
Certolizumab
Cetuximab
Daclizumab
Daratumumab
Denosumab
Dinutuximab
Eculizumab
Efalizumab
Elotuzumab
Evolocumab
Gemtuzumab
Golimumab
Ibritumomab
Idarucizumab
Infliximab
Ipilimumab
Ixekizumab
Mepolizumab
Muromonab-CD3
Natalizumab
Necitumumab
Nivolumab
Obinutuzumab
Ofatumumab
Olaratumab
Omalizumab
Palivizumab
Panitumumab
Pembrolizumab
Pertuzumab
Ramucirumab
Ranibizumab
Reslizumab
Rituximab
Secukinumab
Siltuximab
Tocilizumab
Tositumomab & Iodine[131]
Trastuzumab
Ustekinumab
Vedolizumab

mTOR inhibitor
Everolimus
Temsirolimus
Zotarolimus

Muscarinic antagonist
Amitriptyline
Amoxapine
Atropine Sulfate
Benactyzine
Benztropine
Biperiden
Chlorpheniramine
Chlorpromazine
Cinnarizine
Clidinium
Clomipramine
Darifenacin
Dicyclomine
Diphenhydramine
Disopyramide
Doxepin
Fesoterodine
Flavoxate
Glycopyrrolate
Hydroxyzine
Hyoscyamine
Imipramine
Ipratropium
Maprotiline
Mepenzolate
Olanzapine
Orphenadrine
Oxybutynin
Phenelzine
Prochlorperazine
Procyclidine
Propantheline
Scopolamine
Solifenacin
Tiotropium
Tolterodine
Trihexyphenidyl
Trospium
Umeclidinium

Muscarinic cholinergic agonist
Bethanechol
Carbachol
Cevimeline
Methantheline
Pilocarpine

Non-depolarizing neuromuscular blocker
Atracurium
Cisatracurium
Doxacurium
Pancuronium
Pipecuronium
Rapacuronium
Rocuronium
Vecuronium

Non-nucleoside reverse transcriptase inhibitor
Delavirdine
Efavirenz
Emtricitabine/Rilpivirine/Tenofovir Alafenamide
Etravirine
Nevirapine
Rilpivirine

Non-steroidal anti-inflammatory (NSAID)
Aceclofenac
Acemetacin
Aspirin
Benzydamine
Bromfenac
Celecoxib
Dexibuprofen
Dexketoprofen
Diclofenac
Diflunisal
Etodolac
Etoricoxib
Fenbufen
Fenoprofen
Flurbiprofen
Ibuprofen
Indomethacin
Ketoprofen
Ketorolac
Meclofenamate
Mefenamic Acid
Meloxicam
Metamizole
Methyl salicylate
Nabumetone
Naproxen
Nepafenac
Nimesulide
Oxaprozin
Phenylbutazone
Piroxicam
Pranoprofen
Rofecoxib
Salsalate
Sulindac
Tenoxicam
Tolmetin
Valdecoxib

Nucleoside analog reverse transcriptase inhibitor
Abacavir
Cobicistat/Elvitegravir/Emtricitabine/Tenofovir Alafenamide
Cobicistat/Elvitegravir/Emtricitabine/Tenofovir Disoproxil
Didanosine
Emtricitabine
Emtricitabine/Rilpivirine/Tenofovir Alafenamide
Lamivudine
Stavudine
Telbivudine
Tenofovir Disoproxil
Zalcitabine
Zidovudine

Oligonucleotide
Defibrotide
Fomivirsen

Opiate agonist
Codeine
Heroin
Hydrocodone
Hydromorphone
Loperamide
Meperidine
Methadone
Morphine
Nalbuphine
Oxycodone
Oxymorphone
Pentazocine
Propoxyphene
Sufentanil
Tramadol

Phosphodiesterase inhibitor
- Apremilast
- Avanafil
- Cilostazol
- Inamrinone
- Milrinone
- Roflumilast
- Sildenafil
- Tadalafil
- Vardenafil

Programmed death receptor-1 (PD-1) inhibitor
- Nivolumab
- Pembrolizumab

Prostaglandin
- Alprostadil
- Dinoprostone
- Iloprost
- Treprostinil
- Unoprostone

Prostaglandin analog
- Bimatoprost
- Gemeprost
- Latanoprost
- Tafluprost
- Travoprost

Proton pump inhibitor (PPI)
- Dexlansoprazole
- Esomeprazole
- Lansoprazole
- Omeprazole
- Pantoprazole
- Rabeprazole

Retinoid
- Acitretin
- Adapalene
- Alitretinoin
- Bexarotene
- Clindamycin/Tretinoin
- Isotretinoin
- Tretinoin

Selective estrogen receptor modulator (SERM)
- Chlorotrianisene
- Clomiphene
- Ospemifene
- Raloxifene
- Tamoxifen
- Tibolone
- Toremifene

Selective serotonin reuptake inhibitor (SSRI)
- Citalopram
- Escitalopram
- Fluoxetine
- Fluvoxamine
- Paroxetine Hydrochloride
- Paroxetine Mesylate
- Sertraline

Serotonin
- Buspirone
- Sibutramine

serotonin receptor agonist
- Almotriptan
- Eletriptan
- Frovatriptan
- Lorcaserin
- Rizatriptan
- Sumatriptan
- Vortioxetine
- Zolmitriptan

serotonin receptor antagonist
- Naratriptan
- Vortioxetine

serotonin reuptake inhibitor
- Duloxetine
- Trazodone
- Vortioxetine

serotonin type 3 receptor antagonist
- Alosetron
- Dolasetron
- Granisetron
- Netupitant & Palonosetron
- Ondansetron
- Palonosetron

serotonin type 4 receptor agonist
- Tegaserod

serotonin-norepinephrine reuptake inhibitor
- Desvenlafaxine
- Levomilnacipran
- Venlafaxine
- Vilazodone

Statin
- Atorvastatin
- Fluvastatin
- Lovastatin
- Pitavastatin
- Pravastatin
- Rosuvastatin
- Simvastatin

Sulfonylurea
- Acetohexamide
- Chlorpropamide
- Gliclazide
- Glimepiride
- Glipizide
- Glyburide
- Tolazamide
- Tolazoline
- Tolbutamide

Topoisomerase 1 inhibitor
- Irinotecan
- Topotecan

Topoisomerase 2 inhibitor
- Etoposide
- Teniposide

Trace element
- Arsenic
- Selenium
- Zinc

Tyrosine kinase inhibitor
- Afatinib
- Axitinib
- Bosutinib
- Cabozantinib
- Ceritinib
- Crizotinib
- Dasatinib
- Erlotinib
- Gefitinib
- Imatinib
- Lapatinib
- Leflunomide
- Lenvatinib
- Nilotinib
- Nintedanib
- Pazopanib
- Ponatinib
- Regorafenib
- Sorafenib
- Sunitinib
- Vandetanib

Vaccine
- Anthrax Vaccine
- BCG Vaccine
- Cholera Vaccine
- Diphtheria Antitoxin
- Hemophilus B Vaccine
- Hepatitis A Vaccine
- Hepatitis B Vaccine
- Human Papillomavirus (HPV) Vaccine
- Human Papillomavirus Vaccine (Bivalent)
- Inactivated Polio Vaccine
- Influenza Vaccine
- Japanese Encephalitis Vaccine
- Measles, Mumps & Rubella (MMR) Virus Vaccine
- Meningococcal Group B Vaccine
- Meningococcal Groups C & Y & Haemophilus B Tetanus Toxoid Conjugate Vaccine
- Pandemic Influenza Vaccine (H1N1)
- Pneumococcal Vaccine
- Sipuleucel-T
- Smallpox Vaccine
- Typhoid Vaccine
- Varicella Vaccine
- Yellow Fever Vaccine
- Zoster Vaccine

Vasodilator
- Ambrisentan
- Amyl Nitrite
- Benazepril
- Bosentan
- Captopril
- Cilazapril
- Diazoxide
- Enalapril
- Fosinopril
- Hydralazine
- Iloprost
- Isosorbide Dinitrate
- Isosorbide Mononitrate
- Minoxidil
- Nesiritide
- Nitroglycerin
- Nitroprusside
- Prenylamine
- Quinapril
- Ramipril
- Trandolapril

peripheral
- Cilostazol
- Papaverine
- Pentoxifylline

Vitamin
- Ascorbic Acid
- Beta-Carotene
- Cyanocobalamin
- Ergocalciferol
- Folic Acid
- Niacin
- Niacinamide
- Pantothenic Acid
- Phytonadione
- Pyridoxine
- Riboflavin
- Thiamine
- Vitamin A
- Vitamin E

Vitamin D receptor agonist
- Dihydrotachysterol
- Doxercalciferol
- Paricalcitol

Xanthine alkaloid
- Aminophylline
- Pentoxifylline

CLASSES OF DRUGS THAT CAN CAUSE IMPORTANT INTERACTIONS

ARBs
Angiotensin II receptor antagonists (blockers)
- Candesartan
- Eprosartan
- Irbesartan
- Losartan
- Olmesartan
- Telmisartan
- Valsartan

Anticholinergics
- Amoxapine
- Atropine
- Benztropine
- Biperiden
- Chlorpheniramine
- Clomipramine
- Cyproheptadine
- Desipramine
- Dicyclomine
- Digoxin
- Diphenhydramine
- Disopyramide
- Furosemide
- Glycopyrrolate
- Hyoscyamine
- Oxybutynin
- Propantheline
- Tiotropium
- Tolterodine

Anticoagulants
- Acenocoumarol
- Apixaban
- Aspirin
- Clopidogrel
- Dabigatran
- Dalteparin
- Fondaparinux
- Phenindione
- Rivarobaxan
- Ticlopidine
- Urokinase
- Warfarin

CYP 3A4 inhibitors
- Amiodarone
- Anastrozole
- Azithromycin
- Cimetidine
- Clarithromycin
- Cyclosporine
- Danazol
- Delavirdine
- Dexamethasone
- Diltiazem
- Dirithromycin
- Disulfiram
- Entacapone
- Erythromycin
- Fluconazole
- Fluoxetine
- Fluvoxamine
- Grapefruit juice
- Indinavir
- Isoniazid
- Ketoconazole
- Metronidazole
- Mibefradil
- Nefazodone
- Nelfinavir
- Nevirapine
- Norfloxacin
- Omeprazole
- Paroxetine
- Propoxyphene
- Quinidine
- Quinine
- Ranitidine
- Ritonavir
- Saquinavir
- Sertindole
- Sertraline
- Troglitazone
- Troleandomycin
- Valproic acid

MAOIs
Monamine Oxidase Inhibitors
- Amitriptyline
- Amoxapine
- Atomoxetine
- Benzphetamine
- Brompheniramine
- Bupropion
- Chlorpheniramine
- Citalopram
- Clomipramine
- Cocaine
- Cyclobenzaprine
- Desipramine
- Desvenlafaxine
- Dextroamphetamine
- Dextromethorphan
- Doxepine
- Duloxetine
- Ephedrine
- Escitalopram
- Fentanyl
- Fluoxetine
- Fluvoxamine
- Imipramine
- Ketamine
- Lisdexamfetamine
- Maprotiline
- Mazindol
- MDMA ("Ecstasy")
- Meperidine
- Methadone
- Methamphetamine
- Methylphenidate
- Milnacipran
- Nefazodone
- Nortriptyline
- Paroxetine
- Pemoline
- Phencyclidine
- Phendimetrazine
- Pheniramine
- Phentermine
- Phenylephrine
- Phenylalanine
- Propoxyphene
- Protripyline
- Pseudoephedrine
- Reboxetine
- Sertraline
- Sibutramine
- Tramadol
- Trazodone
- Trimipramine
- Tryptophan
- Venlafaxine

NSAIDs*
Non Steroidal Anti-Inflammatory Drugs
- Aspirin
- Celecoxib
- Diclofenac
- Diflunisal
- Etodolac
- Fenoprofen
- Flurbiprofen
- Ibuprofen
- Indomethacin
- Ketoprofen
- Magnesium salicylate
- Meclofenamate sodium
- Mefenamic acid
- Meloxicam
- Nabumetone
- Naproxen
- Oxaprozin
- Piroxicam
- Rofecoxib
- Salsalate
- Sodium salicylate
- Sulindac
- Tolmetin
- Valdecoxib

Statins
HMG-CoA reductase inhibitors
- Atorvastatin
- Fluvastatin
- Lovastatin
- Pitavastatin
- Pravastatin
- Rosuvastatin
- Simvastatin

* Note that acetaminophen (Paracetamol; Tylenol) is not on this list; unlike other common analgesics such as aspirin and ibuprofen, it has no anti-inflammatory properties, and so it is not a member of the class of drugs known as non-steroidal anti-inflammatory drugs. Acetaminophen relieves pain in mild arthritis but has no effect on the underlying inflammation, redness and swelling of the joint. It belongs to a class of drugs called analgesics (pain relievers) and antipyretics (fever reducers) and is thought to relieve pain by elevating the pain threshold (that is, by requiring a greater amount of pain to develop before it is felt). It reduces fever through its action on the heat-regulating center of the brain; specifically, it tells the center to lower the body's temperature when the temperature is elevated.

CLASS REACTIONS*

ACE INHIBITORS

	B	C	E	F	L	P	Q	R	T	Z	=
SKIN											
Anaphylaxis		[1]	[1]		•	[1]		•			✓
Angioedema	[8]	[45] (15%)	[73]	[3]	[41] (70%)	[6]	[9]	[11]	[3]	[1]	✓✓
Bullous dermatitis		[1]			[1]						
Bullous pemphigoid		[2]	[2]								
Dermatitis		[3]		[1]				[1]			
Diaphoresis	[1]		[1]	•	•	•	[3]	[2]			✓
DRESS syndrome		[2]						[1]			
Edema			[1]	•		•	[4]	[1]	•		✓
Erythema		[1]	[1]		•	•		[1]			✓
Erythema multiforme			•					•			
Erythroderma		[2]	[1]	[1]							
Exanthems	[1]	[19] (10%)	[9]		[4]		[1]	[1]			✓
Exfoliative dermatitis		[4]	•		[2]		•				
Facial edema					[1]	•	[1]				
Jaundice		[1]						[1]			
Kaposi's sarcoma		[2]			[2]		[1]				
Lichen planus pemphigoides		[2]						[3]			
Lichenoid eruption		[12]	[2]		[2]						
Linear IgA	[1]	[5]									
Lupus erythematosus		[8]	[2]		[1]						
Mycosis fungoides		[2]	[1]								
Palmar–plantar pustulosis		[1]				[1]					
Pemphigus	[1]	[23]	[10]	[1]			[1]	[1]	•		✓

B Benazepril; **C** Captopril; **E** Enalapril; **F** Fosinopril; **L** Lisinopril; **P** Perindopril; **Q** Quinapril; **R** Ramipril; **T** Trandolapril; **Z** Zofenopril

These tables concentrate on skin, hair, nails and mucosal reactions.

* The following conventions are followed in these tables:

•	reaction noted (package inserts)
[3]	number of published reports of a reaction
(8%)	highest incidence that has ever been noted or reported
?	20 reports or over or an incidence of 20% or over recorded for this reaction for a minority of drugs in the class
✓	at least half the drugs in the class selection have this reaction noted or reported
✓✓	all drugs in the class selection have this reaction noted or reported
Note:	reactions noted or reported for only one drug in a class selection have been excluded

	B	C	E	F	L	P	Q	R	T	Z	=
Pemphigus foliaceus	[1]	[2]	[2]	[1]	[2]	[1]	[1]	[1]	[1]		✓
Peripheral edema	[3]		[2]		[1]	[3]	[3]				✓
Photosensitivity	•	[3]	[2]	•	•		[2]	[2]			✓
Pityriasis rosea		[6]			[2]						
Pruritus	[1]	[8] (10%)	[3]	[1]	•	(<10%)	[7]	[3]	•		✓
Pseudolymphoma		[2]		[1]	[1]						
Psoriasis		[8]	[3]		[1]	•		[1]			✓
Purpura		[1]	[1]		[2]	•		•			✓
Rash	[1]	[11] (4–7%)	[5]	[1]	[6]	[1] (<10%)	[5]	[4]	•	•	✓✓
Stevens–Johnson syndrome		[1]	•					[1]			
Toxic epidermal necrolysis		[3]	•								
Urticaria	[1]	[9] (7%)	[5]	•	[2]		•	•			✓
Vasculitis		[7]	[2]		[1]		•	[1]			✓
Xerosis		[1]				•					
HAIR											
Alopecia		[4]	[1]		[1]		•	(<10%)			✓
NAILS											
Nail dystrophy		[2]	[1]								
MUCOSAL											
Burning mouth syndrome		[1]	[1]		[1]						
Glossitis		[3]	•								
Glossopyrosis		[1]	[1]								
Oral burn		[1]	[1]								
Oral ulceration		[4]	[2]								
Sialorrhea		[1]						•			
Tongue edema			[2]		[2]	[2]					
Xerostomia		[1]	•	•	•	•	•	•	•		✓

B Benazepril; **C** Captopril; **E** Enalapril; **F** Fosinopril; **L** Lisinopril; **P** Perindopril; **Q** Quinapril; **R** Ramipril; **T** Trandolapril; **Z** Zofenopril

ANTIARRHYTHMICS

	A	Di	Dr	F	I	L	Pn	Pf	Pr	Q	S	=
SKIN												
Acneform eruption								•	[2]	[2]		
AGEP								[1]		[2]		
Anaphylaxis	[2]		[1]			[7]			[1]			
Angioedema	[2]					[3]	[1]	[1]	[2]	•		✓
Bullous dermatitis					[1]				[1]			
Dermatitis		•	(5%)			[27]	[1] (6%)		[2]	[4]		✓
Diaphoresis	[2]			•	[1]	[1]		•				
Eczema			(5%)			[3]			[2]			
Edema	(<10%)	•		•		[2]		•			(5%)	✓
Erythema			(5%)			[3]		[1]	[1]			
Erythema multiforme	[1]					[2]			[1]	[1]		
Erythema nodosum	[2]	[1]				[1]						
Exanthems	[5]	[1] (<5%)	[1]	[1]		[2]	[5] (8%)	[1]	[4]	[6] (17%)		✓
Exfoliative dermatitis	[1]			•		[2]			[1]	[5]		
Fixed eruption				[1]		[2]			[1]	[2]		
Hypersensitivity	[1]		[1]			[9]	[2]			[1]		
Leukocytoclastic vasculitis									[1]		[1]	
Lichen planus							[1]			[7]		
Lichenoid eruption									[3]	[6]	[1]	
Lupus erythematosus	[5] (5%)	[3]				[1]	[175] (15–20%)	[3]	[2]	[35]		✓
Necrosis	[1]								[3]			
Photosensitivity	[41] (10–75%)	[1]	•				[1]		[1]	[21]	•	✓
Phototoxicity	[3]		[1]						[1]	[1]		
Pigmentation	[68] (<10%)					[1]				[3]		?
Pruritus	[2] (<5%)	•	(5%)	•		[3]	•	•	[1]	[3]	(<10%)	✓
Psoriasis	[2]			[2]				[2]	[20]	[5]	[3]	✓
Purpura	[1]	[1]				[1]	[3]	•	[1]	[13]		✓
Rash	[1]	•	[7] (5%)	•		•	•	•	[2] (<10%)	(<10%)	•	✓
Raynaud's phenomenon									[3] (59%)		•	

A Amiodarone; **Di** Disopyramide; **Dr** Dronedarone; **F** Flecainide; **I** Ibutilide; **L** Lidocaine; **Pn** Procainamide; **Pf** Propafenone; **Pr** Propranolol; **Q** Quinidine; **S** Sotalol

	A	Di	Dr	F	I	L	Pn	Pf	Pr	Q	S	=
Sjögren's syndrome							[1]			[1]		
Stevens–Johnson syndrome	•					[1]			[2]			
Toxic epidermal necrolysis	[2]		[1]						[1]	[2]		
Toxicity	[4]	[1]	[1]			[3]		[1]				
Urticaria	[1]			•		[5]	[1] (<5%)	[1]	[3]	[1]		✓
Vasculitis	[5]						[5]			[5]	[1]	
HAIR												
Alopecia	[5]			•				•	[6]	[1]	•	✓
MUCOSAL												
Oral lesions		[1] (40%)						[1]				?
Oral mucosal eruption							[1]			[2]		
Oral ulceration		[1]				[1]			[1]			
Sialorrhea	(<10%)							[1]				
Xerostomia		[2] (40%)		•				•	[1]		•	?

A Amiodarone; **Di** Disopyramide; **Dr** Dronedarone; **F** Flecainide; **I** Ibutilide; **L** Lidocaine; **Pn** Procainamide; **Pf** Propafenone; **Pr** Propranolol; **Q** Quinidine; **S** Sotalol

ANTIBIOTICS, MACROLIDE

	A	C	E	=
SKIN				
Anaphylaxis	[2]	[2]	[2]	✓✓
Angioedema	[1]	[1]	[1]	✓✓
Dermatitis	[1]		[4]	✓
Exanthems	[3]	[1]	[4] (<5%)	✓✓
Fixed eruption		[3]	[6]	✓
Hypersensitivity	[3]	[3]	[3] (<10%)	✓✓
Jarisch–Herxheimer reaction	[2]		[1]	✓
Pruritus	[3]	[1]		✓
Pustules	[1]		[1]	✓
Rash	[6] (2–10%)	[2]	[3]	✓✓
SDRIFE		[1]	[2]	✓
Stevens–Johnson syndrome	[6]	[1]	[7]	✓✓
Toxic epidermal necrolysis		[4]	[7]	✓
Toxicity	[1]	[1]		✓
Urticaria	[2]	[1]	[4]	✓✓
Vasculitis	[1]	[3]	[1]	✓✓
HAIR				
Alopecia		[1]	[1]	✓
MUCOSAL				
Gingival hyperplasia/hypertrophy		[1]	[1]	✓

A Azithromycin; **C** Clarithromycin; **E** Erythromycin

ANTICONVULSANTS

	B	C	G	La	Le	O	Phb	Phy	Ti	To	V	Z	=
SKIN													
Acne keloid		[1]						[2]					
Acneform eruption		[1]	•	[1]		•	[1]	[8]	•	•		•	✓
AGEP		[5]		[1]			[1]	[5]					
Angioedema	•	[5]		[1] (<10%)			•	[2]					
Anticonvulsant hypersensitivity syndrome		[19]	[2]	[17]		[1]	[10]	[10]			[6]		✓
Bullae		[1]					[1]						
Bullous dermatitis		[4]		[1]			[5]	[1]			[1]		
Bullous pemphigoid			[1]		[1]								
Dermatitis		[7]					[1]		•	•			
Diaphoresis		(<10%)		•		•	[1]		•	•	[1]	•	✓
DRESS syndrome		[46] (77%)		[14] (11%)	[7]	[6]	[12] (6%)	[28] (68%)			[7]	[3]	✓
Ecchymoses				•	•	•			(<6%)		[4] (<5%)	•	✓
Eczema		[2]		•					•	•		•	
Edema			[5]		[1]	•	[1]		•	•	[2]	•	✓
Epidermolysis bullosa		[1]						[1]					
Erythema		[1]		[1] (~10%)	[2]								
Erythema multiforme		[16]		[4]	[2]		[7]	[11]			[3]		✓
Erythroderma		[12]			[1]		[2] (16%)	[8] (6%)			[3]		
Exanthems		[35] (17%)	[2]	[18] (20%)	[1]	[4]	[13] (70%)	[22] (71%)	•	[1]	[3] (14%)	•	✓
Exfoliative dermatitis		[24]				[1]	[6]	[15]	•				?
Facial edema		[2]	•	•					•	[1]	•	•	✓
Fixed eruption		[10]		[1]		[1]	[9]	[5]		[2]	[1]		✓
Furunculosis									•		(<5%)		
Hand–foot syndrome								[1]			[1]		
Hot flashes			[1]	(<10%)		•				(<10%)			
Hyperhidrosis				[1]		•							
Hypersensitivity	•	[69]	[1]	[28] (<10%)		[6]	[12]	[46] (23%)			[5]	[4]	✓
Lichen planus		[2]						[1]					
Lichenoid eruption		[7]						[1]					

B Brivaracetam; **C** Carbamazepine; **G** Gabapentin; **La** Lamotrigine; **Le** Levetiracetam; **O** Oxcarbazepine; **Phb** Phenobarbital; **Phy** Phenytoin; **Ti** Tiagabine; **To** Topiramate; **V** Valproic Acid; **Z** Zonisamide

	B	C	G	La	Le	O	Phb	Phy	Ti	To	V	Z	=
Linear IgA		[1]						[8]					
Lupus erythematosus		[35]		[4]			[2]	[19]			[5]	[1]	✓
Lymphadenopathy		[1]				•			•			•	
Lymphoma		[2]						[6]					
Lymphoproliferative disease		[5]						[1]					
Mycosis fungoides		[3]			[1]	[1]		[7]					
Oligohydrosis										[1]		[8]	
Pemphigus		[3]					[1]	[2]					
Peripheral edema		[1]	[11] (8%)				[1]	[1]	•		(<5%)	•	✓
Petechiae		[1]		•					•		[1] (<5%)	•	
Photosensitivity		[9]		[2]			[1]	[1]	•	•	[1]		✓
Pigmentation							[1]	[4]	•	•			
Pruritus		[7]	[1]	[1]	[1]		[1]	[5]	•	[3]	[1]	[1] (2–6%)	✓
Pseudolymphoma		[17]		[1]			[1]	[31]			[2]		?
Psoriasis		[1]			[1]				•				
Purpura		[8]	[1]	[1]		•	[2]	[4]		•	[2]	•	✓
Pustules		[5]					[1]	[3]				•	
Rash		[29] (12%)	[2]	[49] (10–20%)	[4]	[10] (9%)	[4]	[12] (<10%)	[2] (5%)	[3] (6%)	[7] (10%)	[6] (7%)	✓
Scleroderma								[1]			[1]		
Serum sickness		[1]						[2]					
Sjögren's syndrome				[1]			[1]	[1]			[1]		
Stevens–Johnson syndrome		[95] (68%)	[2]	[45] (30%)	[3]	[7]	[20] (15%)	[56] (68%)			[10]	[3]	✓
Toxic epidermal necrolysis		[86] (68%)		[48] (13%)	[2]	[4]	[26] (13%)	[63] (68%)			[7]	[1]	✓
Toxicity		[2]	[1]					[1]					
Toxicoderma		[1]					[1]						
Urticaria		[14] (7%)		[1]	[2]		[1]	[5]	•	[1]		[1]	✓
Vasculitis		[7]	[1]		[1]		[1]	[11]			[3]		✓
Vesiculobullous eruption									•			•	
Xerosis				•					•	[1]		[1]	
HAIR													
Alopecia		[7] (~6%)	[2]	[1]				[3]	•	[2]	[20] (<10%)	•	✓

B Brivaracetam; **C** Carbamazepine; **G** Gabapentin; **La** Lamotrigine; **Le** Levetiracetam; **O** Oxcarbazepine; **Phb** Phenobarbital; **Phy** Phenytoin; **Ti** Tiagabine; **To** Topiramate; **V** Valproic Acid; **Z** Zonisamide

	B	C	G	La	Le	O	Phb	Phy	Ti	To	V	Z	=
Hirsutism		[1] (25%)		•				[8] (13%)	•		[2] (60%)	•	✓
Poliosis							[1]				[1]		
NAILS													
Nail changes								[2]		•			
Nail hypoplasia		[1]					[2]	[3]					
Nail pigmentation								[1]			[1]		
MUCOSAL													
Epistaxis			•			•			•				
Gingival hyperplasia/hypertrophy				•			[3] (16%)	[56] (16-94%)	•	[1]	[7] (42%)	•	✓
Gingivitis			•	•	•				•	•		•	✓
Glossitis									•		(<5%)	•	
Halitosis									•		[1]		
Mucocutaneous eruption		[4]						[2]					
Mucocutaneous lymph node syndrome		[2]						[1]					
Oral ulceration		[2]		[1]		[1]		[1]	•			•	✓
Rectal hemorrhage						•			•			•	
Sialorrhea				•						[1] (4–5%)			
Stomatitis				•					•	•	(<5%)	•	
Ulcerative stomatitis									•			•	
Xerostomia			[1] (5%)	(6%)		•	[1]		[1]	[5] (16%)	[2] (<5%)	•	✓

B Brivaracetam; **C** Carbamazepine; **G** Gabapentin; **La** Lamotrigine; **Le** Levetiracetam; **O** Oxcarbazepine; **Phb** Phenobarbital; **Phy** Phenytoin; **Ti** Tiagabine; **To** Topiramate; **V** Valproic Acid; **Z** Zonisamide

ANTIDEPRESSANTS, TRICYCLIC

	Ami	Amo	C	I	N	T	=
SKIN							
Angioedema	[1]			[1]			
Bullous dermatitis	[1]			[1]			
Dermatitis	[1]		[1]				
Diaphoresis	[1] (<10%)	(<10%)	[2] (43%)	[8] (25%)	(<10%)	[1] (<10%)	✓✓
DRESS syndrome	[2]		[1]				
Edema	[1]	(<10%)	•	[1]			✓
Exanthems		[2]		[6] (6%)	•	•	✓
Fixed eruption	[1]			[1]			
Hypersensitivity	[1]		[2]				
Lichen planus	[1]			[1]			
Lupus erythematosus	[1]			[1]			
Photosensitivity	[3]	•	[3]	[3]	[2]	•	✓✓
Pigmentation	[4]		[1]	[13]			✓
Pruritus	[3]	[1]	[1] (6%)	[6]			✓
Purpura	[2]		•	[3]			✓
Rash		(<10%)	(8%)				
Urticaria		•	[1]	[6]			✓
Vasculitis	[1]	[1]		[1]			✓
HAIR							
Alopecia	[1]	•	•	[2]	•	•	✓✓
Alopecia areata			[1]	[1]			
MUCOSAL							
Stomatitis	[1]			[2]			
Xerostomia	[15] (79%)	[1] (14%)	[6] (84%)	[16] (21%)	[9]	[2]	✓✓

Ami Amitriptyline; **Amo** Amoxapine; **C** Clomipramine; **I** Imipramine; **N** Nortriptyline; **T** Trimipramine

ANTIHISTAMINES (H1)

	Ce	Chl	Des	Dy	Fex	H	Lev	Lor	O	P	=
SKIN											
AGEP	[1]			[1]	[1]	[3]					
Anaphylaxis	[2]	[1]		[4]		[2]		•		[1]	✓
Angioedema	•	(<10%)		[1]		[3]		[1]		•	✓
Bullous dermatitis	•									•	
Dermatitis	•	[4] (<10%)		[4]		[1]	[1]	•		[3]	✓
Desquamation	[1]					[1]					
Diaphoresis	•							•			
Eczema				[2]						[1]	
Edema				•		•					
Erythema multiforme						[2]		•		[2]	
Exanthems	[1]			[1]		[3]				[1]	
Fixed eruption	[6]			[4]		[3]	[3]	[3]	[1]	[1]	✓
Hypersensitivity						[1]				[1]	
Palmar erythema	[1]					[1]					
Photosensitivity	•	(<10%)		[3]		•		•		[12]	✓
Phototoxicity	•			[1]		[1]				[1]	
Pruritus	[1]	[1]		[2]				[1]			
Purpura	•			[1]		[1]		•		[2]	✓
Rash	•			•		•		[1]		[1]	✓
Toxic epidermal necrolysis				[3]						[2]	
Toxicity				[2]		[1]					
Urticaria	[8]		[1]		[3]	[3]	[1]	[4]		[3]	✓
Xerosis	•							•			
HAIR											
Alopecia	•							•			
MUCOSAL											
Oral ulceration			[1]							[1]	
Sialorrhea	•							•			
Stomatitis	•							•			
Xerostomia	[2] (6%)	(<10%)	[3]	[1] (<10%)		[2] (12%)	•	[9]		[2] (<10%)	✓

Ce Cetirizine; **Chl** Chlorpheniramine; **Des** Desloratadine; **Dy** Diphenhydramine; **Fex** Fexofenadine; **H** Hydroxyzine; **Lev** Levocetirizine; **Lor** Loratadine; **O** Olopatadine; **P** Promethazine

ANTIMALARIALS

	Amo	A/L	Art	A/P	C	H	M	P	Quc	Qud	Qun	S	=
SKIN													
Acneform eruption										[2]	[2]		
AGEP				[1]	[1]	[22] (25%)		[1]		[2]			?
Anaphylaxis						[1]	[2]	•					
Angioedema	[1]				[1]	•		[2]		•	•	[1]	✓
Bullous dermatitis						[2]		[2]				[1]	
Dermatitis		[1]			[2]	[1]		•		[4]	[6]		✓
DRESS syndrome						[2]		[2]			[1]		
Erythema							[2]	[1]				[1]	
Erythema annulare centrifugum					[2]	[3]							
Erythema multiforme				[2]	•	[1]		[4]		[1]	[2]	[3]	✓
Erythema nodosum						[1]			[1]				
Erythroderma					[3]	[2]							
Exanthems				[1]	[3] (<5%)	[4] (<5%)	[1] (30%)	[3]	[3] (80%)	[6] (17%)	[3] (<5%)	[1]	✓
Exfoliative dermatitis					[4]	[3]	[1]	[2]	[3] (8%)	[5]	[2]	[3]	✓
Fixed eruption	[1]				•	•		[3]	[3]	[2]	[12]	[2]	✓
Hypersensitivity		[1]						[1]		[1]	[1]	•	
Lichen planus						[1]				[7]	[3]		
Lichenoid eruption					[6]	[4]		[2]	[6] (12%)	[6]	[3]		✓
Livedo reticularis										[6]	[3]		
Lupus erythematosus										[35]	[1]		?
Lymphoproliferative disease						[1]		[1]		[1]			
Ochronosis									[2]		[1]		
Pemphigus					[1]	[1]							
Photosensitivity					[8]	[6]		[3]	[1]	[21]	[19]	[2]	✓
Phototoxicity				[1]	[1]	[3]				[1]			
Pigmentation					[15]	[17] (<10%)		[5]	[9]	[3]	[6]		✓
Pruritus	[3]	[2]	[3]	(<10%)	[36] (47%)	[12] (47%)	[2] (4–10%)	[2]	•	[3]	[1]	[2]	✓✓
Psoriasis					[18]	[12]	[2]		[1]	[5]			
Purpura		[1]					[1]	[1]		[13]	[13]	[1]	✓

Amo Amodiaquine; **A/L** Artemether/Lumefantrine; **Art** Artesunate; **A/P** Atovaquone/Proguanil; **C** Chloroquine; **H** Hydroxychloroquine; **M** Mefloquine; **P** Pyrimethamine; **Quc** Quinacrine; **Qud** Quinidine; **Qun** Quinine; **S** Sulfadoxine

	Amo	A/L	Art	A/P	C	H	M	P	Quc	Qud	Qun	S	=
Pustules		[1]			[1]	[1]		[1]		[1]			
Rash		[6] (11%)			[1]	[4] (<10%)	[1] (<10%)	•	[1]	(<10%)	[1]	•	✓
Stevens–Johnson syndrome				[1]	[4]	[1]	[2]	[25] (<10%)			[2]	[24] (<10%)	✓
Thrombocytopenic purpura						[2]					[8]		
Toxic epidermal necrolysis					[5]	[3]	[2]	[15]		[2]	[3]	[17]	✓
Toxicity					[2]	[1]							
Urticaria	[1]	[2]	[1]	[1]	[4]	[2]	[1]		[1]	[1]	[2]	•	✓
Vasculitis						[1]	[3]			[5]	[5]		
HAIR													
Alopecia				[1]		[1]	•		[2] (80%)	[1]			?
Hair pigmentation					[10]	[7] (<10%)							
NAILS													
Discoloration					[1]	[1]							
Nail pigmentation					[2]	[3]			[2]				
MUCOSAL													
Aphthous stomatitis	[1]		[1]					[1]				[1]	
Gingival pigmentation					[1]	[1]							
Glossitis								•				•	
Oral edema			[1]					[1]				[1]	
Oral mucosal eruption										[2]	[1]		
Oral pigmentation					[12]	[7]			[4]	[1]			
Oral ulceration				[3] (6%)	[1]							[1]	
Stomatitis					•	[2]						[1]	

Amo Amodiaquine; **A/L** Artemether/Lumefantrine; **Art** Artesunate; **A/P** Atovaquone/Proguanil; **C** Chloroquine; **H** Hydroxychloroquine; **M** Mefloquine; **P** Pyrimethamine; **Quc** Quinacrine; **Qud** Quinidine; **Qun** Quinine; **S** Sulfadoxine

BENZODIAZEPINES

	A	Cln	Clo	D	L	M	O	=
SKIN								
Acneform eruption	[1]			[1]				
Anaphylaxis				[1]		[1]		
Angioedema	[1]	[1]		[1]		[1]		✓
Bullous dermatitis		[2]		[1]				
Dermatitis	[5]	(<10%)	(<10%)	[3] (<10%)	(<10%)		(<10%)	✓
Diaphoresis	(16%)	[1]	•	•	•		•	✓
DRESS syndrome		[1]					[1]	
Edema	(5%)					[2]		
Erythema multiforme		[1]			[1]		[1]	
Exanthems	[1]	[1]	[1]	[6]				✓
Exfoliative dermatitis		[1]		[2]				
Fixed eruption				[2]	[1]		[1]	
Peripheral edema				[1]		•		
Photosensitivity	[4]		[1]					
Pruritus	[2] (<10%)			[1]		[3]		
Pseudolymphoma	[1]	[2]			[2]			
Purpura		[1]		[4]				
Rash	[4] (11%)	•	•	[2]	•	•	•	✓✓
Urticaria			[1]	[1]		[1]		
Vasculitis			[1]	[1]				
MUCOSAL								
Sialopenia	(33%)	•	•		•		•	✓
Sialorrhea	•	(<10%)	(<10%)		[1]	•	(<10%)	✓
Xerostomia	[6] (15%)	[1]	•	•	•		•	✓

A Alprazolam; **Cln** Clonazepam; **Clo** Clorazepate; **D** Diazepam; **L** Lorazepam; **M** Midazolam; **O** Oxazepam

BETA BLOCKERS

	A	B	C	N	P	S	=
SKIN							
Anaphylaxis	[2]				[1]		
Cold extremities		[1]			[6] (36%)		?
Dermatitis	[1]			[1]	[2]		✓
Diaphoresis		•	[1]				
Edema		[1]				(5%)	
Fixed eruption	[1]	[1]			[1]		✓
Leukocytoclastic vasculitis					[1]	[1]	
Lichenoid eruption	[1]			[1]	[3]	[1]	✓
Lupus erythematosus	[2]		[1]		[2]		✓
Necrosis	[3]				[3]		
Peripheral edema		(<10%)		•			
Photosensitivity					[1]	•	
Pruritus	(<5%)				[1]	(<10%)	✓
Psoriasis	[7]	[1]			[20]	[3]	✓
Rash	[1]	(<10%)		•	[2] (<10%)	•	✓
Raynaud's phenomenon	[2]	(<10%)			[3] (59%)	•	✓
Urticaria	[2]				[3]		
Vasculitis	[1]					[1]	
HAIR							
Alopecia	[1]				[6]	•	✓
MUCOSAL							
Xerostomia		•			[1]	•	✓

A Atenolol; **B** Bisoprolol; **C** Celiprolol; **N** Nebivolol; **P** Propranolol; **S** Sotalol

BIOLOGICS

	Ald	Alm	Be	Bo	C	D	E	G	Ib	In	Ip	L	P	R	=
SKIN															
Acne keloid			[1]		[1]		[2]								
Acneform eruption			[5] (10%)		[60] (92%)	[1] (<10%)	[26] (73–80%)	[32] (66–85%)	[2]	•		[1]	[17] (81%)		✓
AGEP	[1]						[1]	[1]	[6]						
Anaphylaxis		•			[5] (13%)			[1]				[1]	[1]	[7]	
Angioedema	[2]	•	[1]							[3]			[1]	[4] (11%)	
Bullae	[1]					•									
Bullous dermatitis	[1]	•					[1]			[4]				[1]	
Bullous pemphigoid	[1]						[1]								
Cellulitis		•	[1]									(5%)		[1]	
Dermatitis	[2]		[1]	[1]	[4] (80%)	(<10%)	[2] (14%)			[1] (6%)	[11] (12%)	[1]		[2]	✓
Dermatomyositis									[1]	[1]					
Desquamation	[1]		[1] (8%)		[3] (89%)			[2] (39%)					[3] (13%)		?
Diaphoresis									(13%)	[1]		(8%)		[2] (15%)	
DRESS syndrome							[2]		[3]			[2]			
Ecchymoses				[1] (16%)								[1] (16%)			
Eczema					[1]	(<10%)	[1]	[1]		[6] (39%)			[2]		?
Edema	[3] (47%)		[1] (15%)	(23%)		[5] (23%)	[1]		[33] (80%)	[2] (15%)		[1] (10%)	[1] (15%)	[1]	✓
Embolia cutis medicamentosa (Nicolau syndrome)				[1]						[1]					
Erythema	[5] (41%)	•		[2]	[3] (14%)	[1]	(18%)	[1]	[5] (<10%)	[2]	[1]	(5%)	[5] (65%)	[1] (16%)	✓
Erythema multiforme	[1]			[1] (16%)					[1]		[1]	[1] (16%)			
Erythema nodosum	[3]					•				[1]					
Erythroderma	[4]								[3]						
Exanthems	[5]		[1]	[1] (16%)	[5]		[3] (8%)	[3] (21%)	[8]	[3]	[5] (20%)	[3] (16%)		[1]	✓

Ald Aldesleukin; **Alm** Alemtuzumab; **Be** Bevacizumab; **Bo** Bortezomib; **C** Cetuximab; **D** Dasatinib; **E** Erlotinib; **G** Gefitinib; **I** Imatinib; **I** Interferon Alfa; **I** Ipilimumab; **L** Lenalidomide; **P** Panitumumab; **R** Rituximab

	Ald	Alm	Be	Bo	C	D	E	G	Ib	In	Ip	L	P	R	=
Exfoliative dermatitis	[1] (18%)							[1]	[3]			[1]	[2] (25%)		?
Facial edema		•					[1]		[2] (<10%)					[1]	
Fissures					[4] (14%)		[1]						[4] (21%)		?
Folliculitis				[2]	[12] (83%)		[9] (11%)	[4]				[2]	[3]		?
Graft-versus-host reaction	[1]					[1]					[1] (14%)	[2] (43%)			?
Granulomas		[1]								[1]	[3]				
Hand–foot syndrome			[11] (57%)		[5] (6%)		[3] (30–60%)	[2]	[3]	[1] (10%)	[1]		[3] (23%)		✓
Hematoma		•	[1]		[1]										
Herpes simplex		[2] (6%)								[2]				[2]	
Herpes zoster		[3] (9%)		[12] (10–15%)										[6]	
Hyperhidrosis			[1] (8%)			(<10%)			[1]			[2] (11%)			
Hypersensitivity				[1] (7%)	[8]	•				[1]	[1]			[5]	
Kaposi's sarcoma	[1]									[2]				[3]	
Lesions									[1]	[1] (8%)					
Lichen planus									[5]	[8]					
Linear IgA	[4]									[3]					
Livedo reticularis								[1]		[2]					
Lupus erythematosus	[1]		[1]	[1]		[1]				[17]				[1]	
Malignancies										[1]		[6]			
Necrolysis								[1]	[1]						
Necrosis	[2]		[2]				[1]			[6]				[1]	
Neutrophilic eccrine hidradenitis					[1]				[2]						
Panniculitis						[3]			[2]						
Papulopustular eruption					[6] (83%)		[7] (29%)	[3] (21%)					[4] (21–41%)		?
Pemphigus	[2]									[2]				[1]	
Peripheral edema	(28%)	(13%)	[1] (8%)	[5] (83%)	[1] (40%)	[3] (44%)		•	[5] (75%)			[3] (83%)	[1] (12%)	[1] (14%)	✓
Petechiae	•								(<10%)						

Ald Aldesleukin; **Alm** Alemtuzumab; **Be** Bevacizumab; **Bo** Bortezomib; **C** Cetuximab; **D** Dasatinib; **E** Erlotinib; **G** Gefitinib; **I** Imatinib; **I** Interferon Alfa; **I** Ipilimumab; **L** Lenalidomide; **P** Panitumumab; **R** Rituximab

	Ald	Alm	Be	Bo	C	D	E	G	Ib	In	Ip	L	P	R	=
Photosensitivity	[1]					•	[1]		[1] (<10%)	[2]					
Pigmentation			[1]	[1] (16%)		•		[1]	[9] (60%)	[3] (21%)		[2] (16%)	[1]		✓
Pityriasis rubra pilaris			[1]						[1]						
Pruritus	[7] (24%)	(14–24%)	[1] (91%)	[1] (11%)	[9] (40%)	[3] (14%)	[8] (21%)	[4] (61%)	[3] (10%)	[4] (30%)	[17] (47%)	[3] (42%)	[9] (91%)	[8] (14%)	✓✓
Pseudo-lymphoma	[1]								[3]	[1]					
Psoriasis	[4]				[1]				[2]	[22]				[3]	?
Purpura	[1]	(8%)	[1]	[2]			[3]	[1]	[1]	[2]		[1]		[1]	✓
Pustules					[1]			[1]					[1]		
Radiation recall dermatitis			[1]		[1]		[1]			[1]					
Rash	[2] (42%)	[5] (13–40%)	[15] (91%)	[9] (67%)	[46] (89%)	[9] (34%)	[105] (80%)	[59] (66–85%)	[23] (69%)	[5] (11%)	[24] (61%)	[15] (36%)	[28] (91%)	[12] (58%)	✓✓
Rosacea					[1]		[2]		[1]	[1]					
Sarcoidosis	[1]									[47]	[2]			[1]	?
Scleroderma	[2]									[1]					
Seborrheic dermatitis	[1]						[1]			[2]					
Serum sickness												[1] (8%)		[22] (<17%)	?
Skin reactions				[1]			[1]								
Squamous cell carcinoma		[1]						[1]	[2]		[1] (7%)				
Stevens–Johnson syndrome	[1]				[1]				[11]		[1]	[5]		[5]	
Sweet's syndrome	[1]			[7]		•			[1]		[1]	[3]			
Telangiectasia					[1]		[1]		[1]	[1]			[1]		
Thrombo-cytopenic purpura		[9]	[1]							[2]					
Toxic epidermal necrolysis	[2]				[2]			[1]	[1]		[1]	[1]		[3]	✓
Toxicity	[6]		[9] (16%)	[3] (38%)	[18] (63%)	[6] (36%)	[7] (84%)	[9] (68%)	[8] (30–44%)	[4]	[3] (35%)	[6] (75%)	[25] (95%)	[2] (12%)	✓
Transient acantholytic dermatosis					[1]						[1]				
Tumor lysis syndrome				[2] (17%)		[1] (<5%)					[1]	[3] (<5%)			

Ald Aldesleukin; **Alm** Alemtuzumab; **Be** Bevacizumab; **Bo** Bortezomib; **C** Cetuximab; **D** Dasatinib; **E** Erlotinib; **G** Gefitinib; **I** Imatinib; **I** Interferon Alfa; **I** Ipilimumab; **L** Lenalidomide; **P** Panitumumab; **R** Rituximab

	Ald	Alm	Be	Bo	C	D	E	G	Ib	In	Ip	L	P	R	=
Tumors												[5] (11%)		[1] (11%)	
Ulcerations			[3]	[1]	[1]	•		[2]		[1]					
Urticaria	[3]	[2] (16–30%)				(<10%)		[1]	[1]	[3]	[2]	[1]		[5] (8%)	✓
Vasculitis	[1]			[4]			[1]	[1]	[1]	[7]				[3]	✓
Vitiligo	[3]									[9]	[3]				
Xerosis	(15%)		[1]	[1] (16%)	[14] (49%)	(<10%)	[11] (56%)	[11] (53%)	[1] (<10%)	[1]		[2] (16%)	[12] (62%)		✓
HAIR															
Abnormal hair growth					[2]							[1]			
Alopecia	[2] (10%)		[5] (43%)		(5%)	[1] (<10%)	[10] (14%)	[6]	[1] (10–15%)	[16] (48%)	[1]		[3] (54%)	[1]	✓
Hair changes					[3]		[3]						[2] (9%)		
Hair pigmentation						[2]				[3] (18%)					
Hirsutism							[1]			[1]					
Hypertrichosis					[3]		[4]	[2]		[3]					
NAILS															
Nail changes					[1] (21%)		[2] (17%)	[1] (17%)					[2] (9–29%)		?
Nail disorder					[2]	•									
Nail pigmentation								[1]	[1]						
Paronychia			[1]		[14] (14%)		[11] (15%)	[13] (14–32%)					[12] (85%)		?
Pyogenic granuloma					[1]		[1]	[2]					[1]		
MUCOSAL															
Aphthous stomatitis	[1] (5%)				[1]		[1]		[1]	[2]	[1]				
Epistaxis			[5] (17%)					[1]		[1] (17%)		(15%)	[1]		
Mucocutaneous eruption						[1]			[1]						
Mucosal inflammation			[1]				[1] (18%)			[1]			(6%)		
Mucositis			[9] (75%)	[2] (45%)	[10]	[1] (16%)	[9] (21%)	[4] (6–17%)	[2] (15%)				[4] (75%)		✓
Oral lichenoid eruption									[3]	[1]					

Ald Aldesleukin; **Alm** Alemtuzumab; **Be** Bevacizumab; **Bo** Bortezomib; **C** Cetuximab; **D** Dasatinib; **E** Erlotinib; **G** Gefitinib; **I** Imatinib; **I** Interferon Alfa; **I** Ipilimumab; **L** Lenalidomide; **P** Panitumumab; **R** Rituximab

	Ald	Alm	Be	Bo	C	D	E	G	Ib	In	Ip	L	P	R	=
Oral pigmentation									[3]	[1]					
Oral ulceration	[1]		[2] (18%)	[1]	[1]		[1]	[1]	[3] (15%)						✓
Oropharyngeal pain									[1]					[1]	
Perianal fistula			[1] (67%)								[1]				?
Rectal hemorrhage				[1]		[1]									
Stomatitis	[1] (22%)	[1] (14%)	[8] (75%)	[1] (43%)	[3] (25%)	[1]	[9] (9–19%)	[7] (6–17%)		[1] (30%)			[4] (100%)	[2] (69%)	✓
Xerostomia	[1]				(11%)	[1] (33%)			[1] (44%)	[4] (41%)		(7%)			?

Ald Aldesleukin; **Alm** Alemtuzumab; **Be** Bevacizumab; **Bo** Bortezomib; **C** Cetuximab; **D** Dasatinib; **E** Erlotinib; **G** Gefitinib; **I** Imatinib; **I** Interferon Alfa; **I** Ipilimumab; **L** Lenalidomide; **P** Panitumumab; **R** Rituximab

BISPHOSPHONATES

	A	E	I	P	R	Z	=
SKIN							
Angioedema	[2]	•		•			✓
Candidiasis				(6%)		(12%)	
Eczema	[1] (13%)				[1]		
Edema				•		[3]	
Exanthems				[1]		[1]	
Hypersensitivity	[3] (19%)	•		•	[1]		✓
Peripheral edema	[1]				(8%)	(5–21%)	✓
Pruritus	[1]	[1]	[1] (4–5%)		•		✓
Rash	[5]	•	[1]	[1]	[1] (8%)	[3] (6%)	✓✓
Stevens–Johnson syndrome					[1]	[1]	
Toxic epidermal necrolysis		[1]	[1]				
Urticaria	[1]				[1]		
HAIR							
Alopecia			[1]			[1] (12%)	
MUCOSAL							
Stomatitis	[1]			•		(8%)	✓

A Alendronate; **E** Etidronate; **I** Ibandronate; **P** Pamidronate; **R** Risedronate; **Z** Zoledronate

CALCIUM CHANNEL BLOCKERS

	A	D	F	I	Nic	Nif	Nis	V	=
SKIN									
Acneform eruption		[1]					•	[1]	
AGEP		[21]				[3]			?
Anaphylaxis					[1]	[1]			
Angioedema	[6] (6%)	[3]	[1]		[1]	[2]		[3]	✓
Dermatitis	(<10%)	[1]				[1]			
Diaphoresis	•	[2]	[1]	•		[2]	•	[2]	✓
Ecchymoses		•					•	[1]	
Eczema	[1]	[1]							
Edema	[20] (5–14%)	[4] (<10%)	[1]	[6] (7%)	•	[3]	[1]	[1]	✓✓
Erythema		[2]	•			[2]			
Erythema multiforme	[2]	[11] (31%)				[5]		[4]	✓
Erythema nodosum						[2]		[1]	
Exanthems	[2]	[17] (31%)	[2]	[2]		[9]	[1]	[8]	✓
Exfoliative dermatitis		[6]				[5]	•	[2]	✓
Facial edema			•			•	•		
Hyperkeratosis		[1]						[2]	
Hypersensitivity	[1]	[2]							
Lichenoid eruption		[1]				[3]			
Linear IgA	[1]							[1]	
Lupus erythematosus		[5]				[3]		[2]	
Peripheral edema	[44] (34%)	[1] (5–8%)	[6] (22%)		[2] (7%)	[12] (6%)	[6] (22%)	[1] (<10%)	✓
Petechiae	[1]	•					•		
Photosensitivity		[11]				[5]		[4]	
Pigmentation	[2]	[10]					•		
Pruritus	[3]	[6]	•	[1] (6%)		[3]	•	[6]	✓
Pseudolymphoma	[1]	[1]							
Purpura	[1]	[3]	[1]			[3]		[1]	✓
Pustules		[2]					•		
Rash	(<10%)	[4]	•	•	[3]	[2]	•	[2]	✓✓

A Amlodipine; **D** Diltiazem; **F** Felodipine; **I** Isradipine; **Nic** Nicardipine; **Nif** Nifedipine; **Nis** Nisoldipine; **V** Verapamil

	A	D	F	I	Nic	Nif	Nis	V	=
Stevens–Johnson syndrome	[1]	[4]				[3]		[5]	✓
Telangiectasia	[5]		[2]			[2]			
Toxic epidermal necrolysis	[2]	[4]				[2]			
Toxicity	[2]	[2]						[1]	
Ulcerations						[1]	•		
Urticaria	[1]	[5]	[1]	•	[3]	[7]	•	[5]	✓✓
Vasculitis	[2]	[6]				[4]		[2]	✓
Xerosis	•						•		
HAIR									
Alopecia	•	[2]				[4]	•	[5]	✓
Hair pigmentation						[1]		[1]	
NAILS									
Nail dystrophy		[1]				[1]		[1]	
MUCOSAL									
Gingival hyperplasia/hypertrophy	[28] (31%)	[10] (21%)	[5] (2–10%)	[1]	[2]	[74] (75%)	•	[10] (19%)	✓✓
Oral ulceration		[1]					•	[1]	
Xerostomia	[1]	[2]	[1]	•	•	•	•	•	✓✓

A Amlodipine; **D** Diltiazem; **F** Felodipine; **I** Isradipine; **Nic** Nicardipine; **Nif** Nifedipine; **Nis** Nisoldipine; **V** Verapamil

CEPHALOSPORINS

	Cdxl	Cclor	Ctan	Coxm	Cnir	Cixm	Ctxm	Czim	Caxn	Cpm	CF	Cple	=
SKIN													
AGEP		[2]		[2]			[1]	[1]	[4]	[1]			✓
Anaphylaxis	•	[4]	[3]	[7]		[1]	[1]	[3]	[14]		•		✓
Angioedema	[1]	•		•		•		•	[3]				✓
Candidiasis			•		•			•	[3] (5%)	•			
Dermatitis		[1]							[2]				
DRESS syndrome	[1]					[1]	[4]		[2]				
Erythema	[1]			[1]								(9%)	
Erythema multiforme	•	[6]		•		[1] (13%)	[2]	[1]	[1]				✓
Exanthems	[1]	[9]		[2] (6%)	•		[3]	[1]	[7] (6%)	•			✓
Fixed eruption		[2]				[1]			[1]				
Hypersensitivity			[1]	[4]		[1]	[2]	[1]	[4]	[2]	[2]	[1]	✓
Jarisch–Herxheimer reaction				[1]					[1]				
Lupus erythematosus				[1]						[2]			
Pemphigus	[1]			[1]		[1]			[1]				
Pemphigus erythematodes				[1]				[2]					
Pruritus	[1]	[4]	•	•	•	[1]	[3]	[3]	[2]	[3]	[7]	[1] (9%)	✓✓
Pseudolymphoma				[1]		[1]							
Pustules		[1]		[1]									
Rash	•	[1]	[2]	[1]	•	[2]	[3]	[4]	[5]	[12] (51%)	[7] (10%)	[1]	✓✓
SDRIFE	[1]			[1]									
Serum sickness	•	[31]	•	[2]	•	[1]			[2]				✓
Stevens–Johnson syndrome	•	[1]	•	•	•	[1]	[1]	•	[1]	[1]			✓
Toxic epidermal necrolysis		[1]		[2]		•	[1]	[1]	[1]				✓
Urticaria	[2]	[5]	•	[2]	•	[2] (13%)	•	•	[4]	[1]	•		✓
MUCOSAL													
Glossitis	[1]								[2]				
Oral candidiasis				[1]					[1]	•			
Oral mucosal eruption	[1]								[1]				

1st generation: **Cdxl** Cefadroxil; 2nd generation: **Cclor** Cefaclor, **Ctan** Cefotetan, **Coxm** Cefuroxime; 3rd generation: **Cnir** Cefdinir, **Cixm** Cefixime, **Ctxm** Cefotaxime, **Czim** Ceftazidime, **Caxn** Ceftriaxone; 4th generation: **Cpm** Cefepime; 5th generation: **CF** Ceftaroline Fosamil; **Cple** Ceftobiprole

DISEASE-MODIFYING ANTIRHEUMATIC DRUGS (DMARDS)

	Ab	Ad	Az	Ce	Cy	E	G	H	I	M	P	R	S	=
SKIN														
Abscess		[1]				[2]			[4]	[2]				
Acneform eruption		[2]	[2]		[7] (13%)	[1]			[6]	[1] (67%)				?
AGEP			[2]			[1]		[22] (25%)	[2]				[3]	?
Anaphylaxis		[1]	[1]		[8]	[2]	•	[1]	[10]	[9] (<10%)		[7]	[4]	✓
Angioedema		[3]	[2]	•	[1]	[1]		•	[1]	[1]		[4] (11%)	[2]	✓
Angioma					[1]					[1]				
Atrophy								[1]			[1]			
Basal cell carcinoma	[3]		[1]		[4]		[1]		[1]	[1]				
Bullous dermatitis					[1]			[2]	[1]	[4]	[3]	[1]		
Bullous pemphigoid		[1]				[1]					[6]		[3]	
Burning					[1]					[1]				
Candidiasis		[1]			[2] (16%)				[4] (5%)	[1]	[1]			
Carcinoma		[2]	[3]			[2]				[2]				
Cellulitis	[1]	[2] (<5%)				[2]			[5]	[1]		[1]		
Churg-Strauss syndrome			[1]		[1]									
Cicatricial pemphigoid			[1]								[2]			
Cyst					[5]						[1]			
Dermatitis		[1]	[4]	•		[3]		[1]	[4]	[2]	[4]	[2]	[2]	✓
Dermatomyositis		[5]				[4]		[1]			[14]			
Diaphoresis												[2] (15%)	[1]	
DRESS syndrome								[2]					[31] (7%)	?
Ecchymoses								[1]	[1]	[1]				
Eccrine squamous syringometaplasia					[1]					[1]				
Eczema	[2] (15%)	[2]							[5] (19–30%)				[1]	?
Edema					[1] (5–14%)				[3]	[2]		[1]	[1]	
Erysipelas	[1]	(<5%)												

Ab Abatacept; **Ad** Adalimumab; **Az** Azathioprine; **Ce** Certolizumab; **Cy** Cyclosporine; **E** Etanercept; **G** Golimumab; **H** Hydroxychloroquine; **I** Infliximab; **M** Methotrexate; **P** Penicillamine; **R** Rituximab; **S** Sulfasalazine

	Ab	Ad	Az	Ce	Cy	E	G	H	I	M	P	R	S	=
Erythema		[1]	[1]		[1]				[1]	•		[1] (16%)		
Erythema annulare centrifugum								[3]				[1]		
Erythema multiforme		[1]	[2]					[1]	[2]	[4]	(<5%)		[8]	✓
Erythema nodosum	[1]		[4]	[1]		[1]		[1]			[1]		[2]	✓
Erythroderma								[2]		[2]			[1]	
Exanthems			[10] (5%)		[1]	[2]		[4] (<5%)	[4]	[5] (15%)	[8]	[1]	[23] (23%)	✓
Exfoliative dermatitis			[1]					[3]					[5]	
Facial edema	[1]				[1]				[1]	[1]	[1]	[1]	[1]	✓
Fixed eruption		[1]	[1]			[1]		•	[1]				[7]	
Folliculitis					[8]	[1]			[2]	[2]				
Fungal dermatitis			[1] (42%)		[1]									?
Furunculosis	[1]	[1]								[1]				
Granuloma annulare						[1]			[1]					
Granulomas		[1]				[2]			[1]					
Granulomatous reaction		[5]				[5]			[1]		[1]			
Henoch–Schönlein purpura		[2]				[3]			[1]					
Herpes					[1]				[1]					
Herpes simplex	[3] (<5%)	[1]	[3] (35%)		[4]	[1]			[4] (10%)	[2]		[2]		✓
Herpes zoster	[3]	[9]	[8] (27%)	[2]	[2]	[5]			[10]	[7]		[6]		✓
Hidradenitis		[2]			[1]	[2]			[1]			[1]		
Hyperkeratosis					[1]		[1]							
Hypersensitivity	[2]	[3]	[27]	•	[2]	[1]			[11] (11%)	[2]	[3]	[5]	[16] (<5%)	✓
Kaposi's sarcoma		[1]	[14]		[5]				[1]			[3]		
Keratoacanthoma			[1]		[1]				[1]					
Leprosy		[1]				[2]			[1]					
Leukocytoclastic vasculitis		[1]					[1]		[1]					
Lichen planus						[2]		[1]	[2]		[4]		[3]	
Lichenoid eruption		[5]	[1]		[1]	[3]		[4]	[3]		[7]			✓
Linear IgA					[2]				[1]					
Lupus erythematosus		[16]			[1]	[25]	[3]		[33]		[43]	[1]	[34]	✓
Lupus syndrome		[3]		[2]		[2]			[11]		[1]			

Ab Abatacept; **Ad** Adalimumab; **Az** Azathioprine; **Ce** Certolizumab; **Cy** Cyclosporine; **E** Etanercept; **G** Golimumab; **H** Hydroxychloroquine; **I** Infliximab; **M** Methotrexate; **P** Penicillamine; **R** Rituximab; **S** Sulfasalazine

	Ab	Ad	Az	Ce	Cy	E	G	H	I	M	P	R	S	=
Lymphadenopathy		[1]							[1]	[1]				
Lymphoma		[8]	[1]		[12]	[3]			[9]	[5]		[1]		✓
Lymphomatoid papulosis		[1]			[1]									
Lymphoproliferative disease			[4]		[2]	[1]		[1]	[1]				[1]	
Malignancies	[10] (23%)	[3]	[1]		[2] (8%)	[3]	[5]		[2]	[1]				✓
Melanoma		[6]			[1]	[2]	[1]		[1]	[1]				
Molluscum contagiosum		[1]							[2]	[2]				
Morphea		[1]				[1]					[2]			
Necrosis										[4]		[1]	[1]	
Necrotizing fasciitis					[1]	[1]			[1]	[1]				
Neoplasms		[1]	[2]	[2]	[1]	[2]			[2]	[2]		[1]		✓
Neutrophilic dermatosis	[1]	[1]	[4] (76%)											?
Nevi			[3]			[1]			[2]					
Nodular eruption					[1]	[3]				[15]				
Non-Hodgkin's lymphoma		[1]	[1]							[2]				
Palmar–plantar pustulosis									[3]			[1]		
Pemphigus								[1]			[75]	[1]		?
Pemphigus foliaceus			[1]								[16]			
Peripheral edema	[1]	(<5%)	[1]		[3] (10%)	[1]			[1]		(<10%)	[1] (14%)		✓
Photoallergic reaction								[1]					[1]	
Photosensitivity			[1]					[6]		[9] (5%)			[4] (10%)	
Phototoxicity								[3]		[1]				
Pigmentation			[1] (37%)					[17] (<10%)		(<10%)			[3]	?
Pityriasis lichenoides chronica		[1]				[1]			[2]					
Porokeratosis			[4]		[1]	[1]								
Pruritus	•	[5]	[1]	[1]	[2] (12%)	[2] (14%)		[12] (47%)	[8] (20%)	[1] (<5%)	[2] (44–50%)	[8] (14%)	[7] (10%)	✓
Pseudolymphoma		[1]			[6]	[1]			[2]	[10]			[2]	
Psoriasis	[12]	[38]		[6]	[2]	[19]	[2]	[12]	[51] (19%)		[4]	[3]	[1]	✓
Purpura					[4]						[5]	[1]	[1]	

Ab Abatacept; **Ad** Adalimumab; **Az** Azathioprine; **Ce** Certolizumab; **Cy** Cyclosporine; **E** Etanercept; **G** Golimumab; **H** Hydroxychloroquine; **I** Infliximab; **M** Methotrexate; **P** Penicillamine; **R** Rituximab; **S** Sulfasalazine

	Ab	Ad	Az	Ce	Cy	E	G	H	I	M	P	R	S	=
Pustules		[1]				[2]		[1]	[5]				[2]	
Pyoderma gangrenosum		[1]	[1]											
Rash	[6] (23%)	[4] (12%)	[10] (<10%)	[2] (5%)	[1] (7–12%)	[7] (15%)	[3]	[4] (<10%)	[13] (25%)	[11] (5%)	[6] (44–50%)	[12] (58%)	[19] (6%)	✓✓
Raynaud's phenomenon					[2]					[1]			[3]	
Rosacea		[1]				[1]			[1]					
Sarcoidosis		[6]				[8]			[3]	[1]		[1]	[1]	
Scabies			[5]			[1]				[1]				
Scleroderma		[1]	[1]								[7]			
Serum sickness									[6]		[1]	[22] (<17%)	[3]	?
Sjögren's syndrome	[4]										[1]			
Skin cancer		[1]							[1]					
Squamous cell carcinoma	[5]	[5]	[10]		[12]	[4]	[1]		[1]	[2]				✓
Stevens–Johnson syndrome		[2]	[1]					[1]	[1]	[4]		[5]	[9]	✓
Striae					[1]					[1] (9%)				
Sweet's syndrome			[12]						[1]				[1]	
Thrombocytopenic purpura		[1]			[5]			[2]						
Tinea		[1]	[3]											
Toxic epidermal necrolysis			[1]		[1]			[3]	[2]	[8]	[2]	[3]	[13] (<10%)	✓
Toxicity		[1]	[3] (6%)	[1]	[2]		[1]	[1]	[2] (75%)	[6] (10%)		[2] (12%)		✓
Tumors		[1]	[8] (5%)	[1]	[1]							[1] (11%)		
Ulcerations			[1]		•				[1]	[11]				
Urticaria	[1]	[3]	[5]	•	[2]	[2]		[2]	[6] (17%)	[4]	[2] (44–50%)	[5] (8%)	[10] (<5%)	✓
Vasculitis	[2]	[8] (13%)	[5]	•	[3]	[21] (25%)	•	[1]	[16] (63%)	[9]	[7]	[3]	[4]	✓✓
Vesiculation		[1]								[1]	[1]			
Vitiligo		[2]			[1]				[4]					
Xerosis	[1]										[1]		[1]	
HAIR														
Alopecia		[3]	[9] (54%)	[1]	[2]	[4] (20%)		[1]	[4]	[25] (10%)	[3]	[1]	[6]	✓
Alopecia areata		[7]			[6]	[1]	[1]		[3]					

Ab Abatacept; **Ad** Adalimumab; **Az** Azathioprine; **Ce** Certolizumab; **Cy** Cyclosporine; **E** Etanercept; **G** Golimumab; **H** Hydroxychloroquine; **I** Infliximab; **M** Methotrexate; **P** Penicillamine; **R** Rituximab; **S** Sulfasalazine

	Ab	Ad	Az	Ce	Cy	E	G	H	I	M	P	R	S	=
Follicular mucinosis		[1]							[1]					
Hair pigmentation								[7] (<10%)		[1]				
Hirsutism					[10]						[2]			
NAILS														
Discoloration			[1]					[1]		•				
Leukonychia (Mees' lines)					[2]					[1]	[1]			
Nail pigmentation								[3]		[2]	[4]			
Onychocryptosis		[1]			[1]			[1]						
Onycholysis		[1]								[1]				
Onychomycosis			[2] (5%)						[1] (33%)	[1]				?
Pyogenic granuloma					[1]	[1]								
MUCOSAL														
Aphthous stomatitis			•	•	[2] (9%)					[2]	[2]		[1]	
Cheilitis						[1] (10%)				[1]			[1]	
Gingival hyperplasia/ hypertrophy					[156] (86%)						[1]			?
Gingivitis					•	[1] (7%)				•			[1]	
Glossitis					[1]					•	[1]			
Mucocutaneous reactions						[1]				[2]	[1]	[2]	[2] (6%)	
Mucosal ulceration			[1]								[1]			
Oral candidiasis									[1]	[1] (11%)	[1]			
Oral mucositis			[1]						[1]	[6]				
Oral ulceration			[2]		[2]	[1]				[10] (61%)	[5]		[3]	?
Oropharyngeal pain						[1] (9%)						[1]		
Stomatitis	[3] (24%)		[1]		(5–7%)			[2]		[17] (43%)	[6]	[2] (69%)	[1] (<10%)	✓

Ab Abatacept; **Ad** Adalimumab; **Az** Azathioprine; **Ce** Certolizumab; **Cy** Cyclosporine; **E** Etanercept; **G** Golimumab; **H** Hydroxychloroquine; **I** Infliximab; **M** Methotrexate; **P** Penicillamine; **R** Rituximab; **S** Sulfasalazine

DPP-4 INHIBITORS

	Alog	Lina	Saxa	Sita	=
SKIN					
Anaphylaxis	[1]			[1]	✓
Angioedema	[1]		[1]	[3]	✓
Edema			[1]	[3]	✓
Exfoliative dermatitis		•	•		✓
Hypersensitivity	[2]	[1]	[1]		✓
Peripheral edema	[1]	[1] (10%)	•		✓
Pruritus	[2]	[1]	[1]		✓
Rash	[1]		[1]	[1]	✓
Stevens–Johnson syndrome	[1]			[1]	✓
Urticaria		[1]	•	•	✓

Alog Alogliptin; **Lina** Linagliptin; **Saxa** Saxagliptin; **Sita** Sitagliptin

EGFR INHIBITORS

	C	E	G	L	Nec	Nil	P	Sor	Sun	=
SKIN										
Acneform eruption	[60] (92%)	[26] (73–80%)	[32] (66–85%)	[8] (90%)	[1] (23–43%)	[1] (<10%)	[17] (81%)	[5] (<10%)	[1] (<10%)	✓✓
AGEP		[1]	[1]					[2]		
Anaphylaxis	[5] (13%)		[1]				[1]			
Angioedema							[1]	[1]		
Bullous dermatitis		[1]							[1] (7%)	
Dermatitis	[4] (80%)	[2] (14%)				(<10%)				?
Desquamation	[3] (89%)		[2] (39%)				[3] (13%)	[9] (50%)		?
DRESS syndrome		[2]						[1]		
Eczema	[1]	[1]	[1]			(<10%)	[2]	[1]		✓
Edema		[1]		[2] (29%)		[2]	[1] (15%)	[3] (11%)	[6] (32%)	✓
Erythema	[3] (14%)	(18%)	[1]	[2]		[2] (<10%)	[5] (65%)	[4] (19%)	[5] (7%)	✓
Erythema multiforme						[1]		[10] (17%)		
Exanthems	[5]	[3] (8%)	[3] (21%)	[2]		[1]		[3]		✓
Exfoliative dermatitis			[1]	[2] (14%)		[1]	[2] (25%)	[1] (<10%)	[1] (10%)	✓
Facial edema		[1]				•		[1]	[2]	
Fissures	[4] (14%)	[1]			[1] (22%)		[4] (21%)			?
Folliculitis	[12] (83%)	[9] (11%)	[4]	[2]		(<10%)	[3]	[3]		✓
Hand–foot syndrome	[5] (6%)	[3] (30–60%)	[2]	[16] (76%)			[3] (23%)	[97] (89%)	[61] (45–65%)	✓
Hematoma	[1]					(<10%)				
Hypersensitivity	[8]				[1]			[2]		
Jaundice				[2] (35%)		•		[1]		?
Keratosis pilaris		[1]				[1]		[1]		
Necrosis		[1]							[1]	
Nevi						[1]		[2]	[2]	
Papulopustular eruption	[6] (83%)	[7] (29%)	[3] (21%)				[4] (21–41%)			?
Peripheral edema	[1] (40%)		•			[1] (44%)	[1] (12%)		[1] (17%)	✓

C Cetuximab; **E** Erlotinib; **G** Gefitinib; **L** Lapatinib; **Nec** Necitumumab; **Nil** Nilotinib; **P** Panitumumab; **Sor** Sorafenib; **Sun** Sunitinib

	C	E	G	L	Nec	Nil	P	Sor	Sun	=
Pigmentation			[1]	[2] (18%)			[1]	[2]	[12] (38%)	✓
Pruritus	[9] (40%)	[8] (21%)	[4] (61%)	[6] (33%)	[2] (60%)	[8] (9–21%)	[9] (91%)	[10] (21%)	[3] (<10%)	✓✓
Psoriasis	[1]			[2]		[1]		[2]		
Purpura		[3]	[1]							
Pustules	[1]		[1]				[1]			
Pyoderma gangrenosum			[1]						[4]	
Radiation recall dermatitis	[1]	[1]						[3]	[1]	
Rash	[46] (89%)	[105] (80%)	[59] (66–85%)	[48] (55%)	[7] (53%)	[10] (56%)	[28] (91%)	[46] (30–75%)	[47] (14–38%)	✓✓
Rosacea	[1]	[2]				[1]				
Seborrheic dermatitis		[1]						[1]	[1]	
Skin reactions		[1]						[1]		
Squamous cell carcinoma			[1]			[1]		[7]		
Stevens–Johnson syndrome	[1]							[1]		
Telangiectasia	[1]	[1]					[1]			
Toxic epidermal necrolysis	[2]		[1]							
Toxicity	[18] (63%)	[7] (84%)	[9] (68%)	[12] (46%)	[1] (8%)	[6]	[25] (95%)	[14] (75%)	[20] (67%)	✓✓
Ulcerations	[1]		[2]						[1]	
Urticaria			[1]			(<10%)		•		
Vasculitis		[1]	[1]					[1]		
Xerosis	[14] (49%)	[11] (56%)	[11] (53%)	[2] (29%)	[2] (67%)		[12] (62%)	[6] (14%)	[3] (17%)	✓
HAIR										
Alopecia	(5%)	[10] (14%)	[6]	[4] (33%)		[2] (<10%)	[3] (54%)	[24] (67%)	[3] (5–12%)	✓
Hair changes	[3]	[3]					[2] (9%)			
Hair pigmentation								[1]	[7] (38%)	?
Hypertrichosis	[3]	[4]	[2]							
NAILS										
Nail changes	[1] (21%)	[2] (17%)	[1] (17%)				[2] (9–29%)			?
Nail disorder	[2]			[2] (10%)					[1] (<10%)	

C Cetuximab; **E** Erlotinib; **G** Gefitinib; **L** Lapatinib; **Nec** Necitumumab; **Nil** Nilotinib; **P** Panitumumab; **Sor** Sorafenib; **Sun** Sunitinib

	C	E	G	L	Nec	Nil	P	Sor	Sun	=
Paronychia	[14] (14%)	[11] (15%)	[13] (14–32%)	[6] (27%)			[12] (85%)			✓
Pyogenic granuloma	[1]	[1]	[2]				[1]			
Splinter hemorrhage								[3] (70%)	[1]	?
Subungual hemorrhage								[1]	[3]	
MUCOSAL										
Aphthous stomatitis	[1]	[1]						[1]		
Cheilitis				[2] (14%)				[1]		
Epistaxis			[1]				[1]	[2] (11%)	[2] (13%)	
Glossodynia								(<10%)	[1] (15%)	
Mucosal inflammation		[1] (18%)		[2] (15%)			(6%)		[4] (54%)	?
Mucositis	[10]	[9] (21%)	[4] (6–17%)	[4] (11–35%)			[4] (75%)	[12] (28%)	[16] (~60%)	✓
Oral mucositis			[1] (33%)				(6%)		[1] (20%)	?
Oral ulceration	[1]	[1]	[1]			•		[1] (5%)		✓
Oropharyngeal pain					•			[1] (10%)		
Stomatitis	[3] (25%)	[9] (9–19%)	[7] (6–17%)	[2] (41%)	(11%)	•	[4] (100%)	[11] (28%)	[15] (60%)	✓✓
Xerostomia	(11%)					[1] (11%)		[1] (<10%)	[2] (~60%)	?

C Cetuximab; **E** Erlotinib; **G** Gefitinib; **L** Lapatinib; **Nec** Necitumumab; **Nil** Nilotinib; **P** Panitumumab; **Sor** Sorafenib; **Sun** Sunitinib

FLUOROQUINOLONES

	B	C	L	M	N	=
SKIN						
AGEP		[3]	[1]	[1]		✓
Anaphylaxis		[15]	[5]	[5]	•	✓
Bullous dermatitis		[1]		[2]	[1]	✓
Candidiasis		[2]	•	•		✓
Diaphoresis		[4]	•	•	•	✓
Edema		•	•			
Erythema			[2]		•	
Erythema multiforme		[5]	[1]			
Erythema nodosum		[1]	•			
Exanthems		[4]	[2]	•	[2]	✓
Fixed eruption		[12]			[2]	
Hypersensitivity	[1]	[5]	[5]	[6]		✓
Photosensitivity		[18]	[3]	[5]	[1]	✓
Phototoxicity		[5]	[5]		[4]	✓
Pigmentation		•	[1]			
Pruritus		[10]	[2]	[2]	[1]	✓
Purpura		[4]	[2]			
Radiation recall dermatitis		[1]	[2]			
Rash		[12] (<10%)	[1]	[3]	•	✓
Stevens–Johnson syndrome		[8]	[2]		[1]	✓
Sweet's syndrome		[1]			[1]	
Thrombocytopenic purpura		[1]		[2]		
Toxic epidermal necrolysis		[10]	[5]	[2]	[2]	✓
Toxicity		[2]	[1]			
Urticaria		[8]		[3]	[1]	✓
Vasculitis		[11]	[3]			
MUCOSAL						
Stomatitis		[3]		[1]		
Xerostomia		[3]	•	[1]	•	✓

B Besifloxacin; **C** Ciprofloxacin; **L** Levofloxacin; **M** Moxifloxacin; **N** Norfloxacin

NON-STEROIDAL ANTI-INFLAMMATORY DRUGS (NSAIDS)

	A	C	D	E	F	Ib	In	Ktp	Ktl	Mx	Np	O	P	Su	=
SKIN															
AGEP	[2]	[7]		[1]		[5] (50%)				[1]			[1]		?
Anaphylaxis	[16] (<10%)	[8]	[16] (48%)		[1]	[5] (25%)	•	[4]	[3]	[1]	[2]	•	•	[4]	✓
Angioedema	[64] (22%)	[9]	[2]	[1]	[1]	[8]	[2]	[1]	[1]	[3]	[5]	•	[3]	•	✓✓
Bullous dermatitis	[8]	[1]	[2]			[3]	[2]	[1] (29%)		•	[5]		[1]		✓
Bullous pemphigoid	[2]	[1]	[1]			[2]									
Churg-Strauss syndrome	[2]						[1]								
Dermatitis		[2]	[9]		[1]	[5]	[5]	[29]	(3–9%)				[5]	[1]	✓
Dermatitis herpetiformis	[2]		[2]		[1]	[1]	[2]								
Dermatomyositis	[2]		[1]												
Diaphoresis		•	•			[1]	•	[1]	[2] (<10%)		[3]	•	[1]		✓
DRESS syndrome	[2]	[1]	[1]			[4]					[4]		[1]		
Ecchymoses						[1]	•		•	[1]	(3–9%)	•	•	•	✓
Eczema			•		(3–9%)	[1]	[1]	[3]		[1]					
Edema		[5] (6%)			(3–9%)	[1]	[1] (3–9%)		(<10%)	[1] (6%)	[1] (<9%)	•	•		✓
Embolia cutis medicamentosa (Nicolau syndrome)			[16]			[2]		[1]					[1]		
Erythema		[2] (14%)	[4]					[3] (21%)	[1]	[2]	[1]		[1]	[1]	✓
Erythema multiforme	[18]	[3]	[6]	•	•	[11] (13%)	[1]	[1]		[1]	[2]	[1]	[12]	[8]	✓
Erythema nodosum	[18]		•			[1] (<5%)	[1]				[1]				
Erythroderma	[4]												[2]		
Exanthems	[22] (18%)	[7] (49%)	[6] (<5%)	[2]	[3]	[9]	[7] (11%)	[3]	[1] (3–9%)	[1]	[9] (14%)	[1]	[8]	[9] (<5%)	✓✓
Excoriations						[1] (6%)			[1]						
Exfoliative dermatitis	[2]	[1]	[1]		•	[1]	[1]	•	•			•	[1]	•	✓
Facial edema		[1]	[1]	[2]				•		[1]					
Fixed eruption	[42]	[2]	[4] (18%)	[2]	[2]	[14]	[2]			[1]	[24] (24%)		[15]	[5]	✓
Hematoma	[2]								[2]	[3]					

A Aspirin; **C** Celecoxib; **D** Diclofenac; **E** Etodolac; **F** Flurbiprofen; **Ib** Ibuprofen; **In** Indomethacin; **Ktp** Ketoprofen; **Ktl** Ketorolac; **Mx** Meloxicam; **Np** Naproxen; **O** Oxaprozin; **P** Piroxicam; **Su** Sulindac

	A	C	D	E	F	Ib	In	Ktp	Ktl	Mx	Np	O	P	Su	=
Herpes simplex	[2]	•									[1]				
Herpes zoster		•				[1]									
Hot flashes		•			•	•	•	•		•	[1]		•	•	✓
Hypersensitivity	[10]	[8]	[4]		[4]	[5]	•		[2]	[2] (5%)	[2]			•	✓
Jaundice		[1]			[1]				•					[1]	
Lichen planus							[1]				[3]			[1]	
Lichenoid eruption	[4]										[3]		[5]		
Linear IgA			[6]					[1]			[1]	[1]	[3]		
Lupus erythematosus		[1]				[5]					[2]		[1]		
Pemphigus	[2]		[1]			[1]		[1]					[3]		
Peripheral edema	[2]	[2]	[1]	[1]		[2] (5%)		•		[1]	[1]		[1]		✓
Petechiae							•						•		
Photoallergic reaction		[1]	[1]					[2]							
Photosensitivity		•	[4]	[1]	•	[6]	[1]	[34] (11%)	•	•	[16]	•	[40]	[2]	✓
Phototoxicity											[1]	[1]		•	
Pityriasis rosea	[6]										[1]				
Pruritus	[12]	[6]	[6] (<10%)	[7] (<10%)	[1] (<5%)	[5] (<5%)	[3] (<10%)	[4] (<10%)	[1] (<10%)	[3]	[5] (17%)	(<10%)	[6] (<10%)	[5] (<10%)	✓✓
Pseudolymphoma	[2]		[1]			[1]	[1]	[1]			[1]	[1]		[1]	✓
Psoriasis	[6]		[1]			[2]	[7]	[1]		[1]					
Purpura	[16]	[1]	[2]			[1]	[5]	[1]	[1] (<10%)	•	[4]		[2]	[2]	✓
Purpura fulminans			[2]						[1]						
Pustules		[1]									[2]				
Rash	(<10%)	[11] (40%)	[4] (6%)	[5]	•	[2]	[1]	[1]	[1] (<10%)	[3]	[2] (3–9%)	[2]	[1]	•	✓✓
SDRIFE	[2]	[1]									[1]				
Serum sickness						[1]	[1]					•	•	[1]	
Stevens–Johnson syndrome	[12]	[2]	[5]	•	•	[10] (17%)	•	•	•	[1]	[1]	[2]	[2]	[5]	✓✓
Toxic epidermal necrolysis	[18]	[5]	[4]	•	[1]	[8] (6%)	[6]	[1]	•	[1]	[5]	[4]	[12]	[13]	✓✓
Urticaria	[144] (83%)	[11]	[7]	•	•	[10]	[7]	[6]	[1]	[4]	[6] (<5%)	•	[7]	[4]	✓✓
Vasculitis	[4]	[4]	[3]	[2]	[1]	[8]	[5]		[1]	•	[9]		[3]	•	✓
Vesiculobullous eruption						[2]					[1]				
Wound complications						[1]			[1]						

A Aspirin; **C** Celecoxib; **D** Diclofenac; **E** Etodolac; **F** Flurbiprofen; **Ib** Ibuprofen; **In** Indomethacin; **Ktp** Ketoprofen; **Ktl** Ketorolac; **Mx** Meloxicam; **Np** Naproxen; **O** Oxaprozin; **P** Piroxicam; **Su** Sulindac

	A	C	D	E	F	Ib	In	Ktp	Ktl	Mx	Np	O	P	Su	=
Xerosis		•	[3]					[1]					[1]		
HAIR															
Alopecia	[2]	[3]	•		•	[2]	•	[1]	•	•	[3]		[3]	•	✓
NAILS															
Nail changes		•			•	[1]									
Onycholysis						[1]		[1]							
MUCOSAL															
Aphthous stomatitis	[6]		[1]						[1]		[1]		[4]		
Epistaxis	[2]	•	•						•	[1]					
Glossitis									•					•	
Oral lesions						[1]	[2] (7%)	[1]							
Oral lichenoid eruption					[2]	[1]	[1]							[1]	
Oral mucosal eruption	[6]													[2]	
Oral mucosal fixed eruption											[1]		[1]		
Oral ulceration	[8]		[1]			[1]	[4]				[1]		[1]		
Rectal hemorrhage									•	[1]					
Rectal mucosal ulceration	[2]													[1]	
Stomatitis		[4] (8%)	•					•	(<10%)		•	•	•	[2]	✓
Tongue edema			[1]				[1]		•						
Ulcerative stomatitis							[1]			•					
Xerostomia		•	[2] (26%)		•	•		[1]	[2]	•	[2]		•	[2]	✓

A Aspirin; **C** Celecoxib; **D** Diclofenac; **E** Etodolac; **F** Flurbiprofen; **Ib** Ibuprofen; **In** Indomethacin; **Ktp** Ketoprofen; **Ktl** Ketorolac; **Mx** Meloxicam; **Np** Naproxen; **O** Oxaprozin; **P** Piroxicam; **Su** Sulindac

PROTON PUMP INHIBITORS (PPI)

	D	E	L	O	P	R	=
SKIN							
Acneform eruption	•	•	•		•		✓
AGEP			[1]	[2]			
Anaphylaxis	•	[1]	[6]	[7]	[7]		✓
Angioedema		•		[5]	•		✓
Candidiasis		•	•				
Dermatitis	•	•	[1]	[1]	•		✓
Diaphoresis		•	[1]	[1]	[1]	•	✓
Ecchymoses					•	•	
Eczema				[1]	•		
Edema		•	[1]	[2] (<10%)	•		✓
Erythema multiforme			[2]	[1]	•		✓
Erythroderma			[1]	[2]			
Exanthems		•		[1]	•		✓
Exfoliative dermatitis		[1]	[1]	[3]			✓
Facial edema			[2]	[1]	[1]	•	✓
Fixed eruption		[2]		[1]			
Fungal dermatitis		•			•		
Herpes zoster	•				•	•	✓
Hypersensitivity			[3]	[2]	[1]	[1]	✓
Lichenoid eruption			[1]	[2]	[1]		✓
Lupus erythematosus		[2]	[3]	[5]	[3]		✓
Peripheral edema		•	[2]	[2]	[2]	•	✓
Photosensitivity		[1]			[1]	•	✓
Pigmentation				[1]		•	
Pruritus	•	•	[1] (3–10%)	[8] (<10%)	[1]	[2]	✓✓
Pruritus ani et vulvae		•	[1]				
Psoriasis				[1]		•	
Rash	•	[1]	(3–10%)	[6]	[2]	[2]	✓✓
Stevens–Johnson syndrome			[1]	•	•		✓
Sweet's syndrome		[1]		[1]			
Toxic epidermal necrolysis			[4]	[5]	•		✓

D Dexlansoprazole; **E** Esomeprazole; **L** Lansoprazole; **O** Omeprazole; **P** Pantoprazole; **R** Rabeprazole

	D	E	L	O	P	R	=
Urticaria	•	•	[3]	[8] (<10%)	[2]	•	✓✓
Vasculitis				[2]	[1]		
Xerosis		[1]		[2]	•	•	✓
HAIR							
Alopecia			•	[2]	•	•	✓
MUCOSAL							
Gingivitis					•	•	
Glossitis			[1]		•	•	✓
Oral candidiasis	•			[3]	•		✓
Stomatitis			[2]	[1]	•	•	✓
Tongue edema		•			[1]		
Xerostomia	•	•	•	[2] (<10%)	•	•	✓✓

D Dexlansoprazole; **E** Esomeprazole; **L** Lansoprazole; **O** Omeprazole; **P** Pantoprazole; **R** Rabeprazole

STATINS

	A	F	L	Pi	Pr	R	S	=
SKIN								
Acneform eruption	•						[1] (36%)	?
Dermatomyositis	[3]	[1]	[1]		[2]		[5]	✓
Diaphoresis	•						[1]	
Ecchymoses	•					•		
Eczema	•				[1]		[4] (5%)	
Edema	•		[1] (6%)		•		[1]	✓
Eosinophilic fasciitis	[1]						[2]	
Erythema multiforme					[1]		[2]	
Exanthems			[3] (5%)				[1]	
Herpes zoster	[1]	[1]	[1]		[1]	[1]	[1]	✓
Hypersensitivity			[1]	•			[1]	
Jaundice	[2]						[1]	
Lichenoid eruption	[1]	[1]	[1]		[2]		[1]	✓
Lupus erythematosus	[2]	[2]	[4]		[1]		[5]	✓
Peripheral edema						•	[2] (50%)	?
Petechiae	•						[1]	
Photosensitivity	•				[1]		[7]	
Pruritus	[1]		[2] (5%)		[2]	•	[3]	✓
Purpura			[1]		[1]		[3]	
Radiation recall dermatitis						[1]	[1]	
Rash	[2]	•	[3] (5%)	•	[7] (5–7%)	•	[3] (<10%)	✓✓
Toxicity	[2]					[1]	[1]	✓
Urticaria	[1]			•			[1]	
Vasculitis	[1]						[2]	
HAIR								
Alopecia	[1]		•					
MUCOSAL								
Cheilitis	•						[1]	
Stomatitis	•						[1] (64%)	?

A Atorvastatin; **F** Fluvastatin; **L** Lovastatin; **Pi** Pitavastatin; **Pr** Pravastatin; **R** Rosuvastatin; **S** Simvastatin

TNF INHIBITORS

	A	C	E	G	I	=
SKIN						
Abscess	[1]		[2]		[4]	✓
Acneform eruption	[2]		[1]		[6]	✓
AGEP			[1]		[2]	
Anaphylaxis	[1]		[2]		[10]	✓
Angioedema	[3]	•	[1]		[1]	✓
Basal cell carcinoma				[1]	[1]	
Bullous pemphigoid	[1]		[1]			
Candidiasis	[1]				[4] (5%)	
Carcinoma	[2]		[2]			
Cellulitis	[2] (<5%)		[2]		[5]	✓
Dermatitis	[1]	•	[3]		[4]	✓
Dermatomyositis	[5]		[4]			
Eczema	[2]				[5] (19–30%)	?
Erythema	[1]				[1]	
Erythema multiforme	[1]				[2]	
Erythema nodosum		[1]	[1]			
Exanthems			[2]		[4]	
Fixed eruption	[1]		[1]		[1]	✓
Folliculitis			[1]		[2]	
Granuloma annulare			[1]		[1]	
Granulomas	[1]		[2]		[1]	✓
Granulomatous reaction	[5]		[5]		[1]	✓
Henoch–Schönlein purpura	[2]		[3]		[1]	✓
Herpes simplex	[1]		[1]		[4] (10%)	✓
Herpes zoster	[9]	[2]	[5]		[10]	✓
Hidradenitis	[2]		[2]		[1]	✓
Hypersensitivity	[3]	•	[1]		[11] (11%)	✓
Kaposi's sarcoma	[1]				[1]	
Leprosy	[1]		[2]		[1]	✓

A Adalimumab; **C** Certolizumab; **E** Etanercept; **G** Golimumab; **I** Infliximab

	A	C	E	G	I	=
Leukocytoclastic vasculitis	[1]			[1]	[1]	✓
Lichen planus			[2]		[2]	
Lichenoid eruption	[5]		[3]		[3]	✓
Lupus erythematosus	[16]		[25]	[3]	[33]	✓
Lupus syndrome	[3]	[2]	[2]		[11]	✓
Lymphadenopathy	[1]				[1]	
Lymphoma	[8]		[3]		[9]	✓
Lymphoproliferative disease			[1]		[1]	
Malignancies	[3]		[3]	[5]	[2]	✓
Melanoma	[6]		[2]	[1]	[1]	✓
Molluscum contagiosum	[1]				[2]	
Morphea	[1]		[1]			
Necrotizing fasciitis			[1]		[1]	
Neoplasms	[1]	[2]	[2]		[2]	✓
Nevi			[1]		[2]	
Peripheral edema	(<5%)		[1]		[1]	✓
Pityriasis lichenoides chronica	[1]		[1]		[2]	✓
Pruritus	[5]	[1]	[2] (14%)		[8] (20%)	✓
Pseudolymphoma	[1]		[1]		[2]	✓
Psoriasis	[38]	[6]	[19]	[2]	[51] (19%)	✓✓
Pustules	[1]		[2]		[5]	✓
Rash	[4] (12%)	[2] (5%)	[7] (15%)	[3]	[13] (25%)	✓✓
Rosacea	[1]		[1]		[1]	✓
Sarcoidosis	[6]		[8]		[3]	✓
Serum sickness		•			[6]	
Skin cancer	[1]				[1]	
Squamous cell carcinoma	[5]		[4]	[1]	[1]	✓
Stevens–Johnson syndrome	[2]		•		[1]	✓
Toxicity	[1]	[1]		[1]	[2] (75%)	✓
Tumors	[1]	[1]				

A Adalimumab; **C** Certolizumab; **E** Etanercept; **G** Golimumab; **I** Infliximab

	A	C	E	G	I	=
Urticaria	[3]	•	[2]		[6] (17%)	✓
Vasculitis	[8] (13%)	•	[21] (25%)	•	[16] (63%)	✓✓
Vitiligo	[2]				[4]	
HAIR						
Alopecia	[3]	[1]	[4] (20%)		[4]	✓
Alopecia areata	[7]		[1]	[1]	[3]	✓
Follicular mucinosis	[1]				[1]	

A Adalimumab; **C** Certolizumab; **E** Etanercept; **G** Golimumab; **I** Infliximab

TYROSINE-KINASE INHIBITORS

	Aft	Axt	Cbo	Crz	Dsa	Erl	Gft	Imt	Lpt	Lnv	Nlo	Nnt	Srf	Snt	Vnd	=
SKIN																
Acneform eruption	[24] (92%)				[1] (<10%)	[26] (73–80%)	[32] (66–85%)	[2]	[4] (90%)		[1] (<10%)		[5] (<10%)	[1] (<10%)	[3] (35%)	✓
AGEP						[1]	[1]	[6]					[2]			
Bullous dermatitis	•					[1]								[1] (7%)		
Dermatitis	[1] (21%)				(<10%)	[2] (14%)					(<10%)				[1]	?
Desquamation							[2] (39%)						[9] (50%)			?
Diaphoresis								(13%)					[1] (6%)			
DRESS syndrome						[2]		[3]					[1]			
Eczema					(<10%)	[1]	[1]				(<10%)		[1]			
Edema				[9] (38%)	[5] (23%)	[1]		[33] (80%)	[1] (29%)		[2]		[3] (11%)	[6] (32%)		✓
Erythema		[1]	(11%)		[1]	(18%)	[1]	[5] (<10%)	[1]		[2] (<10%)		[4] (19%)	[5] (7%)		✓
Erythema multiforme				[1]				[1]			[1]		[10] (17%)		[1]	
Exanthems						[3] (8%)	[3] (21%)	[8]	[1]	(21%)	[1]		[3]			✓
Exfoliative dermatitis	•						[1]	[3]	[1] (14%)		[1]		[1] (<10%)	[1] (10%)		✓
Facial edema						[1]		[2] (<10%)			•		[1]	[2]		
Fissures	[2] (12%)					[1]										
Folliculitis	[1]					[9] (11%)	[4]		[1]		(<10%)		[3]		[4] (49%)	✓
Hand–foot syndrome	[2] (10%)	[15] (64%)	[14] (50%)			[3] (30–60%)	[2]	[3]	[8] (76%)	(32%)		[2]	[97] (89%)	[61] (45–65%)	[3] (36%)	✓
Herpes					(<10%)						•					
Hyperhidrosis					(<10%)			[1]			(<10%)	[1] (12%)				
Hyperkeratosis			(7%)							(7%)			[4]			
Hypersensitivity					•								[2]			
Hypomelanosis								[5]						[1]		
Jaundice			(25%)						[1] (35%)		•		[1]			?

Aft Afatinib; **Axt** Axitinib; **Cbo** Cabozantinib; **Crz** Crizotinib; **Dsa** Dasatinib; **Erl** Erlotinib; **Gft** Gefitinib; **Imt** Imatinib; **Lpt** Lapatinib; **Lnv** Lenvatinib; **Nlo** Nilotinib; **Nnt** Nintedanib; **Srf** Sorafenib; **Snt** Sunitinib; **Vnd** Vandetanib

	Aft	Axt	Cbo	Crz	Dsa	Erl	Gft	Imt	Lpt	Lnv	Nlo	Nnt	Srf	Snt	Vnd	=
Keratosis pilaris						[1]					[1]		[1]			
Lesions								[1]						[2] (38%)		?
Necrolysis							[1]	[1]								
Necrosis						[1]								[1]		
Nevi												[1]	[2]	[2]		
Palmar–plantar hyperkeratosis								[1]						[1]		
Panniculitis					[3]			[2]								
Papulopustular eruption						[7] (29%)	[3] (21%)								[1]	?
Peripheral edema				[5] (28%)	[3] (44%)		•	[5] (75%)		[2] (37%)	[1] (44%)			[1] (17%)		✓
Photosensitivity				[2]	•	[1]		[1] (<10%)							[6] (23%)	?
Phototoxicity													[1]		[2]	
Pigmentation					•		[1]	[9] (60%)	[1] (18%)				[2]	[12] (38%)	[4]	✓
Pityriasis rubra pilaris								[1]					[1]			
Pruritus	[2] (13%)	[1] (8%)			[3] (14%)	[8] (21%)	[4] (61%)	[3] (10%)	[3] (33%)		[8] (9–21%)	[1] (19%)	[10] (21%)	[3] (<10%)	[2] (11%)	✓
Psoriasis								[2]	[1]		[1]		[2]			
Purpura						[3]	[1]	[1]								
Pyoderma gangrenosum							[1]							[4]		
Radiation recall dermatitis						[1]							[3]	[1]		
Rash	[43] (92%)	[3] (14%)	[1] (30%)	[4] (16%)	[9] (34%)	[105] (80%)	[59] (66–85%)	[23] (69%)	[24] (55%)	(21%)	[10] (56%)	[4] (41%)	[47] (30–75%)	[14] (14–38%)	[32] (67%)	✓✓
Rosacea						[2]		[1]			[1]					
Seborrheic dermatitis						[1]							[1]	[1]		
Skin reactions						[1]							[1]			
Squamous cell carcinoma							[1]	[2]			[1]		[7]			
Stevens–Johnson syndrome	[1]							[11]					[1]		[2]	
Sweet's syndrome					•			[1]			[1]					
Telangiectasia						[1]		[1]								

Aft Afatinib; **Axt** Axitinib; **Cbo** Cabozantinib; **Crz** Crizotinib; **Dsa** Dasatinib; **Erl** Erlotinib; **Gft** Gefitinib; **Imt** Imatinib; **Lpt** Lapatinib; **Lnv** Lenvatinib; **Nlo** Nilotinib; **Nnt** Nintedanib; **Srf** Sorafenib; **Snt** Sunitinib; **Vnd** Vandetanib

	Aft	Axt	Cbo	Crz	Dsa	Erl	Gft	Imt	Lpt	Lnv	Nlo	Nnt	Srf	Snt	Vnd	=
Toxic epidermal necrolysis							[1]	[1]								
Toxicity	[2]		[2]		[6] (36%)	[7] (84%)	[9] (68%)	[8] (30–44%)	[6] (46%)	[1]	[6]		[14] (75%)	[20] (67%)	[9] (48–50%)	✓
Ulcerations					•		[2]							[1]		
Urticaria					(<10%)		[1]	[1]			(<10%)		•			
Vasculitis						[1]	[1]	[1]					[1]			
Wound complications			[1]										[1]		[1]	
Xerosis	[6] (15%)	(10%)	[1] (23%)		(<10%)	[11] (56%)	[11] (53%)	[1] (<10%)	[1] (29%)	[1] (20%)			[6] (14%)	[3] (17%)	[2] (15%)	✓
HAIR																
Alopecia	[1] (7%)	[2] (6%)	(16%)		[1] (<10%)	[10] (14%)	[6]	[1] (10–15%)	[2] (33%)	(12%)	[2] (<10%)	[2] (71%)	[24] (67%)	[3] (5–12%)	[1]	✓
Hair changes			(34%)			[3]									[1]	?
Hair pigmentation			[2] (34%)		[2]								[1]	[7] (38%)		?
Hypertrichosis						[4]	[2]									
NAILS																
Nail changes	[2] (16%)					[2] (17%)	[1] (17%)									
Nail disorder					•				[1] (10%)					[1] (<10%)		
Nail pigmentation							[1]	[1]								
Paronychia	[9] (33–85%)					[11] (15%)	[13] (14–32%)		[3] (27%)						[3] (7%)	?
Pyogenic granuloma						[1]	[2]									
Splinter hemorrhage													[3] (70%)	[1]	[1]	?
Subungual hemorrhage													[1]	[3]		
MUCOSAL																
Aphthous stomatitis	•					[1]		[1]		(41%)			[1]			?
Cheilitis	[1] (7%)							[1]	[1] (14%)				[1]			
Epistaxis	[3] (17%)	[1] (8%)					[1]			(12%)		[1]	[2] (11%)	[2] (13%)		✓

Aft Afatinib; **Axt** Axitinib; **Cbo** Cabozantinib; **Crz** Crizotinib; **Dsa** Dasatinib; **Erl** Erlotinib; **Gft** Gefitinib; **Imt** Imatinib; **Lpt** Lapatinib; **Lnv** Lenvatinib; **Nlo** Nilotinib; **Nnt** Nintedanib; **Srf** Sorafenib; **Snt** Sunitinib; **Vnd** Vandetanib

	Aft	Axt	Cbo	Crz	Dsa	Erl	Gft	Imt	Lpt	Lnv	Nlo	Nnt	Srf	Snt	Vnd	=
Glossodynia		[1]								(25%)			(<10%)	[1] (15%)		?
Mucocutaneous eruption					[1]			[1]			[1]					
Mucosal inflammation	[6] (69%)	[2] (15%)	[2] (23%)			[1] (18%)			[1] (15%)	[1] (50%)				[4] (54%)	[1] (27%)	✓
Mucositis	[10] (50–90%)		[1]		[1] (16%)	[9] (21%)	[4] (6–17%)	[2] (15%)	[2] (11–35%)				[12] (28%)	[16] (∼60%)	[2] (14%)	✓
Oral mucositis		[1]					[1] (33%)							[1] (20%)		?
Oral ulceration						[1]	[1]	[3] (15%)		(41%)	•		[1] (5%)			?
Oropharyngeal pain								[1]		(25%)			[1] (10%)			?
Rhinorrhea	(11%)												•			
Stomatitis	[17] (50–90%)	[1] (15%)	(51%)	[1] (11%)	[1]	[9] (9–19%)	[7] (6–17%)		[1] (41%)	[2] (41%)	•	[1]	[11] (28%)	[15] (60%)	[2] (33%)	✓
Xerostomia	[1] (20%)				[1] (33%)			[1] (44%)		(17%)	[1] (11%)		[1] (<10%)	[2] (∼60%)		✓

Aft Afatinib; **Axt** Axitinib; **Cbo** Cabozantinib; **Crz** Crizotinib; **Dsa** Dasatinib; **Erl** Erlotinib; **Gft** Gefitinib; **Imt** Imatinib; **Lpt** Lapatinib; **Lnv** Lenvatinib; **Nlo** Nilotinib; **Nnt** Nintedanib; **Srf** Sorafenib; **Snt** Sunitinib; **Vnd** Vandetanib

Concordance of synonyms and trade names with generic names

Synonym/Trade name	Generic
13-cis-retinoic acid	isotretinoin
3,4-methylenedioxymethamphetamine	MDMA
3TC	lamivudine
4-aminopyridine	dalfampridine
4-demethoxydaunorubicin	idarubicin
4-DMDR	idarubicin
5-aminosalicylic acid	mesalamine
5-ASA	mesalamine
5-aza-2'-deoxycytidine	decitabine
5-fluorouracil	fluorouracil
6-mercaptopurine	mercaptopurine
6-MP	mercaptopurine

A

Synonym/Trade name	Generic
A-Acido	tretinoin
A-Gram	amoxicillin
Abaprim	trimethoprim
Abbocillin	penicillin V
Abelcet	amphotericin B
Aberal	tretinoin
Aberela	tretinoin
Abetol	labetalol
Abilify	aripiprazole
Abilitat	aripiprazole
Abraxane	paclitaxel
Abrifam	rifampin
Abstral	fentanyl
Ac-De	dactinomycin
Acaren	vitamin A
Accolate	zafirlukast
AccuNeb	albuterol
Accupril	quinapril
Accuprin	quinapril
Accupro	quinapril
Accuretic	hydrochlorothiazide, quinapril
Accutane	isotretinoin
Acenor-M	fosinopril
Acenorm	captopril
Aceon	perindopril
Acepril	captopril
Acerbon	lisinopril
Acertil	perindopril
Acetazolam	acetazolamide
acetylsalicylic acid	aspirin
Acfol	folic acid
aciclovir	acyclovir
Acid A Vit	tretinoin
Acidulated phosphate fluoride	fluorides
Acifur	acyclovir
Acimox	amoxicillin
Aciphex	rabeprazole
Aclasta	zoledronate
Aclinda	clindamycin
Acnamino	minocycline
Acnavit	tretinoin
Acon	vitamin A
Act-3	ibuprofen
ACT	dactinomycin
Acta	tretinoin
Actacode	codeine
Actemra	tocilizumab
ActHIB	Hemophilus B vaccine
Actigall	ursodiol
Actilyse	alteplase
actinomycin-D	dactinomycin
Actiprofen	ibuprofen
Actiq	fentanyl
Activacin	alteplase
Activase	alteplase
Actonel	risedronate
Actos	pioglitazone
Acuitel	quinapril
Acular	ketorolac
Acupril	quinapril
ACV	acyclovir
Acyclo-V	acyclovir
acycloguanosine	acyclovir
Acyvir	acyclovir
Aczone	dapsone
Adalat	nifedipine
Adalate	nifedipine
Adant	hyaluronic acid
Adapin	doxepin
Adaquin	quinine
Adasuve	loxapine
Adcetris	brentuximab vedotin
Adcirca	tadalafil
Adderall	dextroamphetamine
Addyi	flibanserin
Adempas	riociguat
Adenic	adenosine
Adeno-Jec	adenosine
Adenocard	adenosine
Adenocur	adenosine
Adenoject	adenosine
Adenoscan	adenosine
Adiblastine	doxorubicin
Adipex-P	phentermine
Adipine	nifedipine
Adlyxin	lixisenatide
Adocor	captopril
Adofen	fluoxetine
Adoxa	doxycycline
Adrecar	adenosine
Adrenaclick	epinephrine
Adrenalin	epinephrine

adrenaline	epinephrine
Adriablastine	doxorubicin
Adriacin	doxorubicin
Adriamycin	doxorubicin
Adriblatina	doxorubicin
Adsorbocarbine	pilocarpine
Adumbran	oxazepam
Adursall	ursodiol
Advantan	methylprednisolone
Advicor	lovastatin, niacin
Advil	ibuprofen
Aerolate	aminophylline
Aerovent	aldesleukin
Afaxin	vitamin A
Afinitor	everolimus
Aflodac	sulindac
Aflorix	miconazole
Afluria	influenza vaccine
Afstyla	antihemophilic factor
Aggrenox	aspirin, dipyridamole
Agilect	rasagiline
Agisolvan	acetylcysteine
Agrippal	influenza vaccine
AH3 N	hydroxyzine
Airol	tretinoin
AK-Chlor	chloramphenicol
Ak-Zol	acetazolamide
Akarpine	pilocarpine
Akatinol	memantine
Aknemin	minocycline
Aknemycin Plus	tretinoin
AKTob Ophthalmic	tobramycin
Akynzeo	netupitant & palonosetron
AL-R	chlorpheniramine
Alapril	lisinopril
Alavert	loratadine
Albenza	albendazole
Albiotic	lincomycin
Alcloxidine	chlorhexidine
Alcomicinx	gentamicin
Aldactazide	hydrochlorothiazide, spironolactone
Aldactone	spironolactone
Aldara	imiquimod
Aldoclor	methyldopa
Aldocumar	warfarin
Aldomet	methyldopa
Aldopur	spironolactone
Aldoril	hydrochlorothiazide, methyldopa
Alecensa	alectinib
Alendronic acid	alendronate
Alepsal	phenobarbital
Alercet	cetirizine
Alerid	cetirizine
Alertec	modafinil
Alesse	oral contraceptives
Aleve	naproxen
Alexan	cytarabine
Alfadil	doxazosin
Alfatil	cefaclor
Alferon N	interferon alfa
Alfotax	cefotaxime
Algocetil	sulindac
Alimta	pemetrexed
Alinia	nitazoxanide
Alka-Seltzer	aspirin
Alkeran	melphalan
all-trans-retinoic acid	tretinoin
Allegra-D	pseudoephedrine
Allegra	fexofenadine
Allegron	nortriptyline
Aller-Chlor	chlorpheniramine
Allerdryl	diphenhydramine
Allerglobuline	immune globulin IV
Allermax	diphenhydramine
Allermin	diphenhydramine
Alli	orlistat
Allo 300	allopurinol
Allo-Puren	allopurinol
Alloprin	allopurinol
Allvoran	diclofenac
Almarytm	flecainide
Almatol	spironolactone
Almodan	amoxicillin
Almogran	almotriptan
Aloid	miconazole
Alopexy	minoxidil
Alora	estradiol
Aloxi	palonosetron
alpha tocopherol	vitamin E
Alphagan P	brimonidine
Alphapress	hydralazine
Alprim	trimethoprim
Alprox	alprazolam
Alquingel	tretinoin
Alrheumat	ketoprofen
Alrheumun	ketoprofen
Alsuma	sumatriptan
Altace	ramipril
Alten	tretinoin
Alti-Diltiazem	diltiazem
Alti-Doxepin	doxepin
Alti-Ipratropium	ipratropium
Alti-Minocycline	minocycline
Alti-MPA	medroxyprogesterone
Alti-Trazodone	trazodone
Altocor	lovastatin
Altoprev	lovastatin
Aluvira	lopinavir
Alveolex	acetylcysteine
Amaryl	glimepiride
Ambi	hydroquinone
Ambien	zolpidem
AmBisome	amphotericin B
Amdepin	amlodipine
amethopterin	methotrexate
Ametycine	mitomycin
Amfipen	ampicillin
Amias	candesartan
Amicacina	amikacin
Amicasil	amikacin
Amikacin sulfate	amikacin
Amikal	amiloride

Amikan	amikacin	*antegren*	natalizumab
Amineurin	amitriptyline	Anten	doxepin
Aminophyllin	aminophylline	Antepsin	sucralfate
Amipress	labetalol	Antiflog	piroxicam
Amisalen	procainamide	Antilak	etodolac
Amitiza	lubiprostone	Antilirium	physostigmine
Amjevita	adalimumab	Antipressan	atenolol
Amlodin	amlodipine	Antra	omeprazole
Amlogard	amlodipine	Antrex	leucovorin
Amlopin	amlodipine	Apacef	cefotetan
Amlor	amlodipine	*APAP*	acetaminophen
Amnesteem	isotretinoin	Apatef	cefotetan
Amodex	amoxicillin	Apdormin	hydralazine
Amodopa	methyldopa	Apekumarol	dicumarol
Amoxan	amoxapine	Aphtiria	lindane
Amoxapine	amoxapine	Apidra	insulin glulisine
Amoxil	amoxicillin	APO-Alpraz	alprazolam
amoxycillin	amoxicillin	Apo-Amoxi	amoxicillin
Amphocin	amphotericin B	Apo-Atenol	atenolol
Amphotec	amphotericin B	Apo-Bisoprolol	bisoprolol
Ampicin	ampicillin	Apo-Bromocriptine	bromocriptine
Amprace	enalapril	Apo-Buspirone	buspirone
Ampyra	dalfampridine	APO-Capto	captopril
Amrix	cyclobenzaprine	Apo-Carbamazepine	carbamazepine
Amterene	triamterene	Apo-Cefaclor	cefaclor
Amuno	indomethacin	Apo-Cephalex	cephalexin
Amycil	mebendazole	Apo-Cimetidine	cimetidine
Anacin-3	acetaminophen	Apo-Clomipramine	clomipramine
Anacin	aspirin	Apo-Diclo	diclofenac
Anacobin	cyanocobalamin	Apo-Doxy	doxycycline
Anafranil Retard	clomipramine	Apo-Enalapril	enalapril
Anafranil	clomipramine	Apo-Ethambutol	ethambutol
Anamantle HC	lidocaine	Apo-Famotidine	famotidine
Anamorph	morphine	Apo-Fenofibrate	fenofibrate
Anaprox	naproxen	Apo-Fluoxetine	fluoxetine
Anaspaz	hyoscyamine	Apo-Fluphenazine	fluphenazine
Anatensol	fluphenazine	Apo-Flurbiprofen	flurbiprofen
Anaxanil	hydroxyzine	Apo-Fluvoxamine	fluvoxamine
Anco	ibuprofen	Apo-Folic	folic acid
Andro LA	testosterone	Apo-Furosemide	furosemide
Androcur	cyproterone	Apo-Gain	minoxidil
Androderm	testosterone	Apo-Hydro	hydrochlorothiazide
AndroGel	testosterone	Apo-Imipramine	imipramine
Android	methyltestosterone	Apo-Indomethacin	indomethacin
Andronaq	testosterone	Apo-ISDN	isosorbide dinitrate
Androral	methyltestosterone	Apo-Lorazepam	lorazepam
Andrumin	dimenhydrinate	Apo-Lovastatin	lovastatin
Anectine	succinylcholine	Apo-Metformin	metformin
Aneol	ketoprofen	Apo-Metronidazole	metronidazole
Anergan	promethazine	Apo-Minocycline	minocycline
Anestacon	lidocaine	Apo-Nadolol	nadolol
Angilol	propranolol	Apo-Nicotinamide	niacin
Angiomax	bivalirudin	Apo-Nifed	nifedipine
Angioverin	papaverine	Apo-Nortriptyline	nortriptyline
Anitrim	co-trimoxazole	Apo-Oxazepam	oxazepam
Ansaid	flurbiprofen	Apo-Pen	penicillin V
Ansail	buspirone	Apo-Pentoxifylline	pentoxifylline
Antabus	disulfiram	Apo-Perphenazine	perphenazine
Antabuse	disulfiram	Apo-Piroxicam	piroxicam
Antagonil	nicardipine	Apo-Propranolol	propranolol
Antaxone	naltrexone	Apo-Ranitidine	ranitidine

Apo-Selegiline	selegiline
Apo-Sulfatrim	co-trimoxazole
APO-Sulin	sulindac
Apo-Tamox	tamoxifen
Apo-Temazepam	temazepam
Apo-Trimip	trimipramine
APO-Verap	verapamil
Apocard	flecainide
Aponal	doxepin
Apranax	naproxen
Apresazide	hydralazine
Apresolin	hydralazine
Apresoline	hydralazine
Aprical	nifedipine
Aprovel	irbesartan
Apsifen	ibuprofen
Apsolol	propranolol
Aptiom	eslicarbazepine
Aptivus	tipranavir
Aquachloral	chloral hydrate
Aquamid	hyaluronic acid
Aquamycetin	chloramphenicol
Aquarius	ketoconazole
Aquasol A	vitamin A
Aquasol E	vitamin E
ara-C	cytarabine
Arabitin	cytarabine
Arace	cytarabine
Aracytine	cytarabine
Aragest 5	medroxyprogesterone
Aralen	chloroquine
Aranesp	darbepoetin alfa
Aratac	amiodarone
Arcapta Neohaler	indacaterol
Aredia	pamidronate
Arestin	minocycline
Argesic-SA	salsalate
Aricept Evess	donepezil
Aricept	donepezil
Arimidex	anastrozole
Aristada	aripiprazole
Arixtra	fondaparinux
Aromasin	exemestane
Arovit	vitamin A
Arpamyl LP	verapamil
Arsacol	ursodiol
Artal	pentoxifylline
Artamin	penicillamine
Artecoll	collagen (bovine)
Artha-G	salsalate
Arthaxan	nabumetone
Arthrocine	sulindac
Arthrotec	diclofenac, misoprostol
Artifar	carisoprodol
ARTZ	hyaluronic acid
Arythmol	propafenone
Arzerra	ofatumumab
ASA	aspirin
Asacol	mesalamine
Asacolitin	mesalamine
Asclera	polidocanol
Ascriptin	aspirin
Asendis	amoxapine
Aside	etoposide
Asig	quinapril
Asmaven	albuterol
Aspergum	aspirin
Aspro	aspirin
ASS	aspirin
Assival	diazepam
AsthmaHaler	epinephrine
Astramorph	morphine
Atabrine	quinacrine
Atacand HCT	hydrochlorothiazide
Atacand	candesartan
Ataline	terbutaline
Atarax	hydroxyzine
AteHexal	atenolol
Atelvia	risedronate
Atem	aldesleukin
Atendol	atenolol
Atisuril	allopurinol, salsalate
Ativan	lorazepam
Atosil	promethazine
ATP	adenosine
ATRA	tretinoin
Atragen	tretinoin
Atrenta	artesunate
Atreol	carbamazepine
Atridox	doxycycline
Atripla	efavirenz, emtricitabine, tenofovir disoproxil
Atronase	aldesleukin
Atropine Martinet	atropine sulfate
Atropt	atropine sulfate
Atrovent	ipratropium
Atruline	sertraline
Aubagio	teriflunomide
Audazol	omeprazole
Augmentin	amoxicillin
Autologen	collagen (bovine)
Auvi-Q	epinephrine
Avage	tazarotene
Avalide	hydrochlorothiazide, irbesartan
Avandamet	metformin, rosiglitazone
Avandaryl	glimepiride, rosiglitazone
Avandia	rosiglitazone
Avapro	irbesartan
Avastin	bevacizumab
Avaxim	hepatitis A vaccine
Avelox	moxifloxacin
Aventyl	nortriptyline
Aviane	oral contraceptives
Avinza	morphine
Avipur	vitamin A
Avirax	acyclovir
Avita	tretinoin
Avitcid	tretinoin
Avitene	collagen (bovine)
Avitin	vitamin A
Avitoin	tretinoin
Avloclor	chloroquine
Avlosulfon	dapsone

Avodart	dutasteride
Avonex	interferon beta
Avycaz	ceftazidime & avibactam
Axerol	vitamin A
Axert	almotriptan
Axoban	ranitidine
Aygestin	progestins
Azamedac	azathioprine
Azamune	azathioprine
Azantac	ranitidine
Azasan	azathioprine
AzaSite	azithromycin
Azatrilem	azathioprine
Azenil	azithromycin
azidothymidine	zidovudine
Azilect	rasagiline
Azitrocin	azithromycin
Azitromax	azithromycin
Azol	danazol
Azopt	brinzolamide
AZT	zidovudine
Azucimet	cimetidine
Azulfidine	sulfasalazine
Azupamil	verapamil
Azupentat	pentoxifylline
Azutranquil	oxazepam
Azzalure	botulinum toxin (A & B)

B

Bacille Calmette-Guerin	BCG vaccine
Baclofen	baclofen
Baclon	baclofen
Baclosal	baclofen
Bacomine	hydrocodone
Bactelan	co-trimoxazole
Bactin	trimethoprim
Bactocill	oxacillin
Bactocin	ofloxacin
Bactoscrub	chlorhexidine
BactoShield	chlorhexidine
Bactrim	co-trimoxazole, sulfamethoxazole, trimethoprim
Baklofen	baclofen
BAL5788	ceftobiprole
Balcoran	vancomycin
Balminil	dextromethorphan, pseudoephedrine
Ban-Tuss HC	hydrocodone
Banophen	diphenhydramine
Bantenol	mebendazole
Baraclude	entecavir
Barazan	norfloxacin
Barbilixir	phenobarbital
Barbita	phenobarbital
Barbital	phenobarbital
Barclyd	clonidine
Basaglar	insulin glargine
Basoquin	amodiaquine
Batrizol	co-trimoxazole
Baxan	cefadroxil
Baxo	piroxicam
Baygam	immune globulin IV
Baymycard	nisoldipine
BB	clindamycin
Beatryl	fentanyl
Becenun	carmustine
Beconase AQ	beclomethasone
Begrivac	influenza vaccine
Behapront	phentermine
Beleodaq	belinostat
Belladenal	atropine sulfate
Bellafill	collagen (bovine)
Bellergal-S	atropine sulfate
Beloc-Zoc	metoprolol
Belsomra	suvorexant
Belviq	lorcaserin
Benadryl	diphenhydramine, pseudoephedrine
Benahist	diphenhydramine
Benaxima	cefotaxime
Benaxona	ceftriaxone
Bencid	probenecid
Benecid	probenecid
Benhex Cream	lindane
Benicar	olmesartan
Benuryl	probenecid
Benylin	dextromethorphan, diphenhydramine
Benzaclin	clindamycin
Benzamin	cyclobenzaprine
Benzylpenicillin	penicillin G
Beriglobulin	immune globulin IV
Berkatens	verapamil
Berlthyrox	levothyroxine
Berubigen	cyanocobalamin
Bespar	buspirone
Beta-Adalat	atenolol
Beta-Cardone	sotalol
Betades	sotalol
Betaferon	interferon beta
Betaloc	metoprolol
Betanis	mirabegron
Betapace	sotalol
Betasept	chlorhexidine
Betaseron	interferon beta
Betazok	metoprolol
Betolvex	cyanocobalamin
Betoptic [Ophthalmic]	betaxolol
Betoptic S	betaxolol
Betoptima	betaxolol
Bex	aspirin
Bexsero	meningococcal group B vaccine
BG-12	dimethyl fumarate
Bi-Profenid	ketoprofen
Biaxin HP	clarithromycin
Biaxin	clarithromycin
Bicide	lindane
Biclin	amikacin
BiCNU	carmustine
Bidocef	cefadroxil
Biklin	amikacin
Biliepar	ursodiol
Bilim	tamoxifen
Biltricide	praziquantel
Bimaran	trazodone
Binocrit	epoetin alfa

Binosto	alendronate
Binotal	ampicillin
Bio E	vitamin E
Bio-Well	lindane
Biocet	cephalexin
Biocoryl	procainamide
Biofanal	nystatin
Biosint	cefotaxime
BioThrax	anthrax vaccine
Biozolene	fluconazole
Biron	buspirone
Bismatrol	bismuth
Bismuth Iodoform Paraffin Paste (BIPP)	bismuth
Bismuth subcitrate	bismuth
Bismuth subgallate	bismuth
Bismuth sucralfate	bismuth
Bleminol	allopurinol
Blenoxane	bleomycin
bleo	bleomycin
Bleocin	bleomycin
Bleomycine	bleomycin
Bleomycinum	bleomycin
Blephamide	prednisolone
Blincyto	blinatumomab
BLM	bleomycin
Blocan	cimetidine
Bobsule	hydroxyzine
Bocouture	botulinum toxin (A & B)
Bolutol	gemfibrozil
Bondronat	ibandronate
Boniva	ibandronate
Bonnox	promethazine
Bonzol	danazol
Botox	botulinum toxin (A & B)
Brek	loperamide
Brethine	terbutaline
Brevibloc	esmolol
Brevicon	oral contraceptives
Bricanyl	terbutaline
Bridion	sugammadex
Brilinta	ticagrelor
Brisdelle	paroxetine mesylate
Bristopen	oxacillin
Britiazem	diltiazem
Briviact	brivaracetam
Brocadopa	levodopa
Bromed	bromocriptine
Bromfed	pseudoephedrine
Broncho-Spray	albuterol
Bronitin	epinephrine
Bronkaid	epinephrine
Bronkodyl	aminophylline
Brothine	terbutaline
Brovana	arformoterol
Brufen	ibuprofen
Bucaril	terbutaline
Bufigen	nalbuphine
Busetal	disulfiram
Busirone	buspirone
BuSpar	buspirone
Bustab	buspirone
Butaline	terbutaline
Butibel	atropine sulfate
Bydureon	exenatide
Byetta	exenatide
Bystolic	nebivolol
Byvalson	nebivolol, valsartan

C

Caduet	amlodipine, atorvastatin
Calan	verapamil
Calcicard	diltiazem
calcidiol	calcifediol
Calcidrine	codeine
Calcilat	nifedipine
Calcilean	heparin
Calcimar	calcitonin
Calciparin	heparin
calcipotriene	calcipotriol
Calm-X	dimenhydrinate
Caltine	calcitonin
Calypsol	ketamine
Cambia	diclofenac
Camochin	amodiaquine
Camoquin	amodiaquine
Camoquinal	amodiaquine
Camptosar	irinotecan
Canasa	mesalamine
Cancidas	caspofungin
Candio-Hermal	nystatin
cannabis	marihuana
Caplenal	allopurinol
Capoten	captopril
Capozide	captopril, hydrochlorothiazide
Caprelsa	vandetanib
Caprilon	tranexamic acid
Caprin	aspirin, heparin
Captolane	captopril
Captoril	captopril
Carac	fluorouracil
Carace	lisinopril
Carafate	sucralfate
Carbatrol	carbamazepine
Carbex	selegiline
carbidopa	levodopa
Carbolith	lithium
Carbometyx	cabozantinib
Carboplat	carboplatin
Carbosap	anthrax vaccine
Carbosin	carboplatin
Carcinil	leuprolide
Cardem	celiprolol
Cardene	nicardipine
Cardicor	bisoprolol
Cardigox	digoxin
Cardine	quinidine
Cardiosteril	dopamine
Cardizem	diltiazem
Cardol	sotalol
Cardoxan	doxazosin
Cardoxin	dipyridamole
Cardular	doxazosin

Cardura	doxazosin
Carisoma	carisoprodol
Carmubris	carmustine
Cartia-XT	diltiazem
Casodex	bicalutamide
Cassadan	alprazolam
Cataflam	diclofenac
Catapres	clonidine
Catapresan	clonidine
Caved-S	bismuth
Caverject	alprostadil
CDDP	cisplatin
Cebenicol	chloramphenicol
Cebutid	flurbiprofen
CEC 500	cefaclor
Ceclor	cefaclor
Cedocard	isosorbide dinitrate
Cedrox	cefadroxil
Cefabiocin	cefaclor
cefalexin	cephalexin
Cefamox	cefadroxil
Cefaxim	cefotaxime
Cefaxona	ceftriaxone
Cefaxone	ceftriaxone
Ceforal	cephalexin
Cefotan	cefotetan
Cefotax	cefotaxime
Cefspan	cefixime
Ceftazim	ceftazidime
Ceftenon	cefotetan
Ceftin	cefuroxime
Cefuril	cefuroxime
Celebrex	celecoxib
Celectol	celiprolol
Celexa	citalopram
Celipres	celiprolol
Celipro	celiprolol
CellCept	mycophenolate
Cellmusin	estramustine
Celol	celiprolol
Celsentri	maraviroc
Celupan	naltrexone
Celvapan	pandemic influenza vaccine (H1N1)
Cemidon	isoniazid
Centedrin	methylphenidate
Cepan	cefotetan
Cepazine	cefuroxime
Cephoral	cefixime
Ceporex	cephalexin
Ceporexine	cephalexin
Ceptaz	ceftazidime
Cerdelga	eliglustat
Cerepax	temazepam
Certican	everolimus
Cerubidine	daunorubicin
Cervarix	human papillomavirus vaccine (bivalent)
Cervidel	dinoprostone
Cerviprime	dinoprostone
Cerviprost	dinoprostone
Cesamet	nabilone
Cetrine	cetirizine

Cetrotide	cetrorelix
Cezin	cetirizine
Champix	varenicline
Chantix	varenicline
Chemet	succimer
Cheracol-D	dextromethorphan
Cheracol	codeine
Chibro-Atropine	atropine sulfate
Chibroxin	norfloxacin
Chibroxine	norfloxacin
Chibroxol	norfloxacin
Chinine	quinine
Chlo-Amine	chlorpheniramine
Chlor-Pro	chlorpheniramine
Chlor-Trimeton	chlorpheniramine
Chlor-Tripolon	chlorpheniramine
Chloractil	chlorpromazine
Chloraldurat	chloral hydrate
Chlorate	chlorpheniramine
Chlorazin	chlorpromazine
Chlorhexamed	chlorhexidine
Chloroptic	chloramphenicol
chlorphenamine	chlorpheniramine
Chlorpromanyl	chlorpromazine
Chlorquin	chloroquine
Chol-Less	cholestyramine
Cholacid	ursodiol
Cholbam	cholic acid
Choledyl	aminophylline
Cholestagel	colesevelam
Cholit-Ursan	ursodiol
Cholofalk	ursodiol
Chronovera	verapamil
Cialis	tadalafil
Cibacalcine	calcitonin
Cibace	benazepril
Cibacen	benazepril
Cibacene	benazepril
Ciclosporin	cyclosporine
Cidomycin	gentamicin
Ciflox	ciprofloxacin
Cillimicina	lincomycin
Cillimycin	lincomycin
Ciloxan Ophthalmic	ciprofloxacin
Cimedine	cimetidine
Cimehexal	cimetidine
Cimogal	ciprofloxacin
Cimzia	certolizumab
Cin-Quin	quinidine
Cinqair	reslizumab
Ciplox	ciprofloxacin
Cipramil	citalopram
Cipro	ciprofloxacin
Ciprobay Uro	ciprofloxacin
Cipromycin	ciprofloxacin
Ciproxin	ciprofloxacin
Cisplatyl	cisplatin
Cisticid	praziquantel
Citanest	prilocaine
Citax	immune globulin IV
Citosulfan	busulfan

Citrec	leucovorin
citrovorum factor	leucovorin
Ciuk	cimetidine
Civeran	loratadine
Clacine	clarithromycin
Claforan	cefotaxime
Clamoxyl	amoxicillin
Claragine	aspirin
Claratyne	loratadine
Claravis	isotretinoin
Clarinex	desloratadine
Clarith	clarithromycin
Claritin-D	loratadine
Claritin	loratadine
Claritine	loratadine
Clarus	isotretinoin
Classen	mercaptopurine
Clasynar	calcitonin
Claversal	mesalamine
Cleocin-T	clindamycin
Cleocin	clindamycin
Cleridium	dipyridamole
Clexane	enoxaparin
Climara	estradiol
Clindacin	clindamycin
Clindagel	clindamycin
Clindets	clindamycin
Clinofem	medroxyprogesterone
Clinoril	sulindac
Cloben	cyclobenzaprine
Clofen	baclofen
Clofranil	clomipramine
Clonex	clonazepam
Clont	metronidazole
Clopress	clomipramine
Closerin	cycloserine
Closerina	cycloserine
Closin	promethazine
Clothia	hydrochlorothiazide
Clozaril	clozapine
club drug	MDMA
Coartem	artemether/lumefantrine
Cobex	cyanocobalamin
Cobutolin	albuterol
Codamine	hydrocodone
Codicept	codeine
Codiforton	codeine
Colazal	balsalazide
Colazide	balsalazide
ColBenemid	colchicine
Colchiquim	colchicine
Colcrys	colchicine
Coledos	ursodiol
Colestrol	cholestyramine
Colgout	colchicine
Colo-Fresh	bismuth
Colo-Pleon	sulfasalazine
Combivent	albuterol, ipratropium
Combivir	lamivudine, zidovudine
Cometriq	cabozantinib
Compazine	prochlorperazine
Complera	emtricitabine, tenofovir disoproxil
Compoz	diphenhydramine
Comtan	entacapone
Comtess	entacapone
Comvax	Hemophilus B vaccine, hepatitis B vaccine, influenza vaccine
Concerta	methylphenidate
Concor	bisoprolol
Consolan	nabumetone
Consupren	cyclosporine
Contalgin	morphine
Contigen	collagen (bovine)
Contramal	tramadol
Contrave	naltrexone
Convon	terbutaline
Copaxone	glatiramer
Copegus	ribavirin
copolymer-1	glatiramer
Coracten	nifedipine
Coradur	isosorbide dinitrate
Corax	chlordiazepoxide
Corbionax	amiodarone
Cordarex	amiodarone
Cordarone X	amiodarone
Cordarone	amiodarone
Cordes VAS	tretinoin
Cordiax	celiprolol
Cordilox	verapamil
Coreg	carvedilol
Corflene	flecainide
Corgard	nadolol
Coric	lisinopril
Coricidin D	aspirin
Corifam	rifampin
Corlanor	ivabradine
Corogal	nifedipine
Coronarine	dipyridamole
Corophyllin	aminophylline
Corotrend	nifedipine
Coroxin	dipyridamole
Corsodyl	chlorhexidine
Cortastat	dexamethasone
Cortone	cortisone
Cortosporin	neomycin
Corvert	ibutilide
Corzide	nadolol
Cosentyx	secukinumab
Cosmegen Lyovac	dactinomycin
Cosmegen	dactinomycin
Cosopt	dorzolamide
Cotellic	cobimetinib
Cotrim	co-trimoxazole
Coumadin	warfarin
Coumadine	warfarin
Covera-HS	verapamil
Coversum	perindopril
Coversyl	perindopril
Cozaar	losartan
CPM	cyclophosphamide
Cranoc	fluvastatin
Crasnitin	asparaginase

Cresemba	isavuconazonium sulfate
Crestor	rosuvastatin
Crixivan	indinavir
Cryocriptina	bromocriptine
Cryodoxin	sulfadoxine
Cryptaz	nitazoxanide
Crystamine	cyanocobalamin
Crystapen	penicillin G
Crysti-12	cyanocobalamin
CsA	cyclosporine
CTX	cyclophosphamide
Cubicin	daptomycin
Curantyl N	dipyridamole
Curretab	progestins
Cuvitru	immune globulin sc
Cuvposa	glycopyrrolate
CyA	cyclosporine
Cyanoject	cyanocobalamin
Cyben	cyclobenzaprine
Cycloblastin	cyclophosphamide
Cyclomen	danazol
Cyclomycin	cycloserine
Cyclorine	cycloserine
Cyclostin	cyclophosphamide
Cycosin	cycloserine
Cyklokapron	tranexamic acid
Cymbalta	duloxetine
Cynomel	liothyronine
Cyomin	cyanocobalamin
Cyramza	ramucirumab
Cystrin	oxybutynin
CYT	cyclophosphamide
Cytamen	cyanocobalamin
Cytarbel	cytarabine
Cytomel	liothyronine
Cytosar-U	cytarabine
Cytosar	cytarabine
Cytospaz	hyoscyamine
Cytotec	misoprostol
Cytoxan	cyclophosphamide

D

D-Amp	ampicillin
D-Penamine	penicillamine
D-Zol	danazol
D4T	stavudine
Dacatic	dacarbazine
Dacogen	decitabine
Dagan	nicardipine
Daipres	clonidine
Daklinza	daclatasvir
Daktarin	miconazole
Dalacin C	clindamycin
Dalacin	clindamycin
Dalacine	clindamycin
Daliresp	roflumilast
Dalisol	folic acid
Danocrine	danazol
Danol	danazol
Dantamacrin	dantrolene
Dantrium	dantrolene
Dantrolen	dantrolene
Daonil	glyburide
Dapa-tabs	indapamide
Dapatum D25	fluphenazine
Dapotum D	fluphenazine
Dapson-Fatol	dapsone
Dapson	dapsone
Daraprim	pyrimethamine
Darvocet-N	acetaminophen
Darvon Compound	aspirin
Darzalex	daratumumab
daunomycin	daunorubicin
DaunoXome	daunorubicin
Davedax	reboxetine
Davesol	lindane
Davitamon E	vitamin E
Daxas	roflumilast
Daypro	oxaprozin
Daytrana	methylphenidate
Dazamide	acetazolamide
DDAVP	desmopressin
ddC	zalcitabine
De-Nol	bismuth
Deca-Durabolin	nandrolone
Decadron	dexamethasone
Decentan	perphenazine
Deconsal	pseudoephedrine
Decrelip	gemfibrozil
Dedralen	doxazosin
Defanyl	amoxapine
Defiltran	acetazolamide
Defirin	desmopressin
Defitelio	defibrotide
Deflam	oxaprozin
Dehydrobenzperidol	droperidol
Delatest	testosterone
Delatestryl	testosterone
Delice	lindane
Delsym	dextromethorphan
Delta-Cortef	prednisolone
Delta-Lutin	progestins
Deltasone	prednisone
Deltazen	diltiazem
Delursan	ursodiol
Demadex	torsemide
Demerol	meperidine
Demolox	amoxapine
Demulen	oral contraceptives
Denan	simvastatin
Densul	methyldopa
Dentipatch	lidocaine
Denzapine	clozapine
Depacon	valproic acid
Depade	naltrexone
Depakene	valproic acid
Depakote	valproic acid
Depen	penicillamine
Depo-Provera	medroxyprogesterone
DepoCyt	cytarabine
Deprax	trazodone
deprenyl	selegiline

Derm A	tretinoin
DermaDeep	hyaluronic acid
DermaFlex	lidocaine
Dermairol	tretinoin
DermaLive	hyaluronic acid
Dermalogen	collagen (bovine)
Dermojuventus	tretinoin
Desconex	loxapine
Descovy	emtricitabine, tenofovir alafenamide
Deseril	methysergide
Desernil	methysergide
Deserril	methysergide
Deseryl	methysergide
Desferal	deferoxamine
Desferin	deferoxamine
Desirel	trazodone
Desmospray	desmopressin
Desocol	ursodiol
Desogen	oral contraceptives
Desoxil	ursodiol
Desoxyn	methamphetamine
Destolit	ursodiol
Desyrel	trazodone
Detensol	propranolol
Deticene	dacarbazine
Detimedac	dacarbazine
Detrol	tolterodine
Detulin	vitamin E
Deurcil	ursodiol
Devrom	bismuth
Dexacine	neomycin
Dexambutol	ethambutol
Dexamphetamine	dextroamphetamine
Dexamphetamini	dextroamphetamine
Dexedrine	dextroamphetamine
Dexilant	dexlansoprazole
Dexo	ursodiol
Dexone	dexamethasone
Dextrostat	dextroamphetamine
DHC-Continus	dihydrocodeine
Di-Hydran	phenytoin
Diabeta	glyburide
Diabex	metformin
diacetylmorphine	heroin
Diaformin	metformin
Dialar	diazepam
Diamox	acetazolamide
Diapax	diazepam
Diar-Aid	loperamide
Diarr-Eze	loperamide
Diarrol	triamterene
Diarstop-L	loperamide
Diastat	diazepam
Diatracin	vancomycin
Diazemuls	diazepam
Diazid	isoniazid
Dibloc	carvedilol
Diblocin	doxazosin
Dibrondrin	diphenhydramine
DIC	dacarbazine
Dichlotride	hydrochlorothiazide
Dicolmax	diclofenac
Dicumarol	dicumarol
Dicumol	dicumarol
dideoxycytidine	zalcitabine
Didronate	etidronate
Didronel	etidronate
Diflucan	fluconazole
Diformin	metformin
Difosfen	etidronate
Digacin	digoxin
Digoxine	digoxin
Dilacor XR	diltiazem
Dilanorm	celiprolol
Dilantin	phenytoin
Dilatrate-SR	isosorbide dinitrate
Dilatrend	carvedilol
Dilaudid-HP	hydromorphone
Dilaudid	hydromorphone
Dilocaine	lidocaine
Dilrene	diltiazem
Diltahexal	diltiazem
Diltia-XT	diltiazem
Dimetabs	dimenhydrinate
dimethyl (E) butenedioate	dimethyl fumarate
Diminex	phentermine
Dimitone	carvedilol
Dimodan	disopyramide
Dinol	etidronate
Diocarpine	pilocarpine
Diochloram	chloramphenicol
Diogent	gentamicin
Dionephrine	phenylephrine
Diotame	bismuth
Diovan HCT	hydrochlorothiazide, valsartan
Diovan	valsartan
Diphenylan	phenytoin
diphenylhydantoin	phenytoin
Diphos	etidronate
Dipridacot	dipyridamole
Diprivan	propofol
Diram	spironolactone
Dirythmin SA	disopyramide
Disalgesic	salsalate
Discoid	furosemide
Disonorm	disopyramide
Disprin	aspirin
Distaclor	cefaclor
Distamine	penicillamine
Distocide	praziquantel
Ditropan	oxybutynin
Diu-Melsin	hydrochlorothiazide
Diuchlor H	hydrochlorothiazide
Diuramid	acetazolamide
Diuteren	triamterene
divalproex	valproic acid
Divigel	estradiol
Dixarit	clonidine
Dizac	diazepam
DMSA	succimer
DNR	daunorubicin
Dobetin	cyanocobalamin

Doblexan	piroxicam
Dolac	ketorolac
Dolantin	meperidine
Dolce	vitamin A
Dolestan	diphenhydramine
Dolestine	meperidine
Dolophine	methadone
Dolosal	meperidine
Dom-Baclofen	baclofen
Dom-Fluoxetine	fluoxetine
Domical	amitriptyline
Doneurin	doxepin
Donnagel	atropine sulfate
Donnamar	hyoscyamine
Donnatal	atropine sulfate
Donnazyme	atropine sulfate
Dopaflex	levodopa
Dopamet	methyldopa
Dopamin AWD	dopamine
Dopamin	dopamine
Doparl	levodopa
Dopastat	dopamine
Dormicum	midazolam
Doryx	doxycycline
Dostinex	cabergoline
Dovonex	calcipotriol
Doxil	doxorubicin
Doximed	doxycycline
Doxy-100	doxycycline
Doxycin	doxycycline
Doxytec	doxycycline
Dozic	haloperidol
DPH	phenytoin
Dramamine	dimenhydrinate
Dridase	oxybutynin
Drogenil	flutamide
Droleptan	droperidol
Droperidol	droperidol
Droxia	hydroxyurea
Droxine	levothyroxine
Dryptal	furosemide
Dryvax	smallpox vaccine
DTIC-Dome	dacarbazine
DTIC	dacarbazine
Duboisine	hyoscyamine
Ducene	diazepam
Duexis	famotidine
Dulera	formoterol
Dumirox	fluvoxamine
Dumyrox	fluvoxamine
Dunate	artesunate
Duoneb	albuterol, ipratropium
Duopa	levodopa
Dura-Vent	phenylephrine
Duracef	cefadroxil
Duraclon	clonidine
Duragesic	fentanyl
Duralith	lithium
Duralutin	progestins
Durametacin	indomethacin
Duramorph	morphine
Duraperidol	haloperidol
Duraprox	oxaprozin
Durater	famotidine
Duratest	testosterone
Duratuss	hydrocodone
Durazepam	oxazepam
Durazolam	lorazepam
Durbis	disopyramide
Duricef	cefadroxil
Durlaza	aspirin
Dyazide	hydrochlorothiazide, triamterene
Dyloject	diclofenac
Dymenalgit	naproxen
Dyna-Hex	chlorhexidine
Dynacil	fosinopril
Dynacin	minocycline
Dynacirc SRO	isradipine
DynaCirc	isradipine
Dynatra	dopamine
Dyrenium	triamterene
Dysman	mefenamic acid
Dyspamet	cimetidine
Dysport	botulinum toxin (A & B)
Dytac	triamterene

E

E Perle	vitamin E
E-Mycin	erythromycin
E-Pam	diazepam
E-Vitamin Succinate	vitamin E
E102	tartrazine
E	MDMA
Ebixa	memantine
Ebufac	ibuprofen
Ecalta	anidulafungin
Ecomucyl	acetylcysteine
Ecotrin	aspirin
Ecridoxan	etodolac
ecstasy	MDMA
Ectaprim	co-trimoxazole
Ectasule	ephedrine
ED-SPAZ	hyoscyamine
Edenol	furosemide
Edex	alprostadil
Edisylate	prochlorperazine
Edolan	etodolac
Edronax	reboxetine
EES	erythromycin
Efedron	ephedrine
Eferox	levothyroxine
Effexor XL	venlafaxine
Effexor	venlafaxine
Effient	prasugrel
Efracea	doxycycline
Efudex	fluorouracil
Efudix	fluorouracil
Efurix	fluorouracil
Egacene Durettes	hyoscyamine
Egazil	hyoscyamine
ELA-Max	lidocaine
Elavil	amitriptyline

Eldeprine	selegiline
Eldepryl	selegiline
Elderin	etodolac
Eldopal	levodopa
Elentol	lindane
Elepsia XR	levetiracetam
Elestrin	estradiol
Elidel	pimecrolimus
Eligard	leuprolide
Eliquis	apixaban
Elisor	pravastatin
Elixophyllin	aminophylline
Ellence	epirubicin
Elobact	cefuroxime
Eloctate	antihemophilic factor
Elorgan	pentoxifylline
Eloxatin	oxaliplatin
Elspar	asparaginase
Eltor 120	pseudoephedrine
Eltroxin	levothyroxine
EMB	ethambutol
Embolin	dicumarol
Emcor	bisoprolol
Emcyt	estramustine
Emend	aprepitant
Emeset	ondansetron
Emeside	ethosuximide
EMLA	lidocaine
Emorhalt	tranexamic acid
Empirin	aspirin
Empliciti	elotuzumab
Emquin	chloroquine
Emsam	selegiline
Emselex	darifenacin
Emtriva	emtricitabine
Enablex	darifenacin
Enaladil	enalapril
Enantone	leuprolide
Enapren	enalapril
Enarmon	methyltestosterone
Enbrel	etanercept
Encore	acetylcysteine
Endeavor	zotarolimus
Endep	amitriptyline
Endobulin	immune globulin IV
Endocodone	oxycodone
Endoxan	cyclophosphamide
Endoxana	cyclophosphamide
Ener-B	cyanocobalamin
Engerix B	hepatitis B vaccine
Entex HC	hydrocodone
Entex	pseudoephedrine
Entresto	sacubitril/valsartan
Entumin	clozapine
Entumine	clozapine
Entyvio	vedolizumab
Envarsus XR	tacrolimus
Epanutin	phenytoin
Epaxal	hepatitis A vaccine
Epclusa	sofosbuvir & velpatasvir
Ephedsol	ephedrine
Ephynal	vitamin E
Epi E-Z Pen	epinephrine
Epi-Aberel	tretinoin
Epifrin	epinephrine
Epimorph	morphine
Epipen	epinephrine
Epitol	carbamazepine
Epivir	lamivudine
EPO	epoetin alfa
Epogen	epoetin alfa
Epoxitin	epoetin alfa
Eppy	epinephrine
Eppystabil	epinephrine
Eprex	epoetin alfa
Eprolin	vitamin E
Eptadone	methadone
Epzicom	abacavir, lamivudine
Equagesic	aspirin
Equibar	methyldopa
Eramycin	erythromycin
Eraxis	anidulafungin
Erbaprelina	pyrimethamine
Erbitux	cetuximab
Ercar	carboplatin
Ercoquin	hydroxychloroquine
Erelzi	etanercept
Ergomar	ergotamine
Ergometrine	ergometrine
Ergostat	ergotamine
Erivedge	vismodegib
Ery-Ped	erythromycin
Ery-Tab	erythromycin
Eryc	erythromycin
Erypar	erythromycin
Erypo	epoetin alfa
Erythrocin	erythromycin
erythropoiesis stimulating protein	darbepoetin alfa
erythropoietin	epoetin alfa
Eryzole	erythromycin
Esbriet	pirfenidone
Esclim	estradiol
eserine	physostigmine
Esidrex	hydrochlorothiazide
Eskalith	lithium
Esmino	chlorpromazine
Esperal	disulfiram
Estazor	ursodiol
Esteprim	co-trimoxazole
Estrace	estradiol
Estraderm	estradiol
Estratest	methyltestosterone
Estring	estradiol
Estrogel	estradiol
Estrostep	oral contraceptives
Etapiam	ethambutol
Ethymal	ethosuximide
Etibi	ethambutol
Etopos	etoposide
Etosid	etoposide
Etrafon	perphenazine
Eudigox	digoxin

Eudyna	tretinoin
Euflex	flutamide
Euflexxa	hyaluronic acid
Euglucan	glyburide
Euglucon	glyburide
Euhypnos	temazepam
Eulexin	flutamide
Eulexine	flutamide
Eupen	amoxicillin
Euphyllin	aminophylline
Evamist	estradiol
Evista	raloxifene
Evitocor	atenolol
Evomela	melphalan
Evotaz	atazanavir
Evoxac	cevimeline
Evra	oral contraceptives
Evzio	naloxone
Exacyl	tranexamic acid
Exalgo	hydromorphone
Excedrin	acetaminophen, aspirin
Exelon	rivastigmine
Exforge	amlodipine, valsartan
Exidine Scrub	chlorhexidine
Exjade	deferasirox
Exocine	ofloxacin
Exodus	nicotine
Exomuc	acetylcysteine
Extavia	interferon beta
Eylea	aflibercept
Ezetrol	ezetimibe

F

Fabior	tazarotene
Fabrol	acetylcysteine
Falciquin	artesunate
Famodil	famotidine
Famoxal	famotidine
Famvir	famciclovir
Fanapt	iloperidone
Fansidar	pyrimethamine, sulfadoxine
Fareston	toremifene
Farmablastina	doxorubicin
Farmagard	nadolol
Farxiga	dapagliflozin
Farydak	panobinostat
Faverin	fluvoxamine
Favoxil	fluvoxamine
FazaClo	clozapine
FD&C yellow No.5	tartrazine
Felden	piroxicam
Feldene	piroxicam
Femara	letrozole
Fempatch	estradiol
Fenac	diclofenac
Fentanest	fentanyl
Fentazin	perphenazine
Fenytoin	phenytoin
Feraheme	ferumoxytol
Ferndex	dextroamphetamine
Ferriprox	deferiprone
Fetzima	levomilnacipran
Fevarin	fluvoxamine
Fexmid	cyclobenzaprine
Fibrel	collagen (bovine)
Fibrocit	gemfibrozil
Fiorinal	aspirin
fisalamine	mesalamine
Fisamox	amoxicillin
Fixime	cefixime
Flagyl	metronidazole
Flanax	naproxen
Flavoquin	amodiaquine
Flecaine	flecainide
Flector Patch	diclofenac
Flexeril	cyclobenzaprine
Flexiban	cyclobenzaprine
Flexitec	cyclobenzaprine
Flobasin	ofloxacin
Flodine	folic acid
Flolan	epoprostenol
Flomax	tamsulosin
Florazole	metronidazole
Florid	miconazole
Floxan	ofloxacin
Floxil	ofloxacin
Floxin	ofloxacin
Floxstat	ofloxacin
Fluad	influenza vaccine
Fluarix	influenza vaccine
Flucazol	fluconazole
Flucinom	flutamide
Fluctin	fluoxetine
Fluctine	fluoxetine
Fludac	fluoxetine
Fludara	fludarabine
Fludecate	fluphenazine
Fludex	indapamide
Fluimucil	acetylcysteine
Flukacide	praziquantel
Fluken	flutamide
Flukezol	fluconazole
Flulem	flutamide
FluMist	influenza vaccine
Fluorophosphate	fluorides
Fluoroplex	fluorouracil
Fluorouracil Injection, USP	fluorouracil
Fluoxac	fluoxetine
Fluoxeren	fluoxetine
Flurix	influenza vaccine
Flurofen	flurbiprofen
Flurozin	flurbiprofen
Fluviral	influenza vaccine
Fluxil	fluoxetine
Fluzone	fluconazole, influenza vaccine
Focalin	dexmethylphenidate
Focetria	pandemic influenza vaccine (H1N1)
folacin	folic acid
folate	folic acid
Folina	folic acid
folinic acid	leucovorin
Folinsyre	folic acid

Folitab	folic acid
Folsan	folic acid
Fontex	fluoxetine
Foradil	formoterol
Formula-Q	quinine
Forsteo	teriparatide
Fortamet	metformin
Fortaz	ceftazidime
Forteo	teriparatide
Fortesta	testosterone
Fortipine	nifedipine
Fortum	ceftazidime
Forvade	cidofovir
Fosalan	alendronate
Fosamax	alendronate
Fosinorm	fosinopril
Foxsalepsin	carbamazepine
Fozitec	fosinopril
Fragmin	dalteparin
Fragmine	dalteparin
Fraurs	ursodiol
Frenal	pimozide
Froben	flurbiprofen
Froxal	cefuroxime
Frusid	furosemide
Fugerel	flutamide
Fulcin	griseofulvin
Fulvicin	griseofulvin
Fulvina P/G	griseofulvin
Fulyzaq	crofelemer
Fumaderm	dimethyl fumarate
Funcort	miconazole
Fungarest	ketoconazole
Fungata	fluconazole
Fungilin	amphotericin B
Fungizone	amphotericin B
Fungoid Tincture	miconazole
Fungoral	ketoconazole
Furadantin	nitrofurantoin
Furadantina	nitrofurantoin
Furadoine	nitrofurantoin
Furalan	nitrofurantoin
Furan	nitrofurantoin
Furobactina	nitrofurantoin
Furorese	furosemide
Furoside	furosemide
Fusid	furosemide
Fuzeon	enfuvirtide
Fycompa	perampanel

G

G-Well	lindane
GAB	lindane
Gabbroral	paromomycin
Gabitril	tiagabine
Gablofen	baclofen
Gabrilen Retard	ketoprofen
Gabroral	paromomycin
Galecin	clindamycin
Galedol	diclofenac
Galmax	ursodiol

Gamabenceno	lindane
Gamafine	immune globulin IV
Gamastan	immune globulin IV
Gambex	lindane
Gamene	lindane
Gamikal	amikacin
Gamimune	immune globulin IV
Gamma 16	immune globulin IV
gamma benzene hexachloride	lindane
Gammabulin	immune globulin IV
Gammagard	immune globulin IV
Gammalin	lindane
Gammar PIV	immune globulin IV
Gammer-IV	immune globulin IV
Gammonayiv	immune globulin IV
Gamunex	immune globulin IV
Ganor	famotidine
Garamycin	gentamicin
Garatec	gentamicin
Gardasil	human papillomavirus (HPV) vaccine
Gardenal	phenobarbital
Gastro	famotidine
Gastrodyn	glycopyrrolate
Gastroloc	omeprazole
Gastrosed	hyoscyamine
Gattex	teduglutide
Gazyva	obinutuzumab
GBH	lindane
Geangin	verapamil
Gelnique	oxybutynin
Gelprin	aspirin
Geluprane	acetaminophen
Gemicina	neomycin
Gemlipid	gemfibrozil
Gemzar	gemcitabine
Gen-Baclofen	baclofen
Gen-Fibro	gemfibrozil
Gen-Metformin	metformin
Gen-XENE	clorazepate
Genabid	papaverine
Genahist	diphenhydramine
Genin	quinine
Genoptic	gentamicin
Genora	oral contraceptives
Genoxal	cyclophosphamide
Genpril	ibuprofen
Gentacidin	gentamicin
Gentalline	gentamicin
Gentalol	gentamicin
Genvoya	cobicistat/elvitegravir/emtricitabine/tenofovir alafenamide
Geodon	ziprasidone
Geroxalen	methoxsalen
Gestapuran	medroxyprogesterone
Gesterol 50	progestins
Gevilon Uno	gemfibrozil
Gilenya	fingolimod
Gilex	doxepin
Gilotrif	afatinib
Glatopa	glatiramer
Gleevec	imatinib

Gliadel Wafer	carmustine
glibenclamide	glyburide
Glibenese	glipizide
Glimel	glyburide
Glioten	enalapril
Glipid	glipizide
Glivec	imatinib
Glucagon Emergency Kit	glucagon
Glucal	glyburide
Glucomet	metformin
Glucophage	metformin
Glucotrol	glipizide
Glucovance	glyburide, metformin
Gluquine	quinidine
glybenclamide	glyburide
glyceryl trinitrate	nitroglycerin
glycopyrronium bromide	glycopyrrolate
Glyde	glipizide
Glynase	glyburide
Glypressin	terlipressin
Glyxambi	empagliflozin, linagliptin
GoNitro	nitroglycerin
Goodnight	promethazine
Gopten	trandolapril
Goutnil	colchicine
Gralise	gabapentin
grass	marihuana
Green-Alpha	interferon alfa
Grifulvin V	griseofulvin
Gris-PEG	griseofulvin
Grisefuline	griseofulvin
Griseostatin	griseofulvin
Grisovin	griseofulvin
Guiatuss AC	codeine
Gynodiol	estradiol

H

Habitrol Patch	nicotine
Haemiton	clonidine
Haemopressin	terlipressin
Hairgaine	minoxidil
Halaven	eribulin
Haldol	haloperidol
Halfprin	aspirin
Haloper	haloperidol
Halotussin	codeine
Haltran	ibuprofen
Hamarin	allopurinol
Harkoseride	lacosamide
Harvoni	ledipasvir & sofosbuvir
hashish	marihuana
Havrix	hepatitis A vaccine
Heitrin	terazosin
Helidac	bismuth
Heliopar	chloroquine
Helminzole	mebendazole
Heloxatin	oxaliplatin
Hemangeol	propranolol
Hemi-Daonil	glyburide
Hemovas	pentoxifylline
Henexal	furosemide
Hep-Flush	heparin
Hep-Lock	heparin
Hepalean	heparin
Heparin-Leo	heparin
Heparine	heparin
Hepsera	adefovir
Herceptin	trastuzumab
Herklin	lindane
Heroin	heroin
Herpefug	acyclovir
Hetlioz	tasimelteon
hexachlorocyclohexane	lindane
Hexadrol	dexamethasone
Hexicid	lindane
Hexit	lindane
Hexol	chlorhexidine
Hibiclens	chlorhexidine
Hibident	chlorhexidine
Hibidil	chlorhexidine
Hibiscrub	chlorhexidine
Hibistat	chlorhexidine
Hibitane	chlorhexidine
HibMenCY	meningococcal groups C & Y & Haemophilus B tetanus toxoid conjugate vaccine
HibTITER	Hemophilus B vaccine
Histantil	promethazine
Hitrin	terazosin
Hivid	zalcitabine
Hizentra	immune globulin sc
Holoxan	ifosfamide
Horizant	gabapentin
HPV4	human papillomavirus (HPV) vaccine
Huberplex	chlordiazepoxide
Humagel	paromomycin
Humatin	paromomycin
Humira	adalimumab
Hyalgan	hyaluronic acid
hyaluronidase	hyaluronic acid
Hybloc	labetalol
Hycamtin	topotecan
Hyco	hyoscyamine
Hycosol Sl	hyoscyamine
Hycotuss	hydrocodone
Hydeltrasol	prednisolone
Hydopa	methyldopa
Hydrea	hydroxyurea
Hydrogen fluoride [HF]	fluorides
Hydromet	hydrocodone
Hydrosaluric	hydrochlorothiazide
HydroStat IR	hydromorphone
hydroxycarbamide	hydroxyurea
hydroxydaunomycin	doxorubicin
Hylaform	hyaluronic acid
Hylan G-F 20	hyaluronic acid
Hylutin	progestins
Hynorex Retard	lithium
Hyospaz	hyoscyamine
Hypolar	nifedipine
Hysingla ER	hydrocodone
Hytrin	terazosin
Hytrine	terazosin

Hytrinex	terazosin
Hyzaar	hydrochlorothiazide, losartan

I

IB-Stat	hyoscyamine
ibandronic acid	ibandronate
Ibrance	palbociclib
Idamycin	idarubicin
Idotrim	trimethoprim
Ifex	ifosfamide
IFN	interferon alfa
Ifoxan	ifosfamide
IG Gamma	immune globulin IV
IGIM	immune globulin IV
IGIV	immune globulin IV
Iktorivil	clonazepam
IL-2	aldesleukin
Ilaris	canakinumab
Ilosone	erythromycin
Ilotycin	erythromycin
Imbrilon	indomethacin
Imbruvica	ibrutinib
Imdur	isosorbide mononitrate
Imidol	imipramine
Imigran	sumatriptan
Imipramin	imipramine
Imitrex	sumatriptan
Imlygic	talimogene laherparepvec
Imodium	loperamide
Imossel	loperamide
Imovane	eszopiclone
Imovax	influenza vaccine
Implanta	cyclosporine
Impril	imipramine
Imuprin	azathioprine
Imuran	azathioprine
Imurek	azathioprine
Imurel	azathioprine
Inapsin	droperidol
Inapsine	droperidol
Incivek	telaprevir
Incruse	umeclidinium
Inderal LA	propranolol
Inderal	propranolol
Inderide	hydrochlorothiazide
Indochron	indomethacin
Indocin	indomethacin
Indolar SR	indomethacin
indometacin	indomethacin
Indotec	indomethacin
Inegy	simvastatin
INF	interferon alfa
Infergen	interferon alfa
Inflamase	prednisolone
Inflectra	infliximab
Inflexal V	influenza vaccine
Influsome	influenza vaccine
Infumorph	morphine
Infurin	nitrofurantoin
INH	isoniazid
Inhibitron	omeprazole
Inlyta	axitinib
Innofem	estradiol
Innohep	tinzaparin
Innopran XL	propranolol
Innovace	enalapril
Insomnal	diphenhydramine
Integrex	reboxetine
Integrilin	eptifibatide
Intelence	etravirine
Intercon	oral contraceptives
Interglobin	immune globulin IV
interleukin-2	aldesleukin
Intron A	interferon alfa
Introna	interferon alfa
Introne	interferon alfa
Intropin	dopamine
Invanz	ertapenem
Invega	paliperidone
Invirase	saquinavir
Invivac	influenza vaccine
Invokamet	canagliflozin, metformin
Invokana	canagliflozin
Ionamin	phentermine
Iopidine	apraclonidine
Ipamix	indapamide
Ipolab	labetalol
Ipral	trimethoprim
Ipratropium Steri-Neb	ipratropium
Iquix	levofloxacin
Iremofar	hydroxyzine
Irenor	reboxetine
Iressa	gefitinib
Isavuconazole	isavuconazonium sulfate
Isentress	raltegravir
Ismipur	mercaptopurine
Ismo	isosorbide mononitrate
Ismotic	isosorbide
Isobac	co-trimoxazole
Isoptin	verapamil
Isoptine	verapamil
Isopto Atropine	atropine sulfate
Isopto Eserine	physostigmine
Isopto Pilocarpine	pilocarpine
Isopto-Epinal	epinephrine
Isopto	atropine sulfate
Isordil	isosorbide dinitrate
Isorythm	disopyramide
Isotamine	isoniazid
Isotrex	isotretinoin
Isox	itraconazole
Isozid	isoniazid
Istin	amlodipine
Istodax	romidepsin
Istubol	tamoxifen
Italnik	ciprofloxacin
Itranax	itraconazole
Itrin	terazosin
IV Globulin-S	immune globulin IV
Iveegam	immune globulin IV
IVIG	immune globulin IV
Ixiaro	Japanese encepahlitis vaccine

Izba	travoprost

J

Jacutin	lindane
Jadelle	levonorgestrel
Jadenu	deferasirox
Jalyn	dutasteride, tamsulosin
Janumet	metformin, sitagliptin
Januvia	sitagliptin
Jardiance	empagliflozin
Jenamicin	gentamicin
Jetrea	ocriplasmin
Jezil	gemfibrozil
Jodatum	potassium iodide
Jodid	potassium iodide
Jublia	efinaconazole
Jumex	selegiline
Jurnista	hydromorphone
Juvederm	hyaluronic acid
Juxtapid	lomitapide

K

Kabikinase	streptokinase
Kadcyla	ado-trastuzumab emtansine
Kadian	morphine
Kalcide	praziquantel
Kaletra	lopinavir, ritonavir
Kalium	potassium iodide
Kallmiren	buspirone
Kalma	alprazolam
Kalten	atenolol
Kaluril	amiloride
Kalydeco	ivacaftor
Kanamicina	kanamycin
Kanamycine	kanamycin
Kanamytrex	kanamycin
Kanbine	amikacin
Kanescin	kanamycin
Kannasyn	kanamycin
Kantrex	kanamycin
Kanuma	sebelipase alfa
Kaywan	phytonadione
Kcentra	prothrombin complex concentrate (human)
Keduril	ketoprofen
Kefarol	cephalexin
Keflex	cephalexin
Kefolor	cefaclor
Keftab	cephalexin
Kelac	ketorolac
Kelatin	penicillamine
Kenaprol	metoprolol
Kengreal	cangrelor
Kenzoflex	ciprofloxacin
Kepivance	palifermin
Keppra	levetiracetam
Kerlon	betaxolol
Kerlone	betaxolol
Kerydin	tavaborole
Kessar	tamoxifen
Ketalar	ketamine
Ketalin	ketamine
Ketanest	ketamine
Ketoderm	ketoconazole
Ketoisidin	ketoconazole
Ketolar	ketamine
Ketonic	ketorolac
Keytruda	pembrolizumab
Khedezla	desvenlafaxine
KI	potassium iodide
Kidrolase	asparaginase
Kie	potassium iodide
Kildane	lindane
Kineret	anakinra
Kinidin	quinidine
Klacid	clarithromycin
Klaricid	clarithromycin
Klexane	enoxaparin
Klonopin	clonazepam
Kloramfenicol	chloramphenicol
Klozapol	clozapine
Kodapan	carbamazepine
Koffex	dextromethorphan
Kolkicin	colchicine
Konakion	phytonadione
Konicine	colchicine
Korec	quinapril
Korlym	mifepristone
Kovaltry	antihemophilic factor
KP-E	dinoprostone
Kredex	carvedilol
Krenosin	adenosine
Krenosine	adenosine
Kripton	bromocriptine
Krystexxa	pegloticase
Kwell	lindane
Kwildane	lindane
Kybella	deoxycholic acid
Kyleena	levonorgestrel
Kyprolis	carfilzomib

L

L-asparaginase	asparaginase
L-Cysteine	acetylcysteine
L-deprenyl	selegiline
L-dopa	levodopa
L-DOPS	droxidopa
L-Gent	gentamicin
L-Polamidon	methadone
L-thyroxine sodium	levothyroxine
Labrocol	labetalol
Ladogal	danazol
Lagaquin	chloroquine
lambrolizumab	pembrolizumab
Lamictal	lamotrigine
Lamisil	terbinafine
Lamocot	diphenoxylate
Landsen	clonazepam
Lanicor	digoxin
Lanoxin	digoxin
Lantarel	methotrexate
Lantus	insulin glargine

Lapole	flurbiprofen
Laraflex	naproxen
Larapam	piroxicam
Largactil	chlorpromazine
Lariam	mefloquine
Laricam	mefloquine
Laroferon	interferon alfa
Laroxyl	amitriptyline
Lartruvo	olaratumab
Lasilix	furosemide
Lasix	furosemide
Laspar	asparaginase
Lastet	etoposide
Latisse	bimatoprost
Latuda	lurasidone
Laubeel	lorazepam
LCZ696	sacubitril/valsartan
Lebic	baclofen
Lederfolin	leucovorin
Ledertrexate	methotrexate
Ledoxina	cyclophosphamide
Lenal	temazepam
Lencid	lindane
Lenoxin	digoxin
Lentizol	amitriptyline
Lentorsil	ursodiol
Lenvima	lenvatinib
Leponex	clozapine
Leptanal	fentanyl
Leptopsique	perphenazine
Lescol	fluvastatin
Letairis	ambrisentan
Leucovorin	leucovorin
Leukerin	mercaptopurine
Leukosulfan	busulfan
Leunase	asparaginase
Leuprorelin	leuprolide
Leustatin	cladribine
Levanxene	temazepam
Levaquin	levofloxacin
Levate	amitriptyline
Levbid	hyoscyamine
Levemir	insulin detemir
Levitra	vardenafil
Levlen	oral contraceptives
Levlite	oral contraceptives
Levo-T	levothyroxine
Levodopa-Woelm	levodopa
Levora	oral contraceptives
Levothyroid	levothyroxine
Levothyrox	levothyroxine
Levoxyl	levothyroxine
Levsin/SL	hyoscyamine
Levsin	hyoscyamine
Levsinex	hyoscyamine
Lexapro	escitalopram
Lexin	carbamazepine
Lexinor	norfloxacin
Lexiva	fosamprenavir
Lexpec	folic acid
Lexxel	enalapril
Lialda	mesalamine
Libritabs	chlordiazepoxide
Librium	chlordiazepoxide
Lidaprim	trimethoprim
Lidifen	ibuprofen
Lidodan	lidocaine
Lidoderm	lidocaine
Lidoject-2	lidocaine
Lifaton B_{12}	cyanocobalamin
lignocaine	lidocaine
Likudin M	griseofulvin
Limbitrol	amitriptyline, chlordiazepoxide
Lin-Amnox	amoxicillin
Lincocin	lincomycin
Lincocine	lincomycin
Linzess	linaclotide
Liocarpina	pilocarpine
Lioresal	baclofen
Lipex	simvastatin
Lipitor	atorvastatin
Liponorm	simvastatin
Lipostat	pravastatin
Liptruzet	atorvastatin, ezetimibe
Lipur	gemfibrozil
Liquemin	heparin
Liquiprin	acetaminophen
Liroken	diclofenac
Lisino	loratadine
Lismol	cholestyramine
Litalir	hydroxyurea
Litanin	ursodiol
Lithicarb	lithium
Lithizine	lithium
Lithobid	lithium
Lithonate	lithium
Lithotabs	lithium
Litocure	ursodiol
Litoff	ursodiol
Litursol	ursodiol
Livalo	pitavastatin
Lo/Ovral	oral contraceptives
Locion-V	lindane
Locol	fluvastatin
Lodales	simvastatin
Lodimol	dipyridamole
Lodine	etodolac
Lodosyn	carbidopa
Loestrin	oral contraceptives
Lofene	atropine sulfate, diphenoxylate
Logastric	omeprazole
Logen	atropine sulfate, diphenoxylate
Lomaira	phentermine
Lomanate	atropine sulfate, diphenoxylate
Lomarin	dimenhydrinate
Lomir SRO	isradipine
Lomir	isradipine
Lomotil	atropine sulfate, diphenoxylate
Lomper	mebendazole
Lonazep	clonazepam
Lonine	etodolac
Loniten	minoxidil

Lonolox	minoxidil
Lonoten	minoxidil
Lonox	diphenoxylate
Lonsurf	trifluridine & tipiracil
Lop-Dia	loperamide
Loperhoe	loperamide
Lopid	gemfibrozil
Lopirin	captopril
Lopressor	hydrochlorothiazide, metoprolol
Lopril	captopril
Lorastine	loratadine
Lorcet	acetaminophen
Lorexane	lindane
Lortab	hydrocodone
Losec	omeprazole
Lotensin HCT	benazepril, hydrochlorothiazide
Lotensin	benazepril, hydrochlorothiazide
Lotrel	amlodipine, benazepril
Lovalip	lovastatin
Lovenox	enoxaparin
Low-Quel	diphenoxylate
Loxapac	loxapine
Loxen	nicardipine
Loxitane	loxapine
Lozapin	clozapine
Lozide	indapamide
Lozol	indapamide
Lucassin	terlipressin
Lucentis	ranibizumab
Lucrin	leuprolide
Lugol's solution	potassium iodide
Lukadin	amikacin
Lumigan	bimatoprost
Luminal	phenobarbital
Luminaletten	phenobarbital
Lunelle	medroxyprogesterone, oral contraceptives
Lunesta	eszopiclone
Lupron Depot-Ped	leuprolide
Lupron	leuprolide
Lustra	hydroquinone
Luvox	fluvoxamine
Luzu	luliconazole
Lyeton	ursodiol
Lynparza	olaparib
Lyovac	dactinomycin
Lyple	alprostadil
Lyrica	pregabalin
Lyrinel	oxybutynin
Lysalgo	mefenamic acid
Lysatec rt-PA	alteplase
Lyxumia	lixisenatide

M

M-KYA	quinine
M-M-R II	measles, mumps & rubella (MMR) virus vaccine
Maalox Anti-Diarrheal	loperamide
Maalox	loperamide
Mablin	busulfan
MabThera	rituximab
Macladin	clarithromycin
Macrobid	nitrofurantoin
Macrodantin	nitrofurantoin
Macugen	pegaptanib
Malarivon	chloroquine
Malarone	atovaquone/proguanil
Malocide	pyrimethamine, sulfadoxine
Maloprim	dapsone
Mamofen	tamoxifen
Mapap	acetaminophen
Marax	ephedrine, hydroxyzine
Marcillin	ampicillin
Mareen	doxepin
Marevan	warfarin
marijuana	marihuana
Marinol	dronabinol
Marmine	dimenhydrinate
Marthritic	salsalate
Masmoran	hydroxyzine
Maveral	fluvoxamine
Mavik	trandolapril
Maxalt	rizatriptan
Maxcef	cefepime
Maxidone	hydrocodone
Maxiphed	pseudoephedrine
Maxipime	cefepime
Maxitrol	neomycin
Maxtrex	methotrexate
Maxzide	hydrochlorothiazide, triamterene
Mazepine	carbamazepine
Measurin	aspirin
Mebensole	mebendazole
Med-Glibe	glyburide
Medamor	amiloride
Medianox	chloral hydrate
MedihalerEpi	epinephrine
Medilium	chlordiazepoxide
Medimet	methyldopa
Medipren	ibuprofen
Medispaz	hyoscyamine
Medrol	methylprednisolone
Mefac	mefenamic acid
Mefic	mefenamic acid
Megace	progestins
Megacillin	penicillin G
Mekinist	trametinib
Meladinine	methoxsalen
Melizide	glipizide
Menabol	stanozolol
Menhibrix	meningococcal groups C & Y & Haemophilus B tetanus toxoid conjugate vaccine
Menostar	estradiol
mepacrine	quinacrine
Mephaquin	mefloquine
Mephaquine	mefloquine
Mephenon	methadone
Mephyton	phytonadione
Merabis	spironolactone
Merlit	lorazepam
Meronem	meropenem
Merrem IV	meropenem
mesalazine	mesalamine
Mesasal	mesalamine

Mestacine	minocycline
Mestatin	nystatin
Mestinon	pyridostigmine
Metadate CD	methylphenidate
Metadon	methadone
Metaglip	glipizide, metformin
Metandren	methyltestosterone
Metex	methotrexate
Metforal	metformin
Methadose	methadone
Methipox	sulfadoxine
Methoprim	trimethoprim
Methylin	methylphenidate
methylmorphine	codeine
Meticorten	prednisone
Metomin	metformin
Metrocream	metronidazole
MetroGel	metronidazole
Metrolotion	metronidazole
Metrolyl	metronidazole
Mevacor	lovastatin
Meval	diazepam
Mevinacor	lovastatin
Mevinolin	lovastatin
Miacalcic	calcitonin
Miacalcin	calcitonin
Miacin	amikacin
Miaquin	amodiaquine
Micardis	hydrochlorothiazide, telmisartan
Micotef	miconazole
Micronase	glyburide
Micronor	progestins
Microzide	hydrochlorothiazide
Midamor	amiloride
Midol 220	ibuprofen
Midoride	amiloride
Mifeprex	mifepristone
Miglucan	glyburide
Mindiab	glipizide
Mindol	mebendazole
Minidiab	glipizide
Miniprostin E(2)	dinoprostone
Minirin	desmopressin
Minitran	nitroglycerin
Minobese-Forte	phentermine
Minocin	minocycline
Minoclir 50	minocycline
Minodiab	glipizide
Minogalen	minocycline
Minomycin	minocycline
Minoximen	minoxidil
Minprog	alprostadil
Minurin	desmopressin
Miocarpine	pilocarpine
Miracol	miconazole
Mirapex	pramipexole
Mircette	oral contraceptives
Mirena	levonorgestrel
Mirvaso	brimonidine
Misulban	busulfan
mitomycin-C	mitomycin

Mitomycin	mitomycin
Mitomycine	mitomycin
Mitoxana	ifosfamide
Mitran	chlordiazepoxide
Mobic	meloxicam
Mobilin	sulindac
Modamide	amiloride
Modecate	fluphenazine
Modicon	oral contraceptives
Moditen	fluphenazine
Moduretic	amiloride, hydrochlorothiazide
Molelant	cefotaxime
Molipaxin	trazodone
molly	MDMA
Monazole-7	miconazole
Monistat	miconazole
Mono-Gesic	salsalate
Monocor	bisoprolol
Monodox	doxycycline
Monoflam	diclofenac
Monofluorophosphate [MFP]	fluorides
Monoket	isosorbide mononitrate
Mononate	artesunate
Monopril	fosinopril
Monotrim	trimethoprim
Mopral	omeprazole
Morcomine	hydrocodone
Moronal	nystatin
Morphabond	morphine
Morphine-HP	morphine
MOS	morphine
Moscontin	morphine
Motiax	famotidine
Motifene	diclofenac
Motrin	ibuprofen
Movantik	naloxegol
Movergan	selegiline
Moxacef	cefadroxil
Moxeza	moxifloxacin
MS Contin	morphine
MS-IR	morphine
MS/S	morphine
MSIR Oral	morphine
MST Continus	morphine
MTC	mitomycin
MTX	methotrexate
Mucofillin	acetylcysteine
Mucolit	acetylcysteine
Mucolitico	acetylcysteine
Mucoloid	acetylcysteine
Mucomiste	acetylcysteine
Mucomyst-10	acetylcysteine
Mucomyst	acetylcysteine
Mucosil-10	acetylcysteine
Multaq	dronedarone
Multipax	hydroxyzine
Multum	chlordiazepoxide
Murelax	oxazepam
Muse	alprostadil
Mustargen	mechlorethamine
Mustine Hydrochloride Boots	mechlorethamine

mustine	mechlorethamine
Mutamycin	mitomycin
Myambutol	ethambutol
Mycamine	micafungin
Myciguent	neomycin
Mycobax	BCG vaccine
Mycobutin	rifabutin
Mycol	metoprolol
Mycology-II	nystatin
mycophenolate mofetil, mycophenolate sodium	mycophenolate
Mycostatin	nystatin
Myfortic	mycophenolate
Mylanta AR	famotidine
Myleran	busulfan
Mylocel	hydroxyurea
Mynocine	minocycline
Myobloc	botulinum toxin (A & B)
Myolax	carisoprodol
Myrbetriq	mirabegron

N

N-acetylcysteine	acetylcysteine
Nabuser	nabumetone
NAC	acetylcysteine
Nadic	nadolol
Nalcryn SP	nalbuphine
Nalorex	naltrexone
Nalpin	naloxone
Namenda	memantine
Naplin	indapamide
Naprelan	naproxen
Naprogesic	naproxen
Napron X	naproxen
Naprosyn	naproxen
Naprosyne	naproxen
Narcan	naloxone
Narcanti	naloxone
Narcotan	naloxone
Narilet	aldesleukin
Narol	buspirone
Nascobal	cyanocobalamin
Natesto	testosterone
Natrilix	indapamide
Nauseatol	dimenhydrinate
Nausicalm	dimenhydrinate
Navelbine	vinorelbine
Naxen	naproxen
Nazoltec	ketoconazole
Nebilet	nebivolol
NebuPent	pentamidine
Necon	oral contraceptives
NEE	oral contraceptives
Nelova	oral contraceptives
Nemasol	mebendazole
Nemexin	naltrexone
Neo-Synephrine	phenylephrine
Neomicina	neomycin
Neomycine Diamant	neomycin
Neopap	acetaminophen
Neoral	cyclosporine
Neosar	cyclophosphamide
Neosporin	neomycin
Neosulf	neomycin
Neotigason	acitretin
NEPA	netupitant & palonosetron
Nephronex	nitrofurantoin
Nergadan	lovastatin
Nesina	alogliptin
Neupro	rotigotine
Neurap	pimozide
Neurobloc	botulinum toxin (A & B)
Neurontin	gabapentin
Neurosine	buspirone
Nexavar	sorafenib
Nexiclon	clonidine
Nexium	esomeprazole
Nia-Bid	niacin
Niac	niacin
Niacels	niacin
Niacinamide	niacinamide
Niacor	niacin
Niaspan	niacin
Nicabate	nicotine
Nicardal	nicardipine
Nico-Vert	dimenhydrinate
Nicobid	niacin
Nicobion	niacin
Nicodel	nicardipine
Nicoderm	nicotine
Nicolan	nicotine
Nicorette Plus	nicotine
Nicorette	nicotine
Nicotibine	isoniazid
nicotinamide	niacinamide
Nicotinell-TTS	nicotine
Nicotinex	niacin
nicotinic acid	niacin
Nicotrans	nicotine
Nicotrol	nicotine
Nicovital	niacin
Nicozid	isoniazid
Nida Gel	metronidazole
Nifecor	nifedipine
Nifedipress	nifedipine
Nikofrenon	nicotine
Ninlaro	ixazomib
Niotal	zolpidem
Nirulid	amiloride
Nistaquim	nystatin
Nitro-Dur	nitroglycerin
NitroBid	nitroglycerin
Nitrocap	nitroglycerin
Nitrocine	nitroglycerin
Nitrodur	nitroglycerin
nitrogen mustard	mechlorethamine
Nitroglin	nitroglycerin
nitroglycerol	nitroglycerin
Nitrolingual	nitroglycerin
Nitromist	nitroglycerin
Nitronal	nitroglycerin
Nitrospan	nitroglycerin
Nitrostat	nitroglycerin

Nitrumon	carmustine
Nivemycin	neomycin
Nizoral	ketoconazole
Nobegyl	salsalate
Nocbin	disulfiram
Noctec	chloral hydrate
Nodine	ketorolac
Nolvadex	tamoxifen
Nor-QD	progestins
Norboral	glyburide
Norco	hydrocodone
Nordette	oral contraceptives
Norebox	reboxetine
Norethin	oral contraceptives
Norfenon	propafenone
Norgesic	aspirin
Norinyl	oral contraceptives
Noritate	metronidazole
Noritren	nortriptyline
Norlutate	progestins
Norlutin	progestins
Normison	temazepam
Normorytmin	propafenone
Normozide	labetalol
Noroxin	norfloxacin
Norpace	disopyramide
Norphyl	aminophylline
Norplant	levonorgestrel
Norpress	nortriptyline
Northera	droxidopa
Nortrilen	nortriptyline
Norvas	amlodipine
Norvasc	amlodipine
Norvir	ritonavir
Noten	atenolol
Novahistine DH	codeine
Novahistine	phenylephrine
Novamin	prochlorperazine
Novamoxin	amoxicillin
Novantrone	mitoxantrone
Novapen-VK	penicillin V
Novasen	aspirin
Novazam	diazepam
Novitropan	oxybutynin
Novo-Atenol	atenolol
Novo-AZT	zidovudine
Novo-Chlorpromazine	chlorpromazine
Novo-Cycloprine	cyclobenzaprine
Novo-Digoxin	digoxin
Novo-Dipiradol	dipyridamole
Novo-Doxepin	doxepin
Novo-Doxylin	doxycycline
Novo-Flutamide	flutamide
Novo-Furan	nitrofurantoin
Novo-Hylazin	hydralazine
Novo-Ipramide	ipratropium
Novo-Keto	ketoprofen
Novo-Lexin	cephalexin
Novo-Medrone	medroxyprogesterone
Novo-Metformin	metformin
Novo-Naprox	naproxen
Novo-Pramine	imipramine
Novo-Purol	allopurinol
Novo-Selegiline	selegiline
Novo-Semide	furosemide
Novo-Spiroton	spironolactone
Novo-Sundac	sulindac
Novo-Zolamide	acetazolamide
Novochlorhydrate	chloral hydrate
Novocimetine	cimetidine
Novoclopate	clorazepate
Novofen	tamoxifen
NovoLog	insulin aspart
Novomit	prochlorperazine
Novopen-G	penicillin G
Novopoxide	chlordiazepoxide
NovoRapid	insulin aspart
Novotriptyn	amitriptyline
Novoxapam	oxazepam
Noxafil	posaconazole
NTG	nitroglycerin
Nu-Alprax	alprazolam
Nu-Amoxi	amoxicillin
Nu-Atenol	atenolol
Nu-Baclo	baclofen
Nu-Buspirone	buspirone
Nu-Capto	captopril
Nu-Cimet	cimetidine
Nu-Clonidine	clonidine
Nu-Diclo	diclofenac
Nu-Diltiaz	diltiazem
Nu-Doxycycline	doxycycline
Nu-Famotidine	famotidine
Nu-Flurprofen	flurbiprofen
Nu-Gemfibrozil	gemfibrozil
Nu-Hydral	hydralazine
Nu-Indo	indomethacin
Nu-Loraz	lorazepam
Nu-Medopa	methyldopa
Nu-Naprox	naproxen
Nu-Nifed	nifedipine
Nu-Pirox	piroxicam
Nu-Ranit	ranitidine
Nu-Temazepam	temazepam
Nu-Verap	verapamil
Nubain SP	nalbuphine
Nubain	nalbuphine
Nucala	mepolizumab
Nucofed	codeine
Nucynta ER	tapentadol
Nucynta	tapentadol
Nulev	hyoscyamine
Nulojix	belatacept
Nuplazid	pimavanserin
Nuprin	ibuprofen
Nuvigil	armodafinil
Nyaderm	nystatin
Nystacid	nystatin
Nystan	nystatin
Nystex	nystatin
Nytol	diphenhydramine

O

Ocaliva	obeticholic acid
Octagam	immune globulin IV
Octocaine	lidocaine
Octostim	desmopressin
Ocuflox	ofloxacin
Ocumycin	gentamicin
Ocusert Pilo	pilocarpine
Odefsey	emtricitabine/rilpivirine/tenofovir alafenamide
Odomzo	sonidegib
Odrik	trandolapril
Ofev	nintedanib
Ofirmev	acetaminophen
Oflocet	ofloxacin
Oflocin	ofloxacin
Oforta	fludarabine
Oftalmotrisol-T	tobramycin
Oleomycetin	chloramphenicol
Oleptro	trazodone
Olmetec	olmesartan
Olysio	simeprevir
Omed	omeprazole
Omnicef	cefdinir
OmniHIB	Hemophilus B vaccine
OMS Oral	morphine
Onbrez Breezhaler	indacaterol
Oncaspar	pegaspargase
Onco-Carbide	hydroxyurea
Oncocarbin	carboplatin
Oncoden	ondansetron
oncovin	vincristine
Onglyza	saxagliptin
Onicit	palonosetron
Onivyde	irinotecan
Onmel	itraconazole
Onzetra Xsail	sumatriptan
Opana	oxymorphone
Opdivo	nivolumab
Ophthochlor	chloramphenicol
Opistan	meperidine
Opizone	naltrexone
Opsumit	macitentan
Optenyl	papaverine
Optipres	betaxolol
Optovit-E	vitamin E
Oracea	doxycycline
Oracefal	cefadroxil
Oramorph SR	morphine
Oranor	norfloxacin
Oranyst	nystatin
Orap	pimozide
Oravig	miconazole
Orbactiv	oritavancin
Orencia	abatacept
Orientomycin	cycloserine
Oritaxim	cefotaxime
Orkambi	lumacaftor/ivacaftor
Ormazine	chlorpromazine
Ornade	chlorpheniramine
Ornidyl	eflornithine
Oroken	cefixime
Ortho Tri-Cyclen	oral contraceptives
Ortho-Cept	oral contraceptives
Ortho-Cyclen	oral contraceptives
Ortho-Novum	oral contraceptives
Orthovisc	hyaluronic acid
Orudis	ketoprofen
Oruvail	ketoprofen
Osiren	spironolactone
Ospen	penicillin V
Ospexin	cephalexin
Osphena	ospemifene
Osteum	etidronate
Otarex	hydroxyzine
Otezla	apremilast
Otrexup	methotrexate
Otrivine	xylometazoline
Ovcon	oral contraceptives
Ovral	oral contraceptives
Ovrette	progestins
Oxiklorin	hydroxychloroquine
Oxpam	oxazepam
Oxsoralen	methoxsalen, psoralens
Oxsoralon	methoxsalen
Oxtellar XR	oxcarbazepine
Oxyban	oxybutynin
Oxybutyn	oxybutynin
OxyContin	oxycodone
Oxydess	dextroamphetamine
OxyIR	oxycodone
Oxytrol	oxybutynin
Ozoken	omeprazole
Ozurdex	dexamethasone

P

Pacerone	amiodarone
Pacifen	baclofen
Paclimer	paclitaxel
Palaron	aminophylline
Palexia	tapentadol
Palladone	hydromorphone
Palmitate A	vitamin A
Palux	alprostadil
Pameion	papaverine
Pamelor	nortriptyline
Pamid	indapamide
Pamprin	ibuprofen
Panadol	acetaminophen
Panbesy	phentermine
Panbesyl	phentermine
Pandemrix	pandemic influenza vaccine (H1N1)
Panglobulin	immune globulin IV
Panoral	cefaclor
Pantelmin	mebendazole
Panuric	probenecid
Papaverine 60	papaverine
Papaverini	papaverine
paracetamol	acetaminophen
Paraplatin	carboplatin
Paraplatine	carboplatin
Parilac	bromocriptine
Parizac	omeprazole

Parkemed	mefenamic acid
Parlodel	bromocriptine
Parvolex	acetylcysteine
Pasmex	hyoscyamine
Pasotomin	prochlorperazine
Pataday	olopatadine
Patanol	olopatadine
Pavabid	papaverine
Pavagen	papaverine
Pavased	papaverine
Pavatine	papaverine
Paveral	codeine
Paxene	paclitaxel
Paxil CR	paroxetine hydrochloride
Paxil	paroxetine hydrochloride
Paxistil	hydroxyzine
Paxtibi	nortriptyline
PCC	prothrombin complex concentrate (human)
PCE	erythromycin
PCV	pneumococcal vaccine
Pedi-Dri	nystatin
Pediapred	prednisolone
Pediatrix	hepatitis B vaccine
Pediazole	erythromycin
PedivaxHIB	Hemophilus B vaccine
Pegasys	PEG-interferon
PegIntron	PEG-interferon
Penbeta	penicillin V
Penbritin	ampicillin
Pendramine	penicillamine
Pennsaid	diclofenac
Penstabil	ampicillin
Pentacarinat	pentamidine
Pentaglobin	immune globulin IV
Pentam 300	pentamidine
Pentamycetin	chloramphenicol
Pentasa SR	mesalamine
Pentasa	mesalamine
Pentazine	promethazine
Pentoxi	pentoxifylline
Pentoxil	pentoxifylline
Pepcid	famotidine
Pepcidine	famotidine
Pepdul	famotidine
Pepeom Amide	niacin
Peptard	hyoscyamine
Peptaron	ursodiol
Pepto-Bismol	bismuth
Peptol	cimetidine
Peratsin	perphenazine
Percocet	acetaminophen, oxycodone
Percogesic	acetaminophen
Perforomist	formoterol
Peridex	chlorhexidine
Peridol	haloperidol
PerioChip	chlorhexidine
Periogard	chlorhexidine
Periostat	doxycycline
Perlane	hyaluronic acid
Perlutex	medroxyprogesterone
Perphenan	perphenazine
Persantin	dipyridamole
Persantine	dipyridamole
Pertussin	dextromethorphan
Petar	ketamine
pethidine	meperidine
Petidin	meperidine
Petnidan	ethosuximide
Pexal	pentoxifylline
PGE	alprostadil
Phenaemal	phenobarbital
Phenaphen	acetaminophen
Phenazine	promethazine
Phenergan	promethazine
Phenetron	chlorpheniramine
Phenhydan	phenytoin
phenobarbitone	phenobarbital
Phenoxymethylpenicillin	penicillin V
phenylethylmalonylurea	phenobarbital
Phenytek	phenytoin
phenytoin sodium	phenytoin
Pheryl-E	vitamin E
Phyllocontin	aminophylline
Phyllotemp	aminophylline
Phytomenadione	phytonadione
Picato	ingenol mebutate
Pidilat	nifedipine
Pilo Grin	pilocarpine
Pilogel	pilocarpine
Pilopine	pilocarpine
Pilopt	pilocarpine
Pimodac	pimozide
Pink Bismuth	bismuth
Pirimecidan	pyrimethamine
Pitocin	oxytocin
Pitressin	vasopressin
Placil	clomipramine
Plan B	levonorgestrel
Planphylline	aminophylline
Planum	temazepam
Plaquenil	hydroxychloroquine
Plaquinol	hydroxychloroquine
Plasmotrim	artesunate
Plasticin	cisplatin
Platiblastin	cisplatin
Platinex	cisplatin
Platinol-AQ	cisplatin
Platinol	cisplatin
Platistil	cisplatin
Plavix	clopidogrel
Plegridy	interferon beta
Pletal	cilostazol
Plurimen	selegiline
PMS-Baclofen	baclofen
PMS-Cholestyramine	cholestyramine
PMS-Isoniazid	isoniazid
PMS-Lindane	lindane
PncOMP	pneumococcal vaccine
Pneumovax II	pneumococcal vaccine
Pnu-Immune	pneumococcal vaccine
Polinal	methyldopa
Poly-Pred	neomycin

Polygam S/D	immune globulin IV
Polygris	griseofulvin
Polytrim	trimethoprim
Pomalyst	pomalidomide
Ponstan	mefenamic acid
Ponstel	mefenamic acid
Ponstyl	mefenamic acid
Portrazza	necitumumab
pot	marihuana
Potiga	ezogabine
PPV	pneumococcal vaccine
Pradaxa	dabigatran
Praluent	alirocumab
Prandin E2	dinoprostone
Pravachol	pravastatin
Pravasin	pravastatin
Pravasine	pravastatin
Pravidel	bromocriptine
Praxbind	idarucizumab
Praxiten	oxazepam
Prazite	praziquantel
Pre-Par	ritodrine
Precaptil	captopril
Pred-G	gentamicin
Prefrin Liquifilm	phenylephrine
Prelone	prednisolone
Premphase	medroxyprogesterone
Prempro	medroxyprogesterone
Prepidil	dinoprostone
Pres	enalapril
Prescal	isradipine
Presinol	methyldopa
Presoken	diltiazem
Presolol	labetalol
Prestalia	amlodipine, perindopril
Pretz-D	ephedrine
Prevacid	lansoprazole
Prevalite	cholestyramine
Preveon	adefovir
Prevnar	pneumococcal vaccine
Prevpac	amoxicillin
Prexum	perindopril
Prezcobix	darunavir
Prezista	darunavir
Priadel	lithium
Prialt	ziconotide
Pridemon	tranexamic acid
Prilosec	omeprazole
Primacor	milrinone
Primafen	cefotaxime
Primatene Mist	epinephrine
Primatene	epinephrine
Primiprost	dinoprostone
Primonil	imipramine
Primosept	trimethoprim
Primsol	trimethoprim
Principen	ampicillin
Princol	lincomycin
Prinil	lisinopril
Prinivil	lisinopril
Prinzide	hydrochlorothiazide, lisinopril

Pristiq	desvenlafaxine
Pro-Amox	amoxicillin
Pro-Ampi	ampicillin
Pro-Cure	finasteride
Pro-Depo	progestins
Pro-Trin	co-trimoxazole
Probalan	probenecid
Probuphine	buprenorphine
Procan SR	procainamide
Procan	procainamide
Procanbid	procainamide
Procardia	nifedipine
Procid	probenecid
Procoralan	ivabradine
Procren Depot	leuprolide
Procrin	leuprolide
Procrit	epoetin alfa
Procytox	cyclophosphamide
Prodac	nabumetone
Prodopa	methyldopa
Prodox	progestins
Profen	ibuprofen
Proflex	ibuprofen
Progestaject	progestins
Progevera	medroxyprogesterone
Prograf	tacrolimus
ProHIBIT	Hemophilus B vaccine
Prolaken	metoprolol
Proleukin	aldesleukin
Prolex-D	phenylephrine
Prolex-DH	hydrocodone
Prolia	denosumab
Prolift	reboxetine
Prolixin	fluphenazine
Promacta	eltrombopag
Prometh-50	promethazine
Promine	procainamide
Pronestyl	procainamide
Propachem	hydrocodone
Propaphenin	chlorpromazine
Propecia	finasteride
Propess	dinoprostone
Prorazin	prochlorperazine
Proscar 5	finasteride
Proscar	finasteride
prostaglandin E_1	alprostadil
Prostaphlin	oxacillin
Prostarmon	dinoprostone
Prostigmin	neostigmine
Prostin E2	dinoprostone
Prostin VR	alprostadil, dinoprostone
Prostin	dinoprostone
Prostine VR	alprostadil
Prostine	dinoprostone
Prostivas	alprostadil
Prothiazine	promethazine
Protium	pantoprazole
Protogen	dapsone
Protonix	pantoprazole
Protopam	pralidoxime
Protopic	tacrolimus

Proventil	albuterol
Provera	medroxyprogesterone, progestins
Provigil	modafinil
Prozac	fluoxetine
Prozin	chlorpromazine
Pryleugan	imipramine
Psicofar	chlordiazepoxide
Pulmicort Turbuhaler	budesonide
Punktyl	lorazepam
Puri-Nethol	mercaptopurine
Purinethol	mercaptopurine
Purinol	allopurinol
Puvasoralen	methoxsalen
Pyknolepsinum	ethosuximide
Pyoredol	phenytoin
Pyrethia	promethazine

Q

Q-Vel	quinine
Qnasl	beclomethasone
Qsymia	phentermine, topiramate
Qualaquin	quinine
Quantalan	cholestyramine
Qudexy	topiramate
Quellada	lindane
Quensyl	hydroxychloroquine
Querto	carvedilol
Questran Lite	cholestyramine
Questran	cholestyramine
Quibron	aminophylline
Quiess	hydroxyzine
Quinalan	quinidine
Quinate	quinidine
Quinazil	quinapril
Quini Durules	quinidine
Quinoctal	quinine
Quinora	quinidine
Quinsan	quinine
Quinsul	quinine
Quintasa	mesalamine
Quiphile	quinine
Quixin	levofloxacin
Qvar	beclomethasone

R

Ra-223 dichloride	radium-223 dichloride
Radiesse	calcium hydroxylapatite
Ralovera	medroxyprogesterone
Ralozam	alprazolam
Ramicin	rifampin
Randikan	kanamycin
Ranexa	ranolazine
Raniben	ranitidine
Raniplex	ranitidine
Ranisen	ranitidine
Ranvil	nicardipine
Rapaflo	silodosin
Rapamune	sirolimus
rapamycin	sirolimus
Rapivab	peramivir
Rasuvo	methotrexate
Rayaldee	calcifediol
Razadyne	galantamine
Reactine	cetirizine
Rebetol	ribavirin
Rebetron	interferon alfa, ribavirin
Rebif	interferon beta
Reclast	zoledronate
Recombivax HB	hepatitis B vaccine
Rectiv	nitroglycerin
Redisol	cyanocobalamin
Redusa	phentermine
Refobacin	gentamicin
Refolinin	leucovorin
Refusal	disulfiram
Regaine	minoxidil
Regitin	phentolamine
Regitine	phentolamine
Regonol	pyridostigmine
Relafen	nabumetone
Relenza	zanamivir
Relief	tretinoin
Relif	nabumetone
Relifex	nabumetone
Relpax	eletriptan
Remeron	mirtazapine
Remethan	diclofenac
Remicade	infliximab
Reminyl	galantamine
Renitec	enalapril
Reniten	enalapril
Renova	tretinoin
Repatha	evolocumab
Reposans-10	chlordiazepoxide
Requip	ropinirole
Rescufolin	leucovorin
Rescuvolin	leucovorin
Resmin	diphenhydramine
Respirol	terbutaline
Respontin	ipratropium
Restasis	cyclosporine
Restoril	temazepam
Restylane Fine Lines	hyaluronic acid
retigabine	ezogabine
Retin-A Micro	tretinoin
Retinoic Acid	tretinoin
Retinova	tretinoin
Retrovir	zidovudine
Revapole	mebendazole
Revatio	sildenafil
ReVia	naltrexone
Revimine	dopamine
Reviten	triamterene
Revlimid	lenalidomide
Revolade	eltrombopag
Revonto	dantrolene
Rexulti	brexpiprazole
Reyataz	atazanavir
Rezine	hydroxyzine
rFVIIIFc	antihemophilic factor
Rheumatrex	methotrexate

Rhinocort	budesonide
Rhodacine	indomethacin
Rhodis	ketoprofen
Rhonal	aspirin
Rhotrimine	trimipramine
Rhovail	ketoprofen
Rhythmin	procainamide
Ride	amiloride
Ridene	nicardipine
Rifadin	rifampin
Rifaldin	rifampin
Rifamate	isoniazid
Rifamed	rifampin
rifampicin	rifampin
Rifater	isoniazid
Rilatine	methylphenidate
Rimactane	rifampin
Rimpin	rifampin
Rimycin	rifampin
Rinatec	ipratropium
Riomet	metformin
Risperdal Consta	risperidone
Risperdal	risperidone
Ritalin	methylphenidate
Ritmocamid	procainamide
Ritmolol	metoprolol
Rituxan	rituximab
Rivotril	clonazepam
RMS	morphine
Roaccutan	isotretinoin
Roaccutane	isotretinoin
Roacutan	isotretinoin
Roacuttan	isotretinoin
Robaxisal	aspirin
Robidrine	pseudoephedrine
Robimycin	erythromycin
Robinul	glycopyrrolate
Robitussin AC	codeine
Robitussin-CF	pseudoephedrine
Robitussin	dextromethorphan
Rocefin	ceftriaxone
Rocephalin	ceftriaxone
Rocephin	ceftriaxone
Roceron-A	interferon alfa
Rofact	rifampin
Roferon-A	interferon alfa
Rogaine	minoxidil
Rogal	piroxicam
Rogitene	phentolamine
Rogitine	phentolamine
Rotarix	rotavirus vaccine
RotaTeq	rotavirus vaccine
Roubac	co-trimoxazole
Rovacor	lovastatin
Rowasa	mesalamine
Roxanol	morphine
Roxicodone	oxycodone
Rozerem	ramelteon
Rtsun	artesunate
Ru-Tuss	hydrocodone
Rubesol-1000	cyanocobalamin
Rubex	doxorubicin
rubidomycin	daunorubicin
Rubifen	methylphenidate
Rubramin	cyanocobalamin
Rufen	ibuprofen
Ryanodex	dantrolene
Rybix ODT	tramadol
Rydene	nicardipine
Rynatan	phenylephrine
Rynatuss	ephedrine
Rytary	levodopa
Rythmex	propafenone
Rythmol	propafenone
Rytmonorm	propafenone
Ryzodeg	insulin aspart, insulin degludec

S

S-1	tegafur/gimeracil/oteracil
S-2	epinephrine
Sabril	vigabatrin
Sacbexyl	lindane
Saccharin	saccharin
Saflutan	tafluprost
Salagen	pilocarpine
salazopyrin	sulfasalazine
Salbulin	albuterol
salbutamol	albuterol
Salflex	salsalate
Salgesic	salsalate
salicylazosulfapyridine	sulfasalazine
Salina	salsalate
Salisulf	sulfasalazine
Salmagne	labetalol
Salofalk	mesalamine
Sandimmun	cyclosporine
Sandimmune	cyclosporine
Sandoglobulin	immune globulin IV
Sandoglobulina	immune globulin IV
Sandoglobuline	immune globulin IV
Sandostatin	octreotide
Sandostatina	octreotide
Sandostatine	octreotide
Sanoma	carisoprodol
Sansert	methysergide
Saphris	asenapine
Sarafem	fluoxetine
Sarconyl	lindane
Saridine	sulfasalazine
Saroten	amitriptyline
SAS-500	sulfasalazine
Savaysa	edoxaban
Savella	milnacipran
Savlon	chlorhexidine
Saxenda	liraglutide
Scabecid	lindane
Scabene	lindane
Scabex	lindane
Scabi	lindane
Scabisan	lindane
SCH 619734	rolapitant
SCIG	immune globulin sc

Sebomin	minocycline
Sebvio	telbivudine
Sedanazin	gentamicin
Sediat	diphenhydramine
Seebri Neohaler	glycopyrrolate
Selectin	pravastatin
Selectol	celiprolol
Selektine	pravastatin
Selipran	pravastatin
Seloken-Zok	metoprolol
Selozok	metoprolol
Selzentry	maraviroc
Sendoxan	cyclophosphamide
Septra	co-trimoxazole, sulfamethoxazole, trimethoprim
Ser-Ap-Es	hydralazine
Serax	oxazepam
Serenace	haloperidol
Serepax	oxazepam
Serocryptin	bromocriptine
Seromycin	cycloserine
Seroquel	quetiapine
Seroxat	paroxetine hydrochloride
Serozide	etoposide
Setamine	hyoscyamine
Sevredol	morphine
Sideril	trazodone
Sigacefal	cefaclor
Sigafam	famotidine
Silenor	doxepin
Silgard	human papillomavirus (HPV) vaccine
Silicofluoride	fluorides
Simatin	ethosuximide
Simcor	niacin, simvastatin
Simovil	simvastatin
Simplene	epinephrine
Simponi	golimumab
Simulect	basiliximab
Sinaplin	ampicillin
Sinemet	levodopa
Singulair	montelukast
Sinomin	sulfamethoxazole
Sinosid	paromomycin
Sinquan	doxepin
Sintodian	droperidol
Sinutab	acetaminophen
Siran	acetylcysteine
Sirdalud	tizanidine
Sirtal	carbamazepine
Sirturo	bedaquiline
Sitavig	acyclovir
Sivastin	simvastatin
Sivextro	tedizolid
Sizopin	clozapine
Skelaxin	metaxalone
Sklice	ivermectin
Slo-Bid	aminophylline
Slo-Niacin	niacin
SMX-TMP	co-trimoxazole
SMZ-TMP	co-trimoxazole
Sno Pilo	pilocarpine
Sobelin	clindamycin

Sodium fluoride [NaF]	fluorides
Sodium monofluorophosphate	fluorides
Sodol	carisoprodol
Solage	tretinoin
Solaraze Gel	diclofenac
Solcodein	codeine
Solesorin	hydralazine
Solfoton	phenobarbital
Solgol	nadolol
Soliris	eculizumab
Solis	diazepam
Solium	chlordiazepoxide
Solodyn	minocycline
Solpurin	probenecid
Solu-Medrol	methylprednisolone
Solutrat	ursodiol
Solvex	reboxetine
Soma Compound	aspirin
Soma	carisoprodol
Somadril	carisoprodol
Somatuline Autogel	lanreotide
Somatuline Depot	lanreotide
Somatuline LA	lanreotide
Somavert	pegvisomant
Sominex 2	diphenhydramine
Somnox	chloral hydrate
Somophyllin	aminophylline
Sonata	zaleplon
Soolantra	ivermectin
Sopamycetin	chloramphenicol
Sorbitrate	isosorbide dinitrate
Soriatane	acitretin
Soridol	carisoprodol
Sorine	sotalol
Sostril	ranitidine
Sotacor	sotalol
Sotahexal	sotalol
Sotalex	sotalol
Sotilen	piroxicam
Sotret	isotretinoin
Sovaldi	sofosbuvir
Spectro Gram	chlorhexidine
Spersacarpine	pilocarpine
Spinax	baclofen
Spiriva	tiotropium
Spiroctan	spironolactone
Spirosine	cefotaxime
Splenda	sucralose
Sporacid	itraconazole
Sporal	itraconazole
Sporanox	itraconazole
Sprycel	dasatinib
SSKI	potassium iodide
Stable	hydralazine
Stalevo	entacapone, levodopa
Stamaril	yellow fever vaccine
Stambutol	ethambutol
Stangyl	trimipramine
Stannous fluoride [SF]	fluorides
Stapenor	oxacillin
Staril	fosinopril

Starlix	nateglinide
Statex	morphine
SteiVAA	tretinoin
Stelara	ustekinumab
Stella	prochlorperazine
Stemetil	prochlorperazine
Stendra	avanafil
Stieva-A	tretinoin
Stilnoct	zolpidem
Stilnox	zolpidem
Stimate	desmopressin
Stiolto Respimat	olodaterol, tiotropium
Stomedine	cimetidine
Stopit	loperamide
Storzine	pilocarpine
Strattera	atomoxetine
Strensiq	asfotase alfa
Streptase	streptokinase
Streptomycin	streptomycin
Stribild	cobicistat/elvitegravir/emtricitabine/tenofovir disoproxil
Striverdi Respimat	olodaterol
Stromba	stanozolol
Stromectol	ivermectin
Strumazol	methimazole
Stubit	nicotine
Sublimaze	fentanyl
Suboxone	buprenorphine, naloxone
Subutex	buprenorphine
Sucrabest	sucralfate
Sucrets	dextromethorphan
Sudafed	pseudoephedrine
Sular	nisoldipine
Sulcrate	sucralfate
Sulene	sulindac
sulfamethoxazole-trimethoprim	co-trimoxazole
Sulfatrim	co-trimoxazole
Sulfazine	sulfasalazine
Sulfona	dapsone
Sulfur hexafluoride [SF6]	fluorides
Sulic	sulindac
Sulmidine	clonidine
Suloril	sulindac
Suloton	triamterene
Sumacef	cefadroxil
Sumavel DosePro	sumatriptan
Sumontil	trimipramine
Supartz	hyaluronic acid
Supeudol	oxycodone
Suppress	dextromethorphan
Supradol	naproxen
Supran	cefixime
Suprax	cefixime
Suprenza	phentermine
Supressin	doxazosin
Suretin	tazarotene
Surmontil	trimipramine
Sustiva	efavirenz
Sutent	sunitinib
suxamethonium	succinylcholine
Sweet'N Low	saccharin
Sylatron	PEG-interferon
Symbicort	budesonide, formoterol
Symbol	misoprostol
Symbyax	fluoxetine, olanzapine
Syn-Minocycline	minocycline
Syn-Nadolol	nadolol
Synagis	palivizumab
Syndros	dronabinol
Synflex	naproxen
Synjardy	empagliflozin, metformin
Synribo	omacetaxine
Synthroid	levothyroxine
Syntocinon	oxytocin
Syraprim	trimethoprim
Syscor	nisoldipine
Sytobex	cyanocobalamin

T

T-20	enfuvirtide
T-DM1	ado-trastuzumab emtansine
T-VEC	talimogene laherparepvec
T_3 sodium	liothyronine
T_3	liothyronine
T_4	levothyroxine
Tabalom	ibuprofen
Tabco	flecainide
Tabrin	ofloxacin
Tacex	ceftriaxone
Tachydaron	amiodarone
Tadol	tramadol
Tafil	alprazolam
Tafinlar	dabrafenib
Taflutan	tafluprost
Tagal	ceftazidime
Tagamet	cimetidine
Tagrisso	osimertinib
Taks	diclofenac
Taloken	ceftazidime
Taltz	ixekizumab
Talwin Compound	aspirin
Talwin-NX	naloxone
Tamaxin	tamoxifen
Tambocor	flecainide
Tamiflu	oseltamivir, pandemic influenza vaccine (H1N1)
Tamofen	tamoxifen
Tamoxan	tamoxifen
Tanzeum	albiglutide
Tapazole	methimazole
Tapros	leuprolide
Taravid	ofloxacin
Tarceva	erlotinib
Targiniq	naloxone, oxycodone
Targocid	teicoplanin
Targretin	bexarotene
Tarka	trandolapril, verapamil
Taro-Ampicillin Trihydrate	ampicillin
Taro-Atenol	atenolol
Tasigna	nilotinib
Taucor	lovastatin
Tavanic	levofloxacin
Tavor	lorazepam

Taxagon	trazodone
Taxol	paclitaxel
Taxotere	docetaxel
Taxus	tamoxifen
Tazicef	ceftazidime
Tazorac	tazarotene
Tecentriq	atezolizumab
Tecfidera	dimethyl fumarate
Technivie	ombitasvir/paritaprevir/ritonavir
Tecoplanin	teicoplanin
Tecprazin	praziquantel
Teczem	diltiazem, enalapril
Tedolan	etodolac
Tefamin	aminophylline
Teflaro	ceftaroline fosamil
Tega-Cert	dimenhydrinate
Tega-Vert	dimenhydrinate
Tegretol XR	carbamazepine
Tegretol	carbamazepine
Teichomycin-A2	teicoplanin
Tekamlo	amlodipine
Tekturna HCT	hydrochlorothiazide
Telachlor	chlorpheniramine
Teldrin	chlorpheniramine
Temazepam	temazepam
Tementil	prochlorperazine
Temesta	lorazepam
Temgesic	buprenorphine
Temodar	temozolomide
Tenif	atenolol, nifedipine
Teniken	praziquantel
Tenolin	atenolol
Tenoret 50	atenolol
Tenoretic	atenolol
Tenormin	atenolol
Tenormine	atenolol
Tensin	spironolactone
Tensipine MR	nifedipine
Tensopril	lisinopril
Teralithe	lithium
Teril	carbamazepine
Terlipressin	terlipressin
Ternalax	tizanidine
Ternelin	tizanidine
Tertroxin	liothyronine
Tesavel	sitagliptin
Testandro	testosterone
Testim	testosterone
Testoderm	testosterone
Teston	methyltestosterone
Testopel	testosterone
Testotonic 'B'	methyltestosterone
Testovis	methyltestosterone
Testred	methyltestosterone
Tetradin	disulfiram
tetrahydrocannabinol	dronabinol
Teveten HCT	hydrochlorothiazide
Teveten	eprosartan
Texate	methotrexate
Teysuno	tegafur/gimeracil/oteracil
Thacapzol	methimazole

THC	dronabinol
Theo-Dur	aminophylline
theophylline ethylenediamine	aminophylline
Thevier	levothyroxine
Thiamazol	methimazole
thiamazole	methimazole
Thinex	lindane
Thioprine	azathioprine
Thorazine	chlorpromazine
Thyroid-Block	potassium iodide
Thyronine	liothyronine
Thyrozol	methimazole
tiabendazole	thiabendazole
Tiamate	diltiazem
Tiazac	diltiazem
Tibinide	isoniazid
TICE BCG	BCG vaccine
Tidocol	mesalamine
Tiempe	trimethoprim
Tifomycine	chloramphenicol
Tilazem	diltiazem
Tildiem	diltiazem
Timonil	carbamazepine
Titus	lorazepam
Tivicay	dolutegravir
TMP-SMX	co-trimoxazole
TMP-SMZ	co-trimoxazole
TOBI	tobramycin
Tobra	tobramycin
TobraDex	tobramycin
Tobrex	tobramycin
Tofranil	imipramine
Tolak	fluorouracil
Toloxim	mebendazole
Topadol	ketorolac
Topamax	topiramate
Topicort	desoximetasone
Toprol XL	metoprolol
Toradol	ketorolac
Torem	torsemide
Toremonil	hydroxychloroquine
Torental	pentoxifylline
Torisel	temsirolimus
Torolac	ketorolac
Torvin	ketorolac
Totacillin	ampicillin
Totapen	ampicillin
Toviaz	fesoterodine
tPA	alteplase
Tracleer	bosentan
Tradjenta	linagliptin
Tradol	tramadol
Tramal	tramadol
Tramed	tramadol
Tramol	tramadol
Trandate	labetalol
Transderm-Nitro	nitroglycerin
Transene	clorazepate
Transtec	buprenorphine
Tranxal	clorazepate
Tranxen	clorazepate

Tranxene	clorazepate
Tranxilen	clorazepate
Tranxilium	clorazepate
Trasamlon	tranexamic acid
Travatan Z	travoprost
Travatan	travoprost
Travel Tabs	dimenhydrinate
Trazalon	trazodone
Trendar	ibuprofen
Trental	pentoxifylline
Tresiba	insulin degludec
Trexan	naltrexone
Tri-Levlen	oral contraceptives
Tri-Norinyl	oral contraceptives
Triadapin	doxepin
Triaken	ceftriaxone
Triaminic DM	dextromethorphan
Triaminic	chlorpheniramine
Trian	triamterene
Triasox	thiabendazole
Triavil	perphenazine
Tricodein	codeine
Tricor	fenofibrate
Tridil	nitroglycerin
Tridol	tramadol
Triflucan	fluconazole
Trijodthyronin BC N	liothyronine
Trikacide	metronidazole
Trilafon	perphenazine
Trileptal	oxcarbazepine
Trilifan Retard	perphenazine
Trimopan	trimethoprim
Trimox	amoxicillin
Trimzol	co-trimoxazole
Trinalin	pseudoephedrine
Trintellix (formerly Brintellix)	vortioxetine
Triomin	perphenazine
Triostat	liothyronine
Triphasil	oral contraceptives
Triprim	trimethoprim
Triptone	dimenhydrinate
Trisoralen	psoralens
Trisulfa	co-trimoxazole
Tritace	ramipril
Triumeq	abacavir, dolutegravir, lamivudine
Trivora	oral contraceptives
Triz	cetirizine
Trizivir	abacavir, lamivudine, zidovudine
Trobalt	ezogabine
Trocal	dextromethorphan
Trokendi XR	topiramate
Tronoxal	ifosfamide
Tropax	oxybutynin
Tropium	chlordiazepoxide
Tropyn Z	atropine sulfate
Troxyca	naltrexone, oxycodone
Trulicity	dulaglutide
Trumenba	meningococcal group B vaccine
Truphylline	aminophylline
Trusopt	dorzolamide
Truvada	emtricitabine, tenofovir disoproxil
Tryptanol	amitriptyline
Tryptizol	amitriptyline
TS-1	tegafur/gimeracil/oteracil
Tussar-2	codeine
Tussgen	hydrocodone
Tussi-12D	phenylephrine
Tussi-Organidin	codeine
Tussionex	hydrocodone
Tussogest	hydrocodone
Twinrix	hepatitis B vaccine
Tykerb	lapatinib
Tylenol	acetaminophen
Tylox	oxycodone
Typherix	typhoid vaccine
Typhim Vi	typhoid vaccine
Tysabri	natalizumab
Tyzeka	telbivudine

U

UDC Hexal	ursodiol
UDC	ursodiol
UDCA	ursodiol
Udrik	trandolapril
Uducil	cytarabine
Ulcar	sucralfate
Ulcedine	cimetidine
Ulcogant	sucralfate
Ulcol	sulfasalazine
Ulcyte	sucralfate
Uloric	febuxostat
Ulsen	omeprazole
Ultra-MOP	methoxsalen
Ultracet	tramadol
Ultram	tramadol
Umbradol	salsalate
Umine	phentermine
Unasyn	ampicillin/sulbactam
Unat	torsemide
Uniflox	ciprofloxacin
Unimazole	methimazole
Unimetone	nabumetone
Uniparin	heparin
Uniretic	hydrochlorothiazide
Unithroid	levothyroxine
Unitrim	trimethoprim
Unituxin	dinutuximab
Unizuric	allopurinol
Uptravi	selexipag
Urbal	sucralfate
Urdox	ursodiol
Urem	ibuprofen
Urex	furosemide
Urief	silodosin
Urised	atropine sulfate, hyoscyamine
Uritol	furosemide
Uro-cephoral	cefixime
Urobak	sulfamethoxazole
Urocid	probenecid
Urofuran	nitrofurantoin
Uromax	oxybutynin
Uroxatral	alfuzosin

Urozide	hydrochlorothiazide
Urso 250	ursodiol
Urso Forte	ursodiol
Urso Heumann	ursodiol
Urso Vinas	ursodiol
Ursochol	ursodiol
ursodeoxycholic acid	ursodiol
Ursofal	ursodiol
Ursofalk	ursodiol
Ursoflor	ursodiol
Ursogal	ursodiol
Ursolac	ursodiol
Ursolism	ursodiol
Ursolvan	ursodiol
Urson	ursodiol
Ursoproge	ursodiol
Ursosan	ursodiol
Ursotan	ursodiol
USCA	ursodiol
Utibron Neohaler	glycopyrrolate, indacaterol
Utinor	norfloxacin
Utradol	etodolac

V

V-cillin K	penicillin V
Vacanyl	terbutaline
Vagifem	estradiol
Valadol	acetaminophen
Valcyte	valganciclovir
Valdrene	diphenhydramine
Valium	diazepam
Valni XL	nifedipine
Valodex	tamoxifen
valproate sodium	valproic acid
Valtrex	valacyclovir
Valturna	valsartan
Vamate	hydroxyzine
Vanatrip	amitriptyline
Vanceril	beclomethasone
Vancocin	vancomycin
Vancotil	loperamide
Vandazole	metronidazole
Vaniqa	eflornithine
Vanmicina	vancomycin
Vanquish	aspirin
Vaprisol	conivaptan
Vaqta	hepatitis A vaccine
Varilrix	varicella vaccine
Variquel	terlipressin
Varithena	polidocanol
Varivax	varicella vaccine
Varsan	lindane
Varubi	rolapitant
Vascal	isradipine
Vaseretic	enalapril, hydrochlorothiazide
Vasopril	fosinopril
Vasostrict	vasopressin
Vasotec	enalapril
Vaxchora	cholera vaccine
Vaxigrip	influenza vaccine
Veclam	clarithromycin
Vectibix	panitumumab
Velban	vinblastine
Velbe	vinblastine
Velcade	bortezomib
Veletri	epoprostenol
Velodan	loratadine
Velsar	vinblastine
Velsay	naproxen
Veltassa	patiromer
Vemlidy	tenofovir alafenamide
Venclexta	venetoclax
Venoglobulin	immune globulin IV
Ventolin	albuterol
Ventoline	albuterol
VePesid	etoposide
Vepeside	etoposide
Veraken	verapamil
Verelan	verapamil
Vermicol	mebendazole
Vermox	mebendazole
Versed	midazolam
Vertab	dimenhydrinate
Vertigon	prochlorperazine
Vesanoid	tretinoin
Vesicare	solifenacin
Vestra	reboxetine
Vfend	voriconazole
Viadur	leuprolide
Viaflex	heparin
Viagra	sildenafil
Viberzi	eluxadoline
Vibra-Tabs	doxycycline
Vibramycin-D	doxycycline
Vicapan N	cyanocobalamin
Vicard	terazosin
Vicks Formula 44	dextromethorphan
Vicks Vatronol	ephedrine
Vicodin	acetaminophen, hydrocodone
Vicoprofen	hydrocodone, ibuprofen
Victoza	liraglutide
Victrelis	boceprevir
Vidaza	azacitidine
Videx	didanosine
Vidopen	ampicillin
Viekira Pak	ombitasvir/paritaprevir/ritonavir
Viekira XR	dasabuvir/ombitasvir/paritaprevir/ritonavir
Viekirax	ombitasvir/paritaprevir/ritonavir
Viibryd	vilazodone
Vimizim	elosulfase alfa
Vimpat	lacosamide
Vincasar	vincristine
Viracept	nelfinavir
Viramid	ribavirin
Viramune	nevirapine
Virazid	ribavirin
Virazole	ribavirin
Viread	tenofovir disoproxil
Virilon	methyltestosterone
Virlix	cetirizine
Viromone	methyltestosterone
Vistabel	botulinum toxin (A & B)

Vistacarpin	pilocarpine
Vistaril	hydroxyzine
Vistide	cidofovir
Visudyne	verteporfin
Vita Plus E	vitamin E
Vita-E	vitamin E
Vitak	phytonadione
Vitamin B_{12}	cyanocobalamin
vitamin B_3	niacin, niacinamide
vitamin B_9	folic acid
vitamin K_1	phytonadione
Vitamin K	phytonadione
Vitatropine	atropine sulfate
Vitec	vitamin E
Vitrase	hyaluronic acid
Vivaglobin	immune globulin sc
Vivatec	lisinopril
Vivelle-Dot	estradiol
Vivelle	estradiol
Vividyl	nortriptyline
Vivitrex	naltrexone
Vivitrol	naltrexone
Vivol	diazepam
Vivotif	typhoid vaccine
Vogan	vitamin A
Volibris	ambrisentan
Volmax	albuterol
Voltaren	diclofenac
Voltarene	diclofenac
Voltarol	diclofenac
Vomacur	dimenhydrinate
Vomex A	dimenhydrinate
Vomisen	dimenhydrinate
Vonum	indomethacin
Vozet	levocetirizine
VP-TEC	etoposide
Vraylar	cariprazine
Vytorin	ezetimibe, simvastatin
Vyvanse	lisdexamfetamine

W

Waran	warfarin
Warfilone	warfarin
Waytrax	ceftazidime
Wehamine	dimenhydrinate
Welchol	colesevelam
Wellbutrin	bupropion
Welldorm	chloral hydrate
Wigrettes	ergotamine
Winobanin	danazol
Winstrol	stanozolol
Wintrocin	erythromycin
Wyamicin S	erythromycin

X

X	MDMA
Xalatan	latanoprost
Xalkori	crizotinib
Xanax	alprazolam
Xanef	enalapril
Xarelto	rivaroxaban
Xatral	alfuzosin
Xelevia	sitagliptin
Xeljanz	tofacitinib
Xeloda	capecitabine
Xenical	orlistat
Xeomin	botulinum toxin (A & B)
Xgeva	denosumab
Xifaxan	rifaximin
Xifaxanta	rifaximin
Xigduo XR	dapagliflozin, metformin
Xiidra	lifitegrast
Xofigo	radium-223 dichloride
Xolair	omalizumab
Xomolix	droperidol
Xozal	levocetirizine
Xtampza ER	oxycodone
Xtandi	enzalutamide
Xtoro	finafloxacin
Xusal	levocetirizine
xylocaine	lidocaine
Xylocard	lidocaine
Xyzal	levocetirizine

Y

Yamatetan	cefotetan
Yasmin	oral contraceptives
Yaz	oral contraceptives
Yectamid	amikacin
Yentreve	duloxetine
Yervoy	ipilimumab
YF-VAX	yellow fever vaccine
Yosprala	aspirin, omeprazole
Yuma	hydroxychloroquine
Yurelax	cyclobenzaprine

Z

Zaltrap	aflibercept
Zanaflex	tizanidine
Zanosar	streptozocin
Zantab	ranitidine
Zantac-C	ranitidine
Zantac	ranitidine
Zantic	ranitidine
Zantryl	phentermine
Zapex	oxazepam
Zaponex	clozapine
Zariviz	cefotaxime
Zarondan	ethosuximide
Zarontin	ethosuximide
Zavedos	idarubicin
Zebeta	bisoprolol
Zebinix	eslicarbazepine
Zecuity	sumatriptan
Zedolac	etodolac
Zefone	ceftriaxone
Zeftera	ceftobiprole
Zelapar	selegiline
Zelboraf	vemurafenib
Zenapax	daclizumab

Zentropil	phenytoin
Zeos	loratadine
Zepatier	elbasvir & grazoprevir
Zerbaxa	ceftolozane & tazobactam
Zerit	stavudine
Zestoretic	hydrochlorothiazide, lisinopril
Zestril	lisinopril
Zetia	ezetimibe
Zeto	azithromycin
Ziac	bisoprolol, hydrochlorothiazide
Ziagen	abacavir
Zimovane	eszopiclone
Zinacef	cefuroxime
Zinacet	cefuroxime
Zinat	cefuroxime
Zinbryta	daclizumab
Zinnat	cefuroxime
Zinplava	bezlotoxumab
Zioptan	tafluprost
Zipan	tramadol
Zipsor	diclofenac
Zirtin	cetirizine
Zithromax	azithromycin
Zitromax	azithromycin
ziv-aflibercept	aflibercept
Zmax	azithromycin
Zocor	simvastatin
Zocord	simvastatin
Zofran	ondansetron
Zofron	ondansetron
Zohydro ER	hydrocodone
Zoldan-A	danazol
Zole	miconazole
zoledronic acid	zoledronate
Zolinza	vorinostat
Zoloft	sertraline
ZoMaxx Drug-Eluting Coronary Stent	zotarolimus
Zometa	zoledronate
Zomig	zolmitriptan
Zonegran	zonisamide
Zontivity	vorapaxar
Zorac	tazarotene
Zoref	cefuroxime
Zoroxin	norfloxacin
Zortress	everolimus
Zorvolex	diclofenac
Zostavax	zoster vaccine
Zosyn	piperacillin/tazobactam
Zovia	oral contraceptives
Zovirax	acyclovir
Zumalin	lincomycin
Zunden	piroxicam
Zuplenz	ondansetron
Zurampic	lesinurad
Zyban	bupropion
Zyclara	imiquimod
Zyclir	acyclovir
Zydelig	idelalisib
Zyderm	collagen (bovine)
Zydone	hydrocodone
Zyflo	zileuton
Zyloprim	allopurinol
Zyloric	allopurinol
Zymerol	cimetidine
Zynox	naloxone
Zyplast	collagen (bovine)
Zyprexa Relprevv	olanzapine
Zyprexa	olanzapine
Zyrtec	cetirizine
Zytiga	abiraterone
Zyvox	linezolid